Localization of Clinical Syndromes in Neuropsychology and Neuroscience

Joseph M. Tonkonogy, MD, PhD, FRSM, is clinical professor of psychiatry and neurology at the University of Massachusetts Medical School in Worcester, Massachusetts. A friend and collaborator of the late A. R. Luria, Dr. Tonkonogy is the author or editor of over 150 books and peer-reviewed journal articles, including the books *Vascular Aphasia* (1986) and *Brief Neuropsychological Cognitive Examination* (1997). Dr. Tonkonogy is a member of numerous professional societies, including the National Academy of Neuropsychology, the International Neuropsychological Society, the American Neuropsychiatric Association, the Behavioral Neurology Society, and The Royal Society of Medicine.

Antonio E. Puente, PhD, is professor of psychology at the University of North Carolina, Wilmington, where he teaches courses on clinical neuropsychological assessment. Previously, he was a staff psychologist at Northeast Florida State Hospital. In addition, Dr. Puente maintains a private practice in the Wilmington, North Carolina, area and provides expert testimony as a forensic neuropsychologist. He is the author of six books and over 150 journal articles. He has served as the editor for the journal *Neuropsychology Review,* as well as series editor for *Plenum's Critical Issues in Neuropsychology*.

Localization of Clinical Syndromes in Neuropsychology and Neuroscience

Joseph M. Tonkonogy, MD, PhD, FRSM
Antonio E. Puente, PhD

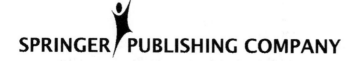

SPRINGER PUBLISHING COMPANY

Springer Publishing Company, LLC
11 West 42nd Street
New York, NY 10036
www.springerpub.com

Acquisitions Editor: Philip Laughlin
Production Editor: Julia Rosen
Cover design: Mimi Flow
Composition: Apex CoVantage

09 10 11/ 5 4 3 2 1

Library of Congress Cataloging-in-Publication Data

Puente, Antonio E.
   Localization in neuropsychology and clinical neuroscience /
Antonio E. Puente, Joseph M. Tonkonogy.
      p. ; cm.
   Includes bibliographical references and index.
   ISBN 978–0–8261–1967–4 (alk. paper)
    1. Clinical neuropsychology.   2. Brain—Localization of
functions.   I. Tonkonogii, I. M. (Iosif Moiseevich)   II. Title.
   [DNLM: 1. Nervous System Diseases.   2. Brain—
physiopathology.   3. Neuropsychological Tests.
4. Neuropsychology—methods. WL 140 P977L 2008]

   RC343.P885   2008
   616.8—dc22   2008038970

Printed in the United States of America by Hamilton Printing Company.

To our families and mentors

To my wife Milla and my children Bella, Milla, and Vitaly
And to my mentors—Aleksandr Luria and Norman Geschwind
  JMT

To my wife Linda and my children Krista, Antonio Nicolas, and Lucas
And to my mentors—L. J. Peacock and Roger W. Sperry
  AEP

Contents

Preface . . . . **xi**

Acknowledgments . . . . **xv**

1 Disturbances of Brain Information
Processing and Localization Studies **1**
Localizationist Approach **1**
Holistic Approach **5**
Modern Approaches: Interfacing Localization
with Holistic Perspectives **7**
Sizes of Lesions and Compensatory Mechanisms
of Brain Information Processing **17**
Types of Lesions **18**
Summary **20**

2 Disorders of Recognition in the Physical
World: Visual Agnosia **21**
Visual Agnosia **22**
Color Agnosia **90**

3 Disorders of Recognition in the Physical
World: Other Types of Agnosia **99**
Visuospatial Agnosia **99**

Loss of Visual Imagery 109
Auditory Agnosia 113
Tactile Agnosia, Astereognosis 129
Somatoagnosia and Disturbances
of Somatic Self-Image 136
Disturbances in the Recognition of Motion
and Action in the Physical World 157

4 Disorders of Recognition in the Physical
   World: Illusions and Hallucinations 187
   Illusions 187
   Hallucinations 191

5 Disturbances of Recognition
   of the Social World 221
   Social Agnosia 221
   Agnosia of Social Actions 254
   Delusions 272

6 Disturbances of Actions 291
   Motor Apraxia 291
   Social Apraxia: Disorganization of Goal-Directed
   Behavior in the Social World 324

7 Communication Disorders 335
   Aphasia Syndromes and Other Language Disorders 335
   Alexia and Agraphia 406
   Amusia 419

8 Memory Disorders: Disturbances
   of the Major Supportive System of Brain
   Information Processing 427
   Amnestic Syndromes 433
   Disturbances of Modular Memory
   for Recognition and Action 455
   Working Memory and Its Disturbances 466

9 Disturbances of Regulatory Activity:
   Impairment of Visually Guided Attention 483
   Disturbances of Visually Guided Attention
   and Visual Agnosia 484

10 Disturbances of Regulatory Activity:
Impairments of Volition. **501**

Avolition, Akinesia, and Negative Symptoms **501**

Apathy, Avolition, Akinesia, and Disturbances
of Brain Information Processing **524**

11 Disturbances of Regulatory Activity:
Impairments of Emotion **529**

Mood Disorders **529**

Anxiety Disorders **566**

Mood Disorders and Disturbances of Brain
Information Processing **599**

12 Generalized Cognitive Disturbances. **607**

Delirium. **607**

Dementia **621**

13 Neuropsychological Testing of
Clinical Syndromes **667**

Neuropsychological Testing and Brain Imaging **667**

Psychometric System Based on Normative
Data of Normal Individuals. **668**

Psychometric Neuropsychological System
Based on Clinical Normative Data **672**

Neuropsychological Testing of Clinical Syndromes. **673**

Use of Diagnostic Algorithms in
Neuropsychological Testing of Clinical Syndromes. **688**

Appendix **693**

References **705**

Preface

Clinical medicine and health care has based its diagnostic decision making on the concept of syndromes—peculiar combinations of signs and symptoms often underlined by common causes, pathogenesis, or localization of lesions. This pattern was, similarly, followed in the early days of neuropsychology. However, a constantly growing number of neuropsychological studies—clinical, experimental, and anatomical—are focusing less on clinical descriptions of major neuropsychological syndromes and are focusing instead on the studies and analyses of simple signs and symptoms, which often reflect impairments of single operations rather than disturbances in particular functional goals manifesting as clinical syndromes. This new approach has resulted in controversies concerning clinical patterns and localization of lesions even in such well-established syndromes as various types of *aphasia, agnosia,* and *apraxia*. The shift in approach is further complicated by discrepancies between the old so-called lesion data and the findings brought to the field of clinical neuropsychology by the explosion of new data obtained through the use of powerful technology such as single-cell recording and functional brain imaging as well as the expansion of the empirical foundation of clinical neuropsychology and neuroscience.

For many years, the clinico-anatomical approach remained one of the major methods in the study of brain information processing in normal and pathological conditions. In many respects, clinico-anatomical data remains pertinent to the new data and to subsequent theoretical explanation based on current methods of cognitive neuroscience, neuropsychology, and neuropsychiatry. The goal of this book is to systematize the historical clinico-anatomical neuropsychological and neuropsychiatric data and to present those data in such a way as to make them more compatible with recent findings based on the modern methods of cognitive neuroscience, especially single-cell recording and brain imaging. It is important to consider both types of data within the frameworks of concepts developed by modern computer science and the construction of artificial cognitive devices. Approaches are also discussed in relation to new types of neuropsychological testing conducted by the authors and their colleagues. This book offers systematic descriptions of the clinical manifestations, anatomical data, and history of studies of the various neuropsychological syndromes; in fact, the text may be used as a frame of reference for clinical signs and syndromes and localization for research and clinical practice in neuropsychology, neuropsychiatry, and cognitive neuroscience.

Also analyzed are findings that exhibit the types of brain information processing that influence the single versus multiple sites of lesion localization that then lead to similar types of disturbances, for example, various sites of lesion that may each cause a similar impairment in one's working memory. These analyses help to present localizationist versus anti-localizationist approaches as perhaps two sides of the same issue. While one side is based on differences in the functional structure of modules for simpler, well-learned, and relatively strictly localized conventional information processing, the other is based on modules for more complicated and unconventional information processing, requiring the use of operations that are localized in several brain areas. It is the entire issue, rather one perspective versus another, that is particularly intriguing, robust and most important. In essence, one cannot leave the role of localization to neuroradiology nor can one simply be content with understanding neuropsychological patterns of performance. It is the interface between localization and functional analysis that is the future of brain study.

The content of this book is based on the taxonomy of neuropsychological syndromes underlined by the functional goals of the various parts of the intermediate and high levels of brain information processing. The text also attempts to incorporate neuropsychological clinico-anatomical syndromes such as agnosia, aphasia, apraxia, and amnesia into the new taxonomy, incorporating a reflection of disturbances in the particular functional goals. Accordingly, the book consists of 13 chapters that describe disturbances of several systems involved in the intermediate and high levels of brain information processing, including recognition, action, communication, and supportive and regulatory functions. These disturbances are described and analyzed within the framework of four major themes explored in the book.

The first theme focuses on the differentiation of syndromes under-lined by disturbances of conventional versus unconventional informa-tion processing, which helps to outline the conventional syndromes in relation to localized circumscribed brain lesions and to bring atten-tion to the localization problems in the unconventional syndromes. Conventional information processing consists of high frequency and well-known items that may be processed using a limited store of rep-resentations as compared to well-learned complex features. Such mod-ules may be tuned to the processing of a particular type of information, for example, the recognition of high frequency objects or faces, or the performance of typical actions. As this processing requires a relatively small amount of brain space, damage to the area may result in the devel-opment of clearly defined clinical syndromes that have been described in detail through years of neuropsychological, behavioral neurological, and neuropsychiatric studies. Conversely, unconventional informa-tion processing deals with more complicated information, including a large number of typically low frequency items that may be completely absent in and/or between the stored representations. Unconventional information processing requires the use of various additional opera-tions to process new items or items with an incomplete set of infor-mation, for example, objects partly occluded by background "noise" or overlapping objects. Processing of such information depends on a wide range of operations performed by multiple structures in various areas of the brain. Damage to these structures may result in disturbances of unconventional information processing, for example, an impairment in the recognition of incomplete objects caused by lesions in multiple different brain sites, lacking a clearly defined, narrow lesion localiza-tion in one specific area of the brain. It is especially important to take this into account as increasingly more sophisticated cognitive tests are often directed toward the evaluation of unconventional information processing, making quite difficult the use of such tests for purposes of localization. Problems arising from studies of single-cell recording are often based on tests directed toward unconventional information processing. Results of these studies have often exhibited a lack of sup-port from the clinico-anatomical cases studied with the use of clinical features of disturbances in conventional information processing.

The second theme presented is related to the information process-ing approach based on the use of features that describe the common invariant properties of the same items, such as a particular object in various positions or actions. The common properties may include sim-ple and complex features as well as the semantic meaning of the item, which may be used for comparison with similar features of represen-tations stored in the memory (Ullman, 1996). This text describes and analyzes disturbances as they are related to the processing of simple and complex features of various types of items in the course of brain information processing, especially the role of the impairment of complex features analysis in the development of the major syndromes of disturbances in the intermediate and high levels of brain information processing.

The third theme gives special attention to disturbances of recognition in both the physical and social worlds. The concepts of agnosia and apraxia as defined in neuropsychological and neurological literature are explored in relation to the physical world, with descriptions and analyses of disturbances in recognition and in social actions being considered. In general, disturbances of recognition and of actions in the social world have been traditionally characterized by vague terms such as social incompetence, and may be better defined and studied within the concepts of *social agnosia* and *social apraxia*. We attempt to systematize these issues in accordance with the already well-studied disturbances of *prosopagnosia* and agnosia of emotions and to outline the current status of the studies and their future directions. The book also includes descriptions of the clinico-anatomical syndromes underlined by disturbances of the *social self* as a module independent from the body image or *somatic self-image;* the book then discusses the roles of disturbances of the somatic self-image and social self in the formation of neuropsychological syndromes.

The fourth theme brings attention to disturbances in the recognition of dynamic components of the world. Agnosia is usually described in relation to disturbances of recognition in the physical world of such static items as objects and space; dynamic actions in the physical world are typically excluded from the major studies of recognition. The text emphasizes the role of impairments of recognition and of actions in the constantly changing dynamic environment via literature-based descriptions of various types of agnosia of action in the physical and social worlds and via an outline of the symptoms of social agnosia and social apraxia. Also discussed are ways to adjust current clinical neuropsychological testing to meet the needs of research and of everyday clinical practice as based on an evaluation of neuropsychological syndromes.

Acknowledgments

The syndromological and localization approaches reflected in this book have been originally discussed by Joseph Tonkonogy with Alexander Luria, one of the founders of neuropsychology. We are grateful to Alexander Luria for his inspiration to continue the efforts in those directions that represented the backbone of the neuropsychology approach at the early stages of its development. The efforts have been later enhanced by help of Ilya Tsukkerman, the eminent physicist and enthusiastic supporter of strong connections between computer science, especially in the area of incomplete information processing, and studies of brain pathology and behavior. We owe a debt of gratitude to Ilya Tsukkerman for his instruction and collaboration.

We benefited enormously from contributions and advice throughout the process of accumulating data, writing, and editing from our colleagues and collaborators including Boris Iovlev, Sofia Dorofeeva, Ludvig Vasserman, Victor Shklovsky, Ludmilla Tonkonogy, James Armstrong, Elizabeth Henrickson, Louise Warren, and especially Yakov Meerson, who presented his data with invaluable advice for the chapter on visual agnosia. Antonio E. Puente would like to acknowledge Griffen Sutton Pollock for her very valuable assistance in editing the manuscript and adding useful commentary to the text.

1

Disturbances of Brain Information Processing and Localization Studies

THE ROLE OF brain scientists and clinicians has historically been focused on localization of brain function. More recently, the advent of sophisticated brain imaging, such as computerized axial tomography and magnetic resonance imaging, has resulted in a significant shift in the understanding of brain structure and function. This shift has resulted in an increasing focus on pattern analysis of cognitive disorder for neurological diseases. However, increasing evidence is suggesting that the correlation between function and neuroradiological studies is weak at best. Thus, interfacing known information about disturbances of brain information processing with localization studies should provide new opportunities for a more robust understanding of brain disorders.

LOCALIZATIONIST APPROACH

AT THE TURN of the nineteenth century, the ideas of undivided mental processes were challenged by suggestions that mental processes might be divided into relatively isolated mental "abilities" with specific locations in the brain. At that time, Gall (Gall & Spurzheim, 1810–1819) tried to suggest the localization of isolated mental abilities in the various regions of the cortex. He was first to point to the localization of speech abilities in the frontal regions of the brain. Though Bouillaud, who by 1825 had reached a position of great influence in the Paris medical community, was a supporter of Gall's ideas, neither Gall nor Bouillaud had any real evidence in support of their point of view.

Such evidence was first presented by Broca, a surgeon and anthropologist, who observed a patient with peculiar speech disturbances related, as Broca stressed, to a lesion in the posterior part of F3. The patient, Leborgne, was able to say only the word "tan" and a few obscenities. However, the muscles needed for speech appeared to be preserved, as the patient was able to eat and to drink, and no disturbances in comprehension of spoken language were observed. Broca concluded that the patient had a specific disorder in his ability to articulate language, a disorder that he termed *aphemie*. Broca presented the patient's brain on April 18, 1861, just one day after the patient's death, at a meeting of the Paris Anthropological Society. During his presentation, Broca (1861a) exhibited his finding of a cerebral infarction in the left hemisphere that extended from the posterior part of the third frontal gyrus, through the lower part of the central gyrus, to the anterior part of the first temporal gyrus. His observations of a sequenced progression of language disturbances in the patient allowed Broca to conclude first that the disturbances were related to the posterior F3 lesion and subsequently that the posterior F3 area represented a center for articulate language. Broca eagerly informed Bouillaud, Broca's teacher and mentor, who supported the idea previously (Bouillaud, 1825) (for details, see chapter 7, section entitled "Aphasia Syndromes and Other Language Disorders").

Several months later, in November 1861, Broca (1861b) presented his second case at a meeting of the Paris Anthropological Society. Lelong, the patient presented, had resided at the Bicetre hospital since 1853, with manifestations of senile dementia. In April 1853, Lelong experienced a stroke; what followed was a development of prominent speech disturbances—the patient was able to utter no more than several words and could do so only with laborious articulation. However, Lelong was able to understand almost everything that was said to him, and no disturbances were observed in the movements of his extremities. On October 27, 1861, Lelong experienced a fall during which he suffered a fracture of the left hip; he died 12 days later. An external overview of the brain revealed the destruction of one half of the posterior F3 in the left hemisphere. This damage was connected with tissue loss in the second F2, an area that was almost completely destroyed. The central gyrus and F1 areas, however, had been completely preserved.

In addition to the clinical significance of lesion localization in patients with speech disorders, the data presented by Broca were probably the first to demonstrate the role of the clinico-anatomical method in the study of isolated mental abilities. Soon after Broca's presentation, similar cases were reported by a number of authors. Later, in 1864, Trousseau pointed out that the word *infamy* in the modern Greek language may be translated as *aphemia,* and suggested the replacement of the word *aphemia* with the word *aphasia.* Despite Broca's objection, Trousseau's suggestion was widely accepted. Thus, the term aphasia became accepted and became widely used in the literature.

Ten years later, in 1874, Karl Wernicke published a book in which he provided 10 case studies and described patients with disturbances in the comprehension of spoken language as well as in expressive speech, naming, reading, and writing. Wernicke called these disturbances sensory aphasia. Following the deaths of two patients, brain autopsies were performed, revealing extensive brain lesions. An autopsy performed in the only case with a circumscribed lesion showed an infarction in the posterior part of T1 and in adjacent areas of T2 in the left hemisphere. Based on these findings, Wernicke attributed the development of sensory aphasia to a lesion in the "auditory speech center" in the posterior T1. He suggested that a lesion in the left posterior T1 resulted in sensory aphasia, while a lesion in the left posterior F3 produced motor aphasia. The interruption of the connection between the centers of "auditory speech images" and "motor speech images" led, according to Wernicke, to the development of conduction aphasia with disturbances of speech repetition.

Lichtheim presented the idea of a "center of concepts" in 1884 and suggested that the development of transcortical motor aphasia was the result of an interruption of the connection between the center of concepts and the motor speech center, while transcortical sensory aphasia occurred when the connections between the center of concepts and the sensory speech center were disturbed. Based on Lichtheim's suggestions, a classification of aphasia was developed (Lichtheim, 1884); it is still currently used (for more details, see chapter 7, section entitled "Aphasia Syndromes and Other Language Disorders").

The studies of Broca and Wernicke may be considered to be important milestones for the series of subsequent works and great successes of localizationists at the end of the nineteenth century and at the turn of the twentieth century. In 1881, Munk showed that following the removal of its occipital lobes, a dog preserved its ability to see but was no longer able to recognize objects. Several years later, Wilbrand (1887) and Charcot (1883) described cases in which visual *agnosia* resulted from cerebral infarctions involving the second occipital gyrus (Wilbrand, 1892). In 1890, Lissauer was the first to describe the apperceptive and associative types of visual object agnosia. Disturbances of writing related to a lesion of the posterior F2 area were reported by Exner in

1881, while in 1877 Kussmaul presented cases of isolated reading disturbances under the name wordblindness, or *Wortblindheit*. Various types of visual spatial agnosia reported at that time included disturbances of topographic disorientation (Wilbrand, 1887) and visual neglect of hemispace (Anton, 1898; Balint, 1909). Tactile agnosia was described and called *astereognosia* by Hoffman in 1885. Motor and sensory *amusia* was observed by Steinhal in 1871 and later by Oppenheim in 1888. In addition to the disturbances of recognition of the outside world, disturbances of recognition in the "somatic Myself" (Pick, 1908), also known as *somatoagnosia*, were defined by cases with *anosognosia* of blindness (Anton, 1898, 1899) and anosognosia of hemiplegia (Babinsky, 1914). The majority of the studies were limited to neurological patients who suffered primarily from circumscribed focal lesions often caused by cerebral infarctions, and in some patients by tumors and head injuries.

The clinico-anatomical approach was more difficult to apply in the field of psychiatry, due to the absence of significant anatomical and localized changes in cases with primary psychiatric illnesses such as schizophrenia and bipolar disorder. However, some cases in which psychiatric manifestations of clearly defined neurological conditions, resulting from head injuries, brain tumors, encephalitis, and degenerative brain diseases, were present allowed for the use of the clinico-anatomical approach.

A classic example is the celebrated case report of Phineas Gage (Harlow, 1868). Gage exhibited profound personality changes following a severe frontal lobe injury caused by an explosion that sent a metal rod through his skull. The rod traveled upward from the left maxilla and through the frontal lobe, exiting to the left of the frontal skull's midline (similar personality changes were later observed in other patients with frontal lobe injuries). Another example is given in a description by Korsakoff (1887) of the peculiar amnestic disorders caused by chronic alcoholism, later found to be related to lesions in the mamillary bodies and medial dorsal nuclei of the thalamus (Gamper, 1928; Victor, Adams, & Collins, 1971).

A series of psychiatric studies based on the clinico-anatomical approach was begun in the 1920s and 1930s during the aftermath of World War I. The main data were provided by evaluations of World War I veterans with various head injuries acquired during battle. Further studies were performed in the 1940s and 1950s involving psychiatric manifestations of brain tumors and epilepsy as well as head injuries sustained in action during World War II. It was demonstrated that *apathy*, or flatness of affect, often developed after frontal lobe injuries, especially following injuries to the dorso-lateral prefrontal cortex, the thalamus, and the globus pallidus (Feuchtwanger, 1923; Kleist, 1934). A melancholic type of depression was frequently observed in cases with temporal lobe tumors (Hécaen & de Ajuriaguerra, 1956). Electrical stimulation of the T1 area led to the development of verbal auditory hallucinations and, in some cases, visual hallucinations (Penfield & Erickson, 1941). Peculiar personality changes were observed and studied in patients with temporal lobe epilepsy (Bear & Fedio, 1977; Waxman & Geschwind, 1975), and caudate and frontal lobe lesions were reported in cases of obsessive-compulsive disorder, and so on.

HOLISTIC APPROACH

F ROM THE EARLY years of localization studies, the idea of strict localization was criticized by anti-localizationists who stressed that mental functions cannot be localized in particular areas of the brain. Flourens (1824, 1842) insisted that the brain is a homogenous substance that is similar to, for instance, the liver in its physiological functioning. Flourens based his ideas on experiments involving the removal of various parts of the cerebral hemisphere in birds. The birds' behaviors were completely restored after a certain amount of postsurgery recovery time, regardless of the localization of the removed parts. Goltz (1876–1884) observed only a transient disturbance of behavior after a surgical removal of various parts of the cerebral hemisphere in dogs, an outcome he considered to be a result of the brain's reaction as a whole. Subsequently, the dogs showed a "general decline of intellect," which Goltz correlated with the size of the removed brain tissue but not with the localization of the lesion.

The idea of a general intellectual decline was explored further by a number of authors. Finkelenburg, in 1870, was probably the first to suggest that damage to the cortex of cerebral hemispheres results in *asymbolia,* a disturbance in one's ability to use symbols, leading to impairments in speech, recognition, and actions. Marie (1906a, 1906b) later brought these ideas to the study of aphasia in 1906, suggesting that the main disturbance in aphasia is a "partial intellectual disturbance" manifesting in impairments of speech comprehension and presenting itself as Wernicke's sensory aphasia—what Marie termed a "true" aphasia.

Subsequently, Head (1926) considered the basic disturbance in aphasia an impairment in "symbol formulation and expression," which represents a part of "general intellectual ability" and cannot be strictly localized in any definite area of the brain. Goldstein (1948) later outlined the differences between the peripheral and central cortices. According to the anatomical principle in which cortical structure leads to disorders of the instrumentalities of speech, such as peripheral motor aphasia and peripheral sensory aphasia, lesions in the periphery result in more elemental neurological manifestations in comparison to more centrally located lesions.

According to Goldstein, the central part of the cortex has the property of equipotentiality. A lesion in any part of this central cortex leads to a disorder in one's ability to form abstractions and to perform categorization; the severity of this disorder depends only on the size of the damaged cerebral tissue. Goldstein considered anomic aphasia to be a typical example of aphasia produced by a disorder of "abstract language." Goldstein's idea was closely linked to Lashley's conception of brain tissue equipotentiality. Lashley (1929) studied the role of extirpations of particular types of cerebral hemispheres on the behavior of rats. He observed that the degree of disturbances in the behavior of rats in the labyrinth did not depend on the localization of the extirpations but rather reflected the size of the removed brain tissue.

Several other studies pointed to the correlation of the development and severity of aphasia with lesion size. Through the years, a series of cases has been described in which small lesions in Broca's area of posterior F3 result in either a transient aphasia or no aphasia at all. Such cases have been collected from both literature and experience, being originally described by Marie (1906a, 1906b), Moutier (1908), Von Meyendorf (1930). Mohr et al. (1978) observed that an infarct limited to the posterior part of the left F3 resulted in transient mutism with subsequent recovery to almost normal speech, though with some mild articulation difficulties, within a few days or weeks following a stroke.

A transient form of Broca's aphasia was also described in cases with symmetrical destruction of Broca's areas in both hemispheres (Tonkonogy & Goodglass, 1981). Tonkonogy (1968b, 1986) demonstrated that in Broca's aphasia the severity and persistence of the deficit is proportionate to the size and distribution of the infarction over the opercular, insular, and adjacent cortical and subcortical regions. The effect of the lesion size on the severity of language impairment was later exhibited by Selnes, Knopman, Niccum, Rubens, and Larson (1983) and Knopman, Selnes, Niccum, and Rubens (1984).

It has also been stressed that the particular symptoms of aphasia, such as a disturbance in comprehension, may be observed in patients with various anterior and posterior lesions within the large perisylvian region in the left hemisphere (Selnes et al., 1983).

Another example against a strict localizationism is a disturbance in one's ability to classify visual stimuli in accordance with a changing target category during the course of testing. For instance, in the Wisconsin Card Sorting Test (WCST), the subject is required to classify the 64 cards according to color, form, number, and again color as the test progresses (Berg, 1948; Grant & Berg, 1948). In Halstead's

Category Test (Halstead, 1947), the subject must classify 208 items into seven sets organized according to different categories—number of objects, ordinal position of an odd stimulus, and so forth. It was suggested that disturbances of categorization revealed by the WCST or by Halstead's Category Test might be related to lesions of the frontal lobe (Halstead, 1947; Milner, 1963; Weinberger, Berman, & Zec, 1988). However, several studies failed to observe any consistent relationship between the results of the category test and any specific location or laterality of brain damage (Doehring & Reitan, 1962; Reitan & Wolfson, 1985), or any differences in WCST performance between groups of patients with local frontal versus nonfrontal lesions (Anderson, Damasio, Jones, & Tranel, 1991; Axelrod et al., 1996). It should be emphasized that Goldstein (1934, 1948), who originally introduced the card sorting tests for studies of "abstract attitude," held that impairments in one's ability to form abstractions cannot be strictly localized in particular cortical areas.

MODERN APPROACHES: INTERFACING LOCALIZATION WITH HOLISTIC PERSPECTIVES

CLINICO-ANATOMICAL STUDIES HAVE been markedly advanced in recent decades by the advent of brain imaging, especially head computerized tomography (CT) scans and brain magnetic resonance imaging (MRI) scans, providing the tools necessary to study the anatomy of lesions in patients. These studies have helped to refine the detection of clinical symptoms, classifications, and anatomical findings in the syndromes previously described using the historical clinico-anatomical approach based on a comparison of clinical and autopsy findings. The new data are discussed and compared with the original findings in this book. The role of functional brain-imaging techniques such as functional magnetic resonance imaging (fMRI) and positron emission tomography (PET) scans in studies of localization is also discussed.

Special attention should be paid to modern approaches based on the theory and models of information processing developed in studies of artificial intelligence. These approaches bring a new dimension to the understanding of brain information processing by outlining the particular goals of recognition and action, the operations needed for the achievement of these goals, and the roles of the supportive and regulatory systems, which may then be compared with the functional structures of corresponding artificial devices. The artificial devices of recognition or action cannot be considered to be identical to the functional structure of brain information processing, but they may be compared, especially in defining some of the important principles and operations required for the successful achievement of particular tasks in the course of such processing. Some of the principles of artificial intelligence have already found their way into modern neuropsychology and neuropsychiatry. They include the application of such terms as *module, circuitry, operation, working memory* (*operational memory* in artificial intelligence), *signal recognition from background noise,* and so forth.

Modularity and Disturbances of Brain Information Processing

General Concept

The term module has been used in the technical description of various devices to outline individual parts with relatively independent tasks and separate functional capabilities that also contribute to the overall goals of the device's function. The conception of modules as the major components of brain information processing represents a further development of the old localizationist approach to brain function. Similar to Gall's "organs" and "centers," the term "module" implies that information processing in the brain is conducted by relatively functionally independent units, each with a special purpose of application. It is reasonable to assume that the system of modules is highly efficient in terms of brain space economy. The system of modules also seems to be reliable, as the particular module processes a certain type of information requiring a relatively small number of stored representations for objects, faces, and actions. The volume of information processed in the course of recognition or action would become prohibitively large and virtually impossible to process without relatively independent modules tuned to a particular type of information.

The conception of modularity was introduced into the modern theory of the mind/brain functions by Fodor in *Modularity and Mind* (1983). Fodor considered the module to be composed of domain-specific, stimulus-driven, autonomous units that assess information via bottom-up processing rather than via top-down processing. According to Fodor, the neural architecture of modules is genetically fixed, hardwired, and prespecified. It is suggested that the independent units are minimally interactive with one another, a view that is reflected in Chomsky's "organology" as well as in Fodor's *Modularity*. This point of view is supported by observations that patients with aphasia suffer from impairments of language, while their cognitive abilities are relatively well preserved; in other words, there is a dissociation of disturbances between the impaired space and preserved object recognition.

The number of such examples may be greatly expanded by the inclusion of the many specific types of agnosia, apraxia, aphasia, and amnesia observed and described since Broca's initial observations. These examples may be considered to reflect impairments in the domain-specific information processing of particular modules. A list of brain modules may thus be composed by using the described types of recognition and action disturbances as confirmation of the existence of certain modules. Such a list may include the modules for recognition and action in the physical world, such as visual object recognition, space orientation, body image orientation, speech production and comprehension, recognition of actions, motor praxis, and other types of modules that have been revealed in clinical and neuropsychological studies based on the strict localizationist approach.

Special attention should be given to the modules that provide recognition of social actions and social praxis, which have been largely omitted from past studies as a target of neuropsychological testing. An example of a module with the purpose of processing social information is facial recognition. A disturbance in this module may be manifested as an impairment in the recognition of known faces or prosopagnosia. Another module may be involved in the recognition of emotional expressions, and disturbances in this condition are known as *sensory aprosodia*. Disturbances of brain information processing in these modules are discussed in subsequent chapters of this book.

The structures of recognition and action modules are based on a set of both simple and complex features. This set is used for descriptions of target objects or actions and their meanings, either in the process of comparison with the stored models for recognition or in the process of evoking a course of action. Other types of modules may be used by supportive and regulatory systems of attention, memory, and emotion, and may be used for central control and support of recognition and action. They may include, for instance, an ability to assign a negative or positive score to the result of an action or an ability to anticipate planned actions using emotions as score indexes. For a module of episodic memory, a special structure is required, probably based on the directory used for selecting the needed information in the memory archive. An attention module helps to direct recognition or action modules to their specific targets.

Modules may have the ability to communicate for the purpose of translating information from the language of one module to the language of another module, for example, from visual to auditory types of languages. Some of the modules may be able to work as multilingual devices able to use different languages of the brain, most likely by translating modality-specific languages into a modality-neutral language. In the studies of present authors and their colleagues, for instance, it was found that parietal lesions were manifested by disturbances of recognition of both visual and auditory sequences, while posterior-superior temporal lobe lesions produced selective impairments in the recognition of auditory sequences, and occipital lesions resulted in disturbances of recognition of visual sequences (for more details, see chapter 2, section entitled "Visual Agnosia").

The most prominent criticism of the claim of modularity has been concentrated on the notion that modular units are informationally independent. Such a criticism may be supported by the findings of informational interdependence in information processing by a particular model: for example, word recognition is markedly improved when a patient with aphasia is asked to point to objects in the same semantic environment, such as the kitchen. Word recognition significantly worsens if the patient is asked to point to objects not found in the kitchen, but rather in a different semantic environment, such as a street scene. Critics also stress their claim that the formation of modules may result from a gradual developmental process rather than from a prespecified modular architecture (Elman et al., 1996; Karmiloff-Smith, 1992; Rose, 1997).

The idea that modules are fully independent in their functions is difficult to imagine, especially since they represent a part of the general system of brain information processing underlying goal-directed behavior. The types and degrees of such interdependency require further exploration, especially for the processing of novel, unconventional information. In addition to bottom-up processing, the role of top-down processing in the functioning of modules warrants further investigation.

Modules for Conventional and Unconventional Information Processing

Based on clinical and neuropsychological studies, it is reasonable to suggest that special modules must exist for the processing of conventional, frequently used information and unconventional, new, and incomplete information processing. The modules for *conventional information processing* are characteristically similar to Fodor's description of modules as units that are domain specific, stimulus driven, and autonomous. The processing of items such as objects or actions that require a short list of predefined features and a limited number of models is represented in memory storage for comparison with a particular set of features. The comparison with features of real items or selection of plan of actions is well learned and may be processed quickly. Such a system allows for substantial conservation through the use of a stable set of features predefined by a learning process and limited in its number of features. The approach also allows for the building of a storage model that consists of a relatively small number of frequently used items and reflects the main features assigned to the modules. The conventional modules are fairly simple, occupy relatively small cortical areas, and may be built with substantial redundancy so as to be protected from brain damage, especially from small lesions. Larger lesions in such areas may lead to the development of a clinical syndrome that reflects a disturbance in the set of operations in a particular domain-specific module, as characterized by the specific localization of the lesion. For example, consider the development of Broca's aphasia as an impairment of a specific module for expressive speech, resulting primarily from a lesion in the inferior-posterior frontal lobe and the inferior central gyri (for more details, see chapter 7, section entitled "Aphasia Syndromes and Other Language Disorders").

Modules for *unconventional information processing* may be connected with the same domain-specific conventional module, but the processing of new or incomplete information requires the use of a more detailed set of features and an extended capacity for memory storage. Furthermore, the speed may be significantly slowed by the increased volume and complexity of information that must be processed. The unconventional module may not satisfy in its structure all of the features included in Fedor's more strict definition of modules as being less autonomous and more interconnected with other modules.

The role of the module in unconventional information processing may be demonstrated via a comparison of the processes of recognition of conventional and unconventional spoken language. This process may be provided by operations based on the alphabet of features that include single phonemes, syllables, words, and even sentences. The program for conventional information processing may be based on a conventional module composed of a limited number of well-known, frequently used words and sentences—the features of the model. Impairments in this conventional module would lead to significant disturbances in the comprehension of conventional language used in everyday conversation, as observed in patients experiencing Wernicke's aphasia. At the same time, recognition of low-frequency words or words of a more complex syntactical structure may be provided by the module for unconventional information processing, based on phonological and semantic analyses of the speech as well as on special operations for streamlining inverted sequences into a more direct order that is much easier to comprehend: for example, "the lion killed the tiger" than "the tiger was killed by a lion."

Conventional information processing for language comprehension may be strictly located in a particular area of the brain, namely, in the posterior T1 of the dominant hemisphere—Wernicke's area. Thus a lesion in the specified area manifests as aphasia with disturbances in the comprehension of conventional spoken language—Wernicke's aphasia. The lesion must certainly involve adjacent areas and must be relatively large to cause disturbances in the set of operations involved in conventional language comprehension. In a case of *unconventional information processing,* such as the comprehension of an inverted and more complicated syntactical structure, the set of operations used for language comprehension is significantly larger and may be localized in many areas around the Sylvian fissure, including the posterior F3, the operculum of the central gyri, and the insula. Thus, lesions in these areas may produce similar disturbances in unconventional language comprehension, for instance, in the comprehension of inverted sentences. While the comprehension of everyday language may be preserved in such cases, the use of special tests, such as inverted sentences and other types of unconventional language, reveals disturbances in this language comprehension (for more details, see chapter 7, section entitled "Aphasia Syndromes and Other Language Disorders"). This observation is often used as evidence against the argument for the strict localization of particular language disturbances.

Similarly, the recognition of real objects based on conventional information processing may be preserved in patients with prominent disturbances in the recognition of incomplete pictures or with decreases in object exposition from less than 2–3 seconds to 100–200 milliseconds. The localization of lesions in such cases may involve the inferior temporal lobe as well as the occipital lobe, as usually observed in patients with visual agnosia of real objects.

Various tasks may require the application of the programs for unconventional information processing. One such task is the recognition of objects or actions with incomplete sets of features, as in cases of object occlusion, in which a part of the object or the entire object is hidden in the midst of background noise. Disturbances in the performance of such tasks may be related to impairments of special programs used for the recognition of signals from noise based on a limited number of features (for more details, see chapter 2, section entitled "Visual Object Agnosia"). Such disturbances may also be observed in the recognition of actions, including social actions, with incomplete sets of features.

Another type of unconventional task requires an ability to overcome the standardized, conventional set of information processing. Such tasks are often described as executive functions and are mainly related to the processing of unconventional information by modules for unconventional sequences recognition. For instance, in the Trail Making Test, Part B (Reitan & Wolfson, 1985), the subject has to alternate between two standard sequences—numbers and letters of the alphabet—thus overcoming the well-learned automatic sequences of 1, 2, 3 . . . and A, B, C. . . . In our test entitled "Number Tracking," the alternation is required between automatic sequences of upward and backward number counting—for example, 1, 12, 2, 11, 3, 10, and so forth (Tonkonogy, 1997).

The ability to overcome the distraction caused by the established type of recognition is also tested by the popular Stroop Test (Stroop, 1935). In this particular test, the subject has to read various color names while simultaneously ignoring the color of the print, which never corresponds with the color names.

Various category tests usually contain two types of unconventional tasks. In the Wisconsin Card Sorting Test (Grant & Berg, 1948), for instance, the first task is to recognize a category or pattern, as predefined by the test procedure, from among sequences of cards with figures composed of different features such as color, form, and number, for example, organization via color. The second task is to overcome the previously learned category once the pattern to be recognized is switched to another leading feature during the course of testing. Finally, the subject is asked to replicate a number of figures as they are displayed on the cards, and then to switch back to organization via color. In such tasks, the main feature of the sequence continues to change throughout the course of testing and is intended to reflect real conditions as they require new actions in the outside world, whether physical or social. It is possible that this ability is interconnected via two different modules—one for the physical world and another for the social world.

Localization of Operations and Syndromes

Operations

Some of the operations performed within the various modules must be similar, if not identical. For instance, operations conducted by working memory are needed for information processing in various modules and thus may be represented in every module. Therefore, similar clinical manifestations of particular operations may be observed as the result of lesions in various sites, giving the impression of the equipotentiality of brain functioning. For example, working memory disturbances have been ascribed to various sites of lesions in the frontal, parietal, temporal, and occipital lobes. On the other hand, auditory working memory disturbances have been observed in patients with temporal lobe lesions, and visual working memory impairments have been attributed to damage to the occipital lobe (for more details, see chapter 8, section entitled "Amnestic Syndromes").

The idea that there exists a wider distribution of operations not strictly localized in one cortical area is further supported by studies of anosognosia. Anosognosia, also known as loss of insight, has been attributed to a wide variety of lesion sites, including lesions in the frontal, parietal, temporal, and occipital areas as well as in subcortical structures. However, anosognosia of paralysis or aphasia was observed in patients with a corresponding right parietal lesion or left temporal lesion, while anosognosia of cortical blindness was found to be related to the presence of an occipital lesion, and loss of insight in psychiatric illnesses is often connected with frontal lobe involvement, and so on.

Particular modules may use the operations provided by specific types of insight typical for that module. It is difficult to imagine that the brain is constructed in such a way that the same operation is performed in many areas of the brain, thus seemingly wasting the large amount of brain tissue needed for so many operations. It is possible that operations such as working memory or insight are included in the set of operations that are performed independently inside the various modules in order to facilitate and speed up the functioning of particular modules. It is further possible that these operations performed by working memory or by insight differ between modules. For instance, visual working memory was found to be disturbed in the task of angle differentiation in patients with occipital lobe lesions and in the task of angle sequences in patients with temporal and parietal lobe lesions. Disturbances of the auditory working memory, as in one's ability to differentiate between single tones and tone sequences, were observed in patients with posterior T1 lesions. Parietal lobe lesions, on the other hand, led to impairments of working memory for tone sequences (Meerson, 1986; Tonkonogy, 1973) (for more details, see chapter 8, section entitled "Amnestic Syndromes").

In some cases, the particular working memory operations may be copied in another site in order to bring the processing closer to the site of subsequent operations, for example, using single-cell recording. Goldman-Rakic, Scalaidhe, and Chafee (2000) showed that in rhesus monkeys, areas in the inferior convexity of the prefrontal cortex were involved in the visual working memory of faces and objects. Selective neuronal activity was recorded following the presentation of a stimulus: a face followed by a delay. This pattern was also observed in the neuronal activity of the inferior temporal cortex, pointing to the possibility that neuronal activity in the prefrontal cortex copied the information transmitted from the primarily sensory temporal cortex areas for further use in the tasks typical for frontal neuronal activity, such as various executive functions in the physical and social worlds.

Rizzolatti, Fogassi, and Gallese (2000) carried out a study further supporting the idea that one area of the cortex may make copies of neuronal activity occurring in another area of the cortex. Using single-cell recording, the authors identified mirrored neuronal activity in the F5 frontal area while a monkey performed or observed hand-object interactions. Mirrored neurons were also found to be active in the superior temporal sulcus (STS) in response to movements with real objects.

It is possible that neuronal activity in the STS closely connected with visual areas in the posterior cortex was transmitted and copied into the F5 area for probable use in the course of motor action initiated by neurons in this area (for more details, see chapter 6, section entitled "Motor Apraxia").

Syndromes

While operations such as working memory may be performed by various modules, there are sets of conventional operations that are specific to particular modules. Lesions in these sets may result in the development of unique clinical syndromes with typical sites of lesion localization. Consider, for example, Broca's aphasia, a clinical syndrome that consists of unique and complex conventional disturbances in expressive speech. These disturbances include difficulties in word finding as well as laborious, effortful speech, which is often characterized by a prevalence of nouns, combined with disturbances of unconventional types of speech comprehension, such as impairments in reading and writing. Broca's aphasia is characterized by a lesion in the posterior F3, the operculum of the central sulci, the insula, and the subcortical nuclei. Another clinical syndrome, known as Wernicke's aphasia, is marked by severe impairments in speech comprehension with a peculiar disorder of expressive speech quite different from Broca's aphasia; contrary to Broca's aphasia, Wernicke's aphasia is characterized by fluency, a prevalence of verbs and functional words, combined with impairments in reading and writing abilities. The syndrome is marked by a lesion both in the posterior T1 and in adjacent structures (for more details, see chapter 7, section entitled "Aphasia Syndromes and Other Language Disorders").

However, some of the symptoms of one particular clinical syndrome may also be present in other syndromes, especially symptoms reflecting disturbances of unconventional information processing. For instance, impairments of more complex types of speech comprehension may be observed in various types of aphasia, both anterior and posterior, thus supporting the holistic approach to the problem of localization. Another example of a single symptom reflecting multiple possible syndromes is *anomia* (also known as *optic aphasia*)—a condition that has been described in cases with lesions found throughout the cortex of the left hemisphere in the frontal, temporal, and parietal lobes as well as far back in the occipital lobe.

In most cases, the presence of anomia is indicative of a part of a particular syndrome, such as Broca's or Wernicke's aphasia, conduction aphasia, transcortical aphasia, and so on. Some differences are indicative of anomia in the various plausible syndromes. For instance, anomia in Wernicke's aphasia is characterized by hyperactive speech, with the production of a series of examples of verbal and literal paraphasia in an attempt to find the proper word. On the other hand, a patient suffering from Broca's aphasia is unable to produce any speech at all while attempting to find the appropriate word. Efforts have been made to identify and categorize differences in the words most often found to be disturbed in patients with anomia and to relate these differences to particular lesion locations.

As in cases of aphasia syndrome, disturbances of auditory or visual working memory may represent a component of a particular clinical syndrome reflecting the malfunction of a corresponding module, as is the case for visual object agnosia, prosopagnosia, spatial agnosia, and auditory agnosia, in which more strictly localized sites of lesions are associated with each of the various syndromes. Conventional and unconventional modules, especially domain-specific modules, may be closely interconnected (e.g., for object recognition).

The modules for conventional information processing may provide the initial stage in the operations of the modules for unconventional information processing, serving as an important component in the hierarchical functional structure for that processing, as in the operations underlying the executive functions.

CIRCUIT AND CIRCUITRY

THE TERMS *circuit* and *circuitry* are typically defined technologically as being part of an electrical scheme. As described in neuropsychiatric literature, the terms were initially used in studies of functional connections between various cortical and subcortical structures. For instance, depression has been described as being the result of lesions in various areas of cortical and subcortical structures and in the diencephalo-hypothalamic region of the brain, with the two areas being connected by cortico-subcortical circuits. It seems possible that the core of the clinical syndrome of depression is underlined by a lesion in the module for emotions and is thus primarily localized in a particular area, namely, the amygdala. This area is turned on via different areas of the brain that receive negative information from both the outside and inside worlds as transmitted through the circuitry, which serves to connect the various regions of the brain involved in the processing of emotions. It is also possible that circuits may be an important part of the operations inside one particular module, or over several connected modules. Specifically, the modules of social recognition and actions include a circuitry of emotion regulating the assessment of situations in the outer and inner worlds so that the various nodes of the emotional circuitry receive input inciting or inhibiting a particular emotion, for example, depression or anxiety (for more details, see chapter 11, section entitled "Mood Disorders").

The circuits and circuitries may very well be an important component in the functional structure of brain information processing, though more in-depth, detailed, definitive descriptions are needed. Still, the words circuit and circuitry are avoided in the major literature related to clinical neuroscience. It has been suggested that electrical schemes of the circuits in computer chips may be used as an initial model for further exploration of the role of circuitry in brain information processing and its disturbances.

SIZES OF LESIONS AND COMPENSATORY MECHANISMS OF BRAIN INFORMATION PROCESSING

CLINICALLY SIGNIFICANT DISTURBANCES of conventional and unconventional information processing are usually observed in cases with relatively large lesions involving the cortical and often subcortical areas of the cerebral hemispheres. For instance, the development of Broca's aphasia is underlined by lesions involving the posterior F3, the lower parts of the central gyri, and the insula, with frequent extensions into the adjacent subcortical areas. Small lesions limited to the parts of those areas such as posterior F3 result only in transient aphasia or do not cause any language disturbances (see review by Tonkonogy, 1986). This effect may be explained by the existence of special mechanisms protecting the uninterrupted functioning of brain information processing. One of the mechanisms may be the presentation and processing of information in a parallel, distributed form, which continues to function even when a portion is damaged by a small lesion. McClelland and Rumelhart (1986) discussed the role of distributed memory in amnesia and suggested a distributed, developmental model for word recognition and naming.

Another mechanism may be related to the possibility that the same functional task may be accomplished by different programs within particular domain-specific conventional and unconventional modules, so that in the event of the impairment of one program, another program may overtake the functional task of the damaged program. A typical example of such a substitution is the use of unconventional information processing when conventional processing is disturbed. A patient with a small posterior T1 lesion may be able to comprehend the language spoken with regular speed, but may show disturbances of comprehension of faster conversational speech, making it impossible to use conventional simplified information processing based on the alphabet of words and phrases. In such cases, comprehension of spoken language may require the use of relatively complex, slow unconventional information processing provided by the alphabet of phonemes and syllables.

Some role may also be played by programs that use probability assessment to restrict the amount of information that has to be processed by the brain. This semantic assessment helps to reduce the number of choices so that the alphabet of the processing message consists of 10–15 items, for instance, when a subject is asked to name an object in the kitchen. In fact, when asked to point to the table and then to the window, the subject makes the determination of a high probability that the next question will be related to objects located in the same room. The same is true for the comprehension of conversational speech dealing with the patient's health or family conditions. However, if the semantic field is suddenly changed, for example, from objects in the room to body parts, a patient with mild aphasia caused by a small lesion will exhibit substantially increased difficulties in comprehension. It is also of interest that the number of errors may increase significantly when the patient is repeatedly asked to show the same objects in the kitchen or office, since probability of such repetitions in questions is, in normal conditions, usually quite low.

TYPES OF LESIONS

CIRCUMSCRIBED LARGE LESIONS AND GENERALIZED EXTENDED LESIONS

VARIOUS TYPES OF aphasia, agnosia, and apraxia have been described in studies of patients with circumscribed but large lesions caused by stroke or, in some cases, by tumors and head injuries. In such cases, the brain tissue is destroyed in particular areas, resulting in the loss of certain operations and leading to the development of specific clinical symptoms and syndromes reflecting the "minus tissue," or *negative* effect, of brain damage. The severity of the negative functional impairment becomes more prominent when the lesion is larger. Certainly, the localization and the size of lesions as well as other factors influence the clinical manifestations of these circumscribed losses of brain tissue. These factors include brain edema surrounding the destroyed brain area, or the so-called ischemic penumbra, caused by diminishing blood flow in the cortex when the cerebral infarction is primarily in the subcortical region. The particular disturbances are often transient in such cases, developing in the acute period of stroke or head injury and subsiding in the course of recovery.

Disturbances of modules for recognition and action underlined by relatively local and circumscribed loss of brain tissue are clinically manifested as aphasia, agnosia, and apraxia. In addition, the loss of brain tissue in a particular brain region may result in impairments of supportive and regulatory modules such as memory, attention, or emotion in the operations of activation of brain information processing for recognition and action. When the loss of tissue is large, extending through the many areas of cortex and subcortical nuclei and white matter, dementia develops, representing the peculiar multimodular combination of many clinical syndromes attributed to the lesions, with tissue loss in the various areas of the brain underlying the functioning of the various modules.

SMALL EXCITATORY LESIONS

ANOTHER TYPE OF lesion consists of small lesions that cause an excitation of the preserved brain tissue. This is true in cases of epilepsy with the preictal in the course of aura, the ictal, and in some cases the interictal psychiatric manifestations. They may include illusions, hallucinations, delusions, and anger with episodes of rage and other changes in mood and behavior. However, lesions with small tissue loss and with the source of excitation in particular brain areas responsible for those psychiatric manifestations being very often difficult to find, even when using the modern method of brain imaging, and especially in patients with primary psychiatric illnesses such as schizophrenia and bipolar disorder. Such disturbances may be mediated by a neurochemical imbalance, particularly at the synaptic level. The disturbances have been intensively and extensively studied over the course of recent decades, leading to the fascinating series of successes in the treatment of psychiatric patients.

However, some important mechanisms related to the excitatory role of small lesions in the formation of psychiatric syndromes and symptoms have been excluded from mainstream studies of diagnoses and treatments of psychiatric disturbances. These mechanisms are directly related to the understanding of the brain as primarily an electrical device with the crucial participation of neurochemically mediated activity. In such cases, a malfunction of the electrical part of the device per se may be responsible for the development of some of the psychiatric problems that, in turn, require treatment approaches based on understanding that an electrical malfunction may be responsible. For example, the intermittent psychiatric problems caused by excitation resulting in aggressive episodes such as rage outbursts may be underlined by subclinical seizure activity with only an indirect relation to the neurochemical imbalance.

Certainly, further studies may elucidate the importance of the direct role of electrical mechanisms in the development, diagnosis, and treatment of psychiatric disturbances and their relationships to neurochemical abnormalities.

SUMMARY

THE ADDITION OF localization information to neuroradiological and neuropsychological studies provides for the field a newer generation of thinking. Historically, neuropsychological studies existed without reference to brain-imaging studies and vice versa. Over the last decade the two have interfaced, resulting in exciting discoveries and a greater understanding of brain dysfunction. However, the relationship between the two remains relatively weak. The integration of the historic roots of neuropsychology brings an even stronger presence to the role that neuroradiological and neuropsychological studies, alone and combined, may add to the understanding and treatment of neurological and neuropsychological disorders.

2

Disorders of Recognition in the Physical World: Visual Agnosia

RECOGNITION REPRESENTS ONE of the major parts of brain information processing. Disturbances of recognition are reflected in many signs and symptoms of various psychiatric and neurological disorders in the physical and social worlds. Disorders of recognition are divided into two major groups—agnosia and delusions. While agnosia reflects one's difficulty in recognizing real objects, scenes, spatial relations, and actions as well as disturbances of language recognition, both oral and written, hallucinations and perceptual delusions involve the recognition of an experience that does not exist outside the mind of the individual. Elementary sensations are usually preserved: thus often they do not have a direct influence on the clinical manifestation of a recognition disturbance.

Agnosia and hallucinations may develop in one of various modalities—visual, auditory, tactile, or somatic. Though various types of modality-specific agnosia have been researched and explored, special attention is given to the disorders of recognition in the physical and social worlds. Social agnosia has only begun, in recent literature, to be described in a systematic manner.

VISUAL AGNOSIA

DISORDERS IN THE understanding, recognition, and use of learned symbols were first described under the term asymbolia, coined by Finkelnburg in 1870. Using Kant's ideas on *facultas signatrix,* a basic human faculty, Finkelnburg suggested that asymbolia is the loss of one's ability to recognize and utilize signs and symbols of objects. According to Finkelnburg, two other basic human faculties—sensorial and intellectual—remained preserved in asymbolia. Similar ideas were advanced by Hulings Jackson in 1876, described under the term *imperception*—namely, a disorder of object recognition and of actions involving the use of objects.

Munk first supported the concept of human faculties in an animal experiment performed in 1881. Following the bilateral extirpation of the occipital cortex in dogs and monkeys, Munk demonstrated the development of *cortical blindness* (*Rindenblindheit*). He also observed a *psychic blindness* (*Seelingblindheit*) following the partial removal of grey matter in the posterior and superior regions of the two occipital tips. While the dogs either avoided or jumped over any encountered obstacles, they remained indifferent and were generally unresponsive to food, fire, sticks, and their masters. Munk concluded that the dogs were suffering from a *psychic blindness* in which previous perceptions were forgotten and the dogs were thus unable to recognize what they had formerly seen. Several years later, Freud (1891) coined the term agnosia, and the condition was defined as a disorder of visual recognition and as an independent syndrome in patients with local brain pathology (Charcot, 1883; Lissauer, 1890; Wilbrand, 1892).

Visual agnosia was first observed as a disorder in which many types of recognition of visual information were disturbed, while elementary visual sensations remained preserved. In 1883, Charcot described the case of a well-educated man, fluent in several languages, including Greek and Latin, who suffered from a stroke. Following the incident, the patient could no longer recognize well-known objects, was unable to recognize his own face in the mirror, and could not recall the faces of his wife and children. Memories of shapes and colors were completely destroyed, and he was unable to recognize the letters of the alphabet. Visual images were absent from his dreams, while auditory images were preserved. The patient could not recognize streets, buildings, or public monuments, and he exhibited difficulties in orientation in the town where he lived. The disturbances outlined in Charcot's case were later described as relatively independent types of visual agnosia and thus classified primarily based on the differentiation between particular tasks of visual information processing as visual object agnosia, prosopagnosia (or facial blindness), visuospatial agnosia, primary alexia, and loss of visual images.

It has become generally accepted that the goals of visual information processing include two major tasks—the recognition of objects and scenes, and the recognition of space. Accordingly, there are two major types of visual agnosia, classified as (1) visual agnosia of objects and scenes, and (2) visual spatial agnosia. Visual space recognition plays a significant role in some forms of praxis, for example, constructional praxis, often making it difficult to distinguish visual spatial agnosia from some types of apraxia. It has been suggested that visual agnosia of objects and scenes primarily involves a lesion in the inferior, ventral occipito-temporal area, while visual spatial agnosia develops following lesions located in the superior, dorsal occipito-parietal area of both cerebral hemispheres (Kleist, 1934; Poetzl, 1928; Ungerleider and Mishkin, 1982).

Since different areas of the brain that perform different functions are often found to be very close to one another, visual information processing may be damaged by an extensive lesion, for example, an infarction or a tumor, and significant overlaps between various types of visual agnosia may be observed. A lesion that does not occur exclusively in one area related to one specific function may result in the development of two or more types of visual agnosia in one patient, as was observed by Charcot. This overlap may also be related to the nature of visual information processing. An individual will typically recognize an object on the basis of its characteristic shape, for example, a bicycle, a table, a letter, or a face. However, some objects are more difficult to discern based on their shape alone without also knowing other characteristics of the object. For instance, the color of a fruit may be necessary for its recognition (for example, as a tomato, a cucumber, or a banana), while the recognition of a tree or of an animal may be primarily based on the object's texture and color (Ullman, 1996). Thus, disorders of object recognition based on the shape of an object may be partly compensated for or worsened depending on a preservation or disturbance in the ability to recognize color or texture.

VISUAL OBJECT AGNOSIA

THE ABILITY TO recognize real objects, drawings of objects, and written letters is disturbed in those who suffer from visual object agnosia. Though elementary visual functions may be preserved and the patient retains the ability to see, the patient's ability to recognize an object may be affected, even when the length of time in which the object is presented is unlimited.

The process of recognition has to include two major parts:

1. The processing of features and structural aspects of the objects via a code that is compatible with the descriptions of corresponding models in the memory store; and

2. The comparison of structured descriptions with stored models that are organized in a beneficial and strategic way and help to limit and to facilitate the search for a corresponding model and subsequently to activate that model.

Disorders of recognition may involve both of these elements, and the different types of recognition disturbances may largely reflect a malfunctioning of each of the respective parts. In 1890, Lissauer divided object visual agnosia into two categories, based on the ideas of association psychology—*apperceptive agnosia* and *associative agnosia*.

In 1889, Freund described and coined a third disorder—*optic aphasia*. The disorder was considered to be the result of a disconnection between the areas of visual object recognition and those of language, leading to disturbances in the naming of visually recognized objects; this particular type of visual object agnosia is considered by some to be a subtype of associative agnosia. Cortical blindness, a fourth type of visual object agnosia, is more peripheral in nature, but it still covers the cortical disturbances of peripheral vision, and it may be related to disturbances in the recognition of some simple visual features of objects not yet clearly described in the literature.

Clinical Aspects

The term *visual object agnosia* refers to a disturbance in the recognition of real objects and their drawings or photographs, while elementary visual functions (such as visual acuity and brightness discrimination) remain relatively preserved.

Visual object recognition involves two major tasks: the recognition of objects in a conventional and unoccluded view; and the recognition of novel objects, of occluded objects, or of objects seen from an unusual, unconventional viewpoint. Visual object agnosia of a conventional *type* may be underlined by disturbances of conventional information processing based on well-learned features of an entire object, or of its part in hierarchical structures. It is also possible that different sets of predefined features are learned for the purpose of differentiating objects at the basic level (car, bird, chair), the superordinate level (vehicle, animal, furniture), or the subordinate level (Mustang, husky, armchair) (see Rosch, Mervis, Gray, Johnson, & Boyes-Braem, 1976).

Disturbances in the use of masked, fragmented, or briefly presented objects as well as objects in unusual positions are reflected in the clinical manifestations of the unconventional type of visual object agnosia. In the case of unconventional information processing, an object may be partly occluded either by another object or by visual "noise," or the shape of the object may be seen differently as a result of significant changes in the view of the observer or of variations in object

her stroke, we observed disturbances in her capacity to recognize both real objects and drawings of real objects, as well as in her ability to copy and match similar and different drawings. She was able to facilitate the recognition of drawings of objects and geometrical figures through the use of tracing hand movements. Within 2 years of her stroke, the patient's recognition of real objects slowly improved, but she continued to demonstrate difficulties in the recognition of drawings of objects and geometrical figures. The patient ambulated freely, her speech and language were preserved, and she was able to perform her daily activity as housekeeper without any apparent problems. This functional preservation was noted by the disability evaluation team, and the patient's disability status was subsequently terminated, to be restored only after our detailed report concerning the patient's agnosia problems.

A similar, if not better, form of compensation was reported in a follow-up of Schneider's functional status. According to information provided to Critchley by Leonhardt in 1953, Schneider was mayor of a small town in southern Germany at the end of the 1940s, and worked as a ticket cashier at the railway station in 1952–1953. Interest in apperceptive agnosia was rekindled by descriptions of a series of cases in which the development of the disorder primarily followed carbon monoxide poisoning (Abadi, Kulikowski, & Meudell, 1981; Adler, 1944; Alexander and Albert, 1983; Benson & Greenberg, 1969; Campion & Latto, 1985; Efron, 1968; Landis, Graves, Benson, & Hebben, 1982; Milner et al., 1991).

Patients suffering from visual apperceptive agnosia are impaired in their ability to perceive shapes. The ability to visually process the well-learned complex features of the object presented in its conventional unoccluded view is also lost. The patient may try to describe the general shape of an object, for example, "oval," "round," or "elongated," but fails to outline the particular details of complex features of the shape that are important for correct recognition of the object. A pen or a hairbrush may be described by the patient as a long narrow object, but it is not distinguished in its individuality. One of our patients looking at a pot described it as "something round, probably a watermelon." A patient described by Benson and Greenberg in 1969 recognized a rubber eraser as "a small ball."

In some cases of apperceptive agnosia, simple features may be recognized, and patients may try to use a simplified structural reconstruction method for recognition. In 1944, Adler described a patient who recognized the numbers that consisted of straight lines, such as 1, 4, and 7, but not the numbers with curved lines, such as 2, 3, 5, 6, 8, and 9. After 7 months, the patient began to recognize numbers with curved lines by using simple features combination: for example, according to the patient's own observations, the number 6 was recognizable by its lower loop, and the number 3 was distinguished by its lower and upper loops.

The ability to perceive color, size, and depth may be preserved in some cases, and patients may try to use these features as clues in the identification of an object. The case of Mr. S., a young man who developed apperceptive agnosia after suffering carbon monoxide poisoning, was described by Efron in 1968 and again by Benson and Greenberg in 1969. Though the researchers observed that the patient's elementary vision was preserved, they found that he was unable to identify real objects, pictorial representations of real objects, geometrical figures, letters, or numbers. The patient tried to overcome his inadequacies by using color and size cues, for example, recognizing the color of a safety pin as "silver and shiny," but he was still unable to identify the shape and would often attribute the recognized characteristics to another object of similar size and color, such as a watch or a nail clipper. Mr. S. learned to recognize a red toothbrush, but he could not identify a green toothbrush and he confused a red pencil with his own red toothbrush, calling it "my toothbrush." In 1944, Adler observed a patient who tried to use color to compensate for experienced difficulties in the ability to execute object shape recognition. A piece of white soap was recognized by the patient as a piece of paper, and vanilla ice cream was mistaken for scrambled eggs. Mr. X., a patient examined by Landis, Graves, Benson, and Hebben in 1982, recognized the drawing of a lion as an animal, but incorrectly guessed that it was a horse or a dog; however, he successfully recognized the drawing as a lion when yellow color was added to the picture.

To compensate for disturbances in the visual processing of shape, patients with apperceptive agnosia have often been observed to resort to a peculiar tracing strategy. A patient of Goldstein and Gelb in 1918 traced the contours of hard-to-recognize stimuli, letters, and objects via movements of the head and hand; if the patient was prevented from moving his head or body, he was unable to read or to correctly recognize the stimulus. Subsequently, several similar cases were reported in the literature (for a review see Farah, 1990). In 1944, Adler reported a patient who used her index finger to trace the contour of an object in her attempts to recognize objects. In 1982, Landis et al. described the use of head and hand tracing movements by their patients, who exhibited improvement in the recognition of circles and triangles when they were allowed to use such tracing strategies. In some cases, the observation of a tracing motion by the examiner facilitated recognition by the patient (Benson & Greenberg, 1969; Efron, 1968).

Disturbances in the shape recognition of a moving object may be mitigated by adding an important feature to the object image, for example, movement, as in a moving vehicle, a flying bird, or a moving animal.

It appears to be quite difficult for patients with visual agnosia to recognize photographs, especially those of objects, as compared to the actual three-dimensional (3-D) objects, since some important features of a 3-D image may be missing in two-dimensional (2-D) drawings or photographs. Drawings and photographs often outline the 2-D contour of the object, which may or may not be exactly the same shape as that of the actual 3-D object. Also, the color, texture, and surroundings of the object may not be accurately reflected in the drawing or photograph. In many cases, amnesia of a visual object may only be revealed when drawings or photographs are presented, while recognition of real objects may be preserved or only mildly disturbed.

Disturbances at the Semantic Level

Associative Object Agnosia. Associative agnosia is characterized by an inability to identify a visually presented object, while the basic operations of the first descriptive, encoding phase of visual information processing remains relatively preserved. An associative agnosia patient also often retains his or her ability to describe the basic features of an object, including its shape, color, and texture. The patient may correctly match identical objects and effectively draw a picture of the object or copy a drawing of the object, and yet still be unable to recognize the object or to match a visual description with the appropriate model in his or her memory store. In short, the visual perception of the object is alienated from its meaning, in a fashion similar to the alienation of word meaning in aphasia.

In 1890, Lissauer described a case of associative visual agnosia in a patient, a merchant who had suffered a stroke at the age of 80. Lissauer first examined the patient around 6 weeks after the onset of the stroke (see a detailed description of the case as documented by Grüsser & Landis, 1991). The patient demonstrated right-sided homonimous hemianopia with macular sparing. Visual acuity was about 0.6. The patient showed disturbances in the visual recognition of common objects, and was able to recognize them by palpation or sound. The patient preserved his ability to copy simple objects, but he was unable to recognize those objects in his own drawings. He was able to draw from memory only rudimentary sketches of objects. The patient's writing capabilities were preserved, but his reading was affected. He suffered from mild color agnosia but did not exhibit any topographical disorientation.

Examining the patient's ability to discriminate between visual forms of a similar, but not identical, nature, Lissauer stressed disturbances in the patient's symbolic understanding of seemingly identical visual forms. The patient was unable to recognize the object, but since the picture of the real object was more similar to that object than the pictures of the other objects, he eventually, using a step-by-step analysis, correctly indicated the correspondence between object and picture.

In addition to the disturbances in symbolic understanding, Lissauer recognized some impairments in the patient's processing of apperception. He suggested the existence of two stages in the process of recognition from apperception to association, the first stage being the apperception process and the second stage being the association of a content of apperception with other notions.

In later agnosia studies, numerous cases of associative agnosia described the condition as a normal percept stripped of its meaning. However, as in Lissauer's case, apperceptive disturbances were found in many instances. Apperceptive disturbances included extreme slowness when copying and difficulties in the matching of complex patterns with subtle differences (Levine & Calvanio, 1978), impairments in the recognition of objects with partial occlusion, disturbances in the ability to recognize objects fragmented and degraded by visual noise (Levine & Calvanio, 1978) and complications in the ability to distinguish between objects found in overlapping drawings (Riddoch & Humphreys, 1987). These disturbances in apperception are mainly related to unconventional information processing. At the same time, though the ability to perceive objects in their conventional and unoccluded view remains "normal," although "stripped of its meaning" in patients with associative agnosia, disturbances involving the perception of objects in their conventional view are observed in patients suffering from apperception agnosia.

The dichotomy suggested by Lissauer in 1890 has remained widely accepted in visual agnosia studies. In addition, some authors have recognized optic aphasia as a separate syndrome of visual object agnosia.

Optic Aphasia.   This refers to a disturbance in the ability to name visually presented stimuli. An optic aphasic patient may be able to describe an object with gestures or descriptive words but is unable to directly name the object. While a patient suffering from associative agnosia experiences a "normal percept stripped of its meaning," a patient suffering from optic aphasia exhibits an inability to name an object, while perception remains normal and its meaning is preserved. Optic aphasia is a modality-specific condition—no disturbances are observed in the naming of nonvisual modalities, as in the naming of an object via obtained tactile information. The patient is also able to point to an object as named or described verbally by the examiner.

Freund first described the condition of optic aphasia in 1889, differentiating modality-specific disturbances of naming from "mind-blindness." At the time, the distinction between associative agnosia, as described by Lissauer in 1890, and optic aphasia was a relatively vague one. Some authors considered optic aphasia to be a mild form of associative agnosia (Bauer & Rubins, 1985; Kertesz, 1987)—a type of associative agnosia with truly normal perception (Humphreys & Riddoch, 1984, 1985). On the other hand, Geschwind suggested in 1965 that associative agnosia is actually optic aphasia (for a review, see Farah, 1990). Other authors have described cases of optic aphasia with disturbances of naming in both visual and tactile modalities (see De Renzi, Zambolin, & Crisi, 1987).

However, primarily semantic errors have been described in numerous cases of optic aphasia, for example, mistakenly naming a cricket for a grasshopper (L'Hermitte & Beauvois, 1973), a bird cage for an aquarium (L'Hermitte & Beauvois, 1973), a cigarette lighter for a lamp or a bracelet for a necklace (Poeck, 1984). These semantic errors were often found to occur in peculiar patterns, usually not seen in anomia observed in patients with aphasia, leading to the hypothesis that some component of agnosia was present in the answers. For example, L'Hermitte and Beauvois (1973, pages 706–707), asked a patient to identify what a bus was. The patient's answer was "a wagon . . . a form of public transportation since there is a back door . . . a stage-coach. . . . it would be . . . no . . . a city cab . . . not a cab, but a city bus." The patient's attempts to use a structural description of the object to facilitate its recognition resembled the visual information processing that had been observed in patients with visual object agnosia. The similarities were especially apparent when the patient was asked to name an aquarium—"A bird cage, unless it is a pot for flowers, a container, a tank, *the four aspects . . . the walls made of glass and wood. . . . it could be an aquarium if it is made of glass*"—a type of answer that has not been observed in patients with regular types of anomic aphasia.

Further studies are needed to better define the condition. An evaluation of the unconventional types of visual information processing in patients of optic aphasia would be important for a comparison of the condition with that of visual object agnosia. A comparison of typical patterns of semantic errors in optic aphasia and of anomia in patients with aphasia is another important topic of possible inquiry.

Cortical Blindness.   Bilateral lesions of occipital lobes involving area V1 and corresponding to Brodmann's area 17 in both hemispheres may result in a loss of elementary vision, possibly to the degree of total blindness. No changes are observed in either the retina or in reflexes in response to light. An EEG shows a loss of alpha rhythms, replaced by slow rhythms of reduced voltage. Loss of vision may be accompanied by anosognosia of blindness and, in some cases, by visual hallucinations.

According to Poetzl in 1928, several main stages may be observed in the course of recovery from cortical blindness: (1) sensation of darkness; (2) grayness of objects similar to achromatopsia, in which objects may be seen as in a fog; (3) recovery of color, beginning with red and ending with blue; and (4) visual fatigue, or asthenopia, with difficulties in fixation and in control of eye movements. During the final stage, as well as in previous stages of the condition, perception of objects may be quite difficult, simulating visual agnosia.

Lesions are often found to be caused either by bilateral infarctions in the posterior cerebral arteries or by basilar artery occlusions. In some cases, cortical blindness may be caused by bilateral occipital glioblastomas, carbon monoxide poisoning, or mercury poisoning.

Disturbances of Unconventional Information Processing in Agnosia

In patients with perceptive agnosia, many authors described disturbances in tests that may be related to unconventional information processing. These disturbances include difficulties in the recognition of figures composed of dots (Goldstein & Gelb, 1918; Landis et al., 1982), of figures drawn with a discontinuation of lines (Landis et al., 1982), of figures drawn with crosshatching lines (Goldstein & Gelb, 1918), of figures found on the background of masking textures (Warrington & Taylor, 1973), and of overlapping figures (De Renzi, Scotti, & Spinnler, 1969). Our studies, described in the following paragraphs, have shown that disturbances in the processing of visual unconventional information may be observed in cases with no signs of agnosia of object recognition in the object's conventional, unoccluded view. It is also important to stress that disturbances in simple feature discrimination, as in Efron's rectangles or in the differentiation of straight lines from curved lines, may be observed in apperceptive agnosia (Adler, 1944; Benson & Greenberg, 1969; Goldstein & Gelb, 1918).

Disturbances of unconventional information processing may be revealed when the patient attempts to recognize novel objects, objects in their unconventional view as taken from an unusual perspective, or occluded objects, such as incomplete figures with missing salient features, figures degraded by "noise," overlapping figures, figures affected by changes in the illumination of the object, or shadow image projections.

In cases in which an occluded, scrambled, or masked version of the object is presented, the process may be markedly simplified by the isolation of the image of a single object so as to separate the signal from "noise" interference. This image isolation is accomplished in the intermediate stages of perception in order to simplify the subsequent process of object recognition. In the first stage of the separation of a signal from noise, an object is localized from a scene that contains either one single object or several different objects. This is accomplished via the detection of an object that is figure-like in appearance by noting differences between the figure and the background in terms of texture, color, orientation, and luminance. In the second stage, a larger structure is created from, for instance, elements of the contour. The creation of this larger structure is often based on the artificial recognition of devices via the detection of simple features of the image, such as edges and the orientation of lines, with a subsequent grouping of the characteristics into more complex features, such as extended smooth curves based on the rule of curvilinearity; the patient is thus able to extract and measure salient image structures (Ullman, 1996). Though the resulting image may be incomplete, some parts of the image represent coherent units of the entire object, such as eyes or wheels. Using structural descriptions of object models stored in memory, the patient may be able to recognize the object at this stage, though in many such cases further processing is required. Thus, the third stage includes a completion of the image by applying such grouping criteria as smooth continuation and extrapolation of contour behind the occlusion by the use of symmetric contours.

Subsequent object recognition, especially in unconventional conditions such as briefly masked objects, often requires the limitation of choices of target objects by categorizing the object using the low frequencies of global features describing the entire object. Choice limitation may also be accomplished by the facilitation of choices using spatial relationships of targeted objects within the context of surrounding objects, for example, objects in the kitchen or in the office. Several types of unconventional conditions, such as the masking of objects by visual noise, overlapping figures, incomplete images of the objects, and shortened time of object exposition, make it more difficult for a patient to recognize the object.

Detection and Recognition of an Object Masked by Background Noise
Simultaneous Presentation of a Signal and Visual Background Noise. The term *filtration of a signal from noise,* defined as the recognition of a signal that is masked by noise, has been employed in recent studies of brain information processing. This term helps to identify the important goal of brain information processing and to measure it quantitatively as the signal/noise ratio.

In 1973, Warrington and Taylor devised a test of shape recognition on the background of texture, subsequently reporting disturbances in test performance in two patients, one with visual object agnosia and one with prosopagnosia. The test, though originally directed toward the intermittent stage of visual information processing and related to figure-background differentiation based on the grouping of single elements of the shape superimposed on texture, soon became used for the evaluation of visual apperceptive agnosia.

Campion and Latto suggested in 1985 that disorders of elementary perception may result from small scotomata brought about by a number of small disseminated lesions caused by carbon monoxide poisoning, "peppering" the patient's visual field. The patient would, in effect, view objects through a "peppery mask," impairing the recognition of form (Riddoch & Humphreys, 1987). Campion and Latto found that normal subjects preserved their ability to recognize photographed objects and scenes through such a mask. Though such an impairment may be found to be quite rare, masking may disrupt the contour and other features of objects and scenes; thus, difficulties in the detection and recognition of stimuli hindered by background noise may represent one of the more frequent manifestations of disturbances in unconventional visual processing. In 1973, we devised a special test to study in a more systematic manner the "filtration" of an image from background "visual noise" as formed by textures (Tonkonogy, 1973). In this test, an object is occluded by background noise, which is created by the introduction of texture with certain statistical characteristics (Figure 2.1). The texture was first developed by Julesz (1971a, 1971b) and was introduced in our studies as the background noise that could be measured according to the statistical characteristic of the texture (Tonkonogy, 1973). Since the object must be filtered from background noise, a disturbance in such filtration may be called *filtration agnosia*. Probabilities are calculated by the number of black squares in each line and presented to patients as $p = 0.15$, $p = 0.24$, and $p = 0.35$. The signal was represented by dotted contours of 12 objects (house, glasses, hammer, gavel, vase, key, bottle, kettle, etc.) (Figure 2.1).

Prior to testing, the subject was acquainted with drawings of the contours of all 12 objects on cards viewed for an unlimited amount

FIGURE 2.1 "Noisy" pictures of the objects. Probability of background black squares is $p = 0.25$ on the left and $p = 0.45$ on the right.

of time. The patients in the occipital group were unable to recognize some of the drawings of object contours presented without knowledge of the limitation of the number of objects to 12. Recognition markedly improved when the patient observed in advance the drawing of all 12 objects. After having taken as much time as needed to correctly recognize all 12 objects, the subject was presented with drawings of the objects' contours as well as with "noisy" figures on a tachistoscope screen with exposition times of 0.1 to 5000 milliseconds. Thresholds of object detection and recognition were recorded.

Testing was performed in one normal control group and in four groups of patients in which each patient had suffered from a stroke that resulted in local brain lesions. The study was performed in the late 1960s and early 1970s, when brain-imaging capabilities such as CT or MRI scans were not yet available. Clinical neurological and neuropsychological findings were used to assess possible lesion localizations. The first experimental group consisted of 19 subjects with various degrees of visual object amnesia and possible localization of lesion primarily in the occipital region, in some cases with a possible extension to the inferior temporal areas. The groups of patients with lesions outside the occipital region included 14 patients exhibiting elements of Gerstmann's syndrome and with possible lesions in the left inferior parietal region, 15 patients with moderate and mild Wernicke's aphasia with principal lesions found in the left superior-posterior temporal region, and 22 patients with mild or moderate Broca's aphasia and presumed localization of main lesions in the left premotor frontal area. In subsequent studies, we added a group of patients who had suffered from unilateral extirpations of the anterior temporal lobe, including 20 patients who had undergone surgery of the left hemisphere, and 22 patients who had undergone surgery of the right hemisphere. The control group consisted of 18 normal subjects corresponding in age and education level to the experimental groups. The results of the testing are presented in Table 2.1.

The table shows that increases in detection thresholds in tests with "noisy" pictures were not more than twofold in most of the patients with nonoccipital lesions. Those thresholds jumped 10 times with an increase in noise level from absent, $p = 0$, to $p = 0.35$ in the occipital group, pointing to a disturbance in the detection of signals from noise in that particular experimental group. At the same time, thresholds of detection remained at 10 millisecond (msec) for the $p = 0.35$ level of noise for the occipital or occipito-temporal patients; these patients were unable to recognize many of the objects with an exposition time of 5000 msec at the $p = 0.35$ level of noise.

More prominent disturbances are observed in the recognition of an object from a noisy background than in the filtration of a signal from

TABLE 2.1 Time Exposition (msec) at the Thresholds of the Contours Detection and Recognition of Objects Masked by the "Noisy" Background

Background textures black squares probability	$p = 0$	$p = 0.15$	$p = 0.25$	$p = 0.35$
Localization of Lesions	**Object Detection**			
Occipital or occipito-temporal, left or right	1.0 ± 0.2	5.0 ± 0.9	7.0 ± 1.8	10.2 ± 2.1
Temporal, superior-posterior, left	0.8 ± 0.3	1.2 ± 0.3	2.0 ± 0.7	2.8 ± 0.8
Parietal, inferior, left	0.7 ± 0.9	1.0 ± 0.4	1.7 ± 0.05	2.5 ± 0.5
Frontal, premotor, left	0.6 ± 0.2	0.8 ± 0.2	1.0 ± 0.2	1.0 ± 0.4
Normal control	0.5 ± 0.1	0.3 ± 0.1	0.6 ± 0.2	1.0 ± 0.3
	Object Recognition			
Occipital or occipito-temporal, left or right	102 ± 15	5000*	5000*	5000 **
Temporal, superior-posterior	6.2 ± 1.1	12.0 ± 1.2	85.0 ± 3.2	185.0 ± 15.0
Parietal	6.5 ± 1.3	9.0 ± 1.0	45.0 ± 0.6	150.0 ± 10.0
Frontal, premotor	2.3 ± 0.2	3.2 ± 0.0	12.0 ± 1.0	58.0 ± 4.0
Normal control	2.0 ± 0.2	2.2 ± 0.2	5.0 ± 0.8	50.0 ± 3.7

*Number of recognized objects: 6–9 out of 12
**Number of recognized objects: 3–6 out of 12

noise. In normal controls, mean thresholds for object recognition increased slightly, from 2.0 msec for $p = 0$ (complete absence of noise) to 2.2 msec for $p = 0.15$ (a mild level of noise), and 10.0 msec for $p = 0.25$ (a moderate level of noise) while markedly increasing to 50 msec when the level of noise reached $p = 0.35$. At the same time, the threshold of object recognition from background noise markedly increased even with low levels of noise in the group of patients with occipital lesions. In that group of patients, a mild $p = 0.15$ level of noise resulted in a significant increase in the threshold to 5000 msec for object recognition, while recognition was still impossible for a significant percentage of the objects—3–6 objects out of 12. The inability to recognize reached 6–9 objects at the high level of noise $p = 0.35$ level of noise. Patients with other lesion sites exhibited a moderate increase in the mean threshold with higher levels of noise, especially those groups of patients with lesions of the inferior parietal and superior-posterior temporal. The increase in threshold in the premotor frontal group yielded data comparable to that of the normal control group. In a separate study of patients who had previously undergone an anterior-inferior temporal lobectomy for the treatment of epilepsy, the number of errors was higher following surgery of the right hemisphere than the number of errors following surgery of the left hemisphere. In general, however, the disturbances were mild and did not exceed the level of impairment observed in the posterior-superior temporal group (Meerson, 1986).

Delayed Presentation of Signal and Visual Noise.   Disturbances in the filtration of a signal from noise are also observed in experiments employing the use of forward and backward masking (Meerson, 1986). In tests with forward masking, the masking signal lasted for 250 msec and consisted of overlapping figures followed by the object image on the tachistoscope screen. During tests of backward masking, the same figures were used, but were presented during the 250 msec after the object image appeared on the screen.

For the control group, the mean threshold of object recognition increased in forward masking from 2 msec to 20 msec and in backward masking to 60 msec. When the time of exposition was increased, the process of recognition by the participants in the control group began with discerning the approximate shape of the object, as, for example, "something round," or "something elongated," followed by the correct classification of the object as an animal, dishes, or utensils. During forward masking, the signal began to fade away when the test signal was presented, but in backward masking the signal overlapped the fading object image in the immediate memory. Therefore, recognition with backward masking probably required more time of object exposition.

The masking effect resulted in a marked increase in the mean threshold of recognition for forward masking to 940 msec in patients with mild visual object agnosia (Group 1) and to 1500 msec in patients with more prominent visual object agnosia (Group 2). Backward masking produced a more prominent increase of mean thresholds, with an increase to 3800 msec in Group 1, and an inability to recognize more than 50% of the objects even with exposition of more than 5000 msec in Group 2. The method of recognition employed by occipital patients in masking conditions also differed from that of normal controls. The patients *relied* on the reconstruction of the objects from the full or almost full account of the details. Thus, the exhibited difficulties could not be explained only by problems with immediate memory. Disturbances at higher levels of the recognition process in patients with occipital lobe lesions were apparent in these experiments. At the same time, patients with lesions localized in areas other than the occipital lobe showed only a mild increase in object recognition thresholds compared to normal controls; the thresholds for forward masking were at mean levels of 20 msec for controls, 26 msec for the frontal premotor group, 45 msec for the left parietal group, and 55 msec for the left upper-posterior temporal group.

Disturbances in the Recognition of Objects With Overlapping Contours.
One type of picture that causes increased difficulties in object recognition is a figure with overlapping contours of several objects.
Poppelreuter first introduced such figures in 1917 for the study of visual
agnosia in patients injured in the course of World War I (Figure 2.2).

A series of different types of overlapping figures was subsequently
used by many authors. DeRenzi, Scotti, and Spinnler (1969) used Ghent's
overlapping figures task to study the impairments suffered by brain-
damaged patients. The test was originally devised to assess the development of perception in children. Some of the patients in the DeRenzi
study were unable to recognize a majority of the overlapped objects
but had retained the ability to recognize non-overlapping drawings of
the same figures.

Difficulties in Poppelreuter's figures present themselves in the patient's need to trace the contour of each object in spite of the mislead-
ing directions imposed by the overlapping contours of other objects.
In some sense, the incomplete object contour has to be detected and
traced from the background noise of other contours by locking one's
attention along the contour of the targeted object and shifting it to
another contour when the previous contour is recognized. The conditions are similar to the situation in natural scenarios in which an
object is seen against a backdrop of other objects, such as a fork among
other types of utensils in a drawer.

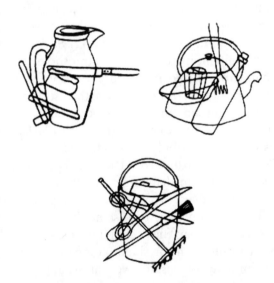

FIGURE 2.2 Overlapping figures. At the left upper corner, the figure originally
introduced for testing by Poppelreuter, 1917.

*Short Time of Object Exposition and Disturbances in Assessing
the Shape of the Entire Object and Its Parts*

Significant disturbances in object recognition may be found when the time of object exposition is shortened by tachistoscope presentation without application of backward or forward masking. According to Meerson in 1986, thresholds of recognition of object drawings were in the range of 1.8–2.5 msec in 10 normal controls. The control subjects were able to detect the presence of "something" on the screen at an exposition time of 0.4–0.5 msec, and to notice approximately the general shape of the objects with an exposition 0.7–1.0 msec, for example, "something round" for a cow or a globe, or "something elongated" for a spade or a pen. Normal controls recognized a class of objects, such as the class of tool for a shovel, or the class of dishes for a pot, at 1.3–1.5 msec of exposition, and correctly recognized most of the objects at an exposition time of 1.8–2.5 msec. Similar results were recorded in 42 patients with a unilateral extirpation of the anterior temporal lobe, where the minimal time for the recognition of object drawings did not exceed 2–2.5 msec. In groups of patients with left superior-posterior temporal lesions and left parietal lesions, the thresholds of object recognition were at 6–8 msec.

In patients with occipital or occipito-temporal lesions and mild visual agnosia for object drawings (12 patients) or with a complete absence of agnosia (11 patients), the thresholds increased to 85–120 milliseconds. The patients with occipital or occipito-temporal lesions detected "something" on the screen at an exposition time of 1.0 msec, a slightly longer time than normal controls. However, they were unable to outline the shapes of object features and to correctly recognize the parts of the objects until the time of exposition reached 120–130 msec. One of the patients, while trying to recognize a bicycle, said "something" at 1 msec, "a wheel" at 10 msec, "a saddle" at 18 msec, "a steering wheel and a lamp" at 20 msec, "no, that is a steering bar, this is not a car" at 30 msec, "two wheels, a saddle, and a steering bar like a scooter" at 50 msec, "a pedal, now I recognize, two wheels, a saddle, a steering bar, this is a scooter" at 70 msec, "I see spikes in the wheels and their connections, this is a bicycle" at 90 msec, and, "yes, this is a race bicycle for men" at 100 msec.

Thus, as in the cases of visual agnosia of object shape with an unlimited length of presentation, the recognition of object shape presented with a short time of exposition did not include a correct appreciation of the particular complex feature that includes details of the object shape needed for correct recognition. The complex feature was usually recognized only in general, without particular salient features, and erroneously ascribed to the wrong object. The patient, in an effort to process such fuzzy pictures, picked up single features one by one from the object picture on the screen of the tachistoscope. Lining up the single features, the patient was unable to recognize them as a part of a particular object. When exposition reached 70 msec, the patient erroneously recognized the object as a scooter instead of a bicycle, and reached the correct answer only after an exposition time of around 100 msec. However, this becomes possible only when almost all or all sets of single parts are accounted for by a simplified structural description.

In general, the shortening of exposition time for the object image with and without the forward and backward masking helps to uncover the disturbances in the two stages of the recognition process in patients with occipital lobe lesions. These two stages involve the disturbances in preserving the image in the immediate memory and in reconstruction of the objects from an incomplete image in the immediate memory. It is probable that the well-learned, invariant properties method probably applies for the recognition of unaltered images of objects in their conventional views, but cannot be used in the recognition of incomplete images of the objects.

Such images require a limitation of choices of objects via the use of preserved low frequencies, properties of the object, and reconstruction of the object based on structural descriptions of object parts, and may be partly based on their segmentation and grouping. This processing of unconventional information is both more vulnerable and less reliable than the processing of conventional information by the invariant properties method. Such disturbances in the processing of unconventional information may be seen in cases in which disorders of conventional information processing are mild, if not completely absent.

Agnosia of Object Drawings With Incomplete Features. Unconventional information processing is required when one is presented with drawings in which an object is presented, sometimes intentionally, with incomplete features. Two major types of incomplete figures have been used for the testing of visual agnosia. One type of incomplete figure employs the degradation of the object contour via breaks, or gaps, in the contour lines. The general contour, as well as other salient features of the object drawing, is thus degraded, making the target object similar to the object image in the background noise as described in the previous paragraph. Pictures from the Street Gestalt Completion Test (Street, 1931) provide examples of such incomplete figures. Gollin (1960) employed similar types of incomplete pictures in a test originally devised for children (Figure 2.3). In Gollin's test, the subject is presented with an increasingly complete version of the object drawing until the object is correctly identified. Similar tests employing progressively more degraded, fragmented images of animate and inanimate objects were employed in a study examining impairments of visual object recognition in patients

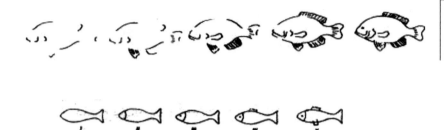

FIGURE 2.3 Upper row: Examples of Gollin's degraded pictures (1960). Lower row:
Heilbronner's pictures with missing features (1904).

suffering from schizophrenia (Doniger et al., 2001). The term *perceptual closure* refers to the filling-in of missing information by the visual system during a partial viewing condition; the term has been used to characterize the ability to recognize objects based on partial and fragmentary information, often as presented in a testing situation (Doniger, Silipo, Rabinowicz, Snodgrass, & Javitt, 2002; Snodgrass & Freenan, 1990).

The use of incomplete figures such as those used by Gollin, by Warrington and James (1967), and later by Warrington and Taylor (1973) showed that patients with posterior hemisphere lesions could recognize only the more complete pictures with a minimum number of missing features. Normal controls, on the other hand, were able to identify drawings of the same objects, but with a larger number of features missing.

In another type of incomplete pictures test, the drawings of the objects were degraded by the omission of some of the salient features, while the general shapes of the object contours were preserved. Such pictures were used in a study of visual object amnesia performed by Heilbronner in 1910. Decreasing numbers of missing salient features were reflected in the decrease in the levels of perceptual degradation from I to V in these pictures (Figure 2.3). Heilbronner's use of incomplete figures is mainly directed toward the general examination of the absence of more and less salient features and its role in the disorders of object recognition. The Street–Gollin's model of incomplete figures, on the other hand, primarily helps to test the way and extent to which a disruption in the shape contour of an object affects patients suffering from visual agnosia of shape.

We used a type of incomplete figures that is similar to that of Heilbronner (Meerson, 1981; Meerson, 1986; Tonkonogy, 1997) and constructed by us to preserve the salient features and to omit the less important details (Figure 2.4). This helped to clarify the role of missing

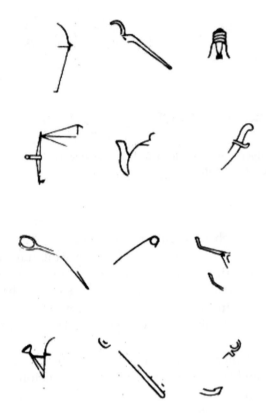

FIGURE 2.4 Examples of incomplete pictures with the preservation of salient features.

secondary features in disturbances of object recognition. Pictures were presented by tachistoscope with an exposition time of 1500 msec.

Drawings of the same 12 objects previously mentioned were included in each series of tests. The attempted recognition of 12 pictures with preserved salient features and with exclusion of the less important details resulted in a significant percentage of errors—4–5 objects were recognized incorrectly by occipital patients, 0–1 objects by patients of the parietal group, compared with zero errors made by the controls. The number of unrecognized objects did not exceed 0–1 for patients with superior-posterior temporal lesions or for patients with a unilateral extirpation of the anterior-inferior temporal lobe.

Disturbances in Recognition of Objects in an Unconventional View, and Disturbances of Alignment of the Object Into Conventional Position. The accurate recognition of an object viewed from an unconventional position may entail special difficulties in the use of well-learned invariant properties methods. According to Ullman (1996), such invariant features as perimeter length, elongation, and shape movements may be significantly altered by changes in viewing position. In response to an impaired ability to achieve recognition of an object via an invariant description of the object, normal subjects may use other compensatory methods, including a structural decomposition and description of the object by its parts, and alignment of the object view to the conventional position of the object.

In cases of the recognition of objects from unconventional viewpoints, several approaches may be applied to normalize an image-based, viewpoint-dependent description of an object with the object-based model (see Ullman, 1996). These approaches include the alignment method, interpolation across the different views (Poggio & Edelman, 1990), and interpolation across different visually similar exemplars of object class (Beymer & Poggio, 1996; Lando & Edelman, 1995).

Several studies have described disturbances in the use of alignment in the recognition of objects from an unusual viewing position. In these studies, patients were unable either to match the photographs of an object in its conventional view to photographs of the object in its unconventional view, or to name the object in its unconventional view (Warrington & Taylor, 1973, 1978). At the same time, patients were able to correctly recognize the object in its conventional view. In 1986, Warrington and James found that, when compared to normal controls, patients required a greater rotation from the unconventional to the conventional perspective to recognize an object. Humphreys and Riddoch (1984) described two patients, both of whom had suffered a lesion in the inferior-posterior parietal region of the right hemisphere, with severe disturbances in the ability to recognize objects photographed from unusual angles.

One method that may be helpful in solving such a problem may be the use of an axis-based description of the object. In 1982, Marr emphasized the role of the major and minor axes of an object in the construction of a coordinate system centered on the object. The object shape is thus described in relation to the coordinate system, making it possible to preserve shape constancies by using an object-centered frame of reference when the viewing position of the object is altered. In 1984 and 1985, Humphreys and Riddoch tested this hypothesis by examining patients' ability to recognize an object with a foreshortened major axis of elongation. They found that four patients with right-hemisphere lesions showed greater disturbances in recognizing the view of the objects foreshortened along the major axis of elongation than in recognizing objects with a reduced number of characteristic features. An opposite pattern of disturbances was found in patients suffering from associative amnesia as a result of bilateral hemisphere lesions. Ullman (1996) argued that in addition to the axis-based structural descriptions, the axis of elongation may be used in alignment. "The problem apparently lies with the ability to compensate for transformations, in general, and not necessarily with the ability to create an axis-based structural description" (p. 185).

Anatomical Aspects

Dorsal and Ventral Pathways of Visual Information Processing

   Neural Correlates of Object Recognition.   Knowledge of the structural organization and function of the visual cortex has been greatly advanced by the use of an electrophysiological technique based on the recording of brain cell activity via intracortical electrodes while animals are presented with different visual tasks. Another modern approach, one of a neuroanatomical nature, involves the application of tracers for intra-axonal anterograde transport from the cell body and dendrites to the axonal terminals where histologically processed brain slices are examined. The most frequently used anterograde tracer is the enzyme horseradish peroxide (HRP). HRP is additionally used for intra-axonal retrograde transport from axonal terminals to the cell body. Fluorescent dyes are also used as tracers in retrograde labeling and may be detected by viewing the brain under specified wavelengths of illumination.

   Using the above-described techniques in studies of primates, it has been shown that visual processing is based on the high functional and architectural organization of the primate visual cortex; two major corticocortical pathways have been shown to begin with the primary visual cortex (Ungerleider & Mishkin, 1982)—the ventral and dorsal processing streams. The ventral pathway, or occipito-temporal stream, is directed from the occipital region to the inferiotemporal region, and includes among its pathway areas V1, V2, and V4 to PIT (the posterior inferotemporal cortex) and AIT (the anterior inferotemporal cortex). The dorsal, occipito-parietal pathway consists of areas V1, V2, V3, MT (middle temporal), and MST (medial superior temporal). The ventral pathway is important for visual object recognition, while the dorsal stream is involved in the processing of visuospatial aspects of the stimuli.

   Lesions in the inferior temporal cortex of monkeys severely impaired their discrimination of visual forms or patterns, and lesions in the posterior parietal cortex resulted in visuospatial deficits (Ungerleider & Mishkin, 1982). Physiological studies have supported this distinction. Neurons along the ventral pathway are activated by shape and color relevant to object identification, while neurons in the dorsal pathway respond to spatial aspects of stimuli (Desimone & Ungerleider, 1989; Maunsell & Newsome, 1987). Some evidence points to the possibility that the ventral pathway extends to the inferior prefrontal convexity, which participates in the short-term memory of an object process-ing for the low frequencies property of the object. That limits the choices of targeted object transferring that information to the lower levels through top-down processing are limited (Bar, 2003). The dorsal pathway extends to the dorsal prefrontal cortex, an area that is im-portant for preserving spatial information about the object (Wilson, O'Scalaidhe, & Goldman-Rakic, 1993). It seems that a third pathway, directed to the rostral superior temporal sulcus, is involved in the in-tegration of object and spatial information (Boussaud, Ungerleider, & Desimone, 1990).

Ventral Pathway and Visual Object Agnosia

 Occipital and Posterior Temporo-Occipital Lesions: Disturbances in Con-ventional Information Processing. One of the first cases of autopsy data involving visual agnosia was presented by Wilbrand in 1892. Wilbrand's patient was a 63-year-old woman who had developed severe visual agnosia following a stroke. Like Charcot's patient, Wilbrand's patient suffered from difficulties in the recognition of faces and of familiar environments. She was unable to orient herself in her own closet and was thus unable to go out alone due to disturbances of orientation. Her ability to invoke visual images of objects and faces, however, was preserved. Some forms of visual illusions and general confusion were also present; for example, the patient believed she saw her commode standing on the street and that there was a street next to her living room. Following the patient's death, an autopsy revealed a relatively new softening in the left hemisphere, which consisted of a small cav-ity in the white matter of the second occipital gyrus attached to the old infarction and extending anterior to the central gyrus. In the right hemisphere, an old infarction of vascular origin was found in the fusi-form gyrus with partial involvement of the cuneus. Wilbrand stressed the role of the bilateral occipital lesions, especially the lesion in the left hemisphere. He did not, however, pay attention to the localization of disturbances in facial recognition including the lesion in the temporal lobe of the right hemisphere.

Stauffenberg (1918) analyzed six cases of object agnosia published in the literature at that time, finding bilateral occipital lesions in all six patients. The lesions, all being more prominent in the left hemisphere, were situated in the white matter under the convexital occipital gyri. The patient experienced a more severe form of object agnosia when the damage was more prominent in the left hemisphere, with the locus of the lesions extending deep into the white matter of the ventral parts of the occipital lobe. Callosal damage was observed in some of the cases.

Nielsen (1937) reviewed and published cases of visual object agnosia that had been verified via autopsy. He then selected 13 cases of patients who had suffered unilateral lesions—9 cases with cerebral infarctions, 3 cases with tumors, and 1 case of abscess. Cerebral infarctions limited to the left or right occipital lobe were observed in 3 cases (Henschen, 1920–1922; Lissauer, 1890). Nielsen stressed that visual object agnosia developed in all 13 cases as a result of unilateral damage to the occipital lobe, in 9 cases with lesions involving the second and third occipital gyri in the left hemisphere, and in 4 cases with similar lesions in the right hemisphere. However, tumors were observed in 2 of the 4 cases with right hemisphere lesions, and in 1 case with a left hemisphere lesion, pointing to the probable role of mass effect produced by the tumor on the occipital lobe of the opposite hemisphere in 3 of the 13 cases. Nielsen discussed the probable role of left-handedness in the reversal of hemisphere dominance in object recognition in cases with right hemisphere lesions; however, no confirmation of left-handedness was available in the cases of right hemisphere lesions. Nielsen stressed that unilateral occipital lesions often led to the development of visual object agnosia when the *genu* of the corpus callosum was damaged. Nielsen did not pay attention to the frequent extension of the lesions to the left temporal lobe in 8 of the 13 cases and to the right temporal lobe in one case. Left and right parietal lobe involvement was noted in 2 and 1 of the 13 cases, respectively.

The roles of occipital and temporal lobe lesions in the development of visual object agnosia were described in a series of recently published cases, with CT or MRI scans being used for verification of the lesion localizations (Jankowiak & Albert, 1994). The authors paid special attention to differences in the localization of lesions in apperceptive and associative agnosia, concluding that associative agnosia is the result of a lesion that interrupts both the inferior longitudinal fasciculus (ILF), which connects the fusiform gyrus to the temporal lobe structures, especially on the left, and the ventral (occipito-temporal) pathway. Lesions resulting in apperceptive agnosia, however, are more diffuse. In order to discuss the localization value of the data assembled by Jankowiak and Albert, Table 2.2 summarizes the data published in the review.

As shown in Table 2.2, an occipital lobe lesion was present in almost all cases with visual object agnosia—in 19 of 21 cases, including 8 of 9 cases of apperceptive agnosia, and 11 of 12 cases of associative agnosia. Temporal lesions were reported in 11 of 12 cases of associative agnosia, but only in 3 of 9 cases of apperceptive agnosia. Thus, lesions of the occipital lobes were involved in apperceptive and associative agnosia, with extensions to the temporal lobes often found in cases of associative amnesia. Lesions were bilateral in 11 of the 12 cases of associative agnosia, and in 4 of the 9 cases of apperceptive agnosia. Instances of bilateral lesions limited to the occipital lobes were observed in only 3 of 9 cases

TABLE 2.2 Summary of CT (17 Cases), MRI (2 Cases), and Autopsy (2 Cases) Verification of Lesions in 21 Cases of Visual Object Agnosia

Localization of lesions	Occipital			Temporal			Parietal		
	Left	Bilateral	Right	Left	Bilateral	Right	Left	Bilateral	Right
Apperceptive visual agnosia									
9 cases	3	4	1	0	1	2	0	0	1
Single lobe lesion	3		0	0		0	0		1
Bilateral lesion of single lobe		3			0			0	
Associative visual agnosia									
12 cases	3	7	1	1	10	0	2	1	1
Single lobe lesion	0		0	0		0	0		0
Bilateral lesion of single lobe		0			1			0	

of apperceptive agnosia, and in only 1 of 12 cases of associative agnosia. Clinical manifestations of the bilateral occipital and occipito-temporal lesions were not limited to object amnesia, but instead frequently included other types of visual agnosia, especially prosopagnosia, color agnosia, and in many cases topographagnosia and alexia.

It is of interest that the anatomo-pathological findings in Lissauer's case with associative agnosia (Hahn, 1895) consisted of a large infarction in the occipito-temporal region of the left hemisphere covering the cuneus, the calcarine fissure, the lingual gyri in the occipital lobe, and the fusiform gyrus in the temporal lobe. The infarction also involved the lower two-thirds of the splenium. No infarction was found in the right hemisphere.

Bilateral occipital lesions following carbon monoxide poisoning, a type of poisoning that usually produces diffuse cortical laminar necrosis, were observed via brain-imaging data in well-studied cases of apperceptive agnosia. The patient R.C. (Abadi, Kulikowski, & Meudell, 1981; Campion & Latto, 1985) underwent a CT scan 3 years after having experienced carbon monoxide poisoning. The CT scan revealed bilateral low-density lesions in the lateral peristriate areas of both occipital lobes. The lesion was much larger in the left occipital lobe, extending from the peristriate to the striate area. In a case of apperceptive agnosia described by Milner et al. (1991), an MRI scan performed 13 months after the onset of the condition revealed extensive bilateral lesions of both lateral occipital cortices extending to the parasagittal parietal region.

Cases of lesions of a single lobe are of special interest in relation to the primary lesion site that results in the syndrome of visual object agnosia. Lesions limited to one of the occipital lobes were found in 2 of 21 cases with apperceptive and associative agnosia, as reviewed by Jankowiak and Albert (1994). As described in Case 2 by Warrington and James (1985), a cyst in the right parietal lobe was found, the etiology of which was thought to be the result of a metastatic squamous cell carcinoma; some additional cerebral metastasis, however, could not be ruled out. These two cases point to the probable role of a left occipital lobe lesion in the development of visual object agnosia. Also, a left occipital lesion with or without an additional lesion in the temporal lobe was found in 6 of the 21 cases, while a similar type of lesion localization in the right occipital lobe was found in only 2 of the 21 cases noted in Jankowiak and Albert's 1994 review.

However, in three cases of visual agnosia resulting from unilateral infarctions limited to the occipital lobe, as reviewed by Nielsen in 1937, the lesion was in the left occipital lobe in one case, and in the right occipital lobe in two cases. The role of callosal degeneration in interrupting the inter-hemisphere connections should be taken into account in two of these three cases. This degeneration of the corpus callosum could have been missed in CT scans in the two recent cases presented in Table 2.2. However, further data collection is needed, especially if taking into account the fact that right hemisphere lesions outside of the occipito-temporo-parietal region were found in two of three cases as verified by autopsy, and in one of two CT-verified cases with isolated left occipital lobe lesions. Also, many of the presented cases of visual object amnesia were accompanied by prosopagnosia or topographagnosia, making the localization specificity of those data less reliable.

Visual object agnosia usually develops as a result of relatively large and bilateral cortical and subcortical lesions in the occipito-temporal region. In cases with unilateral pathology, lesions are frequently localized within the left hemisphere; unilateral lesions of the right hemisphere are relatively infrequent in cases of visual object agnosia. Concerning the localization of lesions within superior or inferior parts of the cortex, the damage in many cases of visual object agnosia involves an area from the inferior parts of the occipital lobe to the posterior parts of the inferior temporal lobe.

Disturbances in Unconventional Information Processing. The data presented in the previous paragraphs showed that patients with occipital lesions, including those without signs of visual agnosia for nonoccluded objects, revealed disturbances in the recognition of occluded objects that were much more prominent than those of patients with non-occipital lesion localizations. These differences were observed in tests with a shortened time of object presentation, the use of incomplete pictures, the use of overlapped figures, and the masking of objects through the use of visual noise. The disturbances were mild or minimal, even in patients with unilateral extirpations of the anterior-inferior temporal areas.

More prominent impairments of the recognition of occluded objects by occipital patients may be explained by the role of disturbances in the intermediate completion stages of conventional information processing. The localization of these disturbances within occipital lobe structures may be investigated using single-cell recording data and the removal of specific brain regions in monkeys.

Activation by "real" and illusory, "subjective" contours defined by edges and lines was recorded in certain neurons of area V2 (part of Brodmann's area 18 in the occipital cortex). (For a review, see von der Heydt, 1995.) Lesions in area V2 may also be related to the disturbances in completion needed for the recognition of simple features masked by noise. Merigan, Nealey, and Maunsell (1993) showed that an isolated lesion of area V2 in monkeys resulted in disturbances of discrimination between three small vertically and horizontally oriented lines masked by orthogonally oriented lines. An increase in threshold was also observed in the discrimination of five co-linear rows of dots masked by randomly distributed dots. Similar disturbances in the discrimination of objects masked by competing stimuli were found in animals following the removal of area V4 (for a review see Pollen, 1999).

Restricted lesions within area V4 in primates resulted in an impaired ability to discriminate between form and pattern, but preserved the achromatic intensity thresholds (Heywood, Cadotti, & Cowey, 1992; Heywood & Cowey, 1987). The lesions also resulted in prominent disturbances of shape discrimination, requiring the use of multiple clues (Merigan & Pham, 1998), while a mild deficit was observed for elemental visual stimuli (Merigan et al., 1993; Merigan & Pham, 1998; for a review, see Pollen, 1999).

These data point to the possibility that lesions in areas V2 and V4 may result in disturbances of the completion needed for contours discrimination and object recognition in patients with visual object agnosia.

Temporal Lobe Lesions

Conventional Information Processing. Temporal lobe structures may participate in the process of matching in the course of recognition of previously well-learned objects. Lesions of those modules in the temporal lobe, especially in posterior parts of the inferotemporal, fusiform, and perihippocampal gyri, may contribute to the development of associative types of visual object agnosia. Such a possibility is supported by the frequent extensions of occipital lesions to the inferior temporal lobe in cases of associative agnosia. Temporal lobe involvement was found in 11 of 12 cases of associative agnosia, and in only 3 of 9 cases of apperceptive agnosia. This points to the probable role of a posterior inferotemporal lesion, together with an occipital lesion, in the development of associative agnosia—a type of agnosia characterized by disturbances in one's ability to match an object description with its meaning. In apperceptive agnosia, the process of object encoding is impaired, an impairment that may be primarily related to a lesion of the occipital lobe.

Unconventional Information Processing. Special consideration should be given to the role of temporal lobe lesions in the development of unconventional types of visual object agnosia. Significant discrepancies exist between the clinico-anatomical data in cases of visual object amnesia and the results of neurophysiological studies, primarily in research based on single-cell recording in response to visual stimuli.

The clinico-anatomical data point to a predominant role of occipital lobe lesions with some involvement of the posterior-inferior temporal lobe in the development of visual agnosia for objects in conventional and unconventional conditions. At the same time, single-cell recording provides ample evidence of the responses of different cells in the inferior temporal (IT) region to particular objects, faces, parts of faces, and hand-like stimuli independent of their orientation, size, color, characteristic of illumination (for a review, see Young, 1995), and changes in viewing positions (Logothetis, Pauls, & Poggio, 1995). Some of the authors stressed that "in primates' IT neuronal network also the spatio-temporal co-operation of manifold different nerve cell classes represents the objects" (Grusser & Landis, 1991, p. 126). Other authors enthusiastically declared "the anterior inferotemporal area of the monkey cortex [to be] the final stage of the visual cortical stream crucial for object recognition" (Fujita, Tanaka, Ito, & Cheng, 1992, p. 343). These discrepancies may be partly explained by the differences in conventional and unconventional visual information processing.

Poetzl (1928) was probably the first to suggest the role of lesion extension to the adjacent areas of the temporal lobe in the development of prominent visual object agnosia, stressing that visual object agnosia develops when lesions are localized in the left occipital lobe, destroying the white matter and spreading to the ventral parts of the occipital lobes. Visual agnosia becomes more pronounced with bilateral lesions and involves the adjacent peristriatal areas, the lingual gyrus in the occipital lobe, the fusiform gyrus in the temporal lobe, and the angular gyrus in the parietal lobe. Poetzl related the development of visual object agnosia to damage to the inferior, ventral region of the "wide visual sphere" located in the occipito-temporal region and consisting of the second and third occipital gyri as well as the lingual and fusiform gyri. Visuospatial agnosia develops, according to Poetzl, as a result of damage to the superior part of the "wide visual sphere," which includes the superior occipital gyrus and the angular gyrus in the parietal lobe.

Ungerleider and Mishkin (1982) proposed the idea of two separate visual systems, ventral and dorsal, for visual information processing. Object recognition is processed by the ventral occipito-temporal system, while spatial location of the object is processed by the dorsal occipito-parietal system. This idea is based on a series of animal experiments that demonstrated the role of the temporal and parietal lobes, as well as the occipital lobe, in visual information processing. However, a review of related data shows that the role of the temporal lobe is mainly related to unconventional information processing.

Disturbances in visual function were found following a bilateral resection of the inferotemporal region, middle and inferior temporal gyri, in monkeys (Chow, 1951; Mishkin, 1966; Mishkin & Pribram, 1954; Wilson, 1957). Visual disturbances were absent or minimal after ablation of the superior temporal gyrus, temporal pole, amygdala, hippocampal or posterior parietal region, frontal cortex, pulvinar, or the dorsomedial nucleus of the thalamus. Medial and posterior inferotemporal lesions did not produce visual field defects or disorders of visual sensitivity (Bender, 1973). At the same time, ablation of the prestriate cortex resulted in disorders of visual acuity, and of the visual field, while visual discrimination tasks were performed better than by monkeys with inferotemporal resections.

Visual discrimination tasks, studied in experiments with monkeys, differ from the recognition of well-known, nonoccluded objects, which is disturbed in patients with conventional visual object agnosia. In visual discrimination tasks, the animal has to learn that food is present if the veil is covered with a circle, while the presence of a triangle signals the absence of food. The task is difficult for normal animals, and requires anywhere from 100 to 200 trials to condition correct and accurate performance on the task. Following a bilateral inferotemporal ablation in a monkey, the number of trials needed to learn the task increases to 900–1000. Thus, the inferotemporal region appears to be involved in learning to process new visual information signaling the presence of food. This learning is mainly directed to the matching of relatively easy to describe signals, such as a circle or a triangle, with memory storage, thus pointing to the presence of food.

Similarly, the prominent role of the learning process in the course of experiments is seen in studies of single-cell responses to objects and their parts in the IT (inferior temporal area), especially in the AIT (anterior temporal area) of the monkeys (Fujita, Tanaka, Ito, & Cheng,

1992) as well as to the different views of previously unknown objects (Logothetis et al., 1995). Logothetis et al. (1995), for example, trained monkeys to respond to the target object and to the distracter by pressing the corresponding right or left levers. Experiments performed by Tanaka et al. (1990), as well as many other similar experiments, required multiple presentations of the same stimuli, reflecting the role of the learning process.

At the same time, the recognition of nonoccluded objects is a conventional and well-learned process and does not require training in the course of recognition. This conventional process may be mediated by operations related to occipital lobe functioning. The functioning is typically disturbed in patients with conventional visual agnosia as a result of an occipital lobe lesion, with a possible extension to the posterior-inferior temporal lobe region. This is especially the case in those suffering from associative agnosia.

Disturbances of unconventional information processing with no signs of conventional visual agnosia have been observed in patients with posterior-inferior and medial temporal lobe lesions; these lesions typically do not involve the occipital lobe. Such cases have been infrequently described in the literature, but one study clearly points to this localization of lesions. In a study of five patients with temporal lobe tumors, Kok (1967) observed no signs of disturbances in the recognition of objects in conventional conditions with an unlimited time of stimulus presentation. Limitation of object exposition time on the tachistoscope screen resulted in a marked increase in thresholds for object recognition. In each of the five cases, tumors damaged the medial and posterior parts of the middle and inferior temporal lobe in the right or left hemisphere, keeping the occipital lobe and anterior temporal lobe from being directly involved. In Case 4, a 14-year-old boy with a history of seizure disorder demonstrated the symptoms of unconventional visual object agnosia, while object recognition in conventional conditions was apparently preserved. The patient died following a surgical procedure related to the treatment of his seizures. The autopsy revealed a calcified mass impressing the inferior-medial region of the right temporal lobe, with extensions to the inferior-posterior areas of that lobe (Figure 2.5).

At the same time, a lesion of the anterior-inferior temporal lobe does not produce any type of object agnosia, conventional or unconventional, contrary to the findings in the anterior temporal region (AIT) of different cell responses to particular objects or their individual parts. Meerson (1986) found that a unilateral ablation of the anterior temporal lobes, a procedure often used for the treatment of epilepsy, resulted in minimal or no interference in the individual's ability to detect and recognize objects presented tachistoscopically for a time

FIGURE 2.5 Autopsy data from Case 4, showing the brain medial surface following the removal of a petrified mass 3.5 cm × 3.0 cm × 2.5 cm from the right side of the interpeduncular cistern. The mass induced pressure onto the inner part of the right interior temporal lobe, thus impressing its medial and partly posterior area. The occipital lobe remained preserved. The patient had no sign of conventional visual object agnosia, but tachistoscopic testing revealed a significant increase in the time needed for object recognition (Kok, 1967).

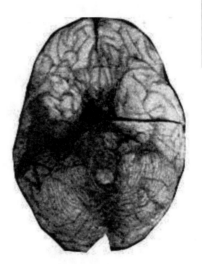

period of 1–1000 msec with a background of visual noise. Patients with occipital lobe lesions exhibited average recognition times as follows: 102 msec ± 15 msec for patients with occipital lobe lesions; 2.2 msec ± 0.04 msec for patients following a unilateral removal of the anterior temporal lobe (including the hippocampus); and 2.0 msec ± 0.02 msec for normal controls (Figure 2.6).

The differences between the lesion data and the findings of the AIT single-cell responses are unclear and require further data collection. It may be of interest to collect cases with occipital lesions and an absence of conventional and unconventional visual object agnosia, as well as cases with isolated temporal lobe lesions and signs of visual agnosia. It is possible that AIT cells are not directly involved in the visual recognition of objects but may participate in some operations that relate to the transformation of the object representation delivered by the occipito-temporal stream to the AIT cells. These transformations may require, for example, the preservation of object features in the visual working memory for effective translation of the visual description of the object to the multimodality description held in common with other modalities, such as the auditory and the tactile. It is of interest that a lesion of the anterior temporal lobe (including the hippocampus) produces disturbances in both visual and auditory working memory for simple features (Meerson, 1986; Milner, 1962, 1967, 1968).

Special attention should be given to the role of the hippocampal lesion. Kluver and Bucy (1937, 1939) found that an ablation of the anterior temporal lobes, including the hippocampus and the amygdala, in rhesus monkeys resulted in specific changes of behavior and visual perception. The monkeys developed and demonstrated

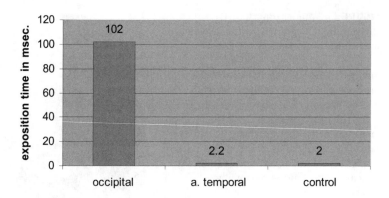

A

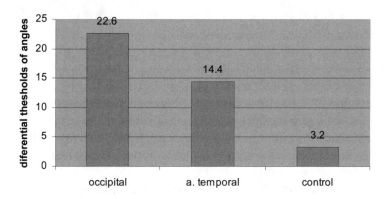

B

FIGURE 2.6 (A) Thresholds of exposition time needed for object recognition in groups of patients with occipital lesions, with anterior inferior temporal lesions (a. temporal), and in a normal control group. (B) The same groups. Differential thresholds of two angles with an interval of 10 seconds between the two stimuli. The group with anterior inferior temporal lesions (after surgery for treatment of temporal lobe epilepsy) exhibits significant differences between preservation of object recognition with a shortening of exposition time and prominent disturbances of angle differentiation. Both tests, however, reveal prominent difficulties in patients with occipital lobe lesions, pointing to the possibility that the role of anterior inferior temporal lobe lesions in the development of visual object agnosia is questionable, in spite of prominent difficulties in the comparison of simple visual features.

tameness, hypersexual behavior, and hypermetamorphosis—an inability to perform object recognition. (The monkeys would examine the objects one after another by putting them into their mouths and then throwing away any noneatable items.) The compulsive act of picking up objects, a behavior known as pica, which is frequently observed in psychiatric patients, may also be considered to be a possible explanation of the hypermetamorphosis exhibited in the experiments of Kluver and Bucy.

From a clinical point of view, the role of a lesion in the anterior temporal lobe, including a lesion of the hippocampus, is quite limited in the development of visual agnosia of objects in their conventional and unconventional views. At the same time, in addition to a main lesion in the occipital lobe, lesions of the middle and, especially, posterior areas of the inferotemporal region seem to play a certain role in both the development of conventional visual object agnosia, especially associative agnosia, and the development of unconventional visual object agnosia.

Disturbances in the recognition of occluded objects may be observed in some cases of patients with lesions in the superior-posterior temporal region. Impairments in the discrimination of complex features had been recorded in some of such cases in our experiments. The role of the posterior T1 area in the processing of visual information is supported by electrical cortical stimulation of the T1 area during the course of surgical treatment of patients with seizure disorders. Such stimulation produces what are called experiential visual responses (Penfield & Jasper, 1954). Recently, Lee, Hong, Seo, Tae, and Hong (2000) observed the complex forms responses consisting of animals, people, landscapes, and scenes from memory, during electrical stimulation of the lateral temporal and occipito-temporal cortex in patients with seizure disorder. Similar responses were recorded following stimulation of the basal occipito-temporal cortex. The role of the superior-posterior temporal lobe in visual information processing was also supported by data from single-cell recording that revealed cellular activation in the V5 area (posterior medial temporal area in monkeys) while monkeys observed motions in their visual fields.

Frontal Lobe Lesions
Unconventional Information Processing. The recognition of real objects and of drawings of objects is usually preserved in patients with frontal lobe lesions. However, disturbances of recognition may appear when an object is presented in an unconventional way, especially in patients with extensive frontal lobe lesions. Examples of such unconventionally presented objects include Poppelreuter's figures (Luria, 1966), as well as Gottschaldt's figures, in which subjects are required to distinguish a certain figure from a complex background design (Figure 2.2) (Teuber & Weinstein, 1956). Similar difficulties were observed in the ability to distinguish shapes, such as a white cross on a chess board (Luria, 1966), as well as in the ability to recognize objects masked by the background noise (Figure 2.1) created by textures (Tonkonogy, 1973). The role of the inferior prefrontal cortex

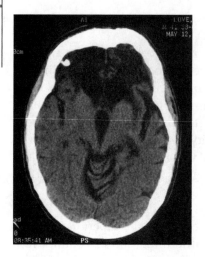

FIGURE 2.7 Head CT scan of a 28-year-old patient who sustained a closed head injury as the result of a motor vehicle accident that had occurred 4 years prior to the brain scan. A left frontal craniotomy was performed following the injury. For 8 weeks, the patient was in a comatose and then semicomatose state and was further hospitalized for another 8 months. Following the accident, he demonstrated symptoms of cognitive impairment, impulse control disorder, and tonic-clonic seizures, and experienced mild weakness in his left extremities. He became hypersexual and was arrested and charged with indecent exposure and assault and battery of a child. The patient's BNCE (Tonkonogy, 1997) total score was 16, indicating the presence of a moderate impairment. He was able to identify only two of four drawings of incomplete objects. When the complete pictures of all four objects were presented, the patient was able to recognize without delay all of the objects, demonstrating no clear signs of conventional visual object agnosia. However, repeated presentation of the incomplete pictures of the same four objects yielded no improvement; the patient was again unable to recognize the same two objects that he could not recognize prior to his exposure to the complete drawings.

in the working memory of single objects, especially faces, was also observed in lesion studies (Freedman, Riesenhuber, Poggio, & Miller, 2001) and in neurophysiological studies (for a review, see Goldman-Rakic, Scalaidhe, & Chafee, 2000).

The recognition of drawings of objects with incomplete features may represent another difficult task for patients suffering from a frontal lobe lesion. One of our patients, with a massive bilateral frontal lobe lesion at the base of the frontal lobes with an extension to the anterior part of the left temporal lobe (Figure 2.7), was able to recognize without difficulty the drawings of objects, but made a series of errors in the attempted recognition of incomplete pictures.

It appears that the anterior temporal lobe did not play a significant role, as lesions in that area typically do not lead to the development of visual object agnosia (Figure 2.7).

Dorsal Pathway and Visual Object Agnosia: Parietal Lobe Lesions

Conventional Visual Object Agnosia. Disturbances in the recognition of objects in their conventional and unoccluded view have been described in single cases with parietal lesions; however, extensions of the lesions to the occipital lobe cannot be completely excluded in these cases.

Unconventional Visual Object Agnosia. The role of parietal lobe lesions in disorders of the relationships of objects in space has been well established since the early studies of neuropsychological syndromes. Recently, the possible role of the parietal lobe in object recognition has been discussed.

Disorders of unconventional recognition of occluded objects—via background noise, figures with missing features, overlapping figures, and shortened time of presentation—are markedly less prominent in patients with parietal lesions than in those with occipital lesions. For example, in our study, the thresholds for the recognition of objects with a shortened time of tachistoscopic presentation reached 150 msec for parietal patients, compared to 5000 msec for occipital patients (see Figure 2.7).

At the same time, parietal patients showed a markedly increased percentage of errors (32% ± 3.3%) compared to that of the occipital group of patients (12% ± 1.7%) (see above) in the recognition of objects divided into several parts and thus requiring a restoration of spatial relations between the parts to recognize the object (Figure 2.8). (Time of object presentation was 1500 msec.) These results point to the role of parietal lesions in disturbances in the ability to use spatial characteristics to effectively reconstruct and recognize an object via unconventional information processing.

Parietal lesions have been also implicated in the increased threshold for the differentiation of angles with different spatial orientations. The thresholds were as follows: 7.6 ± 0.8 for patients with occipital lesions; 13.5 ± 0.85 for patients with left inferior-parietal lesions; 6.3 ± 0.4 for patients with left superior-posterior temporal lesions; and, 6.6 ± 0.6 for patients with left inferior frontal premotor lesions (Figure 2.9).

Kosslyn, Flynn, Amsterdam, and Wang (1990), Kosslyn et al. (1994) and Milner and Goodale (1993) discussed the relationship of the dorsal, parieto-occipital system to the viewpoint-dependent recognition of objects. Some of the recognition disorders in such conditions may be considered to be "unusual view deficits" (Turnbull, Carey, & McCarthy, 1997). It has been suggested that the dorsal system may provide viewer-centered

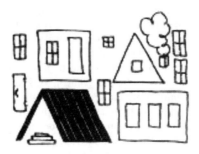

FIGURE 2.8 A picture of a house divided into several parts. The spatial relationships between the parts are disrupted.

information concerning objects in unusual viewing circumstances for use by the ventral, viewer-independent system that is primarily involved in recognition based on the invariant properties of an object (Turnbull et al., 1997).

Disorders of such viewpoint-dependent operations may explain the difficulties in the recognition of objects viewed from an unusual angle, for example, from above or from the bottom (Warrington & Taylor, 1973, 1978). Warrington and James (1986) studied the recognition of objects as rotated from an unconventional to a conventional perspective. They found that the patients, when compared to normal controls, required more of a rotation of the object for the recognition of objects with a preserved or foreshortened axis of elongation. The superimposed reconstruction of the lesion by Warrington and Taylor, (1973) showed the critical site of damage to be in the posterior part of the right hemisphere,

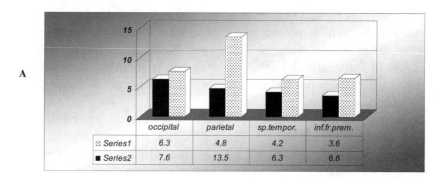

A

	occipital	parietal	sp.tempor.	inf.fr.prem.
▫ Series1	6.3	4.8	4.2	3.6
■ Series2	7.6	13.5	6.3	6.6

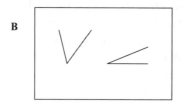

B

FIGURE 2.9 (A) Differential thresholds of angles with different orientations in groups of patients with occipital, inferior-parietal (parietal), superior-posterior temporal (sp.tempor.), and inferior frontal premotor (inf.fr.prem.) lesion localizations in the left hemisphere. (B) Examples of two differently oriented angles presented simultaneously for comparison by the patient. Patients with left inferior-parietal lesions exhibited more than a twofold increase in this particular threshold compared to the differential thresholds for angles with equal orientation. This increase was minimal in other groups, including the group of patients with occipital lesions. Note that an increase to an interval of 10 seconds between the two compared angles with the same orientation resulted in a threefold increase in threshold for the occipital group, with only a 1.4- or 1.5-fold increase in threshold for patients suffering from a left inferior-parietal lesion and for those suffering from a left inferior frontal premotor lesion.

particularly in the inferior parietal lobe. Humphreys and Riddoch (1985) tested four patients with damage to the right hemisphere and found disturbances in the recognition of objects with a foreshortening of the major axis of elongation. No similar deficit, however, was observed in the patients' ability to recognize objects with a reduced number of salient features. The opposite tendency was observed in a patient suffering from associative agnosia.

The recognition of objects as they are presented in an unconventional orientation may be achieved by the use of operations that effectively relay the spatial alignment of the object to a stored model (Ullman, 1996). This may be related to the operations involved in the formation of a combination of views of the object as obtained from multiple different viewpoints (Ullman, 1996). The combination of views may be based on viewer-independent descriptions of object parts, such as ears for faces, wheels or steering wheels for cars, motorcycles, or bicycles, or abstract descriptions of a rooster's crown as some sort of "wiggly" part. Such a description may be provided by the ventral, occipito-temporal visual stream. The next step—the combination of views for such parts, including their spatial relations—may be utilized to recognize a viewer-dependent object as presented in an unusual position. The spatial aspect of this step is most likely related to the dorsal occipito-parietal stream.

However, relevant anatomical data are sketchy, mainly pointing to lesions in the right hemisphere in such cases. At the same time, studies of single-cell responses to novel objects in both canonical and unusual views demonstrated that many cells in the inferior temporal (IT) areas of monkeys prefer a particular view of an object, with the cells responding to only a relatively small range of viewing directions (Logothetis et al., 1995). In the absence of corresponding clinico-anatomical data, these results may be explained by the suggestion that the use of a combination of views in such conditions probably necessitates the participation of the ventral visual occipito-temporal stream, at least during the initial learning stages.

The role of the superior areas of the prefrontal cortex must also be considered as an anterior part of the dorsal pathway. Neurophysiological studies using monkeys have shown that neurons in these areas actively respond to the spatial relationships of objects presented for recognition (Goldman-Rakic et al., 2000).

*Visual Object Agnosia in Various Diseases With Extended
Cortical Lesions*

Visual object amnesia was originally described and studied by examining those who suffered from diseases with relatively circumscribed cerebral lesions caused by strokes, or in some cases by tumors or sstraumatic brain injuries. The disorder was also observed in cases of patients with extended cortical lesions, primarily due to a degenerative dementia of the Alzheimer's type. Benson, Davis, and Snyder (1988) found in some cases that visual object agnosia, especially when accompanied by visuospatial disturbances, represented one of the main clinical manifestations of posterior cerebral atrophy underlined by Alzheimer's disease. A series of cases has also been reported in which visual object agnosia has followed carbon monoxide poisoning (Campion & Latto, 1985; Milner et al., 1991). Disturbances of unconventional information processing in object recognition have recently been reported in cases of schizophrenia. These disturbances have included difficulties in the processing of visual backward masking (Butler, Harkavy-Freedman, Amador, & Gorman, 1996), briefly presented stimuli (Cornblatt & Keilp, 1994), and fragmented, degraded object images (Doniger et al., 2002).

CONCLUSION

1. Disturbances in the ventral and dorsal pathways of visual information processing underline the development of various types of visual object agnosia (Figure 2.10).
2. Visual agnosia of objects and of object drawings in conventional circumstances may often be observed in cases with ventral pathway lesions involving the occipito-temporal region. Though these lesions are frequently bilateral, unilateral lesions in the left hemisphere may underline the development of visual object agnosia not otherwise observed in cases of patients with unilateral right hemisphere lesions.
3. Lesions involved with conventional forms of visual object agnosia are often limited to lesions in the occipital lobes, primarily in cases of apperceptive agnosia. It is possible that disorders of modules with well-learned operations of object descriptions used in the course of recognition underline the development of apperceptive agnosia in cases of patients with occipital lesions, primarily lesions in areas V2 and V4. In cases of associative agnosia, lesions usually extend from the occipital lobe to the ventral pathway in the inferior-posterior parts of the temporal lobes. This particular localization may underline observed disturbances in the module involved in the matching of an object description and its model storage, a condition that often develops in such lesion cases. Data obtained from single-cell recording studies, as well as from animal studies involving the surgical removal of the inferior temporal lobe, point to the more extended involvement of the temporal lobe in the process of visual recognition. This involvement, how-

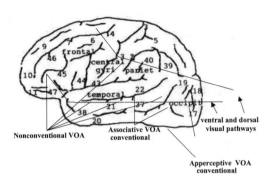

FIGURE 2.10 Localization of left hemispheric lesions in various types of visual object agnosia (VOA), both conventional and unconventional. Numbers indicate Brodmann's cytoarchitectonic areas.

ever, may be primarily related to unconventional conditions and learning processes. On the other hand, it seems that occipital lesions are primarily responsible for disturbances in well-learned invariant processing for the recognition of nonoccluded objects in their conventional view, leading to the development of conventional visual agnosia.

4. It seems that the module for conventional visual object recognition is located in a relatively compact area that includes the occipital lobe and, most likely, the posterior-inferior temporal lobe. A relatively large lesion in this area may result in the development of conventional visual object agnosia. At the same time, unconventional object recognition requires the participation of several areas in various cortical regions. Lesions in these areas, for instance in the inferior frontal region or the medial-posterior temporal region, may lead to the development of unconventional visual object agnosia, with the preservation of conventional visual object recognition. The development of conventional visual agnosia may therefore point to an occipital or occipito-temporal lesion, while unconventional visual object agnosia may result from lesions in several different cortical areas.

5. Disturbances of visual working memory for objects and, especially, simple features may be observed in patients with occipital lesions, as well as in those with lesions localized elsewhere, including anterior and inferior temporal lobe lesions and parietal and inferior premotor frontal lesions. The relationships between these specific types of lesions and disturbances in the recognition of objects in both conventional and unconventional conditions require further evaluation.

6. In cases of reported dorsal pathway lesions involving the parietal lobes and the superior prefrontal areas, disturbances may be primarily related to the spatial aspects of recognition.

VISUAL OBJECT AGNOSIA AND DISTURBANCES OF BRAIN INFORMATION PROCESSING

Role of Processing of the Common Properties of the Object

For a review of the role of the processing of the common properties of the object, see Ullman (1996). A direct approach to object recognition is based on the assumption that the image of an object can be recognized via comparison with images of the object stored in memory. However, the number of images even for one object in multiple different viewing positions and various directions of illumination is prohibitively high, requiring an enormous amount of memory storage; another complication arises from the fact that the image to be recognized may be somewhat different from any similar images seen in the past.

It is reasonable to assume that the system of object recognition may be much more efficient in terms of memory, space, economy, and reliability of the recognition for a particular object if the system is based on the processing of the common properties of the object, which are limited in number and much easier to compare with the object at hand (Ullman, 1996). In order to recognize a table, there is no need to store in one's memory a large number of representative shapes, textures, positions, and colors of various tables in different viewing positions; perhaps it is only necessary that the common properties of tables in any shape, position, color, texture, or size be stored in memory and used in comparison with the similar properties of the object to be recognized.

Stages of Visual Information Processing

Studies of the primate visual system have shown that the visual system processes information reflecting common properties of objects in a hierarchical manner—the common properties are processed in several stages via multiple specialized areas and massive interconnections. It is suggested that these stages are organized in the following hierarchical manner: the processing of elementary visual features, such as luminance, color, and motion, by way of *early vision;* the grouping of these elementary features according to similar attributes into entities and according to the simple features of primitive shapes by way of *intermediate vision;* and the recognition of objects and scenes by way of *higher vision,* using the results of intermediate vision for further processing

(Van Essen, Felleman, DeYoe, Olavarria, & Knierim, 1990). Though disorders at any of the three stages may impair one's visual abilities, the development of visual object amnesia may be predominantly related to the second, and especially third, stages of visual information processing. Disturbances of higher vision processing in object recognition have been described above, and impairments of elementary vision and intermediate vision and their relationships to visual object amnesia are discussed below.

Disturbances at the Elementary Level of Visual Information Processing and Visual Object Agnosia: Incomplete Loss of Elementary Visual Sensations

Some authors have stressed the exclusive role of disturbances in the visual elementary sensation in the development of visual agnosia. Bay (1950, 1953) suggested that subtle disturbances in visual sensation may explain disorders of object identification. He further suggested that dynamic procedures may uncover such elementary disturbances, and subsequently found disorders of local adaptation in normal areas of visual fields in patients with visual agnosia. According to Bay, the stimuli presented in those fields fade away much more quickly in such patients than in normal individuals. Bay postulated the role of dementia and of a reduced level of consciousness as additional factors in the formation of visual agnosia in patients with disturbances of elementary visual sensations.

Ettlinger (1956) showed that elementary disturbances of vision are also often found in patients who do not suffer from the disorder of visual agnosia. In his research, Ettlinger utilized a wide array of elementary visual tests, including brightness discrimination, flicker fusion, acuity for small objects, tachistoscopic acuity, and local adaptation, and found no reliable association between elementary sensory impairment and the presence of visual agnosia in 30 brain-damaged patients. Similar results were reported by Kantimulina (1961), who examined patients with occipital lesions and found evidence of disturbances in brightness discrimination and in local adaptation, but no evidence for the presence of visual agnosia. Though a marked decrease in visual acuity certainly impairs one's ability to extract elementary visual features, these disturbances can be overcome during later stages of visual information processing.

Disturbances at the Intermediate Level of Visual Information Processing and Visual Object Agnosia

Disturbances at the Level of Simple Features Analysis

Neural Correlates of Simple Features Analysis. The classic studies of Hubel and Wiesel (1959, 1968) demonstrated that the early stages of shape encoding, including the processing of line orientations, edges, and gratings, take place in area V1 (Brodmann's area 17) in primates. These early stages of the visual processing of elements that may be used in the analysis of form have also been localized in area V2. These areas prepare information for further processing at the higher level, and this preparation of information has been defined as intermediate-level processing.

Area V1, which occupies primarily the area of the striate cortex corresponding to Brodmann's area 17, contains a lattice of oval patches, or "blobs" and "interlob regions." The neurons in area V1 are sensitive to light within a receptive field, which receives the input from a small part of the retina in one or both eyes via the lateral geniculate nuclei. Area V1 is organized in a columnar orientation and ocular dominance, as was first demonstrated by Hubel and Wiesel (1959, 1968, 1977). The columns are organized in an orderly manner representing, for example, the certain line orientation in a separate colon. Other functional properties of V1 columns include retinotopy, ocular dominance, and color. The cells in V1 receptive fields respond to the orientation of lines, stimulus angular size, the contrast between the borders of contours, contour orientations, grating, movements, and binocular disparity. End-stopped receptive fields have similar preferences for lines and gratings, but their responses are best for short lines and short pieces of edges (for a review, see von der Heydt, 1995). In monkeys, end-stopped cells may be found in areas V1 and V2. Some of the cells in the "blob" region receive a color-coded signal from the cells of the parvocellular lateral geniculus nuclei.

Area V2 is located in the prestriate cortex, occupying part of Brodmann's area 18 and containing different staining patterns of "thick dense," "thin dense," and "pale" bands. A high degree of connectivity exists in area V1/V2 and is likely to be highly divergent and convergent (for a review, see Ts'o and Roe, 1995). Output from area V2 continues to area V4 and then to the cortical area of the MT (middle temporal area). The receptive fields in area V2 are larger than in V1, and retinotopy is thus less precise in area V2 than in V1. Cells in area V2 respond to more integrated features; consider, for instance, disparity cells, which are stimulated by stereoscopic images as formed by optimal retinal disparity between the two eyes, but are silent in response to monocular stimulation. Like V1 cells, V2 cells are activated by line orientation but also exhibit orientation tuning to "real" contrast borders as well as to illusory, "subjective" contours (von der Heydt, Peterhans, & Baumhartner, 1984. These cells are located in the thin pale strips region of area V2 (see Grusser & Landis, 1991; von der Heydt, 1995). Cells in the "thin dense stripes" respond to chromatic stimuli. Area V2 (part of Brodmann's area 18) contains cells that are characterized by strong orientation tuning as well as light-dark bars that indicate a selective spatial frequency tuning that may be interpreted as a first step to texture recognition and spatial frequency tuning in contour detection (for a review, see Grusser and Landis, 1991).

Disturbances in the Differentiation of Simple Features: Preservation of Differential Thresholds for Unlimited Time of Presentation and Short Interstimuli Intervals.   The reviewed data point to the possibility that the recognition of line orientation, angle size, and textures may be performed by the brain during the early stages of object recognition. It was found that impairments may be observed in one's ability to determine whether the slant of two lines is the same or different (Warrington & Rabin, 1970). Special tests were developed (Benton, Varney, & Hamsher, 1978) to assess the ability of patients to match the slant of a line with a "sun ray" line bearing an identical slope from a sample of sun ray lines with orientations from 0 to 180 degrees in relation to the horizontal line, and with differences in orientation in the range of 16 degrees. The length of the line in both the stimulus and the "ray" were equal; in the more difficult version of the test, however, the length of the stimulus line was significantly shorter than that of the ray.

These disturbances may play some role in the development of visual object amnesia. Based on this idea, we examined patients with visual object agnosia and patients with occipital lobe lesions and expected to find disturbances in the recognition of line orientation, the differentiation of angle size, and the differentiation of textures with different statistical characteristics. No significant disturbances were found, however, when the time of stimuli presentation was 2000 msec and the interstimuli interval was 2 sec. The difficulties began to appear when the time of presentation was limited to 200 msec, or when the interstimuli interval was increased to 5 sec or to 10 sec.

We studied 32 patients who had each suffered a stroke (Meerson, 1986; Tonkonogy, 1973) and 42 patients following the removal of each patient's anterior-inferior temporal lobe in the course of surgery for the treatment of temporal lobe epilepsy (Meerson, 1977, 1986). In the group of stroke patients, primarily occipital lesions and possibly occipito-temporal lesions were diagnosed in eight patients, including bilateral lesions in four patients and left occipital lesions in four patients; visual object agnosia was also diagnosed in each patient. Control groups were composed of the following patients: 4 cases of constructional apraxia accompanied primarily by inferior parietal lesions, in 3 cases in the left hemisphere, and in 1 case in the right; 12 cases of Wernicke's aphasia accompanied by superior-posterior temporal lesions in the left hemisphere; and 8 cases of Broca's aphasia, accompanied by right or left hemiplegia as well as left-sided premotor frontal lesions in 6 cases and right-sided premotor frontal lesions in two cases. Clinical criteria for the localization of lesions also included the presence and types of hemianopia. The patients were tested from 5–6 weeks to several months after their stroke.

The group of patients who had undergone the removal of the anterior-inferior temporal lobe was composed of 22 patients with right hemisphere surgery and 20 patients with left hemisphere surgery. The removed parts of the anterior-inferior temporal lobes included the parahippocampal and fusiform gyri as well as mediobasal structures, primarily the hippocampus. Visual object amnesia was not observed in any of these patients. The patients were tested 4–6 weeks following the surgery (Meerson, 1986, pp. 124–125). The ability to differentiate between angles and textures was studied using the same protocol as that used for patients with other localizations of lesions.

The stimuli consisted of lines with orientations toward a horizontal line from 30 to 75 degrees, (Figure 2.11). In the studies of poststroke and postsurgical patients, the angles and lines differed from 5 to 45 degrees and from 1 to 45 degrees respectively.

Another set of stimuli included textures with different statistical characteristics. The textures consisted of small black squares arranged in a linear fashion on a background of a large white square (Julesz, 1971a, 1971b). The textures differed in the frequency of small black squares and appeared in chance order according to the first order statistics ranged from $p = 0.1$ to $p = 0.9$ with differences ranging from $p = 0.05$ to $p = 0.4$.

The stimuli were presented on the screen of a tachistoscope with an exposition time of 2 seconds. For stimuli that were presented simultaneously for comparison, the interval between the two was 0 seconds. After viewing a pair of stimuli, for instance, the subject was instructed to indicate if the two angles of either identical or different degrees were, in fact, "the same" or "different." The mean differential thresholds were calculated following the completion of the tests. We predicted that possible lesions in the V1 and V2 regions studied by Hubel and Wiesel (1968) would manifest themselves in an observed increase in differential thresholds for the discrimination of angles and texture.

The results for angle differentiation showed that differential thresholds in the group of patients with visual object agnosia and occipital or occipito-temporal lesions did not differ significantly from those of the groups of patients with various nonoccipital localizations of lesions (Meerson, 1986). The mean differential thresholds for angles and textures with an exposition time of 2000 msec and the simultaneous presentation of two stimuli for differentiation were similar in all groups of patients (Figure 2.12). For angles, the thresholds for differentiation were slightly higher in the occipital group (6.3) than in the other groups—

A   B

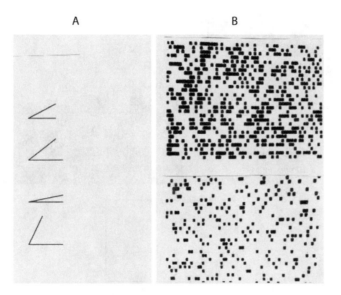

FIGURE 2.11a Change in presentation time affecting response in various localization of lesions.

FIGURE 2.11b Examples of angles and textures used for the differentiation of two stimuli. Probability of black squares $p = 0.2$ for top texture, $p = 0.45$ for bottom texture.

the parietal group (4.8), the superior-posterior temporal group (4.2), the premotor frontal group (3.6), and the anterior-temporal group (3.6).

As in experiments involving angle differentiation, the mean differential thresholds for the simultaneous presentation of two textures for differentiation did not significantly differ between patients with occipital lesions (0.08), parietal lesions (0.075), superior-temporal lesions (0.071), anterior temporal lesions (0.085), and premotor frontal lesions (0.065).

These results point to the possible preservation of the intermediate stages of simple features processing, such as the processing of angle and texture differentiation in patients with various types of local brain pathology, including patients with and without occipital lesions. This preservation effect was observed when signals were presented in conventional conditions with an optimal length of exposition time and interstimuli intervals of 0 seconds, 5 seconds, and 10 seconds. A slight increase in the threshold for angle differentiation noted in the occipital group compared to the other groups of patients is probably related to the relatively mild disturbances demonstrated in the assessment of angle degrees at the low level of visual features processing. The recorded differences between groups of patients with various localizations of lesions became more significant with an increase of interstimuli intervals, as well as with a decrease in exposition time.

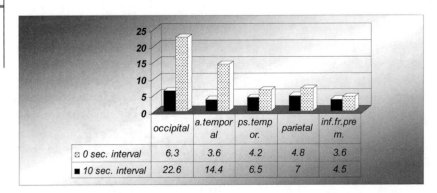

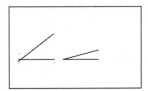

	occipital	a.temporal	ps.tempor.	parietal	inf.fr.prem.
▨ 0 sec. interval	6.3	3.6	4.2	4.8	3.6
■ 10 sec. interval	22.6	14.4	6.5	7	4.5

FIGURE 2.12 Mean differential thresholds for angles in groups of patients with different localizations of cortical lesions. Abbreviations are as follows: a. temporal for anterior temporal; ps.tempor. for posterior-superior temporal; and, inf.fr.prem. for inferior frontal premotor.
Study Design: Two angles, as seen at the bottom of the figure, were presented on a tachistoscope screen with interstimuli intervals of either 0 sec (presented simultaneously) or 10 sec. Each image had an exposition time of 2 sec. The subject was asked to determine whether the two stimuli presented were the same or different.

Increase in Interstimuli Intervals and Disturbances of Visual Working Memory. In the second series of experiments involving angle differentiation, the exposition time for stimuli remained at 2000 msec, while the intervals between two stimuli varied—0 seconds, 5 seconds, and 10 seconds. The results are presented in Table 2.3. The main differential thresholds for angles presented simultaneously were slightly higher in the occipital group than in the other groups of patients. These differences significantly widened with increases in the interstimuli intervals; more specifically, the mean differential threshold for angles increased from 4.6 at 0-second intervals to 8.9 at 10-second intervals for the parietal group, and from 6.3 at 0-second intervals to 22.6 at 10-second intervals for the occipital group. A significant increase in the mean differential thresholds for angles was also prominent for the anterior-temporal group of patients, increasing from 3.6 at 0-second interstimuli intervals to 14.4 at 10-second intervals. (See Table 2.3.)

Similar results were recorded for differential thresholds of textures (Table 2.3). The mean of differential thresholds in the occipital group

TABLE 2.3 Changes in Differential Thresholds for Angles and Textures With Increases of Interstimuli Intervals From 0 Sec (Simultaneous Presentation) to Intervals of 5.0 and 10.0 Sec Between the Two Stimuli

	Interstimuli intervals		
	0 sec	5.0 sec	10.0 sec
Differential thresholds (degree) for angles			
Localization of lesions			
Occipital	6.3 ± 0.37	15.2 ± 3.7	22.6 ± 7.2
Temporal			
anterior-inferior	3.6 ± 0.3	8.2 ± 1.3	14.4 ± 2.3
posterior-superior	4.2 ± 0.66	5.2 ± 0.7	6.5 ± 0.8
Parietal	4.8 ± 0.84	6.3 ± 0.5	7.0 ± 2.1
Frontal, premotor	3.6 ± 0.14	4.0 ± 0.4	4.5 ± 0.4
Differential thresholds (delta p) for textures			
Occipital	0.08 ± 0.02	0.18 ± 0.4	0.23 ± 0.06
Temporal			
anterior-posterior	0.085 ± 0.015	0.10 ± 0.04	0.23 ± 0.09
posterior-superior	0.07 ± 0.015	0.70 ± 0.05	0.10 ± 0.02
Parietal	0.075 ± 0.01	0.09 ± 0.02	0.11 ± 0.02
Frontal, premotor	0.065 ± 0.008	0.07 ± 0.01	0.08 ± 0.06

increased almost threefold, from 0.08 to 0.23, and in the anterior-inferior temporal group they increased from 0.085 to 0.23; the means of the differential thresholds increased only slightly in other groups of patients. These mean thresholds were accompanied by an increase in interstimuli intervals from 0 sec to 10 sec.

Short Time of Exposition. The test procedure, in this case, did not differ from that which was described for the increase in the interstimulus intervals, except that in this case the interstimulus interval remained fixed at 2 sec, while the exposition time decreased from 2000 msec to 500 msec and then to 200 msec. This decrease in exposition time resulted in a marked increase in differential thresholds for the occipital group—from 6.3 ± 0.37 to 9.6 ± 0.85 for 500 msec and to 13.3 ± 2.6 for 200 msec. Differential thresholds did not increase significantly in other groups of patients. In the superior-posterior temporal group, the differential thresholds for angles were 5.3 ± 0.3 for 2000 msec, 5.5 ± 0.66 for 500 msec, and 6.1 ± 0.18 for 200 msec. The anterior-posterior group was not included in this part of the testing.

The results of these tests may be explained as reflecting disturbances in some sort of special operations performed by columns of neurons located in the V1 and V2 areas. It is possible that the operations provided by those neurons include or specifically target the preservation of information concerning line orientation, angle size, and texture properties in the visual working memory for further processing. The operations may thus become disturbed when either an increase in the interstimuli interval or a shortening of the exposition time occurs, presenting a special challenge to the visual working memory. This may be based on the role of low and high spatial frequency features properties in the processing of information. It is possible that low spatial frequency information is better preserved and more difficult to disturb, while the processing of high spatial frequency information is more vulnerable and less protected.

The operations employed to prepare visual information for further processing may be directed to enriching the substantial saving of the volume of information for preservation by scoring or grouping the information into larger chunks. The possible mechanism of such a decrease in informational volume may be related to the process of parsing of the stimuli into chunks for further processing using low and high spatial frequency filters. The parsing of the stimuli into small chunks by high-frequency filters may be disturbed in patients with cortical pathology, while the parsing of the stimuli into large chunks by low-frequency filters may remain preserved in the working memory. For instance, following an initial recording, the angles may be grouped into large chunks with differences of 15 degrees. It is thus possible to divide the stimuli in increments of 5 to 45 degrees into three large chunks, which is easier to process than nine small chunks divided according to increments of 5 degrees (Table 2.3). The parsing and subsequent storage of large chunks in the visual working memory allow reduced storage space, which is easier to protect from disturbances and may be sufficient for well-learned, conventional types of visual information processing. At the same time, the parsing of multiple small chunks requires more time and storage space in the working memory. The smaller chunks of information may, however, be needed in cases of unconventional, novel information processing.

The increases in differential thresholds for angles and textures are limited to those in the visual modality in patients with occipital lesions. An increase in interstimuli intervals did not result in a significant increase in differential thresholds for the differentiation of tones in an occipital group of patients, while the same interval increases resulted in a marked increase in the differential thresholds in visual and auditory modalities for an anterior-temporal group. These results provide evidence for differences in underlying grouping processes in the working memory of the occipital and anterior-inferior temporal areas. It is possible that visual information for simple features is parsed in the visual working memory and then stored in occipital areas for use in subsequent operations of visual information processing. At the same time, the parsing that takes place via visual working memory in the occipital areas and auditory working memory in the superior-posterior temporal areas is used for the translation from unimodal auditory or visual codes to a multimodal code in the anterior-inferior areas. Such a translation may be preserved for information that has been grouped into large chunks but may be divided for multiple numbers of small chunks, leading to an increase in differential thresholds secondary to the lesions of the anterior-posterior temporal areas.

The resulting disturbances of grouping processes in the working memory and the preservation of object recognition observed following the removal of the individual's anterior-inferior temporal lobe point to the possibility that impairments of these processes do not play any significant role in the development of visual object agnosia. There may be an additional factor contributing to the already existing disturbances at the higher level of visual information processing, especially in the course of the learning or recognition of nonconventional views of objects and other types of nonconventional visual information processing.

The mechanisms underlying the parsing of stimuli presented with a short time of exposition may also be related to visual working memory, which in this case would be used to extend the short time of exposition to provide the time needed to parse the stimuli for further processing. This extended time may help to parse the limited number of large chunks of visual information but still may be insufficient for the processing of multiple numbers of small chunks, thus leading to an increase in differential thresholds. Disturbances in the coding of simple features presented over a short period of time may play some role in the formation of visual object agnosia. It is possible that the recognition of objects requires the use of more precise descriptions of simple features and thus may disturb the ability to complete such an operation in a short period of time. However, this may be related primarily to the unconventional types of visual object agnosia, since conventional object agnosia is usually revealed when the time of object presentation is unlimited.

At the same time, more disturbances in the differentiation of line orientation, angle size, and textures presented with an unlimited time exposition may be observed when patients with visual object agnosia are required to differentiate such relatively simple features as parts of more complex features.

Disturbances at the Higher Levels of Visual Information Processing and Visual Object Agnosia

Disturbances at the Level of Complex Features Analysis

Neural Correlates of Complex Features Analysis.   Area V4 occupies the prestriate region of the visual cortex, including parts of the fusiform and lingual gyri (McKeefry & Zeki, 1997) and may be related to higher levels of object recognition processing. A lesion of the V2 or V4 area in the rhesus monkey also interferes with the animal's ability to distinguish stimuli embedded in a dense array of competing stimuli.

Outputs from area V4 continue to the inferotemporal (IT) area, which includes the posterior inferotemporal (PIT) area as well as the anterior inferotemporal (AIT) area. A bilateral ablation of the IT area in a monkey leads to permanent deficits in tasks of visual discrimination and recognition (Gross, 1992; Ungerleider & Mishkin, 1982). Physiological studies examining the AIT demonstrate (for a review, see Young, 1995) better cellular responses to complex stimuli than to simple bars or spots (Fujita et al., 1992; Tanaka et al., 1990). Some of the cells, in response to specific stimuli such as hands (Gross, 1992) or faces (Desimone, Albright, Cross, & Bruce, 1984; Young & Yamane, 1992), remain insensitive to the position, size, color, or spatial frequency of the stimuli. While one group of face-selective cells may respond to complete facial images, others may respond only to facial parts.

Some cells in the IT region seem to prefer and respond to objects only when they are in specific orientations or points of view. Other cells, however, are broadly tuned to the various orientations an object can hold, probably receiving converging information from a number of cells, each tuned to a particular orientation (Logothetis et al., 1995). This may be related to the use of a view-combination approach (Ullman, 1999).

Fujita et al. (1992) found that simplified stimuli representing the more similar components of various objects might excite certain areas close to adjacent cells (Fujita et al., 1992). In vertical penetrations, the cells responded to the same stimulus as the first recorded cell, thus demonstrating an organizational structure of functional columns or modules. These findings led to the suggestion that cells work as a detectors of pattern partials, or "alphabets" of the patterns, providing a basic function for recognition (Stryker, 1992). However, the cells did not respond to the various figures that included the patterns partially preferred by the cells. Thus, the presence of an alphabet feature in an object or figure does not excite corresponding cells, leading to the conclusion that at least the suggested alphabet of basic features does not reflect the alphabet stored in the brain of monkeys.

A detailed review of the data obtained from single-cell recording is presented by Grusser and Landis (1991), Ts'o and Roe (1995), and Parker,

Cummings, Johnston, and Hurlbert (1995). These data represent an important advance in our understanding of the mechanisms of shape analysis and object recognition as performed by the visual system. It remains unclear, however, how the processing of shape evolves from simple features recognition in areas V1 and V2 to complex features and object shape recognition in the IT. This process includes many complex operations related to conventional and unconventional types of visual information processing as reflected in modern theories based on psychological and neuropsychological studies as well as modeling of visual object recognition. Certainly, further studies employing the use of cell recording are needed. It is also of special interest to evaluate the apparent contradictions between the responses of IT cells to visually presented objects and the anatomical findings of primarily occipital and posterior-temporal-occipital lesions in cases of visual object agnosia.

Disturbances in the Formation of Complex Features From Simple Features and Differentiation of Complex Features. Using the complexes of simple features may test the differentiation of complex figures constructed from a set of simple features by one of its simple features. One such test was devised by Efron (1968). The author studied the differentiation of shapes by presenting pairs of rectangles to subjects for comparison. All figures were identical in terms of total light flux and area (Figure 2.13).

The test did not present any difficulties for those in the control group. Using Efron's test, Warrington (1986) studied two patients, J.A.F. and R.B.C., each suffering from visual agnosia for objects and faces. It was found that each patient's performance was a function of the degree of similarity between two rectangles. Performance for each patient significantly worsened when the ratio between the vertical and horizontal sides became too small.

Efron's test eventually became a sort of standard for the examination and evaluation of shape discrimination in patients with visual object agnosia. In actuality, however, the test measures the differentiation of complex features of rectangles that are different from one another in one aspect of their simple features. It would be useful to compare the results of Efron's test with those obtained via the testing of the ability to determine differences in the ratios of the lengths of the vertical and horizontal lines, a simple feature, whether they are equal or different and without the background of other features related to the rectangles. This may help bring to light disturbances in the process of complex feature formation in relation to difficulties in recognition based on simple features processing. Tonkonogy (1973) created a test for such a study.

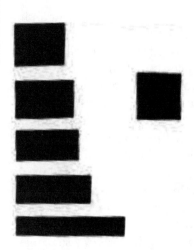

FIGURE 2.13 Effron's figures, as modified by J. Tonkonogy, from McCarthy and Warrington (1990). On the right, the basic figure that was used for comparison with each of the figures on the left. The pairs of figures were identical, or "the same," when the length of the horizontal and vertical sides were equal. The shape remained constant for one of the figures in the "different" pairs, while the ratio of vertical side to horizontal side was progressively increased in the second figure. Each subject was required to compare that ratio against the background of rectangles as matched by the other simple features of flux and area. The subject then had to determine whether the two figures were the same or different.

The groups of subjects included in the testing included 12 patients with visual object agnosia accompanied primarily by occipital lesions, 15 patients with Wernicke's aphasia accompanied by a superior-posterior temporal lesion in each patient's dominant hemisphere, 12 patients with inferior parietal lesions, 18 patients with frontal premotor lesions, and 10 control subjects.

The percentage of errors (Figure 2.14) was 59 ± 13 for patients with visual object agnosia and occipital lobe lesions; patients with frontal premotor lesions and normal controls showed percentages of errors of 10 ± 0.8 and 7.0 ± 0.01, respectively. In comparison, the percentage of errors was more prominent, though still below that of the occipital group, for patients with parietal and superior-posterior temporal lesions—18 ± 2.4 for those in the parietal group, and 23 ± 2.0 for those in the superior-posterior temporal group, in which the patients all suffered from Wernicke's aphasia and exhibited no sign of visual object agnosia. This may be related to the role of the superior-posterior temporal lobe structure and, especially, the parietal lobe areas in the processing of the complex features.

The Role of General Shape Assessment.   Normal controls seem to consider the contours of a complex figure as a single visual structure and to define the general shape of the figure as "elongated" or "round." They also attempt to treat the complexes of the three separated simple features as a single contour interrupted by gaps in the outline (as with illusory contours). The patients, on the other hand, tried to overcome the same difficulties by successively comparing each single feature. Using such a strategy, they were occasionally able to correctly assess whether complexes were the same or different. When the patients were presented with the complexes of three simple features on cards,

A.

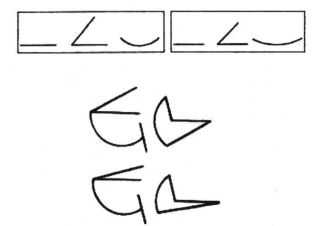

B.

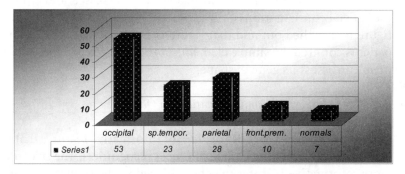

FIGURE 2.14   Differentiation. (A) Each subject was asked to differentiate between complexes consisting of three simple features—line orientation, angle size, and arc degree. Differences between simple features were above the differential thresholds, as established during previous testing, for patients with occipital lesions. The complexes were presented in pairs on a tachistoscope screen. Time length of presentation was 2000 msec. The subject had to determine if the two presented complexes were the same or different. The differences were in one or two elementary features. The three simple features are combined into open and closed geometrical figures in the bottom part of the screen. (B) This presents the percentage of errors in the differentiation of two complexes of three simple features not already combined into geometric figures (top two complexes in part A of Figure 2.14). Abbreviations are as follows: sp.tempor. = superior-posterior temporal; and, front.prem. = inferior frontal premotor.

they tended to place the cards under one another to facilitate recognition via the successive comparison of angles, lines, and arcs. These findings point to the inability of patients to combine simple features into complex features as represented by contour and as needed for the successful processing of object recognition. This impairment in the creation of complex features from simple elements is also observed in studies of object recognition when patients are presented with objects surrounded by visual noise, incomplete objects, or objects presented for only a short amount of time, as previously described.

Disturbances in the construction of complex features may be related to an impairment in the ability to link together the elements of contour, as required in cases in which objects must be recognized while surrounded by background noise. However, according to our studies, this operation does not play a leading role in the differentiation of complex features, with the simple features combined into open and closed geometrical figures (Figure 2.14 A). No improvement was noted in patients with mild visual agnosia primarily accompanied by an occipital lobe lesion in the differentiation of such complex features in comparison to the differentiation of divided complexes of simple features. At the same time, a decrease in the number of errors was observed in normal controls and in patients with temporal and inferior frontal premotor lesions. It is of interest that both the patients with nonoccipital lesions and the normal controls assessed and compared the general configuration of the geometric figures in such ways as "this figure is stretched out and that figure is more round," while occipital patients counted the simple elements of the figure separately and were unable to assess its general shape.

*Role of the Simple and Complex Features in Object
Recognition and Its Disturbances*

There is a limited, well-learned set of informative features that must be processed during the course of object recognition. The selection of more informative features may be achieved in the process of learning by using a neural-network formation that assigns a higher weight to the particular features that co-occur more frequently during the course of the recognition of a particular object and its parts.

Use of Simple Features. Simple features—line orientation, length of line, and edges—may be recognized without the use of special learning by neurons in the V1 and V2 areas during the early stages of visual recognition. The direct use of such simple features seems to be lengthy, thus requiring the description of all or almost all of the simple features of the particular object during the recognition process. In cases involving disturbances of object recognition, such simple features may be used to overcome impairments via the use of complex features. The use of either an almost complete or a complete list of simple features is often required in such cases. As noted above, this approach is often applied in cases of disturbances when the use of complex features becomes difficult, especially for the processing of unconventional information, for example, by shortening the time of object presentation. Control subjects, however, have exhibited no need to use such an approach when the use of complex features in object recognition is preserved.

Use of Complex Features. A substantial amount of memory may be preserved through the use of more complex features when describing the entire object or its parts. In this case, simple features may provide the initial building blocks, or some sort of alphabet, for more complex features; the more complex features would subsequently be used as "syllables" and "words" in the recognition process. The more complex features, such as contours, may be built based on the configurations of the more simple features (Gauthier & Tarr, 1997; Tanaka & Sengco, 1997). An example of such building is used above to study the disturbances of complex feature formation in patients with various localizations of cortical lesions. Such disturbances are especially prominent in patients with occipital lesions; this corresponds to the neurophysiological data. Studies employing the use of single-cell recording techniques have demonstrated cellular responses in the V2 area to contour, both real and illusory, as well as subjective contour. These contours may be included in the predefined set consistent with features used in the process of recognition. In order for a particular object to be recognized, its features are compared with models of different objects that have been built over the course of learning and stored in the individual's memory.

Such a system reflects the ideas of Marr (1982), who considered the goal of the visual system to be the reconstruction of the observed 3-D scene to create the 2-D patterns of light and dark pixels formed by receptive fields in the retina. This is achieved by the combination of simple features into more complex features: for example, lines are grouped into contours, then surfaces, then objects. The final step of the reconstruction process assumes that viewer-centered descriptions of the objects are remade into 3-D object-centered representations. Special emphasis should be placed on the role of expertise, the learning process in the building of features directed toward the recognition of well-known, frequently seen objects in their conventional, unoccluded orientations.

This approach requires the building of a model storage system that consists of relatively small numbers of objects that are frequently seen, often in an unoccluded and conventional view. The system is relatively simple, occupying a rather small cortical area, and may be built with substantial redundancy in order to be protected from brain damage. At the same time, in the case of the presence of a new or occluded object or perhaps the destruction of the system by brain damage, the extensive and less precise system based on simple features may be used in the process of recognition.

Various suggestions may be used in an attempt to outline the exact types of features employed by the system based on complex features. Since they are predefined by a learning process, the features must be invariant to preserve their stability, while possible changes in illumination or relatively small rotations in viewpoint may occur during the course of object recognition. Two types of object descriptions may be suggested (see Ullman, 1996).

One type is based on the invariant features that describe the entire object. The exact types of global features used in this particular type of object recognition remain unknown, but some studies have found evidence for some possibilities. They may be not obviously apparent and may consist, for instance, of the cross-ratio of four co-linear points as a projective invariant (Gibson, 1979). Gibson (1979) also suggested that an additional type related to the higher-order invariant properties may be described as spatial and temporal gradients of texture density. Another approach to selecting features may be based on coefficients in the Fourier transformation. In recognition devices, invariant properties may be based on the measurements of area, elongation, perimeter length, and shape moments (Bolles & Cain, 1982). Invariant features may consist of the total number of the given parts (Ullman, 1996). For instance, a square has four equal straight lines, four vertices, and no free line terminator, while a triangle consists of three vertices and three lines terminated by pairs of lines on those vertices.

This form of entire object description seems to represent the most efficient, simplest, and fastest way to recognize an object in its conventional and unoccluded position, and seems to be impaired in cases of visual object agnosia. In such cases, the patients are unable to correctly describe the general shape of the object, often referring to the object as "something elongated" or "something round." Furthermore, the invariant features of the entire object may not be sufficient to describe the object in its conventional view. Ullman (1996) gave the examples of foxes and dogs, or the set of all possible motorcycles, between which one could not distinguish using such global features as apparent area, perimeter length, or different moments. The construction of an elaborate shape description is needed in such cases.

Another form of object description is based on a breaking down of parts and a subsequent structural description of the object. This method is implemented by the division of an object into its generic parts and then a description of the object as a combination of its parts. Instead of processing the common properties at the level of the entire object, these decomposition methods assume that each object may be described as a combination of small numbers of parts or components. These components are generic elements that are invariant and preserved across different views and orientations of the object—properties that can be immediately identified and recognized first. In the next step, the generic elements may be grouped in different ways to describe an object as a combination of its parts. For instance, a face may be described as being made up of a nose, eyes, ears, cheeks, and a mouth. Following the recognition of its parts, the entire face may be recognized as a combination of these generic components. The features may include, for instance, edges and line segments (Milner, 1974; Sutherland, 1968), cylinders (Brooks, 1981), and contours (Hoffman & Richards, 1984). Biederman (1985) described objects in terms of a small set of primitive parts, which he called "geons." The breaking down of parts may be determined by the relationships between the contours of the image, such as co-linearity of points or lines, symmetry, and skew symmetry. In the schema proposed by Hoffman and Richards (1986), the contours are segmented at curvature minima to form a small "vocabulary," or "codon," of basic parts.

The recognition of parts may be facilitated by a further parsing into simpler low-level parts that subsequently form high-order parts; in this way, a feature hierarchy may be built. For instance, a low-level part may be a straight line, while corners and vertices constitute a high-order part formed on the basis of the straight lines. Disturbances in the use of such an approach may be observed when an object is presented with an incomplete set of features and missing complex features must be reconstructed for recognition to occur. This reconstruction may be based on the rules of symmetry, proximity, or co-linearity as described in gestalt psychology.

The patient with object visual agnosia often tries to use the already existing features in recognition efforts, mistakenly recognizing the scissors as a spoon, or the teapot as a shoe, and thus makes no attempt to reconstruct the image of the original object (Figure 2.15). Often patients do not seem even to try to connect the two parts of the incomplete images, perhaps instead concentrating on the lower part and calling it a "traffic sign." This tendency to jump immediately to the recognition of the complex features of an object without attempting to reconstruct the missing features is probably responsible, at least partly, for erroneous recognition when the object exposition time is shortened. For example, the patient may correctly recognize the parts of a bicycle—the wheels, the steering wheel, and the seat—but may jump to the erroneous conclusion that the object is a motorcycle; a longer presentation of the stimulus, however, yields the correct answer, that it is a bicycle.

Role of Spatial Relations Between Object Features

Structural descriptions of an object may rely on the invariance of the spatial relations between given parts, such as "above," "under," "behind," "longer than," "inside of," "touching," "to the right of," and so forth. In this case, recognition begins with the breaking down of the

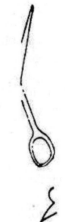

FIGURE 2.15 Incomplete pictures of a pair of scissors and a teapot. The incomplete feature of one left or right half of a pair of scissors may be compensated for by using the symmetrical image of the visible part to mentally account for the missing part. The teapot may be recognized by a continuation of the curvilinear contour of the incomplete drawing of the teapot.

object into simpler parts that are significantly easier to recognize. In the next stage, the entire object is recognized via the utilization of spatial relations between simple parts. This second stage helps to distinguish between objects that are made up of similar parts but differ in the spatial arrangement of those parts.

Meerson (1986) investigated spatial disturbances in the combination of an object's simple features into more complex features using images of objects divided into several parts, including the salient and secondary features of the object, which were placed in various positions that did not correspond to spatial relationships within the object (Figure 2.8).

When presented with an image such as that found in Figure 2.8, the normal subject was able to recognize the object via mental restoration of the spatial relationships between the parts of the object. Each image was presented on a tachistoscope, each with an exposition time of 1500 msec. Disturbances of object recognition as demonstrated through the use of these tests were shown to be less prominent for a group of 23 patients with occipital lesions than for a group of 12 patients with parietal lesions and mild visual spatial amnesia. The observed percentages of error were as follows: 12 ± 1.7 for the occipital group, 32 ± 3.3 for the parietal group, and 4 ± 0.5 for the control group. These results point to the possibility that, in addition to the ventral occipito-temporal stream, the occipito-parietal stream may also participate in the process of object recognition through the use of spatial relationships between features of the objects. This process may be disrupted following a lesion that has primarily affected the parietal portion of the dorsal stream.

Top-Down Processing

Neural Correlates of Feedforward and Feedback Projections. A series of anatomical studies has pointed to the existence of reciprocal projections from limbic structures to the anterior temporal lobe and, through the inferotemporal cortices, back to the extrastriate and then striate areas and the lateral geniculate nuclei. According to tracers and physiological studies, multiple visual areas in the cerebral cortex are interconnected by feedforward and feedback types of projections. Feedforward projections from the lower-order areas, such as V1 and V2, to the higher-order areas in the temporal and parietal cortex originate in layer III and terminate in layer IV, while feedback projections start in layers V and VI and terminate above and below layer IV (Maunsell & Van Essen, 1983; Rockland & Pandia, 1979).

Further studies of such projections between the IT, V5, V4, V3, V2, and V1 areas are summarized by Pollen (1999) and reviewed in detail by Felleman and Van Essen (1991). The deactivation or removal of a lower-order cortical area results in unresponsiveness of the higher-order areas, thus stressing the obligatory role of feedforward projections in the workings of higher-order areas, whereas the cells in the lower-order areas may retain their responsiveness after the deactivation and removal of a high-order area (Pandya & Kuypers, 1969; Sandell & Shiller, 1982). It is believed that feedback projections may provide modulatory influences that play a role in top-down visual information processing.

The idea of bidirectional aspects being involved in the process of object recognition was originally put forward by Sperry (1952) as well as Pribram (1974), who believed in a progressively differentiating feedback loop from an active template within the inferotemporal cortex and projecting back to the striate cortex. Milner (1974) suggested that ascending and descending pathways facilitate the synapses in the complementary pathway. The role of top-down connections has subsequently been explored and extended by many authors. It has been suggested that the backward loop may help to decrease the ambiguity and to increase the reliability of either a pre-attentive separation of the figure from the ground or the selective attention recognition of a complex figure consisting of two patterns. Since communication between the lower-layer units is very limited in permitting parallel processing, the higher-level functions of top-down processing may also be helpful in correlating and synchronizing activity between the lower-layer units.

According to theoretical models developed in recent decades (for a review, see Pollen, 1999), the basic structures of the recognition process include two major layers. The lower, "features" layer extracts and encodes the object's features, which are then compared with the limited number of learned prototypes in the upper, "categories" layer. Grossberg (1976) suggested that neurons forming nodes in various sensory areas of the same modality can establish a steady-state adaptive resonance, or reverberation, between nodes in the upper level ("category nodes") and nodes in the lower level ("visual feature detectors") if the patterns match, and can suppress the resonance if their patterns do not match. Similar models have been developed or extended by many others (for a review, see Pollen, 1999).

According to these models, the tentatively matched category or expectation is conveyed back via top-down processing to modulate, prime, and match the information provided by bottom-up processing (Grossberg, 1976, 1980). This final matching results in the conscious recognition of an object, scene, or movement. Researchers believe that conscious vision or hearing is the result of lower-layer activity, while the upper layer has some sort of modulating or consulting role.

Special attention is given by these authors to the problem of learning without the catastrophic forgetting of previously learned information. Grossberg (1980) ascribed this critical role of preventing the forgetting of information to the top-down process, which "selects and amplifies cells whose activities are confirmed by the hypothesis that is represented by the top-down prototype, and suppresses the activities of the cells that are not.

Top-Down Processing and Visual Object Agnosia: Role of Top-Down Processing in Object Categorization. Classification or categorization may also help to improve recognition in those with apperceptive agnosia by reducing the load of information used at the different stages of object recognition. The objects presented for recognition are placed in separate abstract, superordinate classes (furniture, musical instruments, animals, and vehicles) or less abstract, basic levels of classes (cars, airplanes, and pets). The process requires that the visual features critical for recognition of objects as a member of a particular class be immediately coded. At this particular stage, a limited number of general features of a class of objects may be processed by bottom-up processing and the features later compared with stored models; the classes of objects would be few in number for the processing of conventional information. During the intermediate stage of recognition, the top-down processes transfer the results of object categorization to the level of visual features coding, thus helping to select the critical features needed for the recognition of an individual object within a certain class. This may significantly facilitate and simplify the recognition of individual objects, for instance, in the class of vehicles or within the subclasses of cars, airplanes, or faces. Further facilitation may be achieved by this approach in the recognition of subordinate objects, such as the particular model of a car, the type of bird, or the face of a certain individual.

The role of top-down processing seems to be especially important for unconventional visual object recognition. In such conditions, critical features needed for object recognition via conventional well-learned processing may be partly missing or changed when objects are occluded or presented in unusual positions or are illuminated differently. Top-down processing may be used in such cases to select additional features that may be useful for the recognition of objects with incomplete sets of features used in their conventional recognition process. Based on bottom-up processing, the preliminary categorization of an object on the upper level may also help to reduce the number of choices. The results of such a categorization will then be transferred to a lower level by top-down processing, modulating the coding of visual features needed for the recognition of individual objects. Categorization may also help to facilitate the recognition of novel objects that are members of a certain class. Using some properties that are common to a certain class prototype, such as a class of cars, tables, or faces, a new type of car or an unknown individual face may be identified as a car or a face, even though the model of the new object is not found in storage.

This special role of top-down processing in unconventional visual object recognition points to the possible importance of its disturbance in the development of unconventional forms of visual object agnosia. Bottom-up processing of visual features at the lower level may be preserved in such cases, and no sign of conventional visual agnosia may be demonstrated. Disturbances become apparent only when the patient is confronted with partially occluded or never-before-seen objects as well as objects presented in an unusual view or in different illumination. Classification, or perceptual categorization, may be disturbed in such cases.

Warrington and James (1988) and McCarthy and Warrington (1990) relate the recognition of pictures that are not perceptually difficult to visual sensory analysis, which is similar to what is described in this chapter as a well-learned method of conventional object recognition. The second, and probably parallel, processing route uses perceptual categorization when the "analysis of object structures results in ambiguity and contextual implausibility" (McCarthy & Warrington, 1990, p. 51).

Warrington and James (1988) demonstrated disturbances in the "Unusual View" task in a series of patients with lesions of the splenium. No cases of visual agnosia were found in these patients. These findings confirmed the preservation of visual sensory analysis in the patients, while the main problems appeared to be related to an impairment in perceptual categorization. A similar approach was advanced by Humphreys, Riddoch, and Quinlan (1988).

Since top-down processing originates at a higher level of categories processing, the localization of lesions is expected to differ from those of cases with disturbances of the lower level of visual features processing, a suggestion that is supported by our review of anatomical data. Indeed, as shown in the "Anatomical Aspects" section of this chapter, the localization of lesions in the conventional apperceptive type of visual object agnosia is usually restricted to the occipital lobe, while an extension to the posterior temporal lobe is almost consistently present in patients with associative agnosia. In addition to the splenium of the corpus callosum (Warrington & James, 1988), localization of lesions in unconventional visual object agnosia with disturbances at the higher level of perceptual categorization may involve the posterior temporal and occipital areas, as well as the anterior-temporal, parietal, and frontal regions.

Role of Low and High Frequencies of Object Properties in Top-Down Processing. The role of the prefrontal cortex (PFC) in the activation of top-down facilitation during visual object recognition has been explored by Bar (2003), who suggests that a coarse version of the input image, such as a blurred image, contains the low spatial frequencies of that image and represents global information about the shape, such as general orientation and proportion. During the first stage of processing, this version of the image is projected rapidly from early visual areas directly to the PFC by way of anatomical shortcuts; once at the PFC, the image activates the limited number of possible object models. For example, if the low spatial frequency property extracted from the image is a narrow elongated blob with a circle on one end, the image will activate the high level of representation of objects such as a hockey club, a sunflower, or a pair of scissors.

At the second stage of processing, those initial guesses project back from the PFC to the inferior temporal region (IT) for the activation of a corresponding limited number of object representations; these projections are to be integrated with the bottom-up processes facilitated by a limitation in the number of objects that have to be compared for the choosing and recognition of the target object. The high-frequency property is used during this stage. They "represent abrupt spatial changes (e.g., edges) and generally correspond to configural information and fine detail" (Bar, 2003, p. 601).

In support of these two stages of information processing, Bar (2003) cited recent neurophysiological studies (Sugase, Yamane, Ueno, & Kawano, 1999; Tamura & Tanaka, 2001), which found initially broadly tuned activity in the IT; the recorded activity was found to be representing only the global features of the stimulus, while the fine properties of the image were later represented in the neurons of that region,

51 milliseconds after the onset of the global response (Sugase et al., 1999). The role of the PFC in this processing is supported by data indicating that the ventral PFC is involved in visual object analysis in monkeys (Rainer & Miller, 2000; Wilson et al., 1993). This analysis is elicited by low frequencies, as demonstrated by the PFC's role in distinguishing between objects of different categories; this role of the PFC was not observed, however, in the differentiation of individual objects found in the same category (Freedman et al., 2001).

Through the use of fMRI scans, Bar et al. (2001) observed PFC activation in all recognition conditions, especially in the inferior frontal gyrus and the orbital gyrus. PFC activation was significantly more pronounced in cases of unconventional information processing, both when the images of objects were presented briefly and when they were masked. Bar (2003) stressed that easy recognition may be accomplished via bottom-up analysis, in which case the PFC would be less involved. Activation of the PFC is especially important when recognition is more difficult, for example, for briefly presented or masked objects; here, the PFC is crucial for the processing of coarser and less accurate information reflecting the low-frequency properties of the objects. Such information may be used to limit the number of object choices targeted for recognition. This may be transferred by the top-down process to lower levels, to aid in the recognition of the target object from the limited number of object choices that must be processed.

In cases of visual object agnosia, it is possible that object recognition is disturbed on the lower level, which is based on the use of high-frequency properties of the object image. This is especially prominent in unconventional information processing when object presentation is either brief or masked. In such cases, low-frequency properties of the object may be used. These frequencies are usually rapidly projected to the PFC levels for further processing and are typically preserved in cases of visual object agnosia; patients may be able to recognize, for example, the general shape of an object's general shape as oval, elongated, or round. At the same time, the subsequent stage of top-down processing is disturbed in visual object agnosia. In such cases, a visual object agnosia patient is unable to successfully integrate the general shape of an object with the bottom-up processing of a fine description of the object using the high-frequency property. The patient demonstrates disturbances in assessing the specific details of an object shape, for example, when the time of object image presentation is shortened or the object is masked by noise. For example, the patient is able to recognize the general shape of an object's part as a wheel but unable to recognize the fine details specific to the particular object, thus erroneously identifying the wheel of a bicycle as that of a motorcycle. One of our patients was presented with a "noisy" picture of a pair of glasses and mistakenly identified the object as a sunflower; the patient had missed the specific details of the lenses and the earpieces and was thus unable to use the shapes of the object's parts to correctly identify the glasses.

Top-down processing must play a significant role in the segmentation of figures presented in the midst of background noise formed by overlapping figures. In such pictures, the contour of the particular object is actually represented by low-frequency properties, while the high-frequency properties are hidden by the overlapping figures. Top-down processing based on low-frequency properties of the object's contour may limit the number of object choices and help in the recognition of the targeted contours. Part of the contour may occasionally be recognized as a sign of the class of the object or a particular object, facilitating the tracing of the contour. These processes may be disturbed in patients with mild visual agnosia, leading to difficulties in the recognition of objects presented in overlapping figures; the ability to recognize an object in its conventional and unobstructed view remains preserved in such patients.

Patients would often compensate for these difficulties by using descriptions of all, or almost all, of the features of the targeted object. The patients would often count the parts of the object, often unable to recognize the entire object until all the parts were accounted for. When tested on their ability to recognize an incomplete picture, patients with mild visual object agnosia were unable to recognize the detail of the particular part needed to identify the object. One of our patients recognized a bicycle by counting its parts—"wheels . . . handlebar . . . seat . . . motorcycle," and then after an additional presentation of the image, "Oh, I see pedals. . . . this is a bicycle." Control subjects tended to correctly recognize an object even with the absence of two or three less important parts, and in fact often did not notice that some less important parts were missing. The normal subjects could often recognize the object only by seeing parts of the most salient features, such as the earpiece of a pair of glasses or the handset of a telephone. At the same time, the visual agnosia patients were often unable to recognize the salient features as parts of a particular object, for example, the wheels of a bicycle as they differ from the wheels of a motorcycle.

In order to test the role of top-down processing in disturbances of object recognition, a series of tests was used; it included incomplete figures of four objects followed by the presentation of complete pictures of the same four objects (Tonkonogy, 1997). This allowed for the process of a limitation of the number of object choices, a process usually performed by PFC and important for successful object recognition. The presentation of the complete pictures helped to significantly decrease the volume of information that had to be processed during the course of the recognition of incomplete figures. Following the presentation of the complete pictures of the four objects, the original and incomplete pictures of the four objects were presented to the subjects again. In general, the presentation of complete pictures markedly reduced the number of errors in object recognition observed in the subjects. However, some of the patients continued to experience difficulties in the recognition of some of the objects, for example, the incomplete figure of an anchor and a teapot, each probably requiring the use of completion operations that is commonly disturbed in such cases.

Disturbances in the use of high-frequency properties of object features are also apparent when the time of signal presentation is shortened. In such situations, the patient becomes unable to differentiate the high frequency of the angles degrees when presentation time is shortened, but continues to be able to differentiate correctly the angles with bigger differences in their degrees, representing the low-frequency property. In other words, the differential threshold for angle discernment increases for interval differentiation with the shortening of presentation time from 2000 msec to 0 seconds with angles of 15–30 degrees in the group of patients with mild visual agnosia, but it remains at a statistically insignificant level with angles of 2–3 degrees in the group of patients without agnosia (Meerson, 1986; Tonkonogy, 1973).

Object recognition in the context of scenes may be facilitated by the top-down process that limits the number of possible choices in well-known scenes, such as a kitchen or an office. The recognition of an isolated object may require comparison with a large number of object models in storage to identify the object in a typical scene, for instance, to recognize a desk in an office or a table in a dining room.

Disturbances in the Ability to Apply Completion Operations: Extrapolation to the Missing Parts of the Image

The relative preservation of signal filtration from background noise is sharply contrasted by difficulties in the recognition of an object detected in the noise. This recognition requires a series of completion and grouping operations that may be disturbed in patients with occipital lobe lesions. According to Ullman (1996), one of the operations could include the linking together of local elements of contour detected in the image. The elements are disconnected in the image, and their connection may be achieved by a simple grouping operation based on proximity, curvilinearity, and length of the element. In the following stages, some additional operations to achieve object completion may include the use of vertices to project the other edges of the vertex, to select the symmetric parts not seen in the image (Figure 2.15, incomplete scissors), and to add other parts of the object with occluded shape (Figure 2.15). Such operations may be disturbed when a patient with an occipital lesion does not recognize the drawing of a pair of glasses accompanied by background noise, due to an inability to mentally fill in the missing earpiece on the glasses. This completion and reconstruction of the edges of the lenses may be accomplished via the use of an operation based on co-linearity and symmetry as well as on the projection of the vertex of the glasses.

Similar difficulties have also been observed in the recognition of incomplete pictures of an object. Patients often have difficulty in reconstructing an image using grouping rules of symmetry, continuation, proximity, and co-linearity. They tend to consider each of the parts of the object to be a complete object, and fail to use an extrapolation to complete the object image. Upon seeing the figure of the scissors cut in half (Figure 2.15), for example, a patient with an occipital lobe lesion would recognize it as perhaps a needle or a tennis racquet. The patient in such a case does not seem to be attempting to use the rule of symmetry to find the missing part and to reconstruct the object; in the same way, the part of a teapot that includes the spout may be immediately identified as a shoe without any attempt by the patient to mentally create a continuation of object contour. Two unconnected parts of the same object are treated by the patient as two different objects, "a traffic sign and something else."

Another example is the selection of figure contours from the background of overlapping figures in such tasks, in which case one may group the contour parts into extended smooth curves, or "good continuation" in terms of gestalt psychology and "co-linearity" in terms of modern psychology.

Use of Simple and Complex Features in Decision Making and Assigning a Set of Features to a Particular Object

Since the particular complex and especially simple features are often not unique to a particular object (in clinical terminology, they are not pathognomic for an object) and may have partially overlapping ranges, the concept of *features or properties spaces* has been used in pattern recognition based on invariant properties methods. Each view of the object is considered to be represented by a point in n-dimensional space, where n is a number of measured invariant features. The set of all the views of an object comprises a subspace. When different classes of objects are represented by subspaces that do not overlap, a viewed object will be classified by finding a subspace in which the point of that object lies. Disturbances in this process may underline the development of associative agnosia. However, further studies are needed before we can come to more definite conclusions.

CONCLUSION

THE RESULTS OF the studies reviewed point to the possible existence of at least two types of disturbances in the process of visual object recognition.

1. One type of disturbance is related to conventional information processing, which is based on the well-learned predefined invariant set of complex features of particular objects. In cases of apperceptive agnosia, disturbances of this type culminate in difficulties both in the assessment of high spatial frequencies of object properties and in the recognition of objects in their conventional and nonoccluded views. In cases of apperceptive agnosia, object shape coding operations rely primarily on a description of the general shape of more complex features, which are often insufficient for the correct recognition of a targeted object. Associative agnosia results from a disturbance in the ability to compare and match an object as it is described in its storage model with the observed meaning of the object.

2. Another type of disturbance is related to unconventional information processing and is an impairment in the recognition of objects presented only briefly, of occluded, masked objects, of objects presented in unconventional views, and of novel objects that have not been previously seen. This processing cannot be solely based on well-learned complex and invariant features of nonoccluded objects and their storage in models. Instead, it requires additional higher-level top-down operations based on the use of low-frequency features of an object; in this way, effective categorization can limit the number of object models used in the process of recognition, and top-down processing can guide the structural reconstruction of the object.

3. In disturbances of both conventional and unconventional operation processing, the recognition process is fragmented and based on taking into account the series of generally described low-frequency features of an object and its parts, but without a detailed description of the finer high-frequency parts. This may be compensated for in some cases by the use of all or almost all of the sets of simple and complex features of the object. At the same time, normal subjects may recognize the occluded, masked, or briefly presented object by using a limited set of more precisely described simple features that may be sufficient for object identification.

4. The completion process, or extrapolation, may also be disturbed, and a patient may suffer from an inability both to reconstruct the features of an object using such rules as proximity, co-linearity,

symmetry, and continuity and to appreciate that the image of the object is incomplete and thus requires partial reconstruction from processing of the image as a complete reflection of the object. The disturbances may also be related to an impairment in the use of an axis-based description of an object or of combinations of objects as presented in an unconventional view.

5. The formation and use of complex features represent the main disturbances at the lower, bottom-up level of conventional and unconventional information processing as observed in cases of visual object agnosia.

6. Disturbances of visual working (operational) memory are observed in the processing of simple features in patients with mild visual agnosia. Such disturbances at higher levels of visual information processing in object amnesia require further studies.

7. Many operations involved in the recognition of objects in their unconventional forms and views are connected to the well-learned operations used in the conventional types of recognition. In the course of unconventional information processing, such operations as object completion, sequential descriptions of an object's parts, and alignment are directed to the reconstruction of object description as employed by conventional information processing. At the same time, the storage models are transformed in such a way as to allow for the use of a simplified combination of views. Thus, the disturbances of conventional information processing may contribute to the development of impairments in the recognition of occluded objects, objects observed in unconventional views, and novel objects.

COLOR AGNOSIA

LESIONS AT THE peripheral retinal level of the visual color system may produce a loss of certain sectors of the chromatic spectrum: for example, a loss of middle-wavelength perception results in *achromatopsia,* the loss of chromatic perception, of green color. In patients with cerebral lesions, a prominent achromatopsia is usually spread to all sectors of the light spectrum. This type of achromatopsia was first described in patients with cerebral lesions in the last quarter of the nineteenth century (for a review, see Grusser & Landis, 1991). Quaglino (1867) observed a patient who had developed complete achromatopsia following a stroke; left hemiparesis, left hemianopia, and object agnosia were also noted in the patient. Total color blindness with partial or complete preservation of visual acuity was later described in a patient who regained consciousness following two weeks in a posttraumatic coma (Cohn, 1874), as well as in a professional color printer who had suffered a stroke (Steffan, 1881).

Patients with hemianopia showed complete achromatopsia with the preservation of visual acuity in the remaining hemifield (Samelsohn, 1881; von Seggern, 1881). Verrey (1888) described cases of right-sided hemiachromatopsia. Based on findings of the preservation of light-dark vision in many cases of achromatopsia, early authors concluded that there is a special center for color vision located outside the region for light-dark vision. Wilbrand (1884, 1887) suggested the existence of a separate center for color vision in the occipital cortex along with two other centers—one for light-dark vision and another for shape vision.

Wilbrand (1887) described difficulties in object sorting according to colors as well as disturbances in color naming, subsuming both conditions under the umbrella term "amnestic color blindness." Lewandowsky (1908) was the first to report a patient who, following a stroke, developed several disturbances of the higher level of color information processing, a condition different from that of achromatopsia. These disturbances were later described as relatively independent syndromes, and they included the inability to nominally identify colors, a condition known as *color anomia*; the inability to point to a color when its name was given was termed *sensory color aphasia*. *Color agnosia* was defined as a disturbance in the ability to color a drawing, to differentiate between correctly and incorrectly colored objects, and to match samples of colors with an absent object. A loss in the ability to recall the color of a well-known object was described as a loss of color images. Lewandovsky thought his patient had lost the ability to associate color images with shape images and brightness.

Color agnosia, anomia, and aphasia have since been described in various publications. The term color agnosia was introduced by Sittig (1921). Special research attention was given to examining the differences between color blindness (achromatopsia), color agnosia, and color aphasia (Davidenkoff, 1912; Gelb & Goldstein, 1924; Kok, 1967; Hécaen & Albert, 1978; McCarthy & Warrington, 1990; Sittig, 1921). Other authors have expressed doubts about the existence of color agnosia as a disorder: these include De Renzi (1999), who described its manifestation as "color amnesia."

CLINICAL ASPECTS

Disturbances at the Simple Features Level: Color Blindness (Achromatopsia)

Achromatopsia, or cortical blindness, is defined as a disorder of elementary forms of color perception. Sufferers from achromatopsia will see their visual world become colorless and pale, not unlike images viewed in a black and white movie. In more severe cases, everything is seen in shades of grey. Object recognition in everyday life situations may be preserved for the most part, but difficulties can be observed in patients when the color of an object needs to be used as a main feature in the process of object discrimination, as in differentiation between jars of pickles and jam, or between bronze and silver coins.

Patients with achromatopsia may reach normal limits when evaluated by Ishihara plates (Ishihara, 1983). In this particular test, plates measure discrimination between blue and yellow and between red and green and reveal impairments in some sectors of the color spectrum as observed in patients with retinal colorblindness. Loss of color vision across all spectrums is typical for those suffering from achromatopsia and may be observed using the Farnsworth–Munsell 100 Hue Test (Farnsworth, 1957), which requires the correct arrangement of color patches representing a continuum along the entire color spectrum (McCarthy & Warrington, 1990). Visual acuity may be preserved in patients with severe achromatopsia, as has previously been observed in multiple patients (Meadow, 1974).

Color discrimination deficits may be confined to one-half of the visual field (Albert, Reches, & Silverberg, 1975; Damasio et al., 1980; Verrey, 1888). Achromatopsia is a rare condition and is often associated with prosopagnosia and topographagnosia (Bodamer, 1947; Green & Lessel, 1977; Grüsser & Landis, 1991; Hécaen & de Ajuriaguerra, 1952; Kok, 1967; Levin, Povorinsky, & Tonkonogy, 1961; Meadow, 1974). Object amnesia and pure alexia have also been noted in some cases of achromatopsia.

Disturbances at the Level of Complex Features: Color Agnosia and the Alienation of Color From the Object's Features

Color agnosia has been studied using tasks that concentrate on conventional information processing, in which the object is presented in its unoccluded and conventional view. The term color agnosia is most frequently used to describe nonverbally mediated disorders of color recognition as a feature of an object. Color discrimination is usually preserved in cases of color agnosia.

Patients with color agnosia lose the ability to choose the correct color patch for a specific item in black and white object drawings (tomato, banana, grass, etc.). A similar impairment consists of difficulties in the ability to color such drawings correctly, to assess whether photographs or drawings of an object are correctly colored (e.g., a green elephant or a red banana), and/or to visualize the color of the absent object. These may be considered as a disturbance in the use of color as part of the complex features of an object.

The term color agnosia is also used to denote disturbances in the ability to sort patches with various shades of different colors into more general groups of hues or colors, such as all the shades of green. Such a condition may be defined as a disturbance in the formation of the complex features of colors.

It is unclear, however, whether and if so how these underlying difficulties impair object recognition. Some answers may be obtained via further research into unconventional information processing as performed by patients with color agnosia, for example the recognition of colored objects occluded by noise, with the time of object presentation shortened, and with missing shape features. It would also be of interest to study the recognition of dynamic features of unoccluded objects as reflected by their color, such as ripe versus unripe fruits or vegetables, or trees in different seasons.

Disturbances at the Semantic Level: Color Anomia and Color Sensory Aphasia

The term color anomia is used to characterize disturbances in the naming of the colors of items, such as patches of items and surfaces of objects. Color anomia may be considered to be a disturbance at the semantic level in defining the verbal meaning of a color. Object naming is usually relatively less disturbed than color naming. The term color aphasia, or color sensory aphasia, is applied when a patient demonstrates an inability to correctly point to colors upon verbal command (Davidenkov, 1956; Sittig, 1921). In such cases, the patient may often be able to sort shades of colors or match a specific color with an appropriate object, but will exhibit disturbances in color naming or in the comprehension of color names.

Color anomia and color sensory aphasia have often been observed in the same patients, but cases have also been described in which color anomia and color sensory aphasia have developed independently of one another (Kok, 1967; Mohr, Leicester, Stoddard, & Sidman, 1971; Oxbury, Oxbury, & Humphrey, 1969). Color anomia is often also associated with alexia, anomic aphasia, and space orientation disturbances (Grüsser & Landis, 1991).

Color Agnosia and the Recognition of Scenes, Spatial Relations, and Emotions

The taxonomy of visual agnosia is primarily based on the differentiation between various tasks of visual information processing, such as the recognition of objects, faces, scenes, or spatial relations. Disturbances in the operations underlying these tasks, for example, disorders of shape recognition, are usually analyzed in order to understand and explain the mechanisms of visual agnosia for objects, faces, scenes, and so forth. However, in spite of the clear anatomical and physiological independence of the color processing system, which begins at the retinal level and extends to the cortical structures, the use of the term color agnosia has generally been limited to disturbances of object recognition related to the alienation of color from the object description based on object shape.

However, color as a feature of the visual world seems to play a much greater role in visual information processing and its various disturbances; for example, color agnosia may be implicated in disturbances of the recognition of scenes described by the combination of their textures, colors, and shapes. The inability to recognize the color of landmarks, as needed in such cases as "Turn left when you see a red house" or "a green tag," may impair the topographic memory of patients with color agnosia. Emotions are also connected with the processing of color. For example, the expression "blue mood" is widely used as a description of a depressed mood, and the expression "red faced" may characterize an angry person. Corresponding disturbances may include difficulties in the recognition of emotion or the recognition of personal traits using color as a feature facilitating these processes. Further studies are certainly needed.

Color Agnosia as a Disorder of the Operations of Visual Information Processing

The term color agnosia describes impairment in operations in which color is a feature of the visual word, like shape; the term does not include, however, particular disturbances in the tasks of object or scene recognition. It appears that disorders in the recognition of colors, the sorting of different hues, and the matching of particular objects does not result in any clinically significant deterioration of object or scene recognition. The patient with color agnosia may be unable to differentiate between a tomato and an apple without relying on each object's color features but will be able to recognize most objects using features of their shapes, sizes, and textures. The idea that disturbances of object recognition are amplified or directly related to color agnosia or aphasia has not been supported by research to date. Color disturbances may often accompany other types of visual agnosia, especially prosopagnosia (Green & Lessel, 1977; Meadow, 1974), but they are clinically independent. Disturbances in our life of the colored world have been reflected so little in descriptions of visual agnosia that color agnosia has not yet been included in the leading texts in the field of agnosia (see Farah, 1990; Luria, 1966).

Disturbances of color recognition will require further exploration concerning their role in the functional tasks of visual information processing. We perceive the visual world as colored, and it is difficult to imagine that disorders of colored world recognition are concentrated around the sorting of color patches of different hues and the loss of color images of some fruits and vegetables. Disorders of color recognition may manifest themselves in tasks such as the filtration of a signal from noise or the detection and recognition of objects occluded by a noisy background or by incomplete sets of features, as well as in tasks requiring the use of textures for the recognition of scenes and in tasks related to the spatial orientation of objects. Again, further research into the field is needed.

ANATOMICAL ASPECTS

Neural Correlates of Color Vision

Color is processed by a specific system that starts at the level of the retina and includes three types of cones, or color receptors. The cones differ in peak sensitivity to the pigment of the three wavelength regions of the spectrum—short, middle, and long. Perception of the color blue is mediated by cones tuned to short wavelengths, while perception of the color green is mediated by cones sensitive to middle wavelengths, and the color red is mediated by cones tuned to long wavelengths. Different grades of stimulation of these receptors by light mediate the perception of other colors.

Information from cones is transmitted through the parvocellular system of the lateral geniculate nuclei to the second and third layers of the "blob" cells in area V1. Three different types of cells respond to the chromaticity of the signal in area V1—the red-green, blue-yellow, and black-white systems. The neurons in area V1 then project to the "thin dark stripes" found in area V2. Approximately half of the neurons in these thin stripes are sensitive to the wavelengths, while the remaining neurons are presumably sensitive to shades of grey. Orientation-tuned cells are predominantly found in "thick dense stripes" and exhibit either weak or no responses to the chromaticity of the stimuli (for a review, see Grüsser & Landis, 1991).

Color-sensitive cells in area V4 receive input from the thin stripes of area V2 and receive direct input from the blobs of area V1. While most of the cells in area V4 are sensitive to shape, some of them demonstrate an overlapping sensitivity to chromaticity and spatial properties of visual stimuli (Zeki, 1990), pointing to the probable role of the neurons in area V4 in the integration of chromatic properties with contour and shape (Grüsser & Landis, 1991). Further transmission of the color-specific information may travel via direct input from the V4 area to the visual processing areas of the inferior temporal lobe and to the parahippocampal gyrus, which is related to the limbic system and is located near the V4 area. It seems that area V4 occupies a part of the mesial occipital lobe in the hominid brain.

Role of Occipital and Occipito-Temporal Lesions

Achromatopsia

In cases of achromatopsia, the lesion may be bilateral involving the fusiform and lingual gyri (Meadow, 1974); unilateral lesions, however, have also been suggested. Verrey (1888) was the first to describe achromatopsia limited to the right visual field in a case in which autopsy data provided evidence of a lesion in the left occipito-temporal areas and involving the lingual and fusiform gyri. Kölmel (1988) reported a patient who developed right homonymous hemianopia, mild paresthesia in the right hand, and mild gait unsteadiness. The patient recovered after a few weeks, but a right hemiachromatopsia remained. MRI scans revealed a lesion in the patient's left mesial occipito-temporal region and extending to the parahippocampal gyrus.

Color Agnosia, Anomia, and Aphasia

Most authors attribute the development of color agnosia to lesions of the left occipital lobe with an extension of the lesion to the parietal or temporal lobe (Gloning Gloning, & Hoff, 1968; Hécaen & Angelergues, 1963; Mohr et al., 1971). Gloning et al. (1968) presented 40 cases of color agnosia verified either by autopsy or in the course of surgery for a brain tumor. A unilateral lesion of the left hemisphere was observed in 27 cases, with only two of the patients being left-handed, and a unilateral right hemisphere lesion was observed in only six patients, with three of the six being left-handed; the lesion was bilateral in seven cases. Lesions extended to the temporal lobe in all cases and to the parietal lobe in 20 of the 40 cases. Meadows (1974) reviewed past literature as well as doing his own research, and related color agnosia to lesions of the anterior inferior part of the occipital lobe. Some authors have also stressed the role of bilateral occipital damage (Green & Lessel, 1977).

Difficulties in color naming have been related to a callosal lesion, which disconnects the visual area in the right hemisphere from language areas in the left hemisphere. Geschwind and Fusillo's patient suffered from alexia and difficulties in color naming. The patient's lesion involved the left occipital lobe and the posterior third of the corpus callosum. However, Kinsbourne and Warrington (1962) described a patient with difficulties in color naming who was able to develop a verbal association between names and objects, but could not succeed in the associative learning that was needed to pair color names with objects or color blocks with nonverbal items. Researchers have concluded that difficulties in color naming are associated with an inability to associate color names with objects, while visual-verbal connections remain preserved.

Single-cell recording data points to the possible role of lesions in the V1 and V2 areas in the development of achromatopsia. The destruction of area V4 may be also implicated in such cases (Grusser & Landis, 1991). Since area V1 in humans is probably located in Brodmann's area

17 around the calcarine fissure, and area V2 partly occupies Brodmann's area 18, destruction of these areas may result in the destruction of color-sensitive cells, leading to the development of achromatopsia, an idea that has been supported via evidence obtained from clinico-anatomical cases of achromatopsia. This loss of chromatic vision may be experienced in the visual hemifield contralateral to the side of the lesion (right hemiachromatopsia would be the result of a left hemisphere lesion, and left hemiachromatopsia would be the result of a right hemisphere lesion); a bilateral lesion would produce complete achromatopsia for the entire visual field. This suggestion has been supported by clinical observations. Homonimous hemianopia and cortical blindness are often seen following a stroke or injury in those particular areas of the primary visual cortex. Achromatopsia is usually observed during the course of recovery following an acute vascular or traumatic episode. It remains unclear how the lesion in this area selectively involves cells sensitive to the chromatic properties of the visual signal, while sparing the orientation-tuned cells, but differential vulnerabilities of color and orientation sensitive cells to ischemia may be responsible. Other mechanisms, however, also deserve future consideration and investigation.

The data obtained by single-cell recording also points to the possible role of V4 destruction in the development of color agnosia, as the area includes many cells tuned to shapes as well as cells sensitive to the color of visual stimuli. The chromatic properties of the input may thus be integrated with the system that describes contour and shape. This system could be destroyed by lesions in area V4 that underlie the development of color agnosia, primarily following a lesion of the left hemisphere in right-handed individuals. It is again unclear how a lesion in the same area may produce visual object agnosia in one case and color agnosia in another case. The differences are probably related to the directions of lesion extensions to the various neighboring areas of the temporal and parietal lobes that participate in the process of recognition of visual stimuli based on descriptions of shape, contours, and spatial relationships integrated with color processing in separate areas of the brain. Color agnosia, anomia, and aphasia may result from the extension of a lesion from area V4 to those hypothetical specific areas related to the high level of color processing needed for the development of visual object agnosia in one case and of color amnesia in another case. Further clinico-anatomical and single-cell recording studies are needed to further explore the subject.

CONCLUSION

1. Color agnosia is described as an alienation of color features from object descriptions at the levels of simple and complex features, as well as at the semantic level in color anomia. Further studies

are needed to evaluate the role of color agnosia in the distur-bances of functional tasks in visual information processing such as the recognition of objects, scenes, and spatial relationships, as well as features of emotions and personality traits. Special atten-tion should be given to the study of unconventional types of color processing in the course of recognition.

2. Color agnosia, anomia, and aphasia result from either lesions of the left occipital lobe or bilateral occipital lesions with exten-sions to the temporal lobe and, in many cases, to the parietal lobe (Figure 2.16). Involvement of the corpus callosum has also been re-ported in some cases.

3. In patients with achromatopsia, lesions usually occupy the mesial part of the occipito-temporal region, including the lingual and fusiform gyri. It is possible that unilateral lesions in the V1 and V2 areas result in the development of achromatopsia in the con-tralateral visual field, while bilateral lesions produce complete achromatopsia covering the entire visual field. No anatomical data or single-cell recording data collected thus far has provided an explanation, while the similar lesion site of the V4 area results in visual object agnosia in one case and color agnosia in another case. These differences may perhaps be explained by the exten-sion of the lesion beyond the mesial occipito-temporal region to various areas in the temporal and parietal lobes.

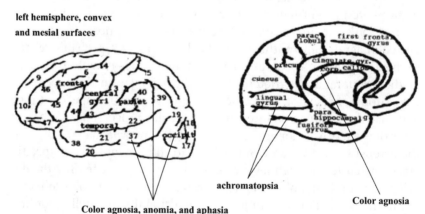

FIGURE 2.16 Localization of lesions on the mesial surface and convexital surface of the left hemisphere in achromatopsia and in color agnosia, anomia, and aphasia.

3

Disorders of Recognition in the Physical World: Other Types of Agnosia

VISUOSPATIAL AGNOSIA

AGNOSIA MAY MANIFEST itself as a visual disorientation in the immediate environment, primarily as agnosia of depth perception. Rare types of visuospatial agnosia include disturbances of stereoscopic vision and visual alloesthesia. *Topographic disorientation* is also considered to be a type of visuospatial agnosia.

VISUAL-SPATIAL DISORIENTATION IN IMMEDIATE SPACE

THE SPACE THAT surrounds us contains multiple objects that form certain relationships within that spatial frame. Orientation in this immediate space is needed to perform many tasks of our daily living activity and represents an important task of information processing performed by our human brains. We must know the locations of single objects and their positions in relation to other objects in space in order to move around, to eat, to wash, and to perform our professional

100

LOCALIZATION
OF CLINICAL
SYNDROMES IN
NEUROPSYCHOLOGY
AND NEUROSCIENCE

activities. The hallmark of *visual-spatial disorientation* consists of difficulties in the visual recognition of the spatial relationships of objects within the immediate environment as seen by the subject; disturbances in topographic disorientation, on the other hand, reflect the loss of one's ability to navigate through space to a certain destination.

A separate syndrome of visual disorientation in space that can be visually screened by the subject was first described in detail by Holmes (1918); the term visual disorientation was later coined by Holmes and Horrax (1919). Similar cases were subsequently reported by Poetzl (1928), Kleist (1934), Riddoch (1935), Lange (1936), Brain (1941), and Critchley (1953). Poetzl (1928) considered the syndrome as a type of "geometric agnosia of the objects," while Kleist (1934) suggested the term "blindness of the space." The disturbances were later described as a "disorder of spatial perception" (Hécaen, 1972; Hécaen & Albert, 1978). The term visual-spatial disorientation seems to be preferable as it points to the specific clinical disturbances of orientation in the surrounding visually appreciated space. "Disorders of spatial perception" often refer to difficulties in the recognition and use of spatial information related to a wider range of disturbances, including *topographic disorientation, constructional apraxia, spatial alexia, acalculia,* and so on.

A series of experimental studies concentrated on examining the role of primary visual sensory disturbances in the formation of visual-spatial disorientation disorders (Bay, 1953; Bender & Teuber, 1947), and the prevalence of deficits of visual localization in the field contralateral to the damaged hemisphere (Ratcliff & Davies-Jones, 1972; Riddoch, 1935). Disturbances of spatial analysis were also investigated with the drawing of lines, objects such as studies of simple figures alignment displaced in horizontal and vertical axis (Paterson & Zangwill, 1944). The paper-pencil tests have subsequently been used in a large number of studies exploring deficits in spatial perception in patients with local brain lesions (for a review, see McCarthy & Warrington, 1990).

Clinical Aspects
Disturbances in 3-D Space Orientation: Agnosia of Depth
Impairments in Conventional Information Processing. The ability to localize objects in 3-D space, especially in the sagittal plane in relation to the patient's position, is disturbed in patients with agnosia of depth; such difficulties are experienced in both the absolute and the relative localization of objects in space. Patients are not able to assess either the absolute distance to an object or the relative localization of two objects in the sagittal plane. They make errors in their attempts to judge which of two objects is nearer to them, to assess the relative height of several objects, and to count objects placed in one line of projection. The location of objects is disturbed in the coronal plane in

101

*Disorders of
Recognition in the
Physical World:
Other Types of
Agnosia*

some cases, and patients experience difficulties in the assessment of an object's location to the right or to the left of the body position (Holmes, 1918; McCarthy & Warrington, 1990). In spite of the preserved ability to recognize objects, patients make errors when trying to touch an object in their field of view or to compare the dimensions of two objects in their sight, and they often bump into objects while walking. In some cases, agnosia of depth is accompanied by disorders of stereoscopic vision (Holmes & Horrax, 1919; Riddoch, 1935).

Disorders of visual orientation are often restricted to the visual modality, and patients tend to demonstrate a preserved ability to locate sources of sounds and to find out which of two objects is closer to the patient by touching the objects with a finger (Holmes, 1918).

Some authors have stressed that disturbances in visual localization may be confined to the visual half-field contralateral to a hemispheric lesion (Riddoch, 1935) or to one portion, usually a single quadrant, of the visual field. However, the role of a primary visual spatial deficit was demonstrated in such cases using special tests (Bay, 1953). Further research into the topic is indeed necessary, as disorders of visual localization have been observed in cases without hemianopic sensory deficits (Riddoch, 1935).

Disturbances in Unconventional Information Processing
Disturbances in the Assessment of Space Features. While clinically diagnosed conventional impairments in visual spatial disorientation have been described in relation to difficulties of visual localization in the surrounding 3-D space, a series of unconventional paper-pencil tests have been used to demonstrate disturbances in the processing of visual spatial information in 2-D space (for a review, see McCarthy & Warrington, 1990). Patients often exhibit preserved orientation in the visual field of real 3-D space, but disturbances may be revealed when they are required to process spatial information in 2-D space as presented on paper. These difficulties include impairments in the assessment of spatial features, such as errors in line bisection tests or in locating the central points of a series of lines (Bisiach, Capitani, Colombo, & Spinnler, 1976), disturbances in the discrimination of relative spatial positions as revealed when the patient must locate a dot in a second square whose position is similar to the position of a dot in a first square (Taylor & Warrington, 1973), or errors made when counting the number of dots in a briefly presented array (Kimura, 1963).

Disturbances in the Transfer of 2-D Space Images to 3-D Space Images. Disturbances in 2-D space orientation may underline the development of various syndromes related to impairments in spatial orientation, such as constructional apraxia, acalculia, or alexia, and may be one

102

LOCALIZATION
OF CLINICAL
SYNDROMES IN
NEUROPSYCHOLOGY
AND NEUROSCIENCE

of the factors that mediates the development of visual disorientation in 3-D space. Other factors are related to the ability to transfer 2-D spatial images into 3-D space. Such a transfer requires special operations, which may be the major factor underlying disturbances in the syndrome of visual disorientation in immediate space.

Anatomical Aspects
Conventional Disturbances in the Assessment of 3-D Space

Most researchers thus far have related the development of agnosia of depth to parieto-occipital lesions (Holmes, 1918; Lange, 1936; Riddoch, 1935). Holmes (1918) noted bilateral inferior hemianopsy in cases of visual disorientation and suggested bilateral lesion localization in the occipito-parietal junctions, while other authors have stressed the role of occipital lesions in such disturbances (Kleist, 1934; Pötzl, 1924). Subsequently, infarctions at the junction of the occipital and parietal lobes were observed in cases and described by Warrington (1986).

Unconventional Disturbances in the Assessment of 2-D Space

The role of parietal lesions in disturbances of visual spatial orientation was demonstrated in our study of the discrimination of angles according to their rotation in space. Discrimination of the angle degree in different spatial rotations of the compared angles (Figure 2.9) was more disturbed in patients with parietal lesions compared to other groups of patients (Meerson, 1986; Tonkonogy, 1973).

In a series of dot-position discrimination studies (Warrington & Rabin, 1970); line orientation (Warrington & Rabin, 1970); and dot counting (Kimura, 1963; Warrington & James, 1967) performance was significantly worse in patients with right posterior lesions compared to both patients with right anterior lesions and patients with lesions in the left hemisphere. Columbo et al. (1976) developed a test that required subjects to match two pairs of rods and determine if the rods were the same or different. The position of one rod in the pair was fixed, while the second rod could be moved in the sagittal plane. The number of errors in comparing the second rod's orientation with the first was highest in patients with right posterior lesions. These results may point to the important role of right hemisphere lesions in the development of agnosia of depth for real 3-D space, but further collection of the quite rare cases of amnesia of depth is needed to test this suggestion.

TOPOGRAPHIC DISORIENTATION

JACKSON (1876) DESCRIBED a patient whose difficulties included finding her way around her neighborhood. Disturbances of topographic

103

*Disorders of
Recognition in the
Physical World:
Other Types of
Agnosia*

orientation were first described as a separate clinical syndrome by Forster (1890). The patient was found to have difficulties in finding his way around familiar environments, while other cognitive functions were relatively preserved. A case of topographic disorientation involving another manifestation of visual agnosia was reported by Wilbrand (1892). Similar cases were subsequently presented by Meyer (1900), Holmes (1918), Holmes and Horrax (1919), Pötzl (1928), Paterson and Zangwill (1945), Hécaen, Penfield, Bertrand, and Malmo (1956), and Hécaen, Tzortis, and Rondot (1980). More recently, special attention has been given to the role of impairment in the recognition of environmental features or topographical landmarks compared to disturbances in the knowledge of spatial relationships (Farrell, 1996; Grusser & Landis, 1991; Levine, Warach, & Farah, 1985). Discussions have also been concentrated around the distinction between topographic agnosia and topographic apraxia (Vighetto & Aimard, 1981; Whiteley & Warrington, 1978). It is difficult, however, to separate disorders in topographic orientation from apraxia, since clinical manifestations of disorders in topographic orientation mainly appear as disturbances of actions or of movements of the body on a particular route to a target; this is not too different from the disturbances of drawing hand movements in constructional apraxia, which used to be called constructional agnosia, or apractognosia. Impairments of recognition play a significant role in the mechanisms of action disturbances and their classifications, especially since diagnosis of agnosia or apraxia are often conditional, depending on the history of the terms and the prevalence of recognition or action disorders in the particular syndrome.

Clinical Aspects

Disturbances in Conventional Information Processing

Disturbances of Topographic Orientation in Real, Familiar Space. In such disturbances, many patients become unable to find the way to their homes, to the store, to the previously well-known and often visited restaurant, or to get back home from a walk around the neighborhood. In more severe cases, patients cannot find the bathroom in their own house or apartment, in hospital settings they often demonstrate difficulties finding their way to the dining room, the bathroom, their own room or their bed.

Sometimes the general direction a patient chooses may be correct, but the ability of the patient to orient his/her own body to particular points on the route may be disturbed. The patient may reach a location in which a turn to the right or to the left is needed, but may find himself/herself unable to figure out the direction that he/she came from and thus to make the appropriate turn. Object recognition is usually preserved in such cases, and to overcome the topographic disorientation,

104

LOCALIZATION
OF CLINICAL
SYNDROMES IN
NEUROPSYCHOLOGY
AND NEUROSCIENCE

patients often try to use some distinctive features, such as tagging their name on the door to indicate their own room or specifying a particular blanket color to help identify their own bed in the room.

Disturbances in General Topographic Self-Orientation. A special type of topographic disorientation concerns the ability to locate oneself in the general topographic coordinates that point to the particular place, town or city, county, and state. A patient suffering from such a disturbance is often unable to figure out where he/she is located at any given moment, for example, whether he/she is in a hospital, school, or apartment, or what city, county, and state he/she is in. This disorder may manifest itself either as a separate syndrome or as accompanied by a topographic disorientation of familiar spaces. These disturbances also represent one of the most important signs of relatively advanced cognitive decline with significant memory impairments, but one's orientation in general topographic coordinates may be preserved, while amnesia for remote and recent events is quite prominent, and vice versa. In some cases of so-called reduplicative paramnesia, the patient may feel that he or she is present in two locations at the same time, for example, in two different cities (for more details, see chapter 8, section entitled "Amnestic Syndromes"). Disturbances in general topographic self-orientation are routinely assessed in the course of mental state evaluation and widely accepted in the regular psychiatric, neurological, and neuropsychological evaluations of patients with dementing illnesses. However, the relationship between these evaluations and the other clinical signs of cognitive decline, including the role of lesion localization, remain unclear.

Disturbances in Unconventional Information Processing
  Impairments in the Ability to Describe or to Draw Topographic Plans. Patients may experience difficulties with topographical coordinates when asked to describe routes and to recall the spatial locations of the streets in town, or to draw or describe the plans of the patient's own apartment or room in the hospital ward. In many cases, disturbances in the drawing and description of routes in one's town or plans of one's own apartment or ward may not be accompanied by disorientation in the real space. In other cases, a patient may be unable to find his/her way to a certain target, but may preserve the ability to accurately describe routes or to draw a map of the town where he/she lives (Landis, Cummings, Christen, Bogen, & Imhof, 1986, Cases 1 and 2; McCarthy, Evans, & Hodges, 1996; Paillas, 1955; Péron, Droguet, & Granier, 1946).

  Disturbances in topographic orientation may be demonstrated when a patient is asked to describe the spatial relations of well-known

105

*Disorders of
Recognition in the
Physical World:
Other Types of
Agnosia*

locations in America using a blank sheet of paper: for example, an examiner outlines with a circle the location of Washington, DC, and the patient is asked to point to the approximate sites of Florida, California, New York, Boston, Texas, Los Angeles, San Francisco, the North, the South, the West, the East, and so on, or to show the appropriate direction of travel from one city to another. Topographic orientation on a real map may also be disturbed in such cases. A patient often finds it especially difficult to extrapolate the position of their own body to the 180-degree change of direction toward the patient on the street map, and the patient must align his imagined orientation of the body to the reverse right-left orientation on the map.

The ability to orient oneself on a map is often disturbed in patients with topographic disorientation in real space but is also often observed in patients without such disturbances (Hécaen, de Ajuriaguerra, & Massonet, 1951; McFie, Piercy, & Zangwill, 1950). Similarly, disturbances in the description of routes and of plans of spaces may be seen without an accompanying disorientation in real space. Thus, topographic disorientation in real space and disturbances in spatial descriptions must be clinically separated as relatively independent syndromes under common names: "topographic disorientation in real space" and "topographic disorientation in virtual space." These syndromes often appear concurrently thus enhancing manifestations of disorientations in real space and impairments in virtual space orientation.

*Topographic Disorientation and Disturbances
of Brain Information Processing*

Disturbances of the two major components of topographic orientation—internal navigation and recognition of familiar landmarks (Farrell, 1996)—may underlie the development of topographic disorientation, and may be termed *topographic apraxia* and *topographic agnosia*, respectively.

Topographic apraxia may be defined as a disorder of internal navigation (Farrell, 1996; Gallistel, 1990), or a disturbance in the ability to use a set of features and memory storage, representing the topographic coordinates and routes in spatial memory, in order to both guide one's own movements into chosen directions and assess one's change in position in the course of such movements by matching the position changes with the topographic coordinates and the route description in memory. This type of topographic disorientation was often described in the literature as topographic amnesia, or a loss of topographic memory (Assal, 1969; Whiteley & Warrington, 1978). However, disturbances in the process of internal navigation may be caused not only by a loss of spatial memory but also by an impairment in one's ability to match the topographic coordinates and the route description in memory with

106

LOCALIZATION
OF CLINICAL
SYNDROMES IN
NEUROPSYCHOLOGY
AND NEUROSCIENCE

an actual position in space; this is quite similar to the disturbances defined by the term apraxia. Actually, spatial memory may be preserved when a patient is able to describe routes or spatial plans but is disoriented in real space, secondary to difficulties in the matching of one's own body position and the representation of space in memory. Remote memory of major events in a patient's life may also be preserved, but recent memory may be disturbed in some cases, with no apparent correlation with topographic disturbances.

Topographic Agnosia of Familiar Landmarks. A patient may be able to recognize a building or a street in general but may experience difficulties in the ability to use a specific set of features and memory storage in the recognition of particular familiar buildings, streets, or well-known city landmarks or public monuments, either on the patient's way home or in other directions. This may enhance the severity of the topographic disorientation (Meyer, 1900; Paterson & Zangwill, 1945; Whitely & Warrington, 1978). Some authors stress that agnosia for topographic landmarks may be the only underlying cause of topographic disorientation, since the patient exhibits an intact ability to draw room plans and pathways to reach the rooms (Farrell, 1996; Landis et al., 1986; Levine, Warach, & Farah, 1985; Paillas, 1955).

Topographic Disorientation and Prosopagnosia

Topographic disorientation is often accompanied by prosopagnosia. Hécaen and Angelergues (1963) observed prosopagnosia in 8 of 11 patients suffering from topographic disorientation. Landis et al. (1986) noted prosopagnosia in 7 of 16 cases of "environmental agnosia," or "loss of topographic familiarities." The major clinical features in both of these syndromes are disturbances in the recognition of individual familiar visual images—of familiar faces in cases of prosopagnosia and of familiar landmarks and routes in topographic disorientation. Difficulties are certainly related to the different types of targets for recognition and the sets of features and model storage used in the course of recognition. Prosopagnosia may persist when topographic disorientation disappears (Assal, 1969), and difficulties in topographic orientation may remain while prosopagnosia is transient (Landis et al., 1986, Cases 4, 8, and 10).

Anatomical Aspects

Disturbances of Conventional Information Processing

Prominent disturbances of topographic orientation in real space were first described in cases with bilateral posterior lesions (Forster, 1890; Holmes & Horrax, 1919; Meyer, 1900; Poetzl, 1928; Wilbrand, 1892).

Since 1876, 15 cases of topographic disorientation and corresponding autopsy results have been reported in literature (Landis et al., 1986, Table 2). Bilateral lesions were found in six of the cases, and unilateral right hemisphere posterior lesions were noted in the remaining nine cases. Cerebral infarctions were reported in six of nine cases with right hemisphere lesions, thus ruling out the role of the mass effect caused by tumor or cerebral hemorrhages. Unilateral lesions of the left hemisphere were not found in any of the 15 cases.

With subsequent advances in brain imaging technology, a series of cases with topographic disorientation have been described in localization studies using head CT or MRI scans (Table 3.1).

Right hemisphere lesions were reported in all 14 cases presented in the table, including three cases with bilateral lesions. No cases with unilateral left hemisphere lesions were noted. The CT, MRI, and surgery data are identical to the autopsy findings in cases with topographic disorientation, firmly confirming the exclusive role of right hemisphere lesions in the development of topographic disorientation. These findings

TABLE 3.1 Localization of Lesions in Cases With Topographic Disorientation Published Since 1969

Published Work	Site of Lesion	Etiology
Aimard et al., 1981		
case 3	CT: right temporo-parietal	infarction
case 4	Surgery: right inferior-posterior temporal	tumor
case 5	CT: right occipito-temporal	tumor
Assal, G., 1969	Surgery: right temporo-parietal	hematoma
Bottini et al., 1990	CT: splenium of corpus callosum extending to the right temporal lobe	glioblastoma
Clarke et al., 1993	MRI: right parietal lobe tumor extending to small portion of left parietal lobe white matter	glioblastoma
Hécaen et al., 1980	CT: right occipital	infarction
Landis et al., 1986*		
case 1	CT: right medial occipital	infarction
case 2	CT: right medial parietal	infarction
case 3	CT: right occipito-temporal	infarction
case 4	CT: bilateral medial occipital	infarction
Levine et al., 1985		
case 2	CT: bilateral occipito-parietal	hemorrhage
Vighetto et al., 1980	CT: right occipito-parietal	infarction
Whitty and Newcombe, 1973	Surgery: right occipito-parietal	abscess

Clinical data and localization of lesions were described in detail in 4 of 16 reported cases.

108

LOCALIZATION
OF CLINICAL
SYNDROMES IN
NEUROPSYCHOLOGY
AND NEUROSCIENCE

may be compared with the high frequency of right hemisphere lesions in prosopagnosia that is characterized by disturbances in the recognition of familiar faces. In cases of topographic disorientation, impairments are noted in the recognition of familiar routes and landmarks, stressing the role of the right hemisphere in the processing of individualized features of objects and scenes.

Posterior regions of the right hemisphere were involved in all 15 autopsy cases as well as the 14 cases presented in the table. From the 15 autopsy cases, occipital lesions were noted in 13 cases, temporal lesions in 9 cases, and parietal lesions in 3 cases. Parietal lesions were seen more frequently in cases with CT, MRI, and surgical lesion verification, as summarized in the table. Occipital lesions were found in seven cases, parietal lesions in seven cases, and temporal lesions in five cases. Since mass effect as produced by a tumor or hemorrhage may involve areas in the vicinity of the main lesion, cases of cerebral infarctions are summarized separately. Out of seven cases with cerebral infarctions, occipital lesions were observed in five cases, parietal lesions in three cases, and temporal lesions in two cases.

Disturbances of Unconventional Information Processing

Right posterior lesions are often seen in cases in which a patient experiences disturbances of topographical concepts, difficulties in the ability to describe or to draw the routes or layout of a space, and problems in indicating the locations of major cities (Hécaen et al., 1951; McFie et al., 1950). Experimental studies with visually or tactually guided maze learning found significant difficulties in the learning of groups of patients with lesions in the posterior parts of the right hemisphere (Elithorn, 1964; Milner, 1965). Posterior parietal damage in the right hemisphere, not left hemisphere damage, was responsible for most observed significant changes in visually guided maze learning (Newcombe, 1969). In cases of the surgical treatment of epilepsy, the inclusion of the hippocampus in the ablation areas as well as large parietal lesions in the right hemisphere has been shown to significantly increase difficulties in maze learning (Milner, 1965).

In summary, of 29 cases of topographic disorientation with verification via autopsy, brain imaging, or surgery, lesions were located in the occipital region in 20 cases, the temporal region in 14 cases, and the parietal region in 10 cases. Lesions in cases of topographic disorientation are thus located in the occipital, temporal, and parietal lobes of the right hemisphere. It seems that in cases with topographic agnosia, the lesions mainly involved occipital and temporal lobes (Landis et al., 1986). More dorsal, occipito-parietal lesions are probably responsible for the development of topographic apraxia.

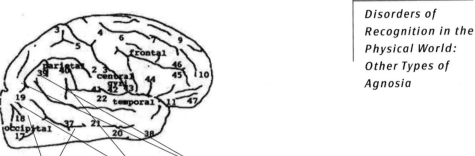

topographic agnosia   topographic apraxia   visual disorientation

FIGURE 3.1 Topographic disorientation. Localization of lesions in patients with right hemisphere lesions. Numbers indicate the corresponding Brodmann's cytoarchitectonic areas.

Lesion localization is similar in cases of disorders of topographical concepts and disorientation in real space. The lesions are usually located in the posterior parts of the right hemisphere. However, the parietal lobe is more frequently involved in cases with disorders of topographical concepts. The role of frontal lobe lesions may be also important in some cases, but further studies are needed for clarification (Figure 3.1).

LOSS OF VISUAL IMAGERY

WEAKNESS OF VISUAL imagery was first described by Charcot (1883) and Wilbrand (1892) as one of the signs of visual agnosia. This type of amnesia was thus known in the old literature as amnesia of Charcot-Wilbrand. Wilbrand's patient suffered difficulties in evoking visual images of objects and scenes and experienced an accompanying peculiar feeling that the entire visible environment was strange. Various cases with loss of visual images were subsequently described in the literature (Brain, 1941; Gelb & Goldstein, 1924; Mehta, Newcombe, & DeHaan, 1992; Semenoff, 1965).

CLINICAL FEATURES

PATIENTS DEMONSTRATE A partial or complete loss of the ability to revisualize, or to evoke from memory the visual images of objects or scenes in the absence of retinal input. They suffer from difficulties in evoking visual images of vegetables, fruits, and animals and are unable

110

LOCALIZATION
OF CLINICAL
SYNDROMES IN
NEUROPSYCHOLOGY
AND NEUROSCIENCE

to evoke images and to describe the peculiar features of an elephant or a cow, for example. Loss of visual images may be often encountered for public buildings and monuments well known to the patient before the onset of the illness. Visual imaging of well-known faces is also disturbed in many cases. In some cases, a feeling of strangeness of surroundings is present.

Weakness of visual imagery often includes an inability to evoke the color of the object. This has often been described in cases of a verbal-visual disconnection syndrome. In such cases, a patient is unable to recall the color of a certain object, for example, a tomato, banana, or cucumber. Color naming and the matching of a color sample with a black and white object picture, however, are usually preserved.

Lately, special attention has been given to the loss of visual spatial imagery compared to the preservation of visual object images. Levine et al. (1985) described a patient with visual disorientation who was unable to describe landmarks or the locations of familiar objects from memory. A second patient (Farah, Hammond, Levine, & Calvanio, 1988) could not describe an object's appearance from memory but was able to perform correctly such spatial tasks as mental rotation, scanning of the visual image, size scaling to assess the distance to the object, and imaging a triad of shapes and reporting which two were closest to one another. Hemispatial neglect may also involve the imaging of the contralateral, usually left, side of the space. Bisiach, Luzzatti, and Perani (1979) described two patients with hemispatial neglect for the left visual field. The patients also neglected the mental images of many landmarks in the well-known main square of Milan, their hometown, while they tended to name more landmarks on the right side of the square.

BRAIN INFORMATION PROCESSING AND LOSS OF VISUAL IMAGERY

Loss of Visual Imagery and Visual Agnosia

Loss of visual imagery is often observed in cases of visual object agnosia, which corresponds to data that demonstrate the role of visual imagery in the facilitation of object perception (Ishai & Sagi, 1997). However, a loss of visual imagery was not accompanied by visual agnosia in many cases. Cases with a loss of visual imagery and a preservation of visual perception were described in the neurological literature (Farah et al., 1988; Goldenberg, 1992; Grossi, Orsini, & Modafferi, 1986; Riddoch, 1990). On the other hand, completely preserved visual imagery was recently reported in a patient with severe agnosia (Behrmann, Winocur, & Moscovitch, 1992).

These findings point to the possible existence of special components and operations in the visual system for image generation that are

111

Disorders of
Recognition in the
Physical World:
Other Types of
Agnosia

relatively independent from visual object recognition. It may be similar to the language system with its relatively independent mechanisms of expressive speech and language comprehension, since visual object imagery requires, as does expressive speech, the ekphorization and decoding of the visual object code that is stored in long-term memory.

In response to a verbal prompt and a volitional attempt, the code of a particular object must be found in visual storage and brought to the special visual buffer (Kosslyn, Flynn, Amsterdam, & Wang, 1990) for further processing, which is aimed at the reconstruction of the object's form and color via the code held in long-term visual storage. The process is different from the description of object features performed in the conventional process of object recognition, but it may employ the same predefined limited set of features that is used for conventional object recognition. It may also be based on processing that is similar to the part decomposition and structural reconstruction of an object that may be used in unconventional types of object recognition. The decoding could start from the reconstruction of the object parts with a subsequent building of the whole object image. Visual object amnesia, especially for unconventional information processing, may thus be accompanied by a loss of visual images. Farah (1995) pointed to many cases in which a subtle visual perceptual disturbance accompanied the prominent imagery impairment. These findings may be further explored by the study of object recognition via unconventional information processing in patients who have suffered a loss of visual imagery and exhibit no signs of conventional visual object amnesia.

On the other hand, a loss of visual object imagery may not be accompanied by visual object amnesia, but lesions in such cases are localized near the cortical occipito-temporal areas involved in the perceptual object processing and damaged in cases with visual object amnesia. This association is even stronger in cases of a loss of visual spatial imagery and visual spatial amnesia. This correspondence was recently demonstrated in fMRI studies of the activation of the same occipito-temporal region during perception and visual imaging of faces and of the parahippocampal place areas in the course of the perception of familiar scenes and their visual imaging (O'Craven & Konvisker, 2000). The magnitude of activation was lower during imaging than during perception. Similar results were reported in the activation of visual motion area MT (middle temporal) during imagery of moving compared to stationary stimuli (Goebel, Khorram-Sefat, Muckli, Haccker, & Singer, 1998). It is possible that visual imagery partly engages the same information processing mechanisms as visual perception, especially at the higher level of processing, while more peripheral stages of object encoding are involved in the recognition of real objects. In some sense, visual imagery is based on the ability to free the visual processing system from

112

LOCALIZATION
OF CLINICAL
SYNDROMES IN
NEUROPSYCHOLOGY
AND NEUROSCIENCE

the control of the stimulus. Visual imagery may act by centrally activating a primarily descending pathway (Farah, 1989), while phenomenal visual experience does so by initial neural activation within input layers of early cortical areas followed by a bidirectional recursive processing, ascending and descending, bottom-up and top-down (Pollen, 1999). This produces a stronger activation of fMRI during perception than during imagery.

Loss of visual spatial imagery requires special consideration, as it seems to be more closely connected to the performance of visual spatial tasks than to visual object recognition. The testing of topographic agnosia and amnesia usually includes items requiring preserved visual imagery, such as drawing from memory the plan of the patient's room in the hospital, of major cities on a map, or of a plan with the correct succession of the side streets located on the right and left sides of the main street in the patient's hometown. Visual disorientation, topographic amnesia thus incorporates disturbances in visual spatial imagery as its important symptom. These disturbances may be also related to the difficulties in ekphorization and in decoding from visual spatial memory storage the coded description of the landmarks and visually coded spatial relations.

ANATOMICAL FINDINGS

LOSS OF VISUAL imagery was described in cases with bilateral occipital and temporal or parietal lesions (Critchley, 1953; Semenoff, 1965; Wilbrand, 1892). Golant (1935) described a case in which a loss of visual imagery followed a stroke. An autopsy revealed a large infarction on the inferior surface of the temporal and occipital lobes in the left hemisphere, extending from the parahippocampal gyrus to the pole of the occipital lobe.

Some of the neurological and neurophysiological data point to the absence of lesions in areas V1 and V2 in cases involving the loss of visual imagery. Bilateral lesions of area V1 result in cortical blindness, but visual imagery usually remains intact. Recently, Goldenberg, Müllbacker, and Novak (1995) described a case of cortical blindness following bilateral infarctions in the posterior cerebral artery. Visual imagery was preserved in this case. MRI findings, however, pointed to the preservation of the occipital cortex in the upper left calcarine lip, and the authors could not completely exclude the role of area V1 in the preservation of visual imagery.

Brain imaging studies performed on control subjects point to the role of posterior parts of the left hemisphere in visual image generation. The tests usually involved a comparison of SPECT, PET scan, even-related potentials (ERPs), or MRI data recorded during the tasks of equal difficulties that did or did not require visual imagery. One such task used by Goldenberg (1992) asked the subject to answer either the question "What is darker green, grass or a pine tree?" which tested the patient's visual imagery, or the question "Is the categorical imperative an ancient grammatical form?" which did not require the use of visual imagery. The results of this and similar studies demonstrated an association between visual imagery and occipital and temporal activation (for a review, see Farah, 1995). Farah et al. (1988) suggested that the left occipito-temporal area may be critical for visual imagery. Activity of the parietal region was reported during map imagery, while color and facial imagery produced the maximum activity over the temporal and occipital regions (Uhl et al., 1990).

In general, lesion localization in patients with a loss of visual imagery usually includes the occipital lobe, probably outside the striate area, extending to the temporal lobe in cases of a loss of visual object imagery, and to the parietal regions in patients with disturbances of spatial visual memory.

AUDITORY AGNOSIA

A*UDITORY AGNOSIA* REFERS to a disorder in the ability to recognize verbal and nonverbal sounds, while one's hearing remains either partially or fully preserved. The human auditory system is primarily used for the processing of verbal information. Disorders in the recognition of spoken language are termed aphasia and will be described in a separate section. Auditory agnosia for nonverbal sounds is observed less frequently than either aphasia or visual agnosia. The term includes agnosia for object sounds, agnosia for sound localization, and amusia.

AGNOSIA FOR OBJECT SOUNDS

ISOLATED AGNOSIA FOR object sounds has been observed in a few patients (Albert, Sparks, von Stockert, & Sax, 1972; Chocolle et al., 1975; Klein & Harper, 1956; Laignel-Lavastine & Alajouanine, 1921; Spreen, Benton, & Fincham, 1965). According to a review by Vignolo (1969), agnosia for object sounds has often been observed in cases of Wernicke's aphasia. Agnosia for object sounds also frequently accompanied word deafness and amusia (Henschen, 1920–1922; Spreen et al., 1965).

In general, the task of auditory recognition of object sounds is different from visual object recognition. The eyes are used to determine the shape, size, and color of an object while sounds travel by going

114

LOCALIZATION
OF CLINICAL
SYNDROMES IN
NEUROPSYCHOLOGY
AND NEUROSCIENCE

around the corner and helping to uncover the occluded object, thus serving as an early warning system. Sounds may also supplement the visually observed scene via a reflection of the energy of the scene produced by a bomb explosion, a car crash, or the blowing of the wind. A number of objects do not produce sounds at all, for example, furniture. The number of choices subjected to the auditory recognition of objects is thus markedly diminished compared to the number of choices for visual object recognition. Even animals that may be easy to visually recognize, such as elephants or camels, may be difficult to recognize via sound. This restriction of choices for auditory object recognition may allow the use of a simplified set of operations in the course of such recognition, markedly decreasing the volume and the complexity of storage memory. Such a system may be less vulnerable to brain damage, which may explain the rarity of cases of auditory agnosia for object sounds.

Object sounds may be considered to be an *auditory stream,* which consists of groups of sound sequences. Selection and recognition of these groups represent the main goal of audition. This process certainly involves the ability to recognize the features and the parts of the auditory stream, in similar fashion to the process of visual object recognition. Auditory features and their combinations may be compared to the models in storage. As in visual agnosia, the process of recognition may be disturbed at different levels, including the detection and description of features and parts, as well as the comparison of the description with the models in storage. This bottom-up process may be facilitated by a top-down process that uses the classification of objects to limit the number of choices. In cases of auditory agnosia, the clinical and experimental data are still quite limited, but some of the findings may be discussed from the point of view of information processing disturbances.

Clinical Aspects

Disturbances of Conventional Information Processing

Agnosia of object sounds includes disturbances at the perceptual level of information processing, or *apperceptive auditory agnosia,* and impairments in the ability to compare the description of an auditory stream with the models in storage—*associative auditory agnosia.*

Disturbances at the Semantic Level: Associative Auditory Agnosia

Consider a case in which the matching of the sound and model sample is disturbed. The patient may hear the sound but is unable to recognize to which object that sound belongs. Hearing may be normal or slightly impaired, but ability to recognize the sounds may be disturbed. The patient cannot identify the voices of animals and birds and

115

*Disorders of
Recognition in the
Physical World:
Other Types of
Agnosia*

is often unable to recognize the noise of wind, a train, a car, crumpling paper, a ringing bell, a tinkling glass, the typical sounds produced by boiling water, the ticking of a watch, and so forth. Certain clues that serve to restrict the choices may be helpful, for example, if the patient is told that a sound belongs to an animal or to a moving object. Albert, Sparks, von Stockert, and Sax (1972) described a patient who was experiencing an inability to attach meaning to nonverbal sounds, while the patient's comprehension of the word meaning remained intact. This patient preserved intact the auditory thresholds for tones. The recognition of word sounds is, however, usually disturbed in patients with auditory agnosia.

To study the identification of meaningful sounds, Spinnler and Vignolo (1966) asked a subject to compare a natural sound, such as the song of a canary, with pictures that gave the subject four choices: the correct source of the sound; a very similar source of sound, acoustically speaking (e.g., a whistling boy); a source of sound from the same semantic category, but acoustically very different (e.g., a cock crowing); and, a source of sound unrelated acoustically or semantically to the original sound-producing event or object. Twenty-six percent of patients with aphasia fell below the normal cutoff score, producing more semantic than acoustical errors; the left or right hemisphere–damaged nonaphasic patients, however, performed within the limits of normal controls. In subsequent studies, the percentage of aphasics with similar difficulties was even higher, reaching 43%–45% (Faglioni, Spinnler, & Vignolo, 1969; Varney, 1980). These data point to the alienation of sounds from their meaning, which may be considered to be a type of auditory agnosia closely connected with aphasia and similar to optic aphasia in patients with visual agnosia.

Disturbances at the Features Level: Apperceptive Auditory Agnosia

Laignel-Lavastine and Alajouanine (1921) described a patient who was unable to differentiate one sound from another. Tinkling glass and the noise of keys resembled a cricket singing. Similar difficulties were reported for the recognition and differentiation of animal voices, laughing, crying, spoken words, and sentences. The patient was able to identify only the intensity of the sound but could not assess the qualitative differences between the sounds. Expressive speech, reading, and writing remained preserved. Such cases may be extremely rare, and further collection of data on similar cases may help to clarify their clinical manifestations.

Disturbances at the Peripheral Level: Cortical Deafness

A bilateral lesion of the primary auditory cortex in the transverse gyri of Heschl may underlie the development of cortical deafness with a complete loss of hearing; such cases, however, are extremely rare. Henschen (1920–1922) reported only nine such cases that had been described in the literature. A vascular lesion in both transverse gyri was found in all cases. L'Hermitte et al. (1971) subsequently noted that deafness in such cases may be related to the involvement of the medial geniculate bodies.

Disturbances of Unconventional Information Processing

Disturbances in Filtration of Sounds From Noise. To the best of our knowledge, there is no literature report of studies that have examined the ability of patients with local brain lesions to detect and recognize nonverbal sounds in noise. The filtration of auditory signals from noise was studied for words only by the dichotic listening test in order to demonstrate the perceptual impairment of the ear contralateral to the hemisphere with temporal lobe lesion.

In our own experiment in which white noise of 50 db above the intensity threshold was masked, we found that absolute thresholds for the low-frequency single tones of 125 Hz and 250 Hz increased by 25–30 db in patients with lesions of the superior-posterior part of the left temporal lobe. This increase did not exceed 10–15 db in cases of parietal or premotor frontal lesions (Tonkonogy, 1973). The intensity thresholds were higher by 5–10 db when signals were delivered to the ear contralateral to the left or right hemispheric side of the lesion compared to the ipsilateral ear of signal delivery. We suggested that the results of these studies could be explained by difficulties in the detection of brief sound intensities, since a long duration signal might be parted to the short duration sounds by noise and summation as a type of *grouping* of the signal is impaired. These results and considerations prompted our study of intensity thresholds for brief signals as described above.

The similar results of both studies point to the role of signal *intensity* assessment in the spatial localization of auditory signals, since the brief signals from the right or the left hemifields are delivered through the corresponding ear to the primary auditory area in the contralateral hemisphere. Certainly, the recognition of auditory signals in noise may involve different mechanisms than the detection and recognition of more complicated auditory images, for example, based on grouping processes.

Recognition of Auditory Images With Incomplete Set of Features. The recognition of words distorted by a low-pass filter leads to the perceptual deficit in the ear contralateral to the side of the temporal lobe tumor (Bocca, Calearo, Cassinori, & Migliavocca, 1955) or to the site of hemispherectomy; using the dichotic listening test with simultaneous presentation of digits, Kimura (1963) found an auditory perception

117

*Disorders of
Recognition in the
Physical World:
Other Types of
Agnosia*

deficit contralateral to the side of the temporal lobectomy performed in the treatment of refractory epilepsy. The deficit was especially prominent when Heschl's gyri were included in the resection. It seems that right-left asymmetry in the described perceptual disturbances may be related to the more elementary underlying problems in the detection of spatial localization of auditory signals.

Auditory Agnosia and Disturbances of Brain Information Processing

Disturbances in the Identification of Simple and Complex Features of Auditory Signals

The sonograms of animal sounds, including human speech sounds, exhibit three patterns based on sound frequencies: constant frequency (CF); noise-burst (NB); and frequency-modulated (FM) components (Suga, 1995). For instance, the sonogram of a vowel consists of several horizontal bars or *formants*—F1 (the lowest), F2, and F3. The formants may be considered to be CF components. The combination of two phonemes to form a monosyllabic word is based on the new components and is called a *transition*. These combinations are FM components and are very important for the identification of a consonant within the words that may be identified by a transition before F1 and F2 of the vowel, as in plosive consonants /k/, /t/, /p/, /g/, /d/, /b/ (Liberman, Delattre, Gerstman, & Cooper, 1956). A vertical bar or band indicates the scatter of sound energy over many frequency-composing NB components, as observed in the fricative consonants /s/ and /sh/. Also, the mustached bat emits many syllable types of non-biosonar sounds that consist of CF, FM, or NB components (Kanwal et al., 1993).

Thus, sound frequencies may be considered one of the main features that must be employed in sound identification by the neural representation of auditory information in the auditory center. Other features may include amplitudes and temporal characteristics of acoustical sounds, including duration and interval. As to the sound frequencies, a tonotopic spatial representation was demonstrated in the primary auditory cortex of bats (Suga & Jen, 1976), cats, and monkeys (Brugge & Merzenich, 1973). Certain neurons in the auditory cortex, called CF-, FM-, and NB-specialized neurons, selectively respond to one of the three different types of frequency features (Suga, 1969; Casseday & Covey, 1992). Disproportional tonotopic representation for the processing of CF-FM sonar signals was also found in the mustache bat's central auditory system (Suga & Jen, 1976). Neurons tuned to a particular amplitude were found to form frequency-amplitude coordinates, which are common in a particular subdivision of the auditory cortex of bats (Suga, 1977), cats (Phillips & Orman, 1984), and monkeys (Brugge & Merzenich, 1973). An amplitopic (amplitude-topic) representation has been found

118

LOCALIZATION
OF CLINICAL
SYNDROMES IN
NEUROPSYCHOLOGY
AND NEUROSCIENCE

in the auditory cortex areas of mustache bats and cats (Shreiner, Mendelson, & Sutter, 1992), and in the human auditory cortex (Pantev, Hoke, Lehnertz, & Lutkenhoner, 1989).

The simple features of auditory signals, such as frequency and intensity, are coded by the auditory periphery. In the mammalian cochlea, including that of primates and humans, the auditory cells are tonotopically arranged along the frequency axis of the basilar membrane. Therefore, the frequency of acoustical signals is expressed by the localization of cells in the cochlea, while the intensity of the signals is reflected by the discharge rate (for a review, see Suga, 1995). Correspondingly, cochlear lesions result in various degrees of hearing loss. Similar types of hearing loss may be caused by a lesion of the auditory nuclei in the brain stem. It seems that a tonotopic representation of frequencies and an ampliotopic representation of amplitudes does not simply record the data coded by the auditory periphery. It remains largely unclear what role the lesions of certain areas of the higher levels of the auditory system have in the identification of both simple and, especially, complex features of auditory signals; this lack of clarity is particularly true for the human auditory cortex, as most reported findings have been from studies of mustache bats. Also, many of the operations related to the feature identification of the auditory signals by humans cannot be fully addressed in animal studies. These include, for instance, the identification of temporal patterns of both nonverbal and, especially, verbal signals, and the processing of a signal by auditory working memory.

Neuropsychological studies of central auditory processing in patients with local cerebral pathology provide some additional information concerning disturbances in the detection and identification of some of the simple and complex features of auditory signals, including impairments in the detection of brief signals, disturbances in the ability to differentiate between simple frequencies and their temporal sequences, and the role of the auditory working memory in that processing.

Disturbances in the Differentiation of Auditory Signals of Various
Frequencies: Role of the Auditory Working Memory

In our studies (Dorofeeva & Kaidanova, 1969; Tonkonogy, 1973; Traugott & Kaidanova, 1975), the testing of auditory working memory began with learning to differentiate between a basic tone of 200 Hz and a tone of 300 Hz. Subjects were instructed to press the button when the tone was 200 Hz, and not to press the button when the tone was 300 Hz. Subjects included three groups with sequelae of stroke: 35 patients suffering from Wernicke's aphasia, with a main lesion in the left superior-posterior temporal lobe; 11 patients suffering from transcortical

119

Disorders of
Recognition in the
Physical World:
Other Types of
Agnosia

sensory aphasia, with a main lesion in the left temporal lobe outside Wernicke's area; and 27 patients suffering from Broca's aphasia, with a main lesion in the premotor frontal area and central gyri at the level of the third frontal gyri. All patients showed absolute thresholds in the normal range for low- and medium-frequency tones. The observed rise in thresholds for high frequencies was within age limits.

The priming of the single signal of 200 Hz occurred after 2–3 trials in all groups of patients. Disturbances were observed in the series of stimuli in which differentiation of the tones was required. Learning to differentiate between the tones of 100 Hz, 200 Hz, and 300 Hz required 7.6 ± 2.4 trials in patients with Wernicke's aphasia, while patients with transcortical sensory aphasia and Broca's aphasia required an average of 2.7 ± 0.8 and 2.7 ± 0.3 trials, respectively. In the subsequent series of stimuli, the basic signal remained at 200 Hz, while the differentiated tone frequencies decreased from 300 Hz to 250 Hz, 230 Hz, 220 Hz, 210 Hz, and 205 Hz. The thresholds of tone differentiation reached only 19.2 ± 3.1 for patients with Wernicke's aphasia, while differentiation thresholds remained at 9–10 Hz and 6–8 Hz for patients with transcortical sensory aphasia and Broca's aphasia, respectively. An increase in the stimulus interval from 1 msec to 10 msec resulted in a prominent increase in differentiation thresholds to 38.5 ± 8.2 for patients with Wernicke's aphasia, while thresholds increased slightly to 10–11 Hz for patients with transcortical sensory aphasia and Broca's aphasia.

It is of interest that the ability to differentiate between tones of 200 Hz and 300 Hz was eventually developed in all 35 patients with Wernicke's aphasia, while the ability to differentiate between tones of 200 Hz and 250 Hz developed in 31 patients, between 200 Hz and 230 Hz in 17 patients, and between 200 Hz and 210 Hz in 7 patients; the ability to differentiate between 200 Hz and 205 Hz developed in only 3 out of the 35 patients with Wernicke's aphasia. All 11 patients with transcortical sensory aphasia developed the ability to differentiate between tones of 300 Hz, 250 Hz, and 230 Hz; 9 of the 11 patients were also able to distinguish between tones of 210 Hz and 200 Hz. Prominent disturbances were noted only in attempts to differentiate between tones of 205 Hz and 200 Hz; in fact, only 5 of the 11 patients successfully achieved such a differentiation. All 27 patients with Broca's aphasia were able to distinguish between tones at levels from 300 Hz to 210 Hz. Difficulties were noted in only 9 of the 27 patients in differentiating between 205 Hz and 200 Hz. At the same time, the differentiation of angles in similar types of testing remained within normal limits in all three groups of patients.

Subsequent studies examined tone differentiation in patients who had suffered from occipital or parietal lesions (Meerson, 1986). The results were as follows: 10.0 ± 2.8 and 15 ± 3.0 for an interval of 1 sec

120

LOCALIZATION
OF CLINICAL
SYNDROMES IN
NEUROPSYCHOLOGY
AND NEUROSCIENCE

between the tones and 15.0 ± 4.0 and 15 ± 3.6 for an interval of 10 sec between the tones for occipital and parietal groups of patients respectively. That result is similar to the results of the group of patients with Broca's aphasia and transcortical sensory aphasia and may be compared with the more prominent increase from 19.2 ± 3.1 for a 1 sec interval and 38.5 ± 8.2 for a 10 sec interval in patients with Wernicke's aphasia (Figure 3.2).

The increase in threshold for tone differentiation is clearly related to disturbances in auditory working memory. These disturbances are manifested when a basic tone has to be memorized either for the purpose and duration of testing as well as in the course of learning or for the time of the interstimuli interval. Thresholds significantly increase in patients suffering from Wernicke's aphasia with posterior-superior temporal lesions in the left hemisphere. In similar fashion to that of patients with disturbances of the visual working memory resulting from occipital lesions, this threshold increase is limited to relatively small differences in tone pitch, thus pointing to the possible existence of two types of auditory working memory. One type of auditory working memory parses tone pitch on the limited number of scores with a wide range of tone pitches that reach at least 15–25 Hz. This type of memory is easier to protect from damage and is fairly reliable. Another type of auditory working memory parses a signal into a large number of small pieces with upper and lower borders differences of 2–3 Hz; this

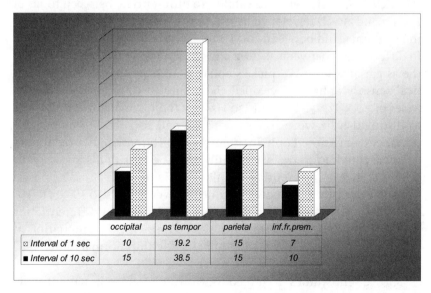

	occipital	ps tempor	parietal	inf.fr.prem.
▨ Interval of 1 sec	10	19.2	15	7
■ Interval of 10 sec	15	38.5	15	10

FIGURE 3.2 Tone differentiation by patients with various cortical localizations of lesions—occipital, posterior temporal, parietal, and inferior frontal premotor.

121

*Disorders of
Recognition in the
Physical World:
Other Types of
Agnosia*

requires more memory space and is difficult to protect from damage. The finer types of auditory working memory seem to be especially important in the process of learning, when a finer description of simple features is needed for the processing of auditory information. Well-learned auditory information may often be processed using a simpler type of auditory working memory.

Differentiation of Sounds Sequences. The recognition of an auditory stream requires the preserved ability to select and group together the tone sequences in the stream, for example, the different sequences of low-pitch and high-pitch tones, or a sequence of tones in which tones either increase or decrease in pitch. The differentiation and recognition of these sequences represent a part of this process that has been studied in brain-damaged patients.

Efron (1963) used click and tone stimuli to study the recognition of temporal order in brain-damaged patients. The author observed that impairment in sequence discrimination may perhaps be seen only in patients with aphasia. Milner (1971), however, did not confirm Efron's conclusions. Milner presented to subjects two sequences of 3–5 tones that were either completely identical or differed by the pitch of several tones. The patient had to compare both sequences and to say whether the sequences were similar or different. The group of patients included cases of right and left unilateral lesions as well as individuals who had suffered from an anterior-medial temporal lobectomy performed for the treatment of temporal lobe epilepsy. The number of errors noted prior to the surgery did not change following the procedure in patients with a left temporal lobectomy. The mean number of errors increased by 23% following the procedure in patients with a right temporal lobectomy.

An increase in differential thresholds for the second tone in the three-tone sequences, however, was reported in a study of patients suffering from Wernicke's aphasia with a lesion in the left hemisphere (Dorofeeva, 1970). The differential threshold was found to be 150 Hz for patients with Wernicke's aphasia, and only 5–10 Hz for patients with Broca's aphasia. The differences in the results yielded by the two studies may be related to the intertone intervals, which were much shorter in Milner's study and may have made the tone sequences sound similar to some type of melody. In this case, the task was similar to the recognition of a melody, which would be more difficult to perform with a lesion in the right hemisphere. Also, the localization of the lesion was different in the two studies. The patients described by Milner had each had an anterior-medial temporal lobectomy, while Dorofeeva's patients suffered from posterior-superior temporal infarctions in the left hemisphere that subsequently led to Wernicke's aphasia.

122

LOCALIZATION
OF CLINICAL
SYNDROMES IN
NEUROPSYCHOLOGY
AND NEUROSCIENCE

In our studies, subjects were asked to compare tone sequences that consisted of two or three tones with either identical or varying orders of succession, for example 200 Hz–1000 Hz–2000 Hz in the first sequence, and 200 Hz–2000 Hz–1000 Hz in the second sequence (Meerson, 1986; Tonkonogy, 1973). Visual sequences consisted of two or three elements of shape, for example, an angle, a curve, and a line. In the first series of testing, each signal in the sequence was presented for 1 sec, and the delay between any two sequences was 2 sec. The delay was increased to 5 sec and 10 sec in the second and third series, respectively. Identical and varying pairs of sequences were presented randomly. Patients with superior-posterior temporal lesions in the left and right hemisphere made a significant number of errors, 15.8% and 12.5% respectively; the errors were observed in a comparison of tone sequences with a delay of 2 sec, while answers were at chance level for a delay of 10 sec. No significant disturbances were observed for visual sequences for all three delays.

The results were reversed for patients with left and right occipital lesions, showing a significant number of errors, 14.8% and 10.6% respectively, for visual sequences with delays of 2 sec, and an increase in errors with delays of 5 sec and 10 sec. The ability to differentiate between tone sequences was preserved, and the number of errors reached only 4.8% and 3.2% for those with lesions of the left and right hemispheres, respectively. In patients with parietal lobe lesions, a significant number of errors was registered for both sequences; errors made in auditory and visual sequences reached 13.6% and 10.6% for sequences of shapes, and 14.3% and 10.5% for tone sequences with delays of 2 sec; an increase to delays of 5 sec and 10 sec did not result in an increase in the number of errors.

These data point to the important role of the left and right temporal lobes in the differentiation of auditory sequences and of both occipital lobes in the differentiation of visual sequences. Within the temporal lobe, it seems that the most prominent disturbances in the differentiation of inharmonious auditory sequences are related to a lesion in the superior-posterior part of the temporal lobe in the left hemisphere. Relatively recent studies have shown that a lobectomy of the right or left anterior-inferior temporal lobe leads to less prominent disturbances of working memory for auditory sequences (Meerson, 1986). However, these disturbances also involve visual sequences, in a fashion similar to patients with parietal lobe lesions. This may be related to differences in the underlying mechanisms of disturbances in sequence differentiation. It is possible that for patients with superior-posterior temporal lesions and occipital lesions, the disorders of sequence differentiation are related to the more perceptual level dependent on difficulties in assessing the single features of sequences,

123

*Disorders of
Recognition in the
Physical World:
Other Types of
Agnosia*

tone pitches in auditory signals, and particular shapes in visual signals. The disturbances may be at the higher level of information processing in anterior-inferior temporal lobe patients and parietal lobe patients. This higher level is concerned with the assessment of the orders of particular signals in the sequence, visual or auditory, as a pattern or specific gestalt. Such a simultaneous type of assessment is probably conducted at the multimodal level. It is possible that a pattern or gestalt type of assessment is also used at the modality-specific levels for auditory signals in the superior temporal lobe, and for visual signals in the occipital lobe.

The role of the working memory in the differentiation of sequences must also be recognized. An increase in interstimulus interval between two compared auditory or visual sequences results in a significant worsening of auditory or visual working memory performance for patients with superior-posterior temporal lesions or occipital lesions, respectively.

Further exploration is certainly needed to understand the role of the described disturbances in differentiation of auditory signals of various frequencies and their sequences in the formation of nonverbal auditory agnosia, especially in relation to the more specific types of frequencies, such as constant frequency (CF), noise-burst (NB) frequency, and frequency-modulated (FM) components. The relation of described disturbances to verbal auditory agnosia is further discussed in chapter 7, section entitled "Aphasia Syndromes and Other Language Disorders."

Disturbances in the Auditory Processing of Brief Signals. Special testing is needed to reveal elementary auditory deficits in patients with unilateral cortical lesions of the primary auditory areas. According to the results of audiometric testing for signals of long duration (1000–2000 msec), such lesions do not result in any clear hearing loss. Using the measurements of pure-tone thresholds of regular, long duration, Karp, Belmont, and Birch (1969) observed hearing loss in the left ear contralateral to the damaged right hemisphere in only 10 of 19 patients, each of whom had developed left hemiplegia following a cerebral infarction in the right hemisphere. These data were not confirmed in subsequent studies (Gershuni, Bary, Karaseva, & Tonkonogy, 1971). However, significant disturbances were found in patients with unilateral lesions in the auditory cortex in the detection of signals presented only briefly (1–4 msec).

In our own series of studies, the white noise threshold was tested using an auditory signal from 1 msec to 1000 msec in duration. The use of a brief signal was based on the anticipated special role of the primary cortical auditory areas in the processing of signals of short duration.

Our first publication on the subject (Baru, Gershuni, & Tonkonogy, 1964) reported the results for 13 patients—eight patients with cerebral infarctions and left superior-posterior temporal lesions, and two patients with lesions of the left parietal lobe, two patients with left inferior premotor lesions, and one patient with a brain stem lesion.

It was found that detection thresholds for white noise with durations of 1000 msec and 100 msec did not differ between the right and left ears in patients with left temporal and left nontemporal cortical lesions. A decrease in signal duration to 1.5 msec and 4 msec resulted in a general increase in thresholds of 26–28 db for the left ear, similar to the increases observed in control subjects. The thresholds for the left ear increased to a mean of 36 db for patients with left superior-posterior temporal lesions, but remained at a normal level of 27–28 db for patients with nontemporal cortical lesions (Figure 3.3). The mean differences between the thresholds of the right and left ears were 9 db, with variations from 6 db to 26 db in individual patients in the temporal group. The study also included one additional patient with a cerebral infarction in the right occipito-temporal region, for which the detection of white noise with a duration of 1000 msec did not differ between the right and left ears, while the thresholds increased by 9 db more for the left ear than the right ear when signal duration was decreased to 1 msec. These results point to a higher increase in thresholds for briefly presented auditory signals in the ear contralateral to the side of the hemisphere lesion. Vasserman (1968) reported similar results in a study of 20 patients, each with a left superior-posterior temporal infarction.

Baru et al. (1964) and Karaseva (1972) observed an asymmetrical increase in the intensity thresholds of brief sounds for the ear contralateral to the side of the lesion in 15 patients with lesions in the right hemisphere and in 22 patients with lesions in the left hemisphere; most of the patients had suffered from temporal lobe tumors. The asymmetric increase in thresholds for brief sounds compared to sounds of longer duration (20–30 db) was not found in nine patients with lesions in the auditory brain stem structures, including one case with a verified lesion of the cochlear nuclei and a significant loss of hearing. The autopsy data in six cases that demonstrated this asymmetrical increase in threshold for brief sounds revealed lesions involving the cortex of the Heschl's gyri and the underlying auditory pathways, as well as retrograde degeneration of the medial geniculate bodies. These areas were intact in two verified cases of temporal lobe tumors, both of which showed an absence of asymmetry for brief sounds.

These data point to the role of the A1, the primary cortical auditory area in humans, in the processing of brief auditory signals delivered to the ear contralateral to the area. Similar results were observed in studies of dogs with a unilateral ablation of the primary auditory area of the

125

*Disorders of
Recognition in the
Physical World:
Other Types of
Agnosia*

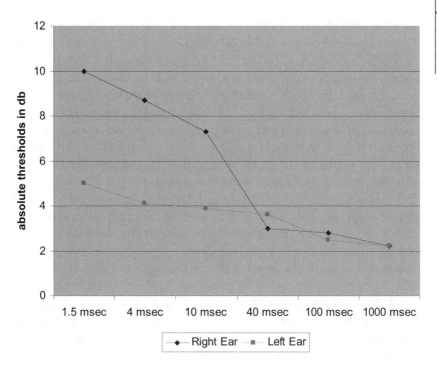

FIGURE 3.3 Absolute thresholds in decibels for white noise of different durations, from 1.5 msec to 1000 msec, in patients with a lesion of the superior-posterior temporal lobe in the left hemisphere.

temporal cortex (Baru, 1966). However, the role of the medial geniculate bodies destroyed by the retrograde degeneration cannot be completely ruled out in such cases. The topic thus requires further exploration.

Albert and Bear (1974) described a patient in which increased interstimulus time was needed for discrimination between two clicks. Lackner and Teuber (1973) found an increase in fusion time for dichotically presented clicks in patients with left-brain damage. Auerbach, Allard, Naeser, Alexander, and Albert (1982) observed similar results in a clicks fusion test in a patient suffering from pure word deafness. The same patient was unable to count the number of clicks presented in the rapid succession.

It seems that the detection and identification of brief signals is especially important in the process of recognition of the complex features of auditory signals, which often include the brief components of frequencies and amplitudes. Further studies of these relationships are needed.

Anatomical Aspects

Localization data in cases of *cortical deafness* point, in some cases, to a bilateral temporal lobe lesion. Mahoudeau, Lemoyne, Foncin, and

126

LOCALIZATION
OF CLINICAL
SYNDROMES IN
NEUROPSYCHOLOGY
AND NEUROSCIENCE

Dubrisay (1958) described a case of cortical deafness with corresponding autopsy findings of bilateral lesions in Heschl's gyri. L'Hermitte et al. (1971) presented anatomical data in two cases with cortical deafness; a bilateral temporal lesion was found in each of the cases. In some cases, however, predominantly or solely right hemisphere lesions were found (Spreen et al., 1965). Spreen et al. (1965) described the only reported case of cortical deafness without an accompanying lesion of the opposite hemisphere. The massive lesion instead involved the frontotemporal region, the insula in the right hemisphere. No lesions were found in either the left hemisphere or the corpus callosum.

A unilateral left hemisphere lesion, however, may often be found in cases of associative auditory agnosia, with disturbances in matching sounds and their meaning. Based on a review of the literature on auditory agnosia, Vignolo (1969) concluded that perceptual, apperceptive discrimination disturbances related to the right hemisphere lesions, while semantic, associative impairments were associated with left hemisphere lesions. This suggestion was based on the study of Faglioni et al. (1969), who compared the results of testing the matching between sounds and their meaning with the ability to discriminate between two successive nondescriptive noises. Aphasics proved to be unimpaired on the second test, while patients with right hemisphere damage showed disturbances on that test. These relationships, however, are likely more complicated. Our own research has shown that prominent disturbances in the differentiation between two tones or between members of a series of three or four tones were usually observed, due to a lesion in the left hemisphere (Meerson, 1986; Tonkonogy, 1973; Traugott & Kaidanova, 1975). It seems that associative auditory object agnosia may have an apperceptive component that is often related to or associated with the development of aphasia in patients with left hemisphere lesions, while the development of a primarily apperceptive auditory object agnosia is not associated with the aphasia and requires bilateral lesions in the primary auditory cortex with a possibility of the predominantly right hemisphere lesion (Figure 3.4).

DISTURBANCES OF SOUND LOCALIZATION IN SPACE: AUDITORY SPACE AGNOSIA

THE LOCALIZATION OF sound may play a role as a supplement to one's visual orientation in space, helping to localize a sound whose source is occluded from view. Sound localization may point to the direction from which a sound is coming, such as an oncoming train, a car, a barking dog, and so forth, and may serve in such cases as an early warning system, directing one's visual attention to the objects producing the sound.

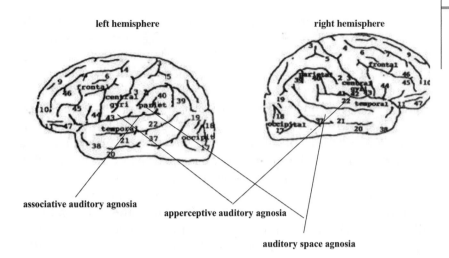

FIGURE 3.4 Localization of lesions in various types of auditory agnosia.

It is reasonable to suggest that disturbances in sound localization may be similar to visual space disorientation, including amnesia of depth. However, sound localization disturbances in humans have been described in only a few studies, most of which have been related to sound localization in the horizontal plane.

Clinical and Anatomical Aspects

The paucity of the literature concerning auditory space agnosia may be related to the difficulty in detecting disturbances in auditory space localization on the basis of conventional clinical observations. Such disturbances may be more easily detected using a special technique similar to that used in studies of visual fields.

Disturbances in sound localization on the left side of the space contralateral to a lesion in the right hemisphere were reported in patients who had been subjected to a right temporal lobectomy for the treatment of a seizure disorder (Penfield & Evans, 1934). The binaural localization of sounds was studied by Teuber and Diamond (1956) using binaural clicks with variable intervals of arrival to the right and left ears. The authors found that patients with right hemispheric lesions were inferior in sound localization to patients with left hemispheric lesions. The probable role of distance was studied by changes in the intensity of both clicks while keeping constant the interval between the clicks. In this condition, the rate of errors was much higher for the side opposite to the damaged hemisphere.

Sanchez-Longo, Forster, and Aut (1957) and Sanchez-Longo and Forster (1958) came to the same conclusion in the study of localization of long duration sounds in the horizontal plane. The researchers placed a sound source on the arc of the perimeter and blindfolded each subject. The subject then had to point to the source of the sound on the perimeter. Disturbances were found in sound localization, especially in the field contralateral to the damaged hemisphere, in 19 of 21 patients with temporal lobe lesions, and in only 4 of 21 patients with other localizations of cortical and subcortical lesions. Similar results were also reported by Wortis and Pfeiffer (1948), and Klingon and Bontecou (1966).

The role of lesions of the auditory cortex in the development of a disturbance in space localization is also supported by animal studies. Sound localization in animals has been recently discussed in a series of papers based on animal research, and it has been demonstrated that the main features of sounds in such systems include the interaural time difference (ITD) and the interaural intensity difference (IID). For a review, see King and Carlile (1995). Initial processing of the ITD and IID takes place in all subsequent levels of auditory pathways, starting with the nuclei of the brain stem. The auditory cortex of carnivores and primates, however, plays a major role in mediating sound localization in space. Unilateral auditory cortical lesions usually produce localization deficits in the contralateral auditory hemifield (Jenkins & Masterton, 1982). Lesions of the auditory cortex in animals result in a loss of the ability to associate the sound with its position in space (Heffner & Heffner, 1990).

A series of works using single-cell recording was directed toward the study of the organization of the cortical auditory space map (King & Carlile, 1995). However, the existence of such a map in the auditory cortex has been questioned. It has been suggested that individual neurons code locations throughout space, while the information about a particular point in space is distributed among a large population of neurons (Middlebrooks, 1999). Another possibility may be related to a mediating role of the parietal cortex in auditory space localization. Studies of patients suffering from auditory sound amnesia, however, have exhibited no direct similarities between those with temporal and those with parietal lesions.

We attempted to make such a comparison in our own study, in which a perimeter was used to study sound localization in 36 patients, including 12 patients with superior-posterior left temporal lesions, 6 patients with inferior parietal lesions, and 18 patients with dorsolateral frontal lobe lesions in either the left or the right hemisphere (Kaidanova, Meerson, & Tonkonogy, 1965). The etiology of the lesions was vascular, and cerebral infarctions were diagnosed in all 36 cases. Lesions were localized based on aphasia type and visual field defects. The mean errors were 19.2 degrees for patients with parietal lobe lesions, 13.3 degrees for those with temporal lobe lesions, and only 8.5 degrees for the dorsolateral frontal group. The mean errors were

129

Disorders of
Recognition in the
Physical World:
Other Types of
Agnosia

much higher when the site of the perimeter was contralateral to the damaged hemisphere: 10.4 degrees for the parietal group; 4.9 degrees for the temporal group; and 3.9 degrees for the frontal group.

These data point to the probable role of both temporal and parietal lesions in the development of disturbances in sound localization. Though only six patients with parietal lobe lesions were observed, and further studies are needed, our data may point to the possible role of the inferior parietal lobe in multimodal space processing. For instance, inferior parietal lobe structures may be involved in a subsequent step in the processing of ITD and IID features initially assessed by the auditory cortex in the temporal lobe, similar to the processing of visual space features assessed by occipital lobe structures.

TACTILE AGNOSIA, ASTEREOGNOSIS

PUCHELT (1844) DESCRIBED five patients who had suffered a partial paralysis of sensation, or a loss in the ability to recognize an object by touch. Hoffman (1885) presented 16 cases of patients with astereognosia, or a disorder of stereognosis. Wernicke (1895) reported two cases of patients with disturbances of object recognition by palpation, and suggested the term "tactile paralysis." Wernicke also divided tactile agnosia into two subcategories: primary agnosia—a loss in the ability to recognize the tactile quality of the object, also known as agnosia of texture; and secondary agnosia—asymbolia with an inability to connect tactile images of objects with their sensory representations.

Similar cases of astereognosis were later described by Raymond and Egger (1906), Goldstein (1916), Gerstmann (1918), Foix (1922), Guillan and Bize (1932), Hécaen and David (1945), Geschwind and Kaplan (1962), Korst (1964), and Sperry and Gazzaniga (1967). Delay (1935) suggested the use of the term "ahylognosia" for disorders in the recognition of the texture, weight, and thermal properties of objects; the term "amorphognosia" was suggested for cases with disturbances of shape differentiation; and the term "tactile asymbolia" was used for cases with a loss of object recognition but with the correct recognition of elementary qualities of objects.

CLINICAL ASPECTS

Disturbances in Conventional Information Processing

Tactile agnosia, or astereognosis, refers to the loss of the ability to recognize objects by touch, while elementary somatosensory sensations are either preserved or only slightly disturbed. The patient suffering from tactile agnosia shows normal two-point thresholds and preservation

130

LOCALIZATION
OF CLINICAL
SYNDROMES IN
NEUROPSYCHOLOGY
AND NEUROSCIENCE

of sensitivity to touch or pressure. Astereognosia is usually restricted to the tactile modalities with a preservation of object discrimination through visual and auditory modalities.

The patient with astereognosis is unable to recognize by palpation objects such as a pen, a key, a paper clip, a coin, or a safety pin. Recognition of an object is often based on one simple feature: for instance, by palpating an elongated key, a patient may recognize the object as a pencil, or the metallic property of a coin may lead to the recognition of the coin as a key. Recognition of 3-D objects, such as models of a chair or a table, and 3-D geometric figures may be especially difficult. Recognition may be facilitated by the top-down process of choice restriction when a patient is informed in advance of the names of three or four objects presented for recognition.

According to a recent detailed examination of patients with tactile agnosia, which is similar to visual object agnosia, various forms of astereognosis or tactile agnosia include apperceptive tactile agnosia, associative tactile agnosia, and tactile aphasia. For a review, see Srivinas and Ogas (1999).

Apperceptive tactile agnosia is characterized by difficulties in shape descriptions of objects with a relative preservation of descriptions of the simple object features. Disturbances may be also observed in the matching of the target object with a set of objects and the selection of an object identical to the target object. As in apperceptive visual object agnosia, the ability to create a drawing of the palpated object is usually disturbed.

Reed and Casseli (1994) and Reed, Caselli, and Farat (1996) recently described a case with a manifestation of apperceptive agnosia—patient E.C. Patient E.C. suffered from an infarction localized in the left inferior parietal region (areas 39 and 40). Tactile amnesia was observed in the patient's right hand. E.C. was able to recognize only approximately 50% of common objects with her right hand, while the recognition of palpated objects with her left hand was fully preserved. The recognition of simple object features was also preserved, including texture, weight, and size discrimination. Mild impairments in discrimination between simple shapes (circles, triangles, and rectangles) showed marked worsening with the presentation of more complex 2-D shapes (diamonds, pentagons, hexagons, and stars) and 3-D shapes (cubes, spheres, eggs, and pyramids). E.C. was also able to identify the shapes of numbers or common objects when traced by a stick on the skin of her right hand. The patient was able to draw only the general outline of the palpated object without any reproduction of the important internal details of the shape. E.C.'s perception of visual shape remained normal.

Associative tactile agnosia manifests itself as an inability to access the meaning of a representation, while the ability to describe shapes and

131

*Disorders of
Recognition in the
Physical World:
Other Types of
Agnosia*

common objects either remains completely intact or is only mildly disturbed. The matching of a palpated object with an identical object in a set of different objects remains intact, as does the ability to draw the shape of the palpated object with subsequent visual recognition of the drawing.

Platz (1996) described a patient, H.K., who suffered from associative tactile agnosia in her left hand as well as from damage to the right supramarginal gyrus (area 40), with the affliction extending to the right postcentral gyrus. The patient demonstrated a preserved ability to perceive light touch, perform two-point discrimination, sense position and vibration, and discriminate between weight, size, and texture. H.K. also demonstrated a preserved ability to discriminate between both common and novel 2- and 3-D shapes. The patient could not, via palpation with his left hand, identify 8 out of 17 common objects, such as a lighter, a paper clip, a battery, and a safety pin. H.K. could not demonstrate the different uses of the unidentified objects but was able to match by palpation with his left hand the sample object with an identical object in a set of various objects.

Similar manifestations of associative tactile agnosia in the right hand were demonstrated by patient Y.K. with damage to the left angular gyri (area 39) (Endo, Makishita, Yangisawa, & Sugishita, 1992). The patient described a button as a "tiny and circular" object; he was able to recognize that the object was plastic, but he could not recognize the identity of the object. Patient Y.K. also suffered from severe disturbances in the naming of palpated objects.

It remains unclear whether patients with associative tactile agnosia suffer from mild perceptual disturbances as do those with associative visual agnosia, and additional studies are needed for further clarification.

In a manner similar to a patient with optic aphasia, a tactile aphasia patient may be able to recognize the texture and shape peculiarities of an object, to describe an object, to demonstrate the use of an object through pantomime gestures, and, in some cases, to draw an object or to match it with an identical object by palpation. The naming of a palpated object, however, is impaired in these patients. At the same time, the naming of the same object when a patient sees it may be completely preserved. Tactile aphasia may often be accompanied by associative tactile agnosia, as in the case of Y.K. (Endo et al., 1992).

Unconventional Information Processing
in Tactile Agnosia

Tactile agnosia is defined as a disorder in the recognition of common objects. This disturbance in conventional information processing is usually accompanied by more prominent difficulties in unconventional

132

LOCALIZATION
OF CLINICAL
SYNDROMES IN
NEUROPSYCHOLOGY
AND NEUROSCIENCE

information processing, for example, in the discrimination of shapes with incomplete sets of features. The test employed by Reed and Caselli (1994) consisted of complex shapes, each with an incomplete set of features due to the elimination of a single part of the shape. The subject was asked to match a sample shape with an identical, but incomplete, copy of the shape. Patient E.C., who suffered from tactile amnesia for common objects, demonstrated prominent difficulties in such matching. It would be of interest to continue the study of unconventional information processing by using overlapping contours of objects, or objects presented on a "noisy" background made up of various textures, and so forth, in a manner similar to that of the studies of patients with visual agnosia.

Stages of Tactile Information Processing and Tactile Agnosia

Disturbances at the Elementary Level of Information Processing

The primary role of disturbances of the elementary sensations in the development of astereognosis has been explored and stressed by several authors (Bay et al., 1949; Déjerine, 1907, 1914; Stein & von Weizsacker, 1926). Bay (1944) analyzed six patients who suffered from difficulties in the tactile recognition of objects and found disturbances in elementary tactile sensory defects in all cases. These defects included an increase in tactile sensitivity thresholds, a loss of finesse in tactile impressions, and a correlation between the degree of so-called tactile agnosia and the degree of impairment of elementary sensitivity. For a review, see Hécaen and Albert (1978).

Subsequent studies, however, showed either complete preservation or only mild disturbances of elementary sensations in patients with astereognosis. Hécaen (1972) described cases of unilateral astereognosis accompanied by the preservation in the affected hand of primary sensations, touch, tactile discrimination, and appreciation of thickness.

Disturbances in elementary sensations not related directly to tactile agnosia also include difficulties in tactile localization, tactile extinction, and alloesthesia.

Disorders of tactile localization, or *atopagnosia*, are characterized by the patient's inability to localize the site of a pinprick. When a pinprick is applied to the patient's extremities, he or she points to the proximal site several centimeters from the original point of the pinprick. The sensation moves to the middle line if a pinprick is applied on the trunk or face.

Tactile extinction may be observed when a pinprick is applied simultaneously to identical points on the left and right side of the body, and the patient only reports the pinprick feeling on one side of the body; the side of reported perception is usually ipsilateral to the side of the

133

*Disorders of
Recognition in the
Physical World:
Other Types of
Agnosia*

cerebral lesion. Sometimes, a pinprick applied to one site results in the simultaneous development of pinprick sensations in several parts of the body, some distance from the original site. When such a sensation develops at the site symmetrical to that of the original pinprick, the phenomenon is called *synesthesia or alloesthesia*. Tactile extinction is similar to unilateral visual neglect, while alloesthesia, as described by Hermann and Pötzl (1928), resembles optic alloesthesia and is characterized by duplication or triplication of the object in the visual field.

Disturbances at the Intermediate Level of Information Processing

The intermediate level of processing includes such basic simple features of tactile information processing as size, shape, texture, substance, and weight, which have recently been defined as "basic somatosensory perception" (Srinivas & Ogas, 1999). The term also includes some more elementary features, such as a two-point threshold, pressure sensitivity, and point localization. It has been shown that a deficit in texture or weight discrimination may be experienced with no other difficulties in shape perception (Caselli, 1991) or disturbances in shape, and substance perception may be not accompanied by deficits in roughness discrimination (Knecht, Kunesh, & Schnitzler, 1996).

Both preservation and mild disturbances of basic somatosensory perception were recently reported in cases with tactile amnesia; the patients examined and reported upon included patient E.C. (Reed & Caselli, 1994), patient H.K. (Platz, 1996), and patient Y.K. (Endo et al., 1992). Preserved or slightly impaired basic somatosensory sensations included discrimination in terms of weight, size, and texture. At the same time, as with patients with visual object amnesia, prominent difficulties were often observed when the patient was required to differentiate between more complex tactile features of objects. For instance, patient E.C., who suffered from apperceptive tactile amnesia, showed marked disturbances in discrimination between figures designed by Efron (1968) and between rectangles with identical surface areas but with different length to width ratios (Reed et al., 1996). Certainly, further systematic studies are needed for the evaluation of such difficulties in discrimination of complex features of an object or grouping problems in patients with tactile agnosia, studies similar to the observations made in studies of patients with visual object agnosia (for more information, see chapter 2, section entitled "Visual Object Agnosia").

ANATOMICAL ASPECTS

FEW ANATOMICAL DATA from cases of tactile agnosia have been collected, but the data already known point to lesions of the inferior parietal area, primarily the supramarginal gyrus, as being responsible for the development of tactile agnosia (Guillan & Bize, 1932; Hécaen & David, 1945; Korst, 1964; Kroll, 1933; L'Hermitte & de Ajuriaguerra, 1938; Platz, 1996; Reed & Caselli, 1994). Astereognosis is bilateral in most cases and may be seen in cases with unilateral lesions in the left or right hemispheres (Foix, 1922; Goldstein, 1916; Korst, 1964; L'Hermitte & de Ajuriaguerra, 1938). Many cases with unilateral tactile agnosia in the right or left hand have been also reported (Delay, 1935; Endo et al., 1992; Hécaen, 1972; Platz, 1996; Reed & Caselli, 1994).

Astereognosis may be also seen in cases of callosal lesions (Geschwind, 1965; Geschwind & Kaplan, 1962; Goldstein, 1916; Raymond & Egger, 1906; Sperry & Gazzaniga, 1967; Stauffenberg, 1918). In such cases, astereognosis is limited to the left hand, and the main problem seems to consist of difficulties in the naming of the palpated object, otherwise known as tactile aphasia. The same objects, however, are recognized and correctly named if placed in the patient's right hand. Geschwind and Kaplan (1962) described this type of tactile agnosia as one of the symptoms of "anterior callosal disconnection syndrome" in a patient who suffered from an infarction of the anterior four-fifths of the corpus callosum. It was suggested that tactile impulses reach the left dominant hemisphere from the right hand, and the object can be correctly named when tactile impulses from the left hand reach the nondominant right hemisphere, where the object can be recognized. A damaged corpus callosum prevents impulses from traveling to the left hemisphere, which is dominant for language, and thus the object cannot be named.

The symptom of tactile extinction is usually observed in patients with lesions of the parietal lobe (Milner & Teuber, 1968), and especially with lesions located in the right parietal lobe (Critchley, 1953).

Disturbances of basic tactile sensations, including the loss of sensitivity to pressure, elevated two-point thresholds, and the loss of point sense and localization, have been correlated with lesions in the contralateral postcentral gyrus, primarily the hand area of Sensory I (Corkin, 1978; Pause, Kunesh, Binkofski, & Freund, 1989; Roland, 1976; Wernicke, 1895). Similar disturbances, though not as severe as in monkeys, have been observed in humans (Corkin, 1978) as a result of lesions in the area Sensory II, including the posterior insula and the parietal operculum (area 43 or area SII from animal work according to Burton, Videen, & Raichle, 1993).

It has also been demonstrated that disturbances in the discrimination of simple features of objects, such as texture and weight, were dissociated with preserved shape perception in two patients, each with a lesion in the parietal operculum and the posterior insula (Caselli, 1991). For a review, see Srinivas and Ogas (1999). An examination of

14 patients also found no correlation between somatosensory deficits and deficits in the discrimination of roughness and shape (Knecht et al., 1996). According to PET studies, the perception of shape and size activates the cortex of the contralateral postcentral gyrus, the anterior parts of the intraparietal sulcus, and the superior parietal lobule (areas 5 and 7) (O'Sullivan, Roland & Kawashima, 1994; Roland, O'Sullivan, & Kawashima, 1998). It seems that elementary tactile perception is processed by the cortex in the posterior central gyrus, while discrimination of simple object features is processed at various different anatomical sites.

CONCLUSION

1. The posterior insula and parietal operculum are involved in the discrimination of simple features of weight and texture, while the interparietal sulcus and adjacent areas are involved in the discrimination of more complex features of size and, especially, shape.
2. It is unclear what differences in localization underlie the development of apperceptive vs. associative tactile agnosia. The development of apperceptive tactile agnosia is probably related to a lesion in the supramarginal gyrus (area 40), with a possible extension to the adjacent areas of the insula and parietal operculum, which are responsible for the discrimination of simpler object features. Associative tactile agnosia probably results from damage to the angular gyrus (area 39), as found in two cases described by Endo, Makishita, Yangisawa, and Sugishita (1992) (Figure 3.5).

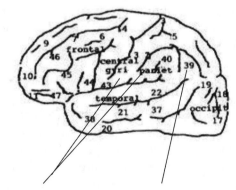

apperceptive tactile agnosia   associative tactile agnosia

FIGURE 3.5 Localization of lesions in the left hemisphere in patients with tactile agnosia.

136

LOCALIZATION
OF CLINICAL
SYNDROMES IN
NEUROPSYCHOLOGY
AND NEUROSCIENCE

SOMATOAGNOSIA AND DISTURBANCES
OF SOMATIC SELF-IMAGE

SELF-IMAGE INCLUDES *MY-NESS,* a subjective feeling of ownership of bodily actions and the ability to exert voluntary control over those actions. Disturbances of my-ness may manifest themselves as a loss of *my* control of *my* body and its actions (Metzinger, 2000). The individual feels as if control over these actions is being exerted from outside, and no longer by *my-self.* Typical examples of such disturbances include the depersonalization and alienation of thoughts. Agnosia of body parts, or autotopagnosia, and somatognosic illusions and hallucinations may also be considered to be impairments in the feeling of my-ness. The feelings in these disturbances, however, are concentrated more on the alienation or estrangement of body parts and the body as a whole than on the individual's actions in relation to the social self-image of *my* mind and *my* volitional act.

Head and Holmes (1911) and Head (1926) considered the body to be a postural scheme serving as a standard against which sensations are measured. This model may be used as a basis for an information processing approach to the understanding of disturbances of self-image in somatoagnosia and social agnosia. In accordance with such an approach, the body scheme, or self-image of the body, represents one of the parts of the system that underlies the process of one's own body recognition, while social self-image underlies the assessment of the self-position in social space. In principle, the task of body recognition, or social self-image assessment, is similar to visual, auditory, or tactile recognition. In all of these cases, the task is to recognize the features of an item, whether somatic or social, in its relation to *myself.* The execution of the task requires the use of the system that is able to transfer a point-to-point description of the item to the more compact description of the features, both simple and complex, that may be matched via a special computational procedure with the models in storage—a body self-image in the case of somatoagnosia, or a self-image in social space in the case of social self-image assessment.

A major input in body self-recognition is provided by the proprioceptive sensation, and the task is greatly facilitated by the presence of one object in the models in storage—a body model. Similar to visual recognition, the model may represent, for instance, the proprioceptive contour of the whole body; the model may also be constructed by a decomposition of the entire body into individual parts and their spatial relations. Features of body parts may include their shape, weight, and size, as in tactile agnosia for objects. In the

137

*Disorders of
Recognition in the
Physical World:
Other Types of
Agnosia*

case of social self-image assessment, the features describing the social environment are compared with the model of the social self-image. The features of social self-image certainly differ from the features of the body model.

Correspondingly, two major types of self-image disturbances have been described. The first type includes disturbances of self-image in its relation to body image, manifesting itself as somatoagnosia, which reflects impairments in the feeling of my-ness and disturbances in the control of body image. The second type consists of disturbances in the self-image in its interactions with the social world, and includes various so-called dissociative disorders (American Psychiatric Association, *Diagnostic and Statistical Manual of Mental Disorders, DSM–IV–TR,* 2000), such as dissociative self-identity disorder, disturbances of self-awareness in social space underlying some of the personality disorders, and dissociative fugue. This second type is further described in chapter 5, section entitled "Social Agnosia."

Somatoagnosia refers to disturbances in the recognition of one's own *body.* Somatoagnosia is primarily based on deep, proprioceptive sensations, the elementary forms of which are usually either fully preserved or only slightly disturbed in patients with somatoagnosia.

Somatoagnosia was originally considered to be the result of a disturbance of the somatopsyche (Wernicke, 1906). Pick (1922) later introduced the term body schema as a spatial image of the body, composed of primary sensory complexes (see Hécaen & Albert, 1978). Schilder (1935) stressed the reflection in body schema of the totality of our internal and external experience resulting from the synthesis of multiple sensory impressions—tactile, visual, and vestibular. Van Bogaert (1924) and L'Hermitte (1922) emphasized the independence of body image from cutaneous and deep sensations.

Based on the information processing approach, three major types of somatoagnosia may be considered. The first type, *autotopagnosia,* refers to the inability to recognize the simple and complex features, location, and spatial relationships of one's body parts. *Anosognosia,* the second type of somatoagnosia, covers the types of agnosia that are related to proprioceptive information processing, for example, the inability to recognize the presence of functional deficits of body parts, such as paralysis of the extremities. The third type of anosognosia refers to a failure to recognize the malfunctioning of other systems related to visual and auditory information processing and manifested as, for example, cortical blindness, hemianopia, aphasia, hallucinations, and so forth. These types of anosognosia are often called loss of insight or limited insight in psychiatry. Somatoagnosia in such cases thus cannot be defined as a pure proprioceptive agnosia, and may be separated from autotopagnosia as well.

138

LOCALIZATION
OF CLINICAL
SYNDROMES IN
NEUROPSYCHOLOGY
AND NEUROSCIENCE

AUTOTOPAGNOSIA

Clinical Aspects

Autotopagnosia refers to the inability to recognize simple and complex features, to locate body parts, and to orient the positions of body parts in relation to the other parts of the body and to the whole body image. Autotopagnosia may affect one's perception of such body parts as the upper extremities, the face, or the left part of the body. The disorder may also be limited to the fingers and hands, in which case the disturbance is known as finger agnosia, or Gerstmann syndrome. Autotopagnosia is similar to visual space disorientation, a type of visual agnosia characterized by difficulties in the absolute and relative localization of objects in immediate space. In autotopagnosia, the agnosia is primarily related to disturbances of the location of body parts and their spatial relations.

Disturbances in Conventional Information Processing

Disturbances at the Level of Complex Features: Disturbances in the Recognition of Body Parts and Their Spatial Locations

Disturbances in the Location of Body Parts Upon Verbal Commands. Disturbances in the ability to name, find, and point to body parts upon verbal command were first described by Pick (1908, 1922). One of Pick's patients could not follow the verbal command to point to her right ear; she then found the left ear, but when asked to point to her left eye, she answered that she had lost it somewhere. Another patient could not find her legs or neck, and decided that the doctor's lower extremities were her own legs. Schilder (1935) stressed the role of left-right disorientation in the development of body image disturbances. De Renzi and Faglioni (1963) described a patient with a preserved ability to name body parts but an inability to point to the body parts on verbal command. Hécaen (1972) observed a patient with a discrepancy between the preserved ability to point to objects and clothes and an inability to point on command to the patient's own body parts. Difficulties in following such commands have often been described in patients with aphasia, pointing to the role of language in the formation of body image (Head, 1926; Tonkonogy, 1986). However, it has been observed that disturbances in the test may be observed in patients who suffer from autotopagnosia while demonstrating no symptoms of aphasia (Ogden, 1985).

Body Parts Alienation and Displacement. In some cases, a patient may feel that his or her head, arms, or legs are separated, alienated from the body. In more severe cases in which some general mental deterioration is also present, a patient may feel that some body parts or perhaps half

139

*Disorders of
Recognition in the
Physical World:
Other Types of
Agnosia*

of the body are absent. The patient may see his hands but may continue to insist that they are lost (Pick, 1908) or perhaps cut off because they were not used (Gerstmann, 1942); a patient may even begin to accuse the doctor of having taken away the patient's hand (Hécaen, 1972).

The patient may feel that certain body parts are displaced, for example, the upper extremity is attached to the lower torso or perhaps to another person entirely. Such corporeal displacement is more frequently related to the extremities, usually the hands, the arms, and so on.

Alien hand syndrome is related to the feeling of a loss of control of the body scheme by the self-image, which guides the volitional movements of the body parts. Patients often report that one of their limbs has been displaying involuntary movements and has felt foreign, as if it did not belong to them. The autonomous movements in the alien hand may include grasping, spontaneous posturing, imitation behavior, and intermanual conflict in goal-directed movements. Geschwind et al. (1995) gave a colorful description of this syndrome in a 68-year-old woman who had suffered from a transient alien hand syndrome that developed on the 8th day after a stroke and lasted for 3 days. The stroke lesion was limited to the middle and posterior parts of the corpus callosum. "According to [the] patient's family, she had complained of loss of control of her left hand, as if the hand were performing on its own. She awoke several times with her left hand choking her, and while she was awake, her left hand would unbutton her gown, crush cups on her tray, and fight with the right hand while she was answering the phone. To keep her left hand from doing mischief, she would subdue it with the right hand. She describes this unpleasant situation as if someone 'from the moon' were controlling her hand" (Geschwind et al., 1995).

Somatic delusions may include beliefs that some parts of the body are ugly (dysmorphophobia) or that certain parts of the patient's body (mouth, skin, rectum, or genitalia) emit a strong unpleasant odor that may be easily sensed by other people. A delusion of infestation or lycanthropy represents another form of somatic delusion, in which a patient believes that his or her skin is infested with small organisms like worms, lice, or various insects, or perhaps that a spider is in the patient's hair.

Finger Agnosia (Autotopagnosia) and Gerstmann Syndrome
Gerstmann (1924) described a 52-year-old woman who, following a stroke, developed a defect in the recognition of finger orientation in relation to her own hand or to those of the examiner. The patient was unable to correctly choose the finger on her hand that was the same as the finger shown by the examiner on his hand. The patient also had difficulties in naming her fingers and in moving the appropriate finger

140

LOCALIZATION
OF CLINICAL
SYNDROMES IN
NEUROPSYCHOLOGY
AND NEUROSCIENCE

in response to a verbal command; movements and sensations, however, were completely preserved. Gerstmann (1927) published accounts of two additional cases of finger agnosia, each accompanied by "pure" *agraphia*, with a disorder of spontaneous writing, literal in one case and verbal in the other; the ability of each patient both to copy written words and sentences and to read was preserved. Finally, Gerstmann (1930) described several such observations and added left-right disorientation and acalculia as covered under the syndrome, considering each to be forms of partial autotopagnosia. This combination of finger agnosia, pure agraphia, left-right disorientation, and acalculia has been called Gerstmann syndrome in the literature.

Finger agnosia represents a specific type of disorientation in body image. No sign of autotopagnosia for other parts of the body is typically seen in cases of finger agnosia. The central feature of finger agnosia is a disturbance in the recognition of one's own fingers and of fingers on the hands of other subjects. The patient is actually disoriented in terms of the relationships of the particular finger and the corresponding hand. With the patient's eyes closed, he or she may move on command a finger other than the one touched by the examiner. When his or her eyes are open, the patient may not be able to touch the finger that is identical to the finger touched by the examiner on his or her hand.

Errors in finger recognition are made more frequently with the three middle fingers than with the thumb and little fingers, perhaps because the thumb and little fingers may be easier to recognize because of their marginal positions on the hands. Difficulties in finger recognition are usually observed on both hands. Finger agnosia is often accompanied by finger anomic aphasia, a condition that is characterized by disturbances in finger naming. At the same time, difficulties in finger recognition in following verbal commands may be secondary to comprehension disorders in aphasia, and the examination of finger recognition should be concentrated on nonverbal commands, especially in patients exhibiting signs of aphasia. The elementary forms of sensation, including position sense, usually either remain completely intact or are only minimally disturbed in patients with finger agnosia.

Other Components of Gerstmann Syndrome. In addition to finger agnosia, Gerstmann syndrome includes right-left disorientation, a pure agraphia of spontaneous writing, and acalculia. Right-left disorientation manifests itself as a disturbance in the ability to recognize which of the two hands, legs, eyes, or ears is on the right side of the body and which of the two is on the left. Right-left disorientation was also frequently present in cases of autotopagnosia for body parts (Pick, 1908,

1922; Schilder, 1935). Primary difficulties in right-left orientation may be similar to the secondary disturbances typically observed in patients with various types of aphasia, especially for more complex types of commands, such as the command to point with the left hand to the right ear or to point to the left hand of the examiner who is facing the patient. Aphasia must be carefully ruled out to confirm the presence of a primary disorder of right-left orientation. It seems quite clear that right-left disorientation may be considered to be a type of autotopagnosia, a disorientation of one's body parts. However, the relationship of agraphia and acalculia to autotopagnosia remains less clear.

After it was originally described, Gerstmann syndrome was found to be frequently accompanied by other deficits, especially constructional apraxia (Brain, 1965; Schilder, 1935) and general autotopagnosia (Gloning et al., 1968). Some authors have stressed that, in some cases, not all of the four types of deficits originally identified may be found. An absence of acalculia was noted in a case described by Lange (1930), Mayer-Gross (1936) presented a patient without agraphia, and no left-right disorientation was noted in a case reported by Conrad (1953).

Benton (1961) questioned the existence of such an isolated syndrome in his paper entitled "Fiction of the 'Gerstmann Syndrome.'" He studied the correlation of four elements of Gerstmann syndrome with disturbances in three additional tests for constructional praxis, reading, and visual memory in two groups—100 subjects with cortical lesions and 100 subjects without such lesions. No significant correlation was found between any of the four elements of Gerstmann syndrome and the three additional tests. Benton showed that the intercorrelations of the four elements of Gerstmann syndrome may be weaker than the correlations of each of them with constructional apraxia, alexia, or disorders of visual memory that are not included in the syndrome. This provides an argument against the role of the "basic disorder" of body image as the underpinning of the whole Gerstmann syndrome. The recognition of finger agnosia as a partial autotopagnosia, however, remains unquestionable.

Benton's study does not exclude the possibility that Gerstmann syndrome existed in some of his cases. The tests used by Benton were also quite complicated and were rather concentrated on unconventional information processing; for example, right-left orientation was examined using Head's test, which requires the subject to point to his or her right ear with the left hand, or to point to the left eye with the right hand. The test may be difficult to perform not only for those with Gerstmann syndrome but also for patients with various types of aphasia, including Broca's aphasia, Wernicke's aphasia, and especially semantic aphasia.

Disturbances in the Recognition of One's Own Body Image

Autoscopic (Heautoscopic) Hallucinations. The term *autoscopic (heautoscopic) hallucination* is used when a patient sees his or her own body image, as if looking into a mirror. The visual image of a double may be transparent, opaque, or colored. The double is usually seen in front of the patient or, in some cases, on one side of the patient's body, more frequently on the left side. Féré (1891) proposed the term autoscopy to describe a patient who saw the reflection of his own image. The term was derived from the instrument called the autoscope, which was used to examine one's own eye. The term heautoscopy was suggested to describe the false perception of one's own form (Menninger-Lerchental, 1935). Many authors have considered the phenomenon as a hallucinatory experience, or as a disorder of body image when one's own body image is projected into the external visual sphere (Critchley, 1950; Lukianowicz, 1958).

Other suggested terms include doppelganger (Mikorey, 1952), or the double (Todd & Dewhurst, 1955). The terms doppelganger and the double stresse projections to the external space as "an awareness of oneself as being both outside, alongside, and inside oneself" (Sims, 1988, p. 156). This may be experienced without an actual visual image mirroring the own body image; it may be cognitive rather than perceptual. In this sense, autoscopy may be considered to be the experience of duplication of one's real self (Damas-Mora et al., 1980).

Autoscopy has been described in such primary psychiatric disorders as schizophrenia, depression, and obsessive-compulsive disorder, as well as in the toxic states of many infectious diseases, such as encephalitis, epilepsy, migraine, posttraumatic cerebral lesions, and subarachnoid hemorrhage. For a review, see Christodoulou (1978) and Damas-Mora et al. (1980).

Feeling of a Presence (FOP). FOP refers to an invisible "stranger" who, a person thinks, is accompanying him or her. The condition is similar to heautoscopy or doppelganger, but without the presence of a visual image. Brugger, Regard, and Landis (1996) reviewed 27 published cases, and added four of their own, of unilateral FOP. We observed a patient with paranoid schizophrenia who reported a presence in the room of many "invisible men of short statue that [were] constantly moving around the room, not representing any threat or causing any feelings" on the part of the patient. That feeling of a presence lasted for many years, being only slightly reduced by various neuroleptics.

Invisible images are most frequently lateralized to the right side of the body and keep a specific distance from the body. FOP is more frequently associated with schizophrenia and epilepsy, but it has been also noted in cases of migraine, depression, head injury, and organic

143

*Disorders of
Recognition in the
Physical World:
Other Types of
Agnosia*

psychosis, as well as following intoxication. For a review, see Brugger et al. (1996).

Phantom Limb. In cases of a perceived phantom limb, the patient continues to experience the presence of a previously amputated or removed limb, reporting its position, weight, and movements. Phantom limb hallucinations often include various sensations such as pain, paresthesia, heat, and cold. The hallucination of a phantom limb develops almost immediately following surgery and may disappear after several days or months but may continue to be present for years, though becoming less vivid and more vague.

The hallucination of a phantom body part is not limited to limb amputation and may be also seen following the amputation of a breast (Weinstein, Vetter, & Sersen, 1970), in cases of congenital absence of limbs (Saadah & Melzack, 1994), and in cases of spinal cord transection or brachial plexus injury.

Disturbances at the Level of Simple Features

Somatic Illusions. Elementary somatognosic illusions may be manifested as misperceptions of simple features of the body parts. Similar to visual elementary illusions, misperceptions are related to the shape and weight of body parts—a patient perceives the size of a particular body part as being either enlarged or reduced. These illusions are called *macrosomatognosia* and *microsomatognosia,* respectively, similar to macropsia and micropsia in visual perception. A patient may experience, for example, a feeling that the size of perhaps the head, the hand, the left side of the body, or even the whole body has become larger or smaller, taller or shorter than usual. This is often accompanied by feelings of the unusually heavy or light weight of the particular body part(s), or that the body parts are empty or filled with foam or water. These feelings are often described as if experienced. They are unreal and uncertain for the patient.

Another type of elementary somatognosic illusion is somatic alloesthesia, a condition in which one's arm, leg, or head, for instance, is perceived to be doubled or perhaps even tripled. As in visual pelopsia, the subject may feel the presence of several hands, three heads, or an extra leg. The sentiment of the doubling of the left hand appears to occur especially frequently.

Disturbances in Unconventional Information Processing

Autotopagnosia of Space Relations of Body Parts and of the Whole Body

Autotopagnosia refers to the inability to properly assess the positions of the parts of the body in relation to the entire body image. The patient may have difficulties, demonstrating multiple errors when trying to copy the position of an examiner's index finger pointing to the external

144

LOCALIZATION
OF CLINICAL
SYNDROMES IN
NEUROPSYCHOLOGY
AND NEUROSCIENCE

or internal eye angle, to the bridge of the nose, to the middle part of the cheek, or to the eardrum, or when the fingers of the left hand point to the palm of the right hand or to the corner of the mouth (Figure 3.6). The patient is sometimes able to point correctly to the eye but is unable to point exactly to the external or internal angle of the eye.

Similar difficulties may be observed when the patient is asked to copy the relative position of two hands or the hand in relation to the face (Figure 3.6). This last-mentioned type of autotopagnosia may be seen even more frequently than finger agnosia or Gerstmann syndrome and has been well studied and described by a number of authors.

Autotopagnosia of body parts in their spatial relations may also be observed as a component of dressing apraxia when the patient is unable to properly adjust the positions of the body parts and particular items of clothing. For example, the patient may have difficulty in adjusting the positions of hands and arms in order to correctly put them into the right and left sleeves.

Autotopagnosia, or agnosia of body parts, has often been described as a paroxysmal or transient phenomenon during an epileptic or migraine aura, or during the course of toxic or infectious illnesses. It may also manifest itself as a more persistent phenomenon in cases of cerebral damage caused by head injury, stroke, or degenerative brain disease.

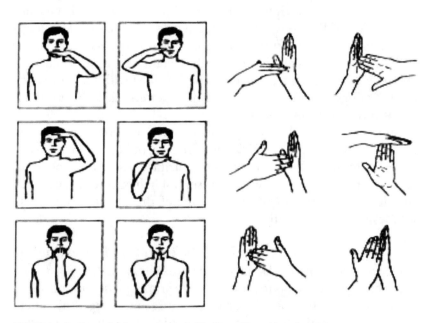

FIGURE 3.6 Examples for testing hand-body and hand-hand positions.

Anatomical Aspects

Lesions in various types of autotopagnosia usually involve the inferior parietal lobe of the left hemisphere. In more severe cases, the lesions are often bilateral (Hécaen & Albert, 1978). The alien hand syndrome was first described by Brion and Jedynak (1972) in patients with tumors of the corpus callosum. A similar syndrome was later described in patients who had experienced transections of the corpus callosum (Bogen, 1993), strokes in the region (Geschwind et al., 1995) or frontal strokes without callosal involvement (Gold, Goodwin, & Chrousos, 1981). In a case described by Geschwind et al. (1995), alien hand syndrome developed in a patient's left hand following a stroke whose damage was limited to the middle and posterior areas of the corpus callosum. Noncallosal frontal lesions usually involved the left supplemental motor area, the mediofrontal cortex, or the anterior cingulate gyrus (Doody & Jankovic, 1992). Kaufer, Mendez, Mishel, Verity, and Benson (1996) recently reported the development of alien hand syndrome in patients with orthochromatic leukodystrophy. An autopsy revealed the involvement of the subcortical white matter and the corpus callosum. The authors suggested that alien hand syndrome had, in this case, resulted from a disconnection between the left and right supplementary motor areas due to a lesion in the corpus callosum, which then led to the loss of motor control of the dominant arm from both supplementary areas.

Somatic delusions have been observed in patients with depression, in some patients with schizophrenia, and in some patients with toxic-metabolic, epileptic, or structural brain disorders. For a review, see Cummings (1985).

Though accurate lesion localization in somatic delusions requires further studies, it is possible that the primary areas damaged in such cases include *temporal and, in some cases, parietal and frontal lesions* (for more details, see chapter 5, section entitled "Disturbances of Self-Image and Social Agnosia").

Hécaen and de Ajuriaguerra (1956) observed somatognosic hallucinations primarily in patients with parietal lobe tumors. The hallucinations were present in 5 of 75 patients with parietal lobe tumors (6.66%), in 1 of 75 patients with temporal lobe tumors (1.33%), and in 1 of 24 patients with occipital lobe tumors (4%).

Menninger-Lerchental (1935) found a high incidence of autoscopy in right parietal focal epilepsy; Hécaen and de Ajuriaguerra (1952) stressed the bilateral involvement, though more frequently on the left, of the occipito-parietal areas. The parietal and temporal lobes were affected in cases reported by Hécaen and Green (1957) and Leishner (1961). Hécaen and de Ajuriaguerra (1952) stressed the role of lesions of the

146

LOCALIZATION
OF CLINICAL
SYNDROMES IN
NEUROPSYCHOLOGY
AND NEUROSCIENCE

basal structures. Conrad (1953) noted autoscopy in patients with tumors of the hypophysis.

The phantom limb phenomenon is related to a lesion of the peripheral nervous system and may disappear following a dissection of the peripheral sympathetic nodules. Phantom hallucinations may disappear in some cases following a cordotomy, the interruption of nerve impulses from the periphery by disconnecting a section of posterior roots. Similar to cases of hallucinations in patients with peripheral lesions of the visual and auditory systems, however, the development of phantom limb hallucinations requires some type of influence of peripheral stimuli on the cortical representation of body image. This idea is supported by cases of the disappearance of a phantom limb following a vascular lesion in the parietal lobe (Head & Holmes, 1911), or surgery on the parietal cortex contralateral to the affected limb (Fredericks, 1969).

Brugger et al. (1996) reviewed 12 autopsy cases previously published in the literature in which patients had experienced the "feeling of a presence" (FOP)—lesions were localized in the left hemisphere in eight cases, and in the right hemisphere in four cases. Parietal lobe involvement has been observed in most of the published cases of FOP, including a right parietal lobe cyst (Kurth, 1941, Case 2); a right parietal meningioma (Nightingale, 1982); a left occipito-parietal glioma (Hécaen & de Ajuriaguerra, 1952, Case 83); and, a left occipito-parietal toxoplasmotic abscess (Brugger et al., 1996, Case 4). Brugger et al. (1996) also noted a case in which a left insular tumor and extensive frontoparietal hypodensity were present, as well as a case in which a right temporo-basal cyst was present.

The recognition of simple features of objects, such as texture and weight, is most likely processed by the posterior insula and posterior operculum, while the processing of size and especially shape involves the interparietal sulcus and adjacent areas of the parietal lobe (for more details, see above, section entitled "Tactile Agnosia, Astereognosis"). It may be suggested that lesions in these areas are also responsible for the development of disturbances in recognition of the size and weight of one's own body parts. Such disturbances have also been reported in patients with mesencephalic lesions. The development of somatic alloesthesia has been also considered to be a symptom of a parietal lobe lesion.

Finger Agnosia

Gerstmann (1930) did not specifically report any anatomical cases of finger agnosia but suggested that the condition is the result of a lesion between the angular gyrus and the second occipital gyrus in the left hemisphere. In the first reported anatomical case of Gerstmann syndrome, Herrmann and Pötzl (1926) observed the syndrome in a patient

147

*Disorders of
Recognition in the
Physical World:
Other Types of
Agnosia*

who was suffering from a tumor in the right occipito-parietal region; the patient, however, was ambidextrous. Based on an analysis of the literature on the subject, Hécaen and Albert (1978) concluded that when the partial or complete syndrome develops in a particular patient, the most probable localization of lesion is the parietal lobe in the dominant hemisphere. Bilateral or left hemisphere lesions are suggested in cases of autotopagnosia.

The effect of a lesion situated between the angular gyrus and the second occipital gyrus was described by Lange (1930) in cases of Gerstmann syndrome with vascular lesions. Nielsen (1946) found that lesions were localized in the area bordering the angular and second occipital gyri in the majority of published finger amnesia cases. Critchley (1953), however, stressed the predominant role of a parietal lesion in the development of finger agnosia.

Strub and Geschwind (1983) summarized the anatomical data on 96 cases of full Gerstmann syndrome published in the literature, from the first publication on the syndrome in 1924 to 1983. Lesions in the left hemisphere were found in 68 of the cases and bilateral lesions in 20 of the cases. Unilateral right hemisphere lesions were reported in only 4 cases. The localization of lesions was limited to the parietal region in 26 of the cases, including 3 cases with the predominant involvement of the angular gyrus. Other sites of lesion localization included occipito-parietal lesions in 7 cases, parieto-temporal and occipito-temporo-parietal lesions in 4 cases, a temporal tumor in 1 case, a temporal hemorrhage in 1 case, and frontotemporal tumors in 2 cases. Bilateral atrophy of the brain was reported in most of the remaining cases. These data provide support for the suggestion that the role of a left parietal lesion in the development of Gerstmann syndrome in a preponderance of the cases. Possible lesion extension to the occipital lobe and, in some cases, to the temporal lobe must also be taken into account (Figure 3.7).

ANOSOGNOSIA

A PATIENT SUFFERING from anosognosia denies the presence of any disturbances, behaving as if no significant changes have occurred concerning the patient's health. In some cases, the patient may only show an indifference to the disturbances, a condition known as anosodiaphoria. Both syndromes in the same patient are often described under the common name anosognosia.

Anosognosia, or a denial of the presence of an illness, was first described by Anton (1898, 1899) in three patients—one patient denied the presence of cortical blindness, one denied cortical deafness, and a third denied left-sided hemiplegia. Babinsky (1914), coining the term anosognosia, described patients who denied the presence of left-sided

148

LOCALIZATION
OF CLINICAL
SYNDROMES IN
NEUROPSYCHOLOGY
AND NEUROSCIENCE

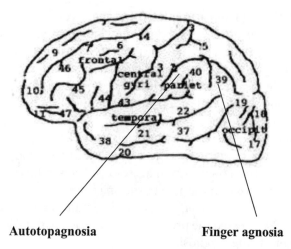

Autotopagnosia **Finger agnosia**

FIGURE 3.7 Localization of lesions in the left parietal lobe in various types of autotopagnosia.

hemiplegia. Similar cases were subsequently published by Pötzl (1924), Nielsen (1946), Hécaen and de Ajuriaguerra (1954), Hécaen (1972), and Levin, Povorinsky, and Tonkonogy (1961).

The term anosognosia has been used by neurologists to describe the denial of such neurological disturbances as hemiplegia, aphasia, hemianopia, and cortical blindness. Psychiatrists generally use the term loss of insight, or limited insight, when such disturbances involve hallucinations, delusions, or the denial of illness related to a mental disorder in general. The neurological term anosognosia and the homologous psychiatric term loss of insight or limited insight actually represent the disturbances that reflect the malfunctioning of brain information processing in various systems: sensory, movement, and language. It is difficult to imagine that malfunction detection may be successfully processed by a unitary device that covers multiple brain systems or modules. This is why the anatomical aspects of anosognosia, which may involve various forms of denial of particular functional disturbances and unawareness of diseases, especially mental illnesses, cannot be limited to one area of the brain.

Anosognosia of Hemiplegia
Clinical Aspects

The patient denies his or her hemiplegia, usually involving a weakness of the left side, insisting that all limbs are functioning properly and that he or she is able to get up and to walk but just does not want to do so at that particular moment. Evidence that the limbs are not moving on the left side of the body may be heeded only briefly, but the

149

*Disorders of
Recognition in the
Physical World:
Other Types of
Agnosia*

patient then promptly returns to his or her denial of the hemiplegia. In less severe cases, a patient may agree that there is a weakness in his or her left extremities, but he or she considers that weakness insignificant and not interfering with his or her ability to stand up and walk. Anosodiaphoria may also be present in some cases in which a patient demonstrates a lack of concern about and an indifference to his or her paralysis. As in cases of visual, auditory, and tactile amnesia, elementary sensations, cutaneous sensations, and deep sensations are often either completely preserved or only mildly disturbed in patients with anosognosia of hemiplegia.

Anosognosia of right-sided hemiplegia is rare and may be most often seen as a paroxysmal or transient disorder. Anosognosia of hemiplegia is frequently seen in the acute stages of a stroke, becoming less prominent in the course of recovery. It is frequently accompanied by states of confusion, reduced levels of consciousness, visual field defects, and signs of parietal lobe lesions such as alexia, acalculia, constructional apraxia, and dressing apraxia (Hécaen, 1972).

Anatomical Aspects

Babinsky (1914) described several cases of patients with anosognosia of left-sided hemiplegia and stroke in the right parietal lobe, suggesting that the lesion in the right parietal lobe might result in the development of amnesia of hemiplegia.

Pötzl (1924) presented two cases of anosognosia of left-sided hemiplegia. In the second of the two cases, anosognosia of hemiplegia was combined with corporeal displacement when the patient perceived his paralyzed left hand as foreign to him and placed it between the right and left halves of his body. In the first of the two cases, an autopsy revealed an infarction of the supramarginal gyrus, which extended backward to the interparietal fissure, and another lesion in the thalamus that had destroyed the thalamoparietal pathways. An almost identical lesion was found in the second case, in which an infarction was destroying the right parietal lobe, the lower lip of the interparietal sulcus, and the right thalamus between the medium and lateral nuclei. Pineas (1926, 1931), however, described anosognosia of hemiplegia in two cases in which the thalamus had been preserved. In the first case, an infarction had destroyed in the right hemisphere the entire inferior parietal lobe, the T1 and T2, the insula, and the subcortical nuclei. In the second case, an infarction in the right hemisphere extended from the anterior and posterior central gyri to the second frontal gyrus. Nielsen (1946) reported anosognosia of hemiplegia in a patient with spongioblastoma of the inferior parietal lobule in the left hemisphere and stressed the role of thalamo-parietal connections in the development of anosognosia of hemiplegia.

150

LOCALIZATION
OF CLINICAL
SYNDROMES IN
NEUROPSYCHOLOGY
AND NEUROSCIENCE

In summary, anatomo-clinical correlations point to lesions in the right inferior parietal region in most cases of anosognosia of hemiplegia. Additional lesions of thalamoparietal connections or direct thalamic involvement may be also required for the development of this particular type of anosognosia.

The rarity of anosognosia of the right hemiplegia may be related to the role of the right parietal lobe in the detection of malfunction in the right and the left extremities, while the left hemisphere is only responsible for the detection of malfunction in the right extremities. In such cases, the detection of malfunction in the right extremities is covered by parietal lobes in both hemispheres and may only be damaged in cases of bilateral lesions or left-handedness. The detection of a malfunction in the left extremities is related only to the right hemisphere and may be vulnerable to lesions of the right hemisphere. This is similar to the prevalence of left visual neglect and may point to the better protection of the right visual field, the right side of the body probably reflecting the more significant role assigned by brain information processing to the right side of space in the visual environment and in the body image.

Anosognosia of Cortical Blindness
Clinical and Anatomical Aspects

Anosognosia of blindness consists of the denial of blindness and often combines with a confabulation of visual images that are perceived by the patient as actual visual images. It is often accompanied by cognitive decline, disorientation, and/or memory disturbances.

Anton (1898, 1899) described three patients suffering from anosognosia—one from anosognosia of central blindness, one from anosognosia of central deafness, and one from anosognosia of left-sided hemiplegia. In the case of anosognosia of cortical blindness, an autopsy revealed a symmetrical ischemic infarction of both occipital lobes, with the lower portion of the corpus callosum disrupting the connections between the occipital lobes. Redlich and Dorsey (1945) also described patients with anosognosia of blindness. Most of the reported cases were accompanied by a cognitive decline, disorientation, and severe amnestic disorders with confabulations, especially in the visual sphere. Bilateral lesions of the occipital lobes and visual radiation were also noted in these cases.

Unawareness of Hemianopia
Clinical and Anatomical Aspects

Hemianopic anosognosia is manifested as an unawareness of a visual field defect. It occurs more frequently in the left visual field but may be present in cases of right hemianopia. Since the loss of vision in the hemianopic visual field is relatively well compensated for by the

151

*Disorders of
Recognition in the
Physical World:
Other Types of
Agnosia*

preserved opposite field of vision, hemianopic anosognosia is more often related to the failure of discovery of deficit. In such cases, the unawareness of hemianopia cannot be considered to be a true anosognosia. However, hemianopic anosognosia may be combined in some cases with anosognosia of motor defect or manifested in cases of apparent disturbances in the recognition of vision difficulties in the right or left hemifield. The development of hemianopic anosognosia may be facilitated either by a patient's cognitive impairment or by visual hemineglect.

Anosognosia of Cortical Deafness

Clinical and Anatomical Aspects

Anton (1899) reported a denial of deafness in one of the three cases described in the previous paragraph. It is probable that the rarity of cases with cortical deafness is responsible for the absence of any similar description in subsequent literature. An autopsy performed on Anton's patient revealed bilateral symmetrical infarctions in the first and second temporal gyri involving their connection with the other cortical and subcortical structures.

Anosognosia of Aphasia

Clinical and Anatomical Aspects

Anosognosia of aphasia refers to the inability of a patient to acknowledge the presence of a language disorder that, in effect, makes his or her speech difficult to comprehend. In spite of the prominent verbal and literal paraphasia that makes the speech incomprehensible, the patient believes that his or her speech is normal and is thus easy for others to comprehend. The patient may become irritated or angry when someone is unable to understand his or her speech. In less severe cases, a patient with mild verbal or literal paraphasia fails to recognize errors made in his or her speech and does not make any effort to correct the errors. Anosognosia of aphasia is usually present in patients with Wernicke's aphasia, while patients with Broca's aphasia tend to make strenuous efforts to overcome their speech disturbances.

Since anosognosia of aphasia is present in all cases of Wernicke's aphasia, it is reasonable to suggest that the lesion typical in cases of Wernicke's aphasia, namely, in the superior-posterior area of the temporal lobe in the left hemisphere, is also responsible for this particular type of anosognosia. It is possible that the frequently observed extension of the lesion to the angular gyrus of the parietal lobe also contributes to the development of anosognosia of aphasia.

Some degree of anosognosia may be also present in patients with transcortical sensory aphasia and conduction aphasia, in which patients are unable to acknowledge the presence of literal and verbal paraphasia in their expressive speech. This may also be related to a

152

LOCALIZATION
OF CLINICAL
SYNDROMES IN
NEUROPSYCHOLOGY
AND NEUROSCIENCE

superior-posterior left temporal lesion with an extension to the parietal lobe. At the same time, anosognosia of aphasia has not been noted in patients with Broca's aphasia, which may be related to the differences in the localization of lesions in Broca's aphasia as against Wernicke's aphasia.

Anosognosia (Asymbolia) for Pain
Clinical and Anatomical Aspects

Asymbolia for pain refers to the absent or incomplete reaction of an individual to pain. Elementary sensations remain preserved, however, and the patient is able to differentiate between a sharp touch and a dull touch.

Asymbolia for pain was first described in patients with cerebral lesions by Schilder and Stengel (1931). Cases of agnosia of pain were subsequently reported by Rubins and Friedman (1948), Hécaen and de Ajuriaguerra (1950), and Weinstein, Kahn, and Slate (1955). For more information, see the review by Hécaen and Albert (1978). The syndrome may be explained by the inability to comprehend painful stimuli related to the body schema (de Ajuriaguerra & Hécaen, 1960), or perhaps as a loss of interconnections between the awareness of pain and the body schema (Brain, 1965).

Patients suffering from anosognosia of pain behave in a way that may be interpreted as a loss in the acknowledgment of pain stimuli, or at least as a significant weakening in reaction to pain. Patients' facial expressions and gestures are either diminished or do not change at all in response to supposedly painful stimuli. Patients may be able to confirm the presence and intensity of the pain stimuli, but the unpleasant feeling accompanying pain is either completely absent or markedly diminished. Vegetative reactions to painful stimuli are not reduced. As in cases of visual, auditory, or tactile agnosia, elementary somatic sensations, such as the differentiation of sharp from dull, are preserved.

According to Hécaen and Albert (1978), anosognosia of pain is often associated with sensory aphasia, apraxia, and autotopagnosia. Geschwind (1965, 1973) stressed the association of the condition with conduction aphasia. These associations point the localization of lesions to the left hemisphere, as was found in most cases. However, lateralization of lesions to the right hemisphere was observed in a small number of cases. The location of the lesion usually includes areas within the inferior parietal region such as the supramarginal gyrus (Schilder, 1935) and the white matter of the parietal operculum (Geschwind, 1965). Weinstein et al. (1955) described eight cases of patients with pain anosognosia accompanied by a parietal lesion in six cases and a temporal lesion in two cases. The role of additional frontal lobe lesions is suggested by Hécaen and de Ajuriaguerra (1950).

153

*Disorders of
Recognition in the
Physical World:
Other Types of
Agnosia*

Anosognosia of Hallucinations
Clinical and Anatomical Aspects

Some people who experience hallucinations—visual, auditory, tactile, or somatic—may not recognize that these hallucinations are not actually real events, and describe the hallucinations without showing an awareness of their artificial nature. Such an uncritical acceptance of hallucinatory images is frequently present in patients with schizophrenia, as well as in the psychiatric manifestation of neurological illnesses. Some of these patients, however, are able to recognize that the hallucinations are foreign and may consider them as a troubling sign of the disease.

Anosognosia of hallucinations, or a lack of insight, is often accompanied by various degrees of cognitive impairments and disorders of reality testing. In cases of *hallucinosis,* reality testing and insight may be preserved; the patient knows that the hallucinations do not represent an external reality. An absence of delirium or dementia is typical for such patients. Hallucinosis may be induced via the chronic use of alcohol, cocaine, and other substances. The *DSM–IV–TR* does not use the term hallucinosis but stresses intact reality testing when a person is aware that the substance induces the hallucinations as well as visual, auditory, or tactile illusions.

There is a tendency to relate anosognosia of hallucination to frontal lobe involvement. However, as with other types of anosognosia, it is possible that anosognosia of various types of hallucinations is the result of lesions in the malfunctioning region originally responsible for the development of that particular type of hallucination.

Anosognosia of Delusions
Clinical and Anatomical Aspects

The definition of delusion includes as a main feature the denial of one's pathological nature. Patients show no doubt that their delusional beliefs are pathological. Reality testing is disturbed, causing patients to lose the ability to compare their grandiose, persecutory, or other type of delusions with reality. As in cases of hallucinations, various types of delusions may be related to the involvement of the different cerebral structures, thus making it possible that the loss of the ability to detect grandiosity as a pathological sign may be related to a frontal localization of the lesion, while a lack of insight in cases of persecutory delusions results from a posterior-superior temporal lesion.

Anosognosia, or Lack of Insight, in Schizophrenia and Bipolar Disorders
Clinical Aspects

A moderate or severe lack of insight in schizophrenia and bipolar disorder is a common clinical problem in the course of an acute

154

LOCALIZATION
OF CLINICAL
SYNDROMES IN
NEUROPSYCHOLOGY
AND NEUROSCIENCE

psychotic episode (Amador et al., 1994; David, 1990; McEnvoy et al., 1989). For more details, see also the review by Ghaemi (1997). Though significantly less severe in depression, a lack of insight is prominent in both schizophrenia and mania (Ghaemi, Stoll, & Pope, 1995; Michalakeas et al., 1994) and may not improve in spite of a resolution of acute psychotic episodes. This represents one of the major obstacles in the treatment of psychiatric patients and its social acceptance, since unawareness of mental illness is correlated with medication noncompliance and poor short-term outcome (McEnvoy et al., 1989). A lack of insight is more prominent for positive symptoms of delusions and formal thought disorders than for negative symptoms of asociality (Amador et al., 1994), but it is actually secondary in many cases to the anosognosia of positive symptoms. An unawareness of tardive dyskinesia is also frequently observed in 50% to 92% of patients with schizophrenia (Alexopoulos, 1979; Smith, Kucharski, Oswald, & Waterman, 1979).

While a lack of insight is often observed in mania, opposite disturbances such as hypochondriasis and somatization may be among the manifestations of depression and/or anxiety. The patient becomes preoccupied with various signs of supposed illness that cannot be confirmed via clinical data or by a number of laboratory studies.

An unawareness of mental illness in schizophrenia cannot be considered a direct result of general cognitive impairment. It has been demonstrated that IQ does not significantly correlate with level of awareness, failing to discriminate between high versus low awareness (Young, Davila, & Scher, 1993). Some studies point to the more complicated curvilinear relationship between IQ and insight, with high and low levels of cognitive functioning characterized by the lowest degrees of insight, while insight is better preserved in cases where there is a moderate level of cognitive impairment (Startup, 1996).

Anatomical Aspects

Unawareness of illness has been described as one of the major manifestations of frontal lobe tumors (Hécaen & de Ajuriaguerra, 1956), Alzheimer's disease, and stroke (Michon, Deweer, Pillon, Agid, & Dubois, 1994; Starkstein et al., 1995). This points to the possibility of frontal lobe dysfunction as a leading cause of lack of insight in patients with schizophrenia. Some neuropsychological data in support of this suggestion have been provided by Young, Davila, and Scher (1993). Young et al. (1993) administered four neuropsychological tests—SUMD (the Scale to Assess Unawareness of Mental Disorder), WCST (the Wisconsin Card Sorting Test), a test of verbal fluency, and trail-making tests A and B—to 31 patients with chronic schizophrenia. The authors found a significant correlation only with the unawareness scale (SUMD) for the percentage of perseverative responses on the WCST, which was considered to be an indication of frontal lobe dysfunction.

155

*Disorders of
Recognition in the
Physical World:
Other Types of
Agnosia*

Cuesta and Peralta (1994), however, found a lack of insight in patients with schizophrenia that did not correlate with frontal and right parietal neuropsychological tests, including fluency, face-matching, and trail-making tests. In addition, an unawareness of delusions may be related to the localization of lesions in other regions underlying their development. This is especially important, considering that the major feature of this type of disturbance is a lack of insight.

Anosognosia of Dementia
Clinical and Anatomical Aspects

Loss of insight is reported as one of the early signs of the onset of Pick's disease, thus pointing to the role of the frontal lobe, whose involvement is more severe in the early stages of Pick's disease. Patients with Alzheimer's disease suffer from a loss of insight that develops with the progression of the disease, most likely reflecting the spread of posterior degeneration to the frontal lobes in the early stages of the condition (Gustafson & Nilsson, 1982; McGlynn & Kasniak, 1991; Reisberg, Gordon, McCarthy, & Ferris, 1985). Unawareness of illness is also described in patients with vascular dementia (Danielczyk, 1983) and Huntington's disease (Caine & Shoulson, 1983; McGlynn & Kasniak, 1991), while insight remains relatively preserved in nondemented patients suffering from Parkinson's disease (Danielczyk, 1983; for a review, see McGlynn & Schacter, 1997).

Hypochondriasis, or a patient's belief that he or she may have serious undiagnosed medical or mental illnesses, is usually described as an overvalued idea that does not reach delusional proportions. In some patients, however, hypochondriasis may reach delusional proportions, becoming unshakable and perhaps even leading to violent action. A mother with schizophrenia, for example, may believe that her children are suffering from incurable illnesses and thus may try to kill them to prevent their suffering (Fish, 1985). Another example of delusional hypochondriasis is a patient who believes that his body is full of water (Sims, 1988) or, as in a case of Cotard's delusions, a patient who believes that he has no stomach and no heart.

Nondelusional hypochondriasis and as other types of preoccupation with nonexisting or minor somatic problems have been described independently from somatic delusions, for example, as various forms of somatoform disorders (American Psychiatric Association, 2000) or in a chapter separate from the treatment of somatic delusions as hypochondriasis and conversion hysteria (Sims, 1988).

Anosognosia and Disturbances of Brain Information Processing

Clinico-anatomical data support the subdivision of anosognosia into a number of separate disturbances of malfunction detection specific to the different systems of brain information processing (Figure 3.8). Anosognosia is probably underlined by right parietal lesions in cases of left-sided hemiplegia, occipital lesions in cortical blindness and hemianopia, superior-posterior temporal lesions in Wernicke's aphasia and auditory hallucinations, and frontal lobe lesions in dementia and schizophrenia. The functional structure of malfunction detection in the various brain information systems remains unclear, but disturbances in this detection may be related to impairments in the ability to correctly assess the outcomes of information processing and to compare the results with their corresponding representations.

The development of anosognosia may be related to lesions in the different brain structures underlying the functioning of certain systems of information processing, such as motion, vision, hearing, kinesthesia, or speech. It remains unclear how malfunction detection may be structured. It is possible that such a malfunction is usually detected when the description of an object or action is compared with the stored model, and a special algorithm distinguishes between the correct and incorrect descriptions at the initial stage of comparison. The wrong description can thus be removed from further processing. When this operation is disturbed, the module continues to process the description of disturbed actions or objects as usual, leading to a denial of malfunction.

This process may be influenced by top-down biases toward a denial of malfunction, especially in cases of delusions. Malfunction may also be detected by the use of several identical channels. The differences in decision making of one or two of those channels would result

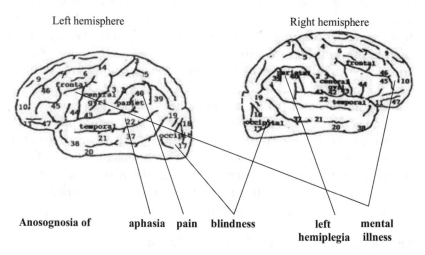

FIGURE 3.8 Localization of lesions in the left and right hemispheres for various types of anosognosia.

157

*Disorders of
Recognition in the
Physical World:
Other Types of
Agnosia*

in heightened attention to the possible malfunction. However, such a system, often used in the past in computer-based devices, may be prohibitively big and does not provide a clear-cut answer concerning the presence and cause of malfunction. In any case, malfunction detection seems to be a task that is quite complicated and which may be performed much more efficiently if processed separately by different brain modules.

DISTURBANCES IN THE RECOGNITION OF MOTION AND ACTION IN THE PHYSICAL WORLD

STUDIES OF VISUAL agnosia have been primarily concentrated on disturbances in the recognition of static environment, including objects and their spatial relations. Under the term *apraxia,* which is defined as a disturbance in the dynamics of the environment, moment-to-moment changes have been studied in relation to actions based on the use of objects and body parts.

Disturbances in the recognition of actions have been investigated predominantly in direct relation to the mechanisms of apraxia, while agnosia of actions as a relatively independent syndrome has remained outside the main scope of clinical research and practice.

The introduction of the term "agnosia of actions" as a recognition disorder may help in the study of large areas of vaguely defined concepts such as "general intellectual ability," "semantic disorders," and "meaning" from the perspective of clearly defined disturbances of operations involved in the recognition of objects and their spatial relations. These operations may include the recognition of signals with incomplete sets of features, the detection and filtration of signals from noise, and the role of bottom-up and top-down information processing. Special attention must also be given to the study of motion recognition, as it represents one of the basic components of action and may be disturbed in cases of agnosia of action.

Interest in this area has only begun to grow in recent years following the studies of action recognition and research has been conducted in cognitive neuroscience primarily via the use of single-cell recording. Research has mainly concentrated on motion recognition and on the studies of so-called mirror neurons, which are activated in monkeys by their observation of a single action, such as a grasp. Some of the neuropsychological findings related to the assessment of general intellectual abilities may also be considered as manifestations of agnosia of actions. Those findings may be divided into two major groups—single actions and complex actions, which consist of sequences of single actions.

158

LOCALIZATION
OF CLINICAL
SYNDROMES IN
NEUROPSYCHOLOGY
AND NEUROSCIENCE

DISTURBANCES IN THE RECOGNITION OF MOTION

Recognition of Direction and Speed of Motion and Its Disturbances

Clinical Aspects

The motion of an object, which adds an additional feature—the ability to move—to the description of the object, usually aids in object and scene recognition in cases of visual agnosia. Motion may also add some additional views to a partially occluded object or scene, further aiding in the recognition process.

Motion recognition includes the assessment of motion direction and speed of motion, which may be disturbed due to two possible underlying impairments of motion recognition—impairments in the assessment of the speed of motion and disturbances in judging the direction of motion.

Disturbances of motion recognition may also lead, in some cases, to difficulties in compensation for impairments caused by visual object or space agnosia. However, disorders of motion detection are noted infrequently, and the preserved detection of fast motion may even be observed in the blind hemifield of patients with hemianopia (Barbur, Watson, Frackoviak, & Zeki, 1993). In rare cases, disturbances of motion recognition may be manifested as an accelerated or decelerated motion effect that may be observed without any sign of agnosia and may be considered a type of illusional experience.

Disturbances in the Recognition of Motion Speed

Accelerated or Decelerated Motion Effect, or Time Acceleration Phenomenon and Time Deceleration Phenomenon. Motion is perceived as accelerated, like the fast forward movements of a tape in a VCR, or like time-lapse cinematography in the past when a special mechanical device was used to accelerate the motion in a film. Since this acceleration device was called a *Zeitraffer* (time accelerator), the term *Zeitrafferphenomen* was coined by the German authors who first described patients with an accelerated motion effect or an accelerated experience of time. For more details, see review by Payk (1977).

According to Hoff and Pötzl (1938), the initial observation of the time acceleration phenomenon was made in 1919 by Klein, who described an 8-year-old boy who was suffering from a fever accompanied by epileptoid attacks, which were characterized by the sensation of accelerated movements in the environment, as well as of speech, both his own and others.

Hoff and Pötzl (1934) presented two cases of the time acceleration phenomenon. An occipital lesion manifested by transient left hemianopia was reported in one of the cases, while an epileptic aura

159

*Disorders of
Recognition in the
Physical World:
Other Types of
Agnosia*

began in the second case with a left deviation of the head and eyes, followed by an accelerated motion effect. A third case described by Hoff and Poetzl (1938) was that of a 62-year-old male who had developed an accelerated time phenomenon during the course of a stroke. While in a coffee shop, the patient had developed a string attack of vertigo. He left the shop, but when he tried to cross the street, he experienced the sensation that cars were rushing, moving with high speed toward him from both left and right. He backed two steps away from the curb and noticed pedestrians moving quickly toward and away from him. When he looked straight ahead, the sensation of deceleration developed; he now saw the cars moving very slowly. Thus, he experienced an acceleration of motion in the periphery of the visual field, and a deceleration of motion in the center of the visual field. The unpleasant sensations disappeared on the fifth day following the initial experience, but left hemianopia remained. No sign of visual amnesia was noted.

A few single cases of accelerated time experiences were subsequently described by Pichler (1943), Wagner (1943), Pötzl (1951), and Gloning, Gloning, and Hoff (1955). Binkofski and Block (1996) recently presented a report on a 66-year-old patient who was experiencing an accelerated time phenomenon. While driving a car, the patient experienced the sensation that external objects were rushing toward him at an incredible rate. He was forced to stop the car, unable to continue to drive. The patient described his sensation as an "accelerated motion" of events, similar to that experienced in a time-lapse film.

In some patients, an accelerated time effect in the visual modality is accompanied by acceleration in other modalities, such as speech or music. In two cases presented by Hoff and Poetzl (1938), auditory stimuli such as speech and music were, at times, perceived by patients as accelerated to the point of incomprehensibility. A similar observation was later reported by Pötzl (1951).

The visual motion effect of deceleration, which is the opposite of the acceleration of motion experience, has also been observed, though in rare cases. Goldstein and Gelb (1918) reported a patient who experienced an apparent standing still of moving people, or an absence of motion perception. The patient perceived objects not in motion but only at the beginning and the end of motion. Hoff and Pötzl (1938) reported a patient who was experiencing a slowness of motion experience, with a suppression of movement speed in the center of the visual field. Deceleration of motion was also reported in cases described by Wilbrand (1892) and Poetzl (1951).

Some of the authors stressed that an accelerated time experience may reflect disturbances in the general ability to estimate a time of short duration. Binkofski and Block (1996) examined that ability in a patient who was experiencing an accelerated motion effect. The patient was asked to say stop when he felt that 60 sec had elapsed since the experimenter said start. Five trials were conducted with an interval of several minutes between each two trials. The mean of the five trials was 286.0 sec for the estimated duration of 60 sec, with marked overestimation of time duration of 226 sec. The estimation of 60-sec time duration by normal elderly subjects yielded a mean of 45.4 sec, with a slight 14.6-sec under-estimation of time duration. However, this marked overestimation or underestimation of time duration may be not directly related to the ac-celeration or deceleration of motion effect, as that effect may be seen in the same patient when the focus of attention moves from the periph-ery of the visual field, in which there is an accelerated motion effect, to the center of the same field, in which there is a decelerated motion phenomenon, as was described by Hoff and Pötzl (1938). It is probable that the experience of an acceleration or deceleration of motion is a transient phenomenon closely related to timing mechanisms that guide the perception of motion, speech, or music. At the same time, a general ability to appreciate short time duration may be relatively separate and not directly connected with the timing of motion perception.

Anatomical and Neurophysiological Aspects

An accelerated time experience was recently described by Binkofski and Block (1996) in a case of left superior frontal lobe glioma. However, descriptions and figures showing CT slices in this case point to a more extended lesion involving the left superior parietal lobe. Most acceler-ated motion effect cases are the result of a lesion in the right occipito-parietal region (Gloning et al., 1955; Hoff & Poetzl, 1938; Pichler, 1943; Pötzl, 1951; Wagner, 1943).

The involvement of the right temporal lobe was noticed via autopsy in a case described by Hoff and Pötzl (1938). A macroscopic study of the brain in this case revealed several foci in the right hemisphere involving the occipito-temporo-parietal region. One of the foci destroyed a small part of the ventral branch of the calcarine tip and the beginning part of the lingual fissure, extending through the deep white matter back-ward and terminating 2 cm from the occipital pole, scarcely involving the visual cortex. The second focus of the cerebral infarction appeared as a long, deep furrow-shaped lesion that spread from the base of the second occipital gyrus to the second temporal gyrus, destroying cortex and white matter dorsally and ventrally from this main line, including the white matter between the second and third temporal as well as part of the inferior parietal lobule. A group of smaller foci was seen in the posterior supratemporal region involving a small part of the plenum temporale. The left hemisphere seemed to have remained intact.

The involvement of the temporal lobe in cases of accelerated mo-tion experience may be compared with recent animal studies, which

161

*Disorders of
Recognition in the
Physical World:
Other Types of
Agnosia*

point to the role of the middle temporal cortical area (MT) in the detection of motion direction and speed in monkeys. The majority of neurons in the visual area of the MT in the posterior bank of the superior temporal sulcus were found to be selective for direction and speed in macaque monkeys (Albright, 1984; Maunsell & Van Essen, 1983). Moving stimuli usually included slits, single spots, and random-dot fields. Direction selectivity was found to be unidirectional and of similar magnitude for all three stimulus types. Direction selectivity was also found in V1 neurons in the striate area of the occipital lobe. V1 responses to moving stimuli were weaker, however, and bidirectional tuning was more common (Albright, 1984). Most MT neurons also demonstrated the orientation selectivity. Similar findings were reported in owl monkeys.

Case studies examining the detection of motion direction and speed in humans were presented by Barbur et al. (1993). The authors described a 36-year-old male who sustained an injury in a car accident at the age of seven. MRI scans revealed massive damage to the medial occipital lobe, involving the cortex and the optic radiation medially and, to a lesser extent, laterally in the left hemisphere. The patient had right-sided homonymous hemianopia with macular spearing. In spite of the hemianopia, the patient was able to detect and localize fast-moving stimuli in his blind hemifield. The stimulus used during testing was a vertical bar that was either stationary or moving at different speeds. The patient detected the moving bar and was able to determine and verbally express its direction of motion; when the target was stationary, however, the patient's performance was at the chance level.

Following a PET scan, Barbur et al. (1993) paid special attention to area V5, which is situated ventrally in the occipital lobe just posterior to the ascending limb of the inferior temporal sulcus. They also took into account two other areas, which included area V3 in the occipital lobe and Brodmann's area 7 in the superior parietal lobe. Both areas had been also shown to be active when subjects during previous studies were asked to view a moving pattern. PET scans performed while subjects were viewing a bar in motion demonstrated increased activation in area V5, the left V3 area, area 7, and the areas of the right middle temporal lobe and the superior vermis. No activity was noted in either the V1 region or the adjoining V2 region. Visual motion detection thus seems to be related to increased activity in the occipital, parietal, and temporal lobe areas. The authors stressed the absence of activity in the V1 area. It is thus possible to suggest that area V5 may be able to mediate conscious visual perception. This possibility is supported by the findings of retinal inputs in monkeys to the V5 area. These retinal inputs bypass the V1 area and include a direct input from the lateral geniculate nucleus (Benevento & Yoshida, 1981; Fires, 1981) as well as an input

162

LOCALIZATION
OF CLINICAL
SYNDROMES IN
NEUROPSYCHOLOGY
AND NEUROSCIENCE

through the superior colliculus and the pulvinar nucleus (Standage & Benevento, 1983), at least in monkeys.

It remains unclear, however, what role the V5 areas in the parietal and temporal lobes, as well as the V1 area in the occipital lobe, have in motion detection and recognition. The detection of direction and speed of motion are likely subserved by different areas in the occipital, parietal, and temporal lobes, but the specific roles of those different areas remain unclear. It is of interest that in a second article describing studies of the 36-year-old male (Ffytche, Guy, & Zeki, 1996), it was found that an early response to fast motion was preserved, but slow motion failed to elicit a response in the patient, pointing to the probable role of area V1 in the detection of slow motion.

It was recently shown that the third dimension, depth, may be provided by motion, helping the individual to recognize 3-D objects and scenes. This is especially important considering that the image created by the retina is flat and 2-D. This effect, known as "structure-from-motion," has been shown to be related to activity in the middle temporal area of macaque monkeys (Maunsell & Van Essen, 1983), the same area as that which is involved in the detection of motion direction. At the same time, agnosia of depth for stationary scenes has usually been described in cases with parietal and occipito-parietal lesions, pointing to the possibility that the detection of depth may be provided by two different mechanisms—motion detection provided by the middle temporal area, and spatial features used for depth recognition by a mechanism located in the occipito-parietal region.

Disturbances in the Recognition of Motion Directions

No systematic clinical studies have been conducted to evaluate such disturbances in patients with brain pathology. However, various neurophysiological studies have been directed toward the evaluation of neuronal activation in several cortical areas in response to observed movements and actions.

Neurophysiological and Anatomical Aspects

Recognition of Nonbiological Motion. Single-cell recording has demonstrated the presence of neurons specialized for the recognition of motion in the dorsal visual pathways, starting from area VI and projecting through area V5/MT (medial-temporal) to the parietal lobe (Andersen, 1997). The MT and MST (medial-superior temporal) areas have been found to be especially important for the recognition of nonbiological motions, such as judging the direction of object motion (Gros, Blake, & Haris, 1998) and differences in the speed of motion (Chen & Berrious, 1998), as well as being a source of important information for the recognition of 3-D shapes of objects (Tittle & Perotti, 1998).

Two types of stimuli have often been used in studies of non-biological motion, coherent motion, and kinetic-boundary motion. For example, Grossman et al. (2000) employed coherently moving stimuli consisting of 100 dots moving at a constant velocity within a circular aperture. Eight strips formed kinetic boundaries with the dots, each moving in the direction to that of its adjacent strips.

Sunaert, Van Hecke, Marchal, and Orban (1999) showed that coherent-motion stimuli caused activation in the MT, with an extension to a sulcus between the lateral-occipital (LO) sulcus and the inferior-occipital sulcus (MT+ region). The kinetic boundary motion activated a large region that is adjacent and posterior to the MT+ and is located along the LO sulcus (Grossman et al., 2000).

AGNOSIA OF ACTION

RECOGNITION OF ACTION may be related to conventional and unconventional information processing. A typical example of conventional information processing is the observation and recognition of such simple actions as kicking, throwing, jumping, and running. Unconventional information processing involves the recognition of more complex actions, especially when presented as in real life but reflected in a static picture or series of pictures, thus perhaps requiring inferences about the actions depicted.

Conventional Action Recognition

Clinical Aspects

Typical pictures of simple actions are often included in the aphasia batteries and are intended to be used for the evaluation of naming; this evaluated ability to name differs from the naming of objects usually employed in the evaluation of anomia. The recognition of an action itself, however, is often considered to be preserved in patients with aphasia and remains beyond the attention of the examiners. It is also apparent from clinical experience that disturbances of simple action recognition may often be seen in cases of severe dementia, while the role of circumscribed local lesions in the impairment of simple action recognition requires further study.

Neurophysiological and Anatomical Aspects

At the same time, single-cell recording and functional neuroimaging open up the possibility of studying the neurophysiological and anatomical aspects of simple action recognition. Single-cell recording has recently been used in studies of so-called mirror neurons, which are involved in the recognition of simple actions in monkeys.

Some of the F5 neurons are active not only when a monkey performs an action but are also strongly activated while the monkey observes a similar action performed by another monkey (Gallese, Fadiga, Fogassi, & Rizzolatti, 1996; Rizzolatti, Faddiga, Fogassi, & Gallese, 1996). These neurons are called mirror neurons and they were seen to be activated by hand actions such as grasping, manipulating, and placing. The activation of more than 50% of the mirror neurons was triggered only by one specific action of the hand, for example, grasping, with some of the neurons selectively firing in response to a particular type of grip, for example, a precision grip or whole-hand prehension. The remaining less than 50% of the neurons responded to two or, rarely, three types of hand action. The neurons did not fire when a second monkey grasped food or ate it. Static object presentation such as that of 3-D solid objects and food did not trigger these same neurons. The response was not influenced by the distance from the object, its precise orientation toward the hand, or the action in two-thirds of the tested neurons, but the size of the object was reflected in the response (for a review, see Rizzolatti, Fogassi, & Gallese, 2000).

Similar responses to observation of hand-object interactions were observed in the neurons located in the lower bank of the superior temporal sulcus (STS) (Perrett et al., 1989; Perrett, Mistlin, Harries, & Chitty, 1990). The mirror neurons in both locations did not respond to pantomimic hand actions without the actual target object. The F5 neurons differed from the STS neurons in that the F5 neurons were activated by the monkey's own active movements, while the STS neurons were activated only during observation of the action.

Another series of experiments using fMRI scans has been directed toward the study of the recognition of *biological motion* in humans. Examples of biological motion as defined in these studies include such simple actions as jumping, kicking, running, and throwing (Ahlstrom, Blake, & Ahlstrom, 1997).

In some studies, point-light animation was used to examine biological motion (Grossman et al., 2000). This point-light animation was created by the placement of 12 dots on the limbs and head of an actor demonstrating various actions, including jumping, kicking, running, and throwing. It was found that, in monkeys, the recognition of biological motions characterized by complex kinematics activates the neurons in area STPa (the superior-temporal-polysensory area), which is located away from the areas that are activated during the recognition of nonbiological motions. Puce, Allison, Bentin, Gor, & McCarthy (1998) demonstrated that, in humans, the viewing of animated sequences of eye and mouth movements activated an isolated region in the right-posterior-temporal sulcus (STS). The same region

165

*Disorders of
Recognition in the
Physical World:
Other Types of
Agnosia*

was activated on positron emission tomography (PET) and fMRI scans when people viewed point-light animations (Bonda, Petrides, Ostry, & Evans, 1996; Grossman et al., 2000; Howard et al., 1996). This activation was either bilateral, involving the superior temporal gyrus anterior to MT (Howard et al., 1996), or primarily in the right hemisphere (Grossman et al., 2000). A small area within the medial cerebellum was also activated while the observer viewed the point-light animation.

The STS areas were not activated by nonbiological coherent motions or by motions outlining kinetic boundaries (Grossman et al., 2000). However, Grossman et al. (2000) found that the MT+ complex was activated during the viewing of point-light animation. The authors discussed the possibility that the MT+ complex provides some feed-forward signals to the STS area.

It must be stressed that biological motions were represented in different studies by incomplete figures. Normal subjects were unable to recognize the figures in the static condition, while the movements of the light-points made it possible to recognize the motions. This helped to exclude the recognition of static figures from the testing procedure.

Rizzolatti et al. (2000) suggest that social interactions in animals and humans require a system that provides the ability to recognize the actions performed by other individuals and to react properly. At the same time, humans have developed an ability to use such observations of actions for learning by mimicking the observed actions, while monkeys remain unable to imitate the actions of other individuals.

Unconventional Action Recognition: The Recognition of Complex Actions as Depicted by Single Pictures and Series of Pictures

Clinical Aspects

Recognition of Basic, Relatively Simple Features of Actions. The recognition of action requires a preserved ability to process the basic component of the actions, the objects and the subjects participating in the action. Similar to the preserved ability to process single features in visual object agnosia, primary agnosia of action is usually characterized by a preserved ability to recognize the basic elementary components of actions and the objects and subjects involved. In cases of visual object agnosia, prosopagnosia, or attention disturbances as in Balint's syndrome, disturbances in the recognition of actions may be manifested as secondary to impairments in the recognition of basic, elementary features of actions. However, agnosia of action becomes primary when the recognition of objects and subjects is preserved, while the ability to recognize the action is disturbed.

Disturbances in the Recognition of the Complex Features of Actions:
Apperceptive Agnosia of Action and Wolpert's Simultanagnosia

The type of primary agnosia of action in which one is unable to recognize a scene was first noted by Wolpert (1924), who described the condition as a disturbance in the recognition of the "whole," with a preserved ability to recognize the "parts of the whole." Wolpert described this disturbance as simultanagnosia. The term primarily refers to disturbances in the recognition of actions depicted in pictures of scenes. Though a picture is static and motionless, it implies motion in the course of actions depicted by the picture. Some of the major features of the action are not shown in the static pictures, however, making it similar recognition in this case similar to the recognition of incomplete pictures of objects in unconventional information processing.

Wolpert's patient was unable to interpret the contents of the actions depicted in images from the Binet-Bobertag series of pictures. In one picture, a man is shown catching one of two boys who has just broken his glass window with a snowball. The patient did not notice the broken window and snowballs near the second boy, who was hiding under the fence. Wolpert suggested that this disturbance in recognition of the content of the scene related to a disorder in the patient's general ability to grasp the scene as a "whole" "simultanagnosia" ("simultanagnosie") independent of the way of its perception, visual, tactile, or auditory. Wolpert defined his patient's simultanagnosia as a difficulty in ability to read words as a "whole"; he did note, however, that the patient's ability to read single letters was preserved. Wolpert stressed that the recognition of words as a "whole" may be disturbed in patients with aphasia, while the recognition of speech sounds is preserved.

The term simultanagnosia was subsequently limited to disturbances in the recognition of situations and events depicted in pictures (Pözl, 1928). Many authors had described similar disturbances in patients with agnosia prior to Wolpert's celebrated case, which stressed that recognition was difficult for the "whole" scene, and while individual components of the scene may be correctly perceived, they cannot be brought together into a meaningful scene by such patients; some of those individual components, however, may also be missed by such patients. Poppelreuter (1917) described a patient who missed the snowball and broken window on the same picture from Binet-Bobertag's series, which led to an inability to correctly recognize the scene in the picture. Wolpert's patient also missed some crucial details in the picture of a dog crossing the street; the patient correctly recognized the dog but did not recognize the dog's action.

Similar observations were later found in studies that were based on the use of so-called thematic pictures. These pictures have primarily been used in the course of the assessment of general intellectual

167

*Disorders of
Recognition in the
Physical World:
Other Types of
Agnosia*

ability in patients with dementia or mental retardation (Rubinstein, 1970; Spreen & Strauss, 1998).

In one such test, the subject must recognize the actions depicted on a static picture. Such pictures have been defined by Luria as "thematic pictures," but the term "action pictures" seems to be more precise in reflecting the actual content of the pictures depicting the various actions. In some sense, the action pictures resemble the incomplete pictures of objects since they do not represent all of the details and dynamics of the actions. The actions have to be reconstructed using the incomplete features of the actions depicted in the picture. For example, the picture of the children's chorus (Figure 3.9) shows the position, though not the actual movements, of the lips typical of actual singing, but the conductor does not move her hands and the contour of a piano is incomplete; the recognition of actions is also much easier when a subject is able to hear sounds typical of a singing chorus accompanied by a piano (Tonkonogy, Vasserman, Dorofeeva, & Meerson, 1977). Such a static picture with an incomplete set of features reflecting the actions may be difficult to recognize for patients with some types of cerebral lesions.

Similar static pictures reflecting actions have also been used to assess simultanagnosia. For instance, in the "telegraph boy" picture (Figure 3.10), widely employed in the assessment of simultanagnosia, it is logical to assume that the front wheel of the bicycle fell off before the boy began to wave for help from the side of the road.

Disturbances in recognition of the actions depicted by such pictures may be secondary to the inability to pick up the complex features of an action in the scene, including unusual details of the action, making the condition similar to apperceptive visual agnosia for objects, and allowing it possibly to be defined as apperceptive agnosia of action.

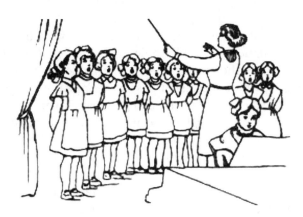

FIGURE 3.9   The picture of the school's chorus (from Tonkonogy et al., 1977).

168

LOCALIZATION
OF CLINICAL
SYNDROMES IN
NEUROPSYCHOLOGY
AND NEUROSCIENCE

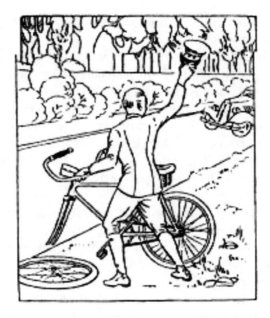

FIGURE 3.10   The picture of the "telegraph boy" (from the Binet-Bobertag series).

Disturbances at the Semantic Level: Associative Agnosia of Action

In other cases, difficulties in action recognition may be similar to associative object agnosia. Typical examples of associative agnosia of action can be found in Luria's description of disturbances in the recognition of "thematic" pictures by patients with frontal lobe lesions (Luria, 1966). One of the pictures shows a man falling through the ice and people who are running to help him. A sign near the pond reads "Danger," and the background of the picture is an outline of a city with church towers. Luria's patient, who had suffered a frontal lobe lesion, recognized that people were running and suggested that the picture depicted a "war" because "people are running," "it shows [a] high-voltage line," or "it warns of wet paint" because of the danger sign. It seems that the patient was able to describe the details of the simple actions depicted by the picture, but being unable to invoke from the model storage of actions the list of possible complex actions typical for a scene including "a man on the ice of a pond" and to bring together the details depicting the actions in the scene, the patient could not connect this observation with its meaning.

Another test assessing recognition of action is the "picture arrangement" (Wechsler, 1955) or "series of thematic pictures" (Luria, 1966; Rubinstein, 1970) test. The test requires the recognition of actions as they are depicted on sets of cartoon-like pictures in a sequentially mixed-up order. The subject is asked to arrange them in an order that properly reflects the actions reflected in the set. The test is usually described as a simple arrangement of pictures in the correct sequential order without defining the test as the recognition of action. However, the test clearly requires the recognition of actions depicted in sequential order in the set of 3–6 pictures. A subject must recognize the action reflected on the cards as well as its important features that may be used to recognize the entire story reflected in the set of cards. The cards may facilitate the recognition of actions presented on a single picture, adding the signs of movements and the direction of actions to the more static picture presented on single cards.

The sequential order of actions depicted by the test may be quite simple, as in the story presented below, which shows, over the course of three cards, a boy climbing a hill and falling from the sled while sliding back down the hill (Figure 3.11).

In the standardized picture arrangement subtest of Wechsler Adult Intelligence Scale (WAIS), there are eight stories of various complexity depicted on sets of 3–6 cards. According to the description given by the WAIS manual (Wechsler, 1955), each card in the series depicts a particular action, for instance, in the NEST item the first card shows that "the bird is building the nest, the next picture shows the eggs which the bird has laid, and the last picture shows the bird feeding its young which have hatched" (Wechsler, 1955, p. 49).

It is apparent that each picture series requires the preservation of the ability to recognize a simple action on a single card and simultaneously tests the subject's ability to correctly arrange the cards in order according to increasingly complex actions. At the same time, the details of the action's dynamics are incomplete, as the action is presented in a series of static pictures, and the subject must mentally reconstruct the action using the incomplete description provided by the pictures. As in tests of the recognition of single pictures, picture arrangement may be characterized as unconventional information processing, similar to the recognition of incomplete drawings of objects.

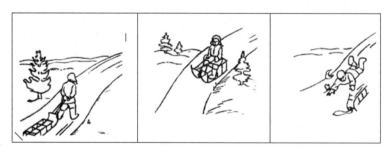

FIGURE 3.11   Picture arrangement test. A series of three cards depicting the story of "the boy falling from the sled" (from Tonkonogy et al., 1977).

170

LOCALIZATION
OF CLINICAL
SYNDROMES IN
NEUROPSYCHOLOGY
AND NEUROSCIENCE

Special attention may be given to the recognition of actions presented via verbal descriptions. Luria (1966) reported a patient with an extensive lesion of the frontal lobe (arachnoid endothelioma) who demonstrated disturbances in the recognition of actions depicted in Tolstoy's *School Stories*. The original story, "The Hen and the Golden Eggs," describes a man who had "a hen laying golden eggs. The man wished to obtain more of the gold at once and killed the hen. However, he found nothing inside. It was just like any other hen." The patient was unable to correctly recognize the actions that took place in the story. After listening to the story three times, the patient said only, "A man had a hen. . . . . it walked around and grew fat." The story was read again and the patient continued to show an inability to recognize the actions depicted in the story: "A man had a hen. . . . . It lived like any other hen, pecked grain, kept busy, and so was able to live" (Luria, 1966, pp. 352–353).

Luria described this inability to recognize the actions depicted in the story as an impairment in the understanding of the *meaning* of the text, in other words, a disturbance in the analysis of semantic structures. It seems that disturbances of meaning *and of* semantic structures may be considered to be a sign of associative agnosia of action.

Anatomical Aspects

Disturbances in the recognition of single-action pictures, whether depicted individually or in a series, have typically been described as a sign of general cognitive impairment. To the best of our knowledge, no systematic anatomical studies of these disturbances have yet been conducted.

Wolpert's simultanagnosia was described in a few rare cases. Nielsen (1946) found in the literature two such cases describing patients with lesions in the left occipital lobe. Kinsbourne and Warrington (1962) point to damage of the anterior part of the left occipital lobe in one of their two cases. Lesions confined to the occipital regions were also suggested by Girotti et al. (1982), while the superior parietal lobe was involved in a case described by Kase, Troncoso, Court, Tapia, and Mohr (1977).

Disturbances in the recognition of more than one object and complex pictures, with an accompanying preservation of the ability to recognize a single object, were originally described by Farah (1990) under the term "ventral simultanagnosia." The ventral occipito-temporal region was suggested as a probable lesion locale. The author noticed similarities between ventral simultanagnosia and "dorsal simultanagnosia," including reading disturbances, the preservation of the ability to recognize objects of different sizes, and the perception of complex visual stimuli in a piecemeal manner. The dorsal occipito-parietal region has been suggested as a lesion locale for dorsal simultanagnosia. Some important differences were also stressed, however, including the

171

*Disorders of
Recognition in the
Physical World:
Other Types of
Agnosia*

preservation of the ability of patients with ventral simultanagnosia to see multiple objects and, if provided with sufficient time, to recognize these objects. Patients with ventral simultanagnosia did not bump into objects while walking around, as did the patients with dorsal simultanagnosia. It seems that the description of ventral simultanagnosia was mainly concentrated on difficulties in the recognition of complex pictures, as with Wolpert's simultanagnosia.

Some authors have pointed to a prominent impairment in understanding of thematic (action) pictures by patients suffering from frontal lobe lesions (Luria, 1966; Zeigarnik, 1961). These findings may be compared with recent data obtained via single-cell recording in monkeys that revealed the activation of so-called mirror neurons in the F5 area when the animal observed an action of grasping by another monkey (Gallese, Fadiga, Fogassi, Luppino, & Murata, 1997; Rizzolatti et al., 1996).

Other areas of the cortex, however, may also be involved in action recognition. It has been demonstrated that mirror neurons might also be found in frontal lobe area F5 and the lower bank of area STS in monkeys (Perrett et al., 1989, 1990). In human studies, Ombredane (1951) and Luria (1966) reported findings that may be compared with the activation of mirror neurons in monkeys. The authors found evidence of difficulties in picture arrangement in patients with various forms of aphasia, which included Broca's aphasia, with premotor frontal lobe lesions, as well as Wernicke's aphasia, with typical superior temporal lobe lesions. Ombredane, however, considered these disturbances as secondary to the impairment of inner speech, which is needed to perform mental picture arrangement, while the ability to recognize a single thematic picture may be preserved, and difficulties may be related only to the verbal formulation of the theme.

In our own experience, picture arrangement has usually been disturbed in patients with Broca's and Wernicke's aphasia, with difficulties being much more prominent for series of pictures rather than single pictures. To clarify the role of language disorders in the development of action agnosia, it would be of interest to study cases of temporal or parietal lesions with an absence of aphasia. It is possible that lesions in the posterior-superior areas of the temporal lobe and adjacent areas of the parietal and occipital lobes in the left hemisphere primarily result in the impairment of recognition of sequences of actions. The role of this occipito-temporo-parietal junction area in such disturbances is supported by recent findings obtained via single-cell recording in monkeys, as well as studies employing the use of fMRI and PET scans. These studies showed neuronal activation in the SPTa areas in monkeys and the STS region in humans while subjects viewed biological motion consisting of single actions (see previous paragraph).

172

LOCALIZATION
OF CLINICAL
SYNDROMES IN
NEUROPSYCHOLOGY
AND NEUROSCIENCE

It is possible that the STS region is primarily involved in perceptual bottom-up information processing in the course of action recognition, which would explain why this area is activated in the course of the recognition of biological motion with an incomplete set of features. At the same time, frontal areas may participate in top-down information processing, helping to limit the number of learned actions that may be chosen from the stored models of actions. The frontal area may also be involved in the breaking down of action sequences into their major components and especially in the process of shifting from one major component to another during sequence recognition. Such a role has been supported by studies of object alternation (Freedman, Black, Ebert, & Bimms 1998), as well as by studies of the vasomotor sequential procedure in monkeys (Hikosaka et al., 2000). The role of frontal lobe structures was also apparent in our studies of probabilistic prognosis. The role of nonfrontal areas of the brain, however, must also be taken into account.

Agnosia of Action and Disturbances of Brain Information Processing

Brain information processing in the course of action recognition has to include two major stages. The first stage is the recognition of the objects, the subjects participating in the action, and the subjects' state in relation to the action. The second stage is composed of the evaluation of sequences of movement and simple actions that form the complex action. Both stages may be combined into one by using the complex feature describing the action as a "whole."

Disturbances in the Recognition of an Image as a "Whole,"
or a "Gestalt," Using the Complex Features of Action Descriptions

Difficulties in the processing of the image as a "whole" as stressed by Wolpert, or in more modern terminology, in describing the image by a complex unique feature, may play an important role in the development of the agnosia of action.

Patients suffering from simultanagnosia may lose the ability to use the more complex visual features in the description of objects simultaneously presented as a "whole" or "gestalt," resorting instead to a strategy based on the successive recognition of single objects, in a manner similar to a strategy employed by patients with visual object agnosia when they are unable to use more complex features for single object recognition. It is apparent that such a strategy leads to a marked increase in recognition time and possible errors due to the unconventional nature of such visual information processing.

In normal subjects, action recognition may be based on the use of general complex features of the action as either the conventional or the

173

*Disorders of
Recognition in the
Physical World:
Other Types of
Agnosia*

unconventional "whole," while patients with simultanagnosia resort to successive recognition of the state of every object of which the action is composed. The latter strategy may lead to the concentration of attention and efforts on the recognition of a scene in general, such as a kitchen, a living room, an office, a street, or a forest, but may be disturbed by an inability to single out the unusual and important details that may help in the recognition of the events and actions reflected in the scene, for example, snowballs and a broken window in the Binet-Bobertag picture used by Wolpert in his description of simultanagnosia. Such cases are similar to the apperceptive form of agnosia and may be defined as apperceptive agnosia of action. Associative agnosia of action may be observed in other cases showing the preserved recognition of some important details of actions, while the patient fails to correctly reconstruct the actions depicted in the thematic (action) pictures.

It should be stressed that disturbances in the processing of the "whole" are not limited to simultanagnosia or agnosia of action. Kinsbourne and Warrington (1962) studied four patients suffering from simultanagnosia of action. The patients were able correctly, though slowly, to depict the objects in the complex pictures, but they were unable to understand the action of the picture as a whole. These patients with reading disorders demonstrated the same pattern of reading the words slowly, letter by letter instead of as a whole (spelling dyslexia), while the ability to read isolated letters was preserved. In the study of these four patients, stimuli were presented on a tachistoscope for a time period of 2.5 msec to 1600 msec. The presented stimuli included letters, geometric figures, contour drawings of known objects, and groups of up to 10 dots. It was found that thresholds of recognition increased markedly with a change from one to two stimuli. Thresholds for the recognition of one to two letters were approximately 4 msec for normal controls, while for patients with nonoccipital cortical lesions the minimal recognition time was 7 msec for one letter and 10 msec for two letters. In patients suffering from simultanagnosia, thresholds increased from 16–25 msec for one letter to 500–1600+ msec for two letters.

This sharp increase in recognition thresholds for two letters compared to one letter was considered by Kinsbourne and Warrington to represent a limitation of the simultaneous perception of visual forms that could not otherwise be explained by disturbances in the shifting of attentional focus from one object to another object as was observed in Balint's syndrome. This same explanation may be used in findings that demonstrate that a decrease of interstimulus interval from 400 msec to 2 msec yielded no change in thresholds. Support for such suggestion was also obtained from the study of dot counting. Patients suffering from simultanagnosia correctly counted the number of dots, which

174

LOCALIZATION
OF CLINICAL
SYNDROMES IN
NEUROPSYCHOLOGY
AND NEUROSCIENCE

was anywhere from 1 to 6, as they were presented on the tachistoscope for 100 msec, and, like normal control subjects, only began to make errors when the number of dots exceeded seven.

Similar results were reported by Levine and Calvanio (1978), who studied three patients with simultanagnosia and found that tachistoscopic recognition thresholds were within normal limits for single letters, even when the letters were masked, and sharply increased when two or three letters were simultaneously presented for recognition. They demonstrated that the visual complexity of the letters plays a significant role. The thresholds were lower when the patient had to recognize two identical letters in a set of three visually dissimilar letters (e.g., OXO) compared to a set of three visually similar letters (e.g., OCO).

Meerson (1986) showed that a sharp increase in recognition thresholds for two objects is usually observed in patients with occipital lobe lesions without the development of simultanagnosia or agnosia of action. These patients suffered from severe, moderate, or even mild visual object agnosia and prosopagnosia. Similar disturbances in the simultaneous processing of the "whole" were observed in our testing of differential thresholds for single angles of various degrees, line orientations, and arcs in comparison with the differentiation of complex figures composed of those single figures. The same group of occipital patients with no agnosia of scene showed prominent disturbances in the differentiation of complex figures as against the differentiation of single figures. The patients typically tried to use the "sequential strategy" of attempting to recognize one single figure after another in an effort to compensate for their inability to use complex features of the "whole" complex figure (for more details, see chapter 2, section entitled "Visual Object Agnosia").

These data support the suggestion first proposed by Wolpert concerning the possibility that many types of simultanagnosia may develop in various types of agnosia—visual, auditory, or tactile. It seems that reading disturbances as described in cases of simultanagnosia are somewhat independent of disturbances in the recognition of complex pictures in simultanagnosia, since some patients with reading disturbances typical of simultanagnosia may be able to recognize complex pictures (Shallice & Warrington, 1980).

It is also important that at least two types of simultanagnosia may be observed. The first type is characterized by apperceptive difficulties in the recognition of some important details of the action picture. The second type, on the other hand, is characterized by associative disturbances in the ability to connect the correct picture description with its meaning.

In some cases, agnosia of action may be related to disturbances in the shifting of the focus of processing, as well as to difficulties in the

175

*Disorders of
Recognition in the
Physical World:
Other Types of
Agnosia*

regulation of the direction of attention from one to another object. Such difficulties constitute one of the three major features of Balint's syndrome and were studied extensively by Luria (1959), Luria, Pravdina-Vinarskaya, and Yarbuss (1963), and Karpov, Meerson, and Tonkonogy (1979).

*Disturbances in the Recognition of Sequences
as the Complex Features of Actions*

Several operations related to sequential information processing could be involved in the recognition of actions. These operations include the recognition of simple actions and the sequences of these simple actions that form the more complex actions. Such sequences may consist of the repetition of a simple action or may be manifested as a shift from one simple action to another action, each often connected with preceding actions and thus reflecting the general pattern of the complex action. The recognition of the general pattern of actions may help to anticipate the following action, in this way facilitating their recognition.

In the course of action recognition, a subject has to divide a sequence into its major components, to establish their relationships to each other in time and space and to compare the simple actions or sequences of actions with models in action storage. No systematic studies of disturbances of these operations have been conducted thus far, but some studies may help to highlight the disturbances while taking into account the fact that they were often conducted according to different conceptual frameworks. Similar operations of the recognition of sequences are also important for visual and auditory gnosis, as well as for speech comprehension. These disturbances are discussed in this chapter, section entitled "Auditory Agnosia" and in chapter 7, section entitled "Aphasia Syndromes and Other Language Disorders."

Neurophysiological Aspects

The Learning of Visuomotor Sequential Procedures. Monkeys were presented with a panel of 16 LED buttons arranged in a 4 × 4 matrix (Hikosaka et al., 2000). At the start of the experiment, 2 of the 16 LED buttons were simultaneously illuminated by the pressing of the start key. The monkey was to press 2 buttons according to a predetermined order; for example, the monkey was to press the key on the upper row (key 1) first, followed by the key in the lower row (key 2). The correct key order had to be discovered via trial and error. After figuring out the correct order, the LED buttons were turned off and another, second, pair of LEDs was illuminated. The correct order in the second set might be the same as that of the first set, or perhaps might be reversed, for example the key on the lower row (key 2) might have to be pressed first, followed by key 1 in the upper row. Five such sets, called a hyperset, were presented during each trial. The predetermined order of such a hyperset might be, for instance, 2,1; 1,2; 1,2; 2,1; 1,2. After successful performance on 10–20 trials, a new "hyperset" was presented, for example, 1,2; 2,1; 2,1; 1,2; 2,1.

During the initial stages, the main part of this visuomotor test, since the monkey has to learn the visually presented order of the illuminated keys, is visual. The initial stage of the test is thus primarily related to the monkey's ability to learn the visuospatial structure of the hyperset sequences, or the order of the upper and lower LED buttons, with key-pressing movements following this learned order. After a few minutes of trial and error, the monkeys learned to correctly perform the sequence, but their performance was slow. In the next stage, performance became skillful and more rapid after the monkey was allowed to practice the same sequence for a month or more. At this stage, the main part of the test is predominantly related to the learning of motor skills needed for speedy performance on the test.

Through the use of single-cell recording in the medial frontal cortex, Nakamura, Sakai, and Hikosaka (1998) observed that many neurons became preferentially active in the pre-SMA compared to the SMA (supplementary motor area) while the monkeys tried to learn new sequences. Following an inactivation of the pre-SMA and the SMA via muscimol injection (Hikosaka et al., 2000), the number of errors increased for new sequences and it was greater than after pre-SMA injections. The effect was observed for both hands, contralateral and unilateral to the injection side. Following the SMA injection, however, the button-press reaction time reflecting the anticipatory movements of the hand was higher for learned sequences and, to some extent, for new sequences.

Differences in learning memory for sequential procedures were also found following an inactivation of the caudate and the putamen via muscimol injections (Miyachi, Hikosaka, Miyashita, Karadi, & Rand, 1997). The inactivation of the anterior striatum (the head of the caudate and the anterior putamen) resulted in an increase in the number of errors made, primarily for new sequences. The inactivation of the midposterior putamen led to a significant increase in errors for learned sequences.

The same task with 2 × 10 and 3 × 10 sequences was used for human studies and supplemented by functional magnetic resonance imaging (fMRI). In the stage of learning (Hikosaka et al., 2000), a region of medial frontal lobe activation was located slightly anterior to the anterior commissure, a human homologue of the pre-SMA (Picard & Strick, 1996). In addition, at least four cortical areas were active in the course of learning (Sakai et al., 1998). The dorsolateral prefrontal cortex was

177

Disorders of
Recognition in the
Physical World:
Other Types of
Agnosia

active in the early stage, the pre-SMA in the early and intermediate stages, the medial parietal cortex in the intermediate phase, and the intraparietal sulcus region in the intermediate and advanced stages. The fMRI studies also pointed to the possibility that the parietal area is involved in the learning of visuomotor sequences, but its activation perhaps largely disappears after extensive learning.

Hikosaka et al. (2000) considered a model for the learning of sequential procedures based on two learning systems—one system codes the sequence in visual coordinates and is associated with the premotor frontal cortex, while the other system codes the sequence in motor coordinates and is related to the SMA. The pre-SMA controls both systems, and the premotor cortex (PM) is a translator from visual to motor coordinates and vice versa. The basal ganglia and the cerebellum are considered to have supportive roles in the reinforcement of the learning system (basal ganglia) and in the refining and coordinating of individual movements based on timing information. The role of the parietal lobe, however, remains unclear in this particular model.

Neuropsychological Aspects
The Recognition of Sequences Formed by the Repetition of the Same Basic Feature and Its Shifting to Another Basic Feature. The old neuropsychological tests involving the sorting of cards or objects may be considered to be examples of the recognition of a main feature in sequences. This feature is repeated in the sequential presentation of the cards or objects, forming a sequence based on the repetition of the same basic feature. For example, the Hanfmann-Kasanin test (Freeman, 1959) consists of 22 blocks of five different colors, six shapes, two heights, and two widths. The subject is asked to divide the blocks into four categories. The categories are determined based on several features, including the four vertical and horizontal sizes of the blocks: tall versus short blocks and wide versus narrow blocks, and tall-wide, short-wide, tall-narrow, and short-narrow blocks. The subject is not privy to this information in advance. Each block contains a nonsense name on its bottom that is repeated on the back of blocks of the same size, for example, *bik* for short-wide size. Each subject typically starts with categorization according to color or shape. After each attempted grouping, the examiner shows the subject one of the wrongly selected colors or shapes by revealing that it has a different name. The testing continues until the subject is able to figure out that the correct classification is based on block sizes and is determined according to the combination of horizontal and vertical measurements.

That task actually consists of finding the feature or the signal masked by the noise formed by the decoys. Such detection requires the ability to differentiate the main feature of the signal from the decoy,

178

LOCALIZATION
OF CLINICAL
SYNDROMES IN
NEUROPSYCHOLOGY
AND NEUROSCIENCE

and is similar to the detection and recognition of objects from the noisy background in the Poppelreiter figures. The operations involved in such recognition require *grouping* of the blocks using their nonsense names as a feature that facilitates the unmasking of the correct signal.

The basic classification feature of the sequences may shift during the course of testing. A series of tests has been developed to study the effects of such a shift. These tests include the Object Alternation Test (OA) and a group of card sorting tests. Shifting is also the main feature among the other tests and is usually employed in the examination of executive functions, for example, in the Stroop Color Test, the Trail-Making Test Part B, and so on. Lately, the Recurrent Figure Test was introduced to study the repetition of more complex basic features, consisting of two or three simple components (Figure 2.14 A). The task is simplified by the absence of masking features (Tonkonogy, 1997). Most such tests require the recognition of the basic feature of a sequence, followed by the recognition of the shifting pattern of the sequence.

Object Alternation Test. In the OA Test, a subject's choice between two objects is rewarded when the subject chooses the second alternating object after receiving a reward for choosing the first object. No reward is provided when the same object continues to be selected from the two objects. The objects cover two wells. When an object is raised, the subject is able to see if the well contains a reward—a penny for humans and food for monkeys. The test was first employed in animal models to study the role of orbitofrontal lesions in disturbances of test performance in monkeys (Mishkin & Manning, 1978; Pribram & Mishkin, 1956).

The test was subsequently used with humans and demonstrated impairments in six patients with bilateral lesions in the orbitofrontal and anterior cingulate regions (Freedman et al., 1998). The researchers suggested the role of the ability to shift sets and the role of working memory in correct test performance. It is important to stress that simple memorizing is not sufficient for uncovering the test structure, and the main challenge of the test is directed toward the recognition of the shift in alternating objects. The idea that the working memory has a small role is also supported by the markedly reduced number of errors in delayed alternation (DA) and delayed response (DR) tests observed in the same group of six frontal lobe patients studied by Freedman et al. (1998). It has been well accepted that in these two tests, DA and DR provide a direct measurement of working memory that is clearly challenged by the delays between two signals (DA) or between signals and responses (DR). Such a delay is not included in the OA test, but some involvement of the working memory is needed to temporarily store information about particular stimuli needed for the recognition of the sequences of alternating signals.

179

*Disorders of
Recognition in the
Physical World:
Other Types of
Agnosia*

Card Sorting Tests. A more complex shifting task may include changes in a basic component or the stimuli when one of the features is used as a decoy, then later becomes a main component of a sequence while the previous main feature is considered as one of the decoys. The ability to switch, or to *shift,* from a recently learned operation to a new task based on similar sets of elementary features in the sequences is thus tested. Such a test in the ability to shift was first introduced by Goldstein and his colleagues in the form of the Gelb-Goldstein Color Sorting Test, the Object Sorting Test, and, relatively recently, the Weigl-Goldstein-Scheerer Color-Form Sorting Test. The idea of a main feature masked by another feature was presented via a hue versus brightness distinction in the Gelb-Goldstein Color Sorting Test and a color versus shape distinction in the Weigl-Goldstein-Scheerer Color-Form Sorting Test.

The concept of shifting reflected in these tests has been further developed in the Wisconsin Card Sorting Test (WCST), which has been widely used over the course of the last decade in studies of executive function. The WCST was developed by Berg and Grant (Berg, 1948; Grant & Berg, 1948) and later standardized by Heaton et al. (1993). The test begins with the matching of two decks of 64 cards each with four stimulus cards, which are placed in front of the subject, according to predetermined classification rules. These predetermined rules are unknown to the subject and change several times during the testing session. The images on the four stimulus cards include a red triangle, two green stars, three yellow crosses, and four blue circles. After the presentation of each response card, the subject is informed by the examiner as to whether his or her choice is "right" or "wrong." The subject is first required to sort according to *color.* Following 10 consecutive correct responses, the sorting principle is changed without warning to *form,* then to *number,* and finally back to *color.* The testing session continues until the subject either successfully completes two sorting sequences according to color, form, and/or number, or has "played" all 128 cards (Spreen & Strauss, 1998). The WCST actually tests the ability to unmask the correct main feature, or sorting principle, of the sequences, which consists of the repeated main features of color, form, and number, as well as the ability to shift from one principle to another.

Milner (1963) studied a series of patients before and after the excision of parts of the dorsolateral frontal cortex, the orbitofrontal cortex, or the anterior temporal cortex in the course of surgical treatment for epilepsy. Milner found that the patients, especially those who had undergone a dorsolateral frontal excision, were unable to shift from one sorting principle to another. However, it was shown that WCST performance did not differ in patients with focal frontal lesions and patients with lesions outside the frontal lobes (Anderson, Damasio,

180

LOCALIZATION
OF CLINICAL
SYNDROMES IN
NEUROPSYCHOLOGY
AND NEUROSCIENCE

Jones, & Tranel, 1991; Axelrod et al., 1996). The test requires the employment of several different operations, including learning to detect and differentiate between main features and decoys, to acknowledge the change and to successfully switch one's attention to a new main signal, and so on. This requires the participation of several cortical areas that are involved in these sets of operations.

Recurrent Figures. Recurrent Figures is a simple test that has been introduced to study the recognition of the major feature of simple visual sequences and their alternating shifting patterns (Luria, 1966; Tonkonogy, 1997). The test requires the subject to copy three sequences: the repetition of a triangular shape; the repetition of alternating triangular and rectangle shapes; and two subsequent triangular shapes alternated with a single rectangle shape (Figure 3.13). The main feature in each of the second and third sequences is actually a shifting of sets that is repeated several times in each sequence. The subject can copy the sequences either via the use of a slavish copy of each triangular or square shape or by recognizing that the set consists of several repetitions of the same main feature. This recognition is especially important when a subject is asked to draw the sequence after the sample and the copy have been removed. The subject is then asked to draw the sequence using his or her memory of the sequence structure.

In our experience, difficulties with test performance may be related to the inability of the subject to recognize the main feature of the sequence. One of our patients, who was suffering from Alzheimer's disease, described the sequence as a combination of horizontal and vertical lines. When his attention was drawn to the triangular and square shapes, the patient corrected the examiner by saying, "not square, but rectangular shape," but continued to describe the sequence according to its horizontal and vertical lines, not taking into account the existence of the main components, which were the triangular and rectangular shapes.

In most cases, the main features of the sequences are recognized, but the patient erroneously alternates them in the sequence, noting, for example, three triangular shapes in a row instead of only one or two, or perhaps two rectangular shapes instead of one (Figure 3.12).

The Recognition of Sequences as Formed by the Shifting of the Order of Their Main Features. This type of sequencing is closely related to real actions, which are usually based on the sequences of simple actions, which, in turn, form the pattern of a more complex action. An example of this type of sequencing is seen in the testing of the differentiation between a series composed of low-, medium-, and high-tone pitches presented in various orders of succession, for example, series 200

181

*Disorders of
Recognition in the
Physical World:
Other Types of
Agnosia*

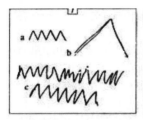 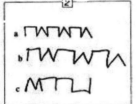 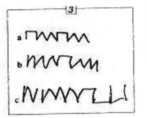

FIGURE 3.12 "Recurrent figures" test. In each picture, (a) samples and (b) copies of the figures as drawn by a patient with mild cognitive decline in the early stages of Huntington's disease; (c) the same patient, drawing the figures from memory after a 2-3 sec delay (from Tonkonogy, 1997).

Hz–2000 Hz–800 Hz versus series 200 Hz–800 Hz–2000 Hz. Similar types of sequences were formed by visual signals, such as angles of varying degrees or colors (for more details, see chapter 2, section entitled "Visual Agnosia," as well as "Auditory Agnosia" in the present chapter). Disturbances in the differentiation of auditory sequences may be observed in patients with posterior-superior temporal lesions, and visual sequencing impairments in patients with occipital lesions. Both types of sequencing were disturbed in patients with parietal lesions as well as in patients with anterior-inferior temporal lesions (Dorofeeva, 1970; Meerson, 1986; Tonkonogy, 1973).

Probability Prognosis of Shifting Patterns of Orders of Main Features. Adjustment to the constantly changing conditions of the physical and social environment requires the ability to predict upcoming events. This may be easier to accomplish when the sequences of events are predetermined with a probability of 1.0. In such circumstances, it is relatively easy to choose the proper, conventional preparation and reaction to the successive events.

However, the chain of events may often be probabilistic and not fully predetermined. The frequencies of particular events may help in predicting an upcoming occurrence in such a chain of events, especially when one of the events is more frequent than another event or other events. However, the knowledge of frequencies requires some additional ability to assess the probability of every upcoming event, since each such probability is less than 1.0. For instance, the probability of encountering a red card in a chain of red and green cards may be 0.8, while the probability of encountering a green card may be 0.2. If the order of the cards is determined according to chance, a green card may appear following another green card in two of eight instances in general, but a particular appearance of the green card may be seen after any number of red cards. In this case, minimization of the number of

182

LOCALIZATION
OF CLINICAL
SYNDROMES IN
NEUROPSYCHOLOGY
AND NEUROSCIENCE

errors made in prediction of the color for the next card requires preservation of special abilities.

We performed a study investigating the reliability of probabilistic prognosis in patients with local brain pathology, in which each subject was instructed to predict the subsequent color or tone pitch in a sequence (Bajhin, Meerson, & Tonkonogy, 1973). The visual sequences included a series of red and green lights, each of which appeared for 1 sec on a tachistoscope screen. The auditory sequences consisted of pure tones at 200 Hz and 2000 Hz of 1 sec duration. After the presentation of the color or tone, the patient was asked to predict whether the following color would be red or green, or whether the following tone pitch would be low or high. In the first testing set, the sequences were composed of a series of two visual or auditory signals, with first order statistics having probabilities of 0.9:0.1; 0.8:0.2; 0.7:03; and, 0.6:04. The second set consisted of first order statistics of 0.5:0.5 but second order statistics of 0.9:0.1 to 0.6:0.4. The learning period for each set included 50 presentations with first order statistics of 0.8:0.2 for the first set, and 50 presentations with first order statistics of 0.5:0.5 and second order statistics of 0.8:0.2. The structure of the sequences is reflected by the textures that have the same orders statistics of black and white squares (Figure 3.13).

Following the conclusion of the learning tasks, the subjects were asked to assess either the relative frequencies of red and green lights (more red than green), or of low- and high-pitch tones (more high than low). When a subject was unable to correctly assess the relative frequencies, he/she was excluded from the testing. Each of the patients in the excluded group had suffered from a massive frontal lobe lesion. The testing of each set included 200 signals with 50 presentations for each probability from 0.9:0.1 to 0.6:0.4. The studied groups included 10 patients with local lesions outside the frontal lobe and four patients with moderate prefrontal lesions. The control group consisted of 10 subjects. The group of non–frontal lobe patients included three individuals with Wernicke's aphasia and posterior-superior temporal

FIGURE 3.13 Simultaneous presentation of the first order statistics for red (black squares), probability $p = 035$, and green (white squares), probability $p = 065$.

183

*Disorders of
Recognition in the
Physical World:
Other Types of
Agnosia*

lobe lesions, three individuals with visual object amnesia and occipito-temporal lesions, and four individuals with parietal lobe lesions.

The number of errors made by control subjects in the study did not exceed 65–70 for the first order statistics, and did not surpass 55–60 for the second order statistics. These numbers reached 75–80 and 55–60, respectively, for the non–frontal lobe group of patients. At the same time, the number reached 95–105 for the first order statistics in the frontal group of patients. While this number decreased for the second order statistics in non–frontal lobe patients, the number remained at the same high level in frontal lobe patients. No significant differences were recorded between the visual and auditory sequences for all groups of patients, including those in the control group. No increase in the number of errors was observed for the auditory sequences in patients with Wernicke's aphasia and for the visual sequences in patients with visual object amnesia (Figure 3.14).

The high number of errors in the frontal group of patients as observed in all types of tests points to the special role of the frontal lobe in probability prediction. It should be stressed that probability predictions as made by all of the groups of patients, as well as by the normal control subjects, were not usually based on the so-called optimal strategy, which consists of a constant prediction of the most frequent

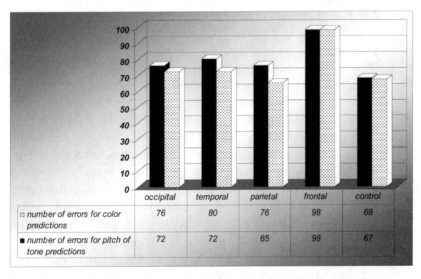

	occipital	temporal	parietal	frontal	control
▨ number of errors for color predictions	76	80	76	98	68
■ number of errors for pitch of tone predictions	72	72	65	98	67

FIGURE 3.14 Number of errors for 200 anticipations of the succeeding signals, red or green in the visual series, and low- or high-pitch tone in the auditory series for sequences of first order statistics. The patients with frontal lobe lesions show the highest number of errors for both types of signal, visual and auditory, pointing to the non–modality specific nature of prediction ability in this type of testing.

184

LOCALIZATION
OF CLINICAL
SYNDROMES IN
NEUROPSYCHOLOGY
AND NEUROSCIENCE

signal. The patients, as well as the subjects in the normal control group, tried to find the particular structure of the signal sequencing in order to correctly predict the subsequent signal. This turned out to be easier for sequences based on second order statistics for both control subjects and non–frontal lobe patients. At the same time, the frontal patients could not use the stronger correlation between the appearance of the same current and subsequent signal in the statistics of the second order. The patients exhibited an absence of differences in the number of errors between the sequences with the first and the second order statistics. It seems that probability prediction is based on one's ability to assess the approximate number of more frequent signal repetitions before the shift to the less frequent signals, and vice versa. This ability may be especially helpful for the second order statistics.

The results of this particular study must certainly be considered preliminary. Their statistical significance requires further confirmation in a larger group of patients, including subjects with both frontal and nonfrontal local brain pathology. A study is also needed to investigate more specifically the tactics used by normal controls as well as patients, both frontal and nonfrontal, in the course of probability predictions.

CONCLUSION

1. Disturbances in the recognition of motion may be manifested in the recognition of the speed and direction of motion.
2. Agnosia of actions may be observed by the testing the recognition of actions depicted either by single pictures or by a series of pictures.
3. Disturbances in the recognition of complex features describing the scene of an action may underline so-called impairments in the recognition of the "whole," or the "gestalt," in cases of Wolpert's simultanagnosia or, in modern terminology, agnosia of action. Such disturbances may also be of the associative type when an individual is able to correctly describe the details of an action scene, but the description cannot be connected to or associated with its meaning. Another type of disturbance in such cases may be related to difficulties in the recognition of a scene's details, which are important for action recognition; this particular type of disturbance is similar to that of apperceptive object agnosia.
4. Agnosia of actions may be underlain by disturbances in the recognition of sequences. Different structures of sequences include repeats of the same basic feature, but masked by "noise" as created by other features. These features become basic following a shifting in the course of testing. Another type of sequences consists of changes in the pattern of succession in the gradation of

185

*Disorders of
Recognition in the
Physical World:
Other Types of
Agnosia*

basic features. The ability to predict the subsequent feature in statistically based sequences represents the type of sequence that is especially disturbed in patients with frontal lobe lesions. It is an important task for future studies to compare impairments in the recognition of sequences with agnosia of action.

5. Further studies are needed to successfully localize the lesions responsible in cases of agnosia of action. Some data point to the role of occipital and occipito-parietal lesions in the development of apperceptive agnosia of action, and to frontal and temporal lobe lesions in the development of associative agnosia of actions.

4

Disorders of Recognition in the Physical World: Illusions and Hallucinations

ILLUSIONS AND HALLUCINATIONS differ from agnosia in that they *produce* the images of objects or actions with a misperception of their simple or complex features. In other words, images are formed without external stimulation, as in hallucinations, when information processing seems to work independently from external stimuli. This was reflected in the old psychiatric literature by the term *productive symptoms,* which was applied to the definitions of illusions, hallucinations, and delusions.

ILLUSIONS

AN ILLUSION IS a conscious misperception of a real external stimulus. Some of the first detailed studies of illusions were reported by Pötzl (1928) and by Hoff and Pötzl (1935). Further studies were reviewed by Critchley (1953) and Hécaen and Albert (1978). In accordance with sensory modalities, illusions may be described as visual, auditory, or somatognostic. *Elementary illusions* are manifested as misperceptions

188

LOCALIZATION
OF CLINICAL
SYNDROMES IN
NEUROPSYCHOLOGY
AND NEUROSCIENCE

of simple features, while *complex illusions* are related to the misperception of objects and scenes.

Illusions are frequently observed as an aura of a seizure and in patients with brain tumors or infections, and, in some cases, following head injury, stroke, and disturbances at the peripheral level of sensory systems.

VISUAL ILLUSIONS

Illusions of Static Features of the Visual World
Clinical Aspects

Elementary Illusions: Metamorphopsia. Illusional perceptions of single features of objects such as shape, size, and color, are termed *metamorphopsia.* Hécaen and Albert (1978) presented a modified version of Critchley's classification of metamorphopsias (Critchley, 1953). According to this classification, elementary illusions have several varieties, including the distortion of size, shape, and color.

Illusions, or distortions of visual perception, otherwise known as metamorphopsia, may be observed during the course of a seizure. They also may be persistent in the acute period of a head injury, as well as in cases of peripheral ophthalmologic problems.

Metamorphopsia of shape is the modification of an object's shape by any one of the following mechanisms: the shape may be stretched in a single dimension, usually in length and less frequently in width; the obliquity of the vertical and/or horizontal component of the object may assume a sinusoidal shape, or perhaps curve in one direction as if it is bending over; the outlines of the shape may be blurred or irradiated; or the object's contour may be fragmented (Hécaen & Albert, 1978).

Metamorphopsia of size is the modification of object size, causing real objects and entire scenes to look either smaller, via *micropsia,* or bigger, via *macropsia,* than their actual size. Lilliputian hallucinations occur when an individual sees images of small human and animal figures (Alexander, 1926; Goldin, 1955; Lewis, 1961). Brobdingnagian hallucinations, on the other hand, are figures that to an individual appear to be larger than normal. Such hallucinations are reported only in a small number of cases (Fleming, 1923, Thomas & Fleming, 1934). While Lilliputian and Brobdingnagian hallucinations have not been described as parts of a seizure event, micropsia and macropsia are mentioned relatively frequently in the course of occipital lobe seizures.

Metamorphopsia of color is a modification of object color, including *achromatopsia,* which is the disappearance of color, and *erythropsia,* or the perception of a uniform tint of a particular, often reddish color.

Complex Illusions. Complex illusions may be similar to visuospatial agnosia and may be manifested as *telescopy, pelopsia,* and a loss of stereoscopic vision. Telescopy, which resembles micropsia, is the perception that those objects that are smaller than reality are moving increasingly farther away. Pelopsia, on the other hand, is a condition in which objects perceived as being larger than in reality, as in macropsia, have the appearance of approaching the subject. A loss of stereoscopic vision is characterized by the perception of 3-D objects in 2-D space. According to Pötzl (1928), the loss of stereoscopic vision may be limited to the vertical meridian of the visual field.

Other types of complex illusions include *polypsia* and *alloesthesia.* Misperceptions in these illusions are related to the presence, number, and position of an object in space. In polypsia, the number of objects may multiply, perhaps doubling, tripling, quadrupling, or infinitely extending the number of objects as perceived in either the sagittal or frontal planes or in a concentric manner (Gloning et al., 1968). Optic alloesthesia is also characterized by the doubling of an image, but in this case the double appears specifically in the symmetrical horizontal position of the visual field.

Pareidolia is a peculiar type of illusion that has often been reported in normal individuals. Subjects have reported to have seen vivid images in fire and in clouds. Sims (1988) described his own pareidolic illusion of the head of a spaniel, which he repeatedly saw on the first paving stone on the path while revisiting the house in which he had lived as a child.

Anatomical Aspects

Visual illusions are more frequently associated with cortical involvement (Hécaen & Albert, 1978). Metamorphopsias have been reported in patients with lesions in the occipito-parietal region (Hoff & Pötzl, 1935, 1937) as well as in the occipital and occipito-temporal regions (Teuber, Battersby, & Bender, 1960). Hécaen and Angelergues (1963) found evidence of metamorphopsia more frequently with occipito-parietal and temporal lesions in the right hemisphere than in the left. These lesions in the right hemisphere involved the occipital, temporal, and occipito-temporal regions and, in some cases, the occipito-parietal region. Hécaen and Angelergues (1963) observed occipital involvement in 11 of 13 cases of patients with metamorphopsia, 3 of whom had suffered from isolated occipital lesions. The authors reported that occipito-parietal lesions seemed to be most common in cases that involved the left hemisphere. Mullan and Penfield (1959) observed metamorphopsias via the electrical stimulation of different areas of the brain, but in most cases the stimulation of the temporal lobe.

190

LOCALIZATION
OF CLINICAL
SYNDROMES IN
NEUROPSYCHOLOGY
AND NEUROSCIENCE

The development of visual illusions may be underlain by lesions localized in the peripheral levels of the visual system. An illusion may be caused by disturbances in ocular motility via an interruption of vestibulocerebellar connections caused by brain stem lesions (Hécaen & Albert, 1978).

Illusions of Dynamic Features of the Visual World. An illusion of movement represents a special type of misperception related to the dynamic features of the visual world, as against misperceptions of static characteristics of objects and scenes. Illusory misperceptions include distortions in the conscious visual assessment of the presence, type, and speed of movements. In a misperception of the presence and type of a movement, a stationary object is incorrectly perceived as being in motion. According to Hécaen and Angelergues (1963), this illusion of movement may, for example, be a flag waving or a poorly adjusted television set. In other cases, subjects have perceived a stationary object as jumping from one place to another, or moving up and down in one place.

The illusory movement may be unidirectional to the right or to the left and is often accompanied by a rotation of the object upon itself. A peculiar phenomenon is that of illusory acceleration and deceleration of movements, which occurs when the real movement of an object that is holding a steady speed is instead misperceived as being in accelerated motion; the opposite can also occur; in this case, it appears as though a moving object reveals instead a decreased or perhaps complete absence of movement (for more details, see chapter 3, section entitled "Disturbances in the Recognition of Motion and Action in the Physical World").

Auditory Illusions

Auditory illusions are similar to visual illusions, or metamorphopsias. Patients perceive sounds as being either louder than reality, a condition known as *hyperacusia,* or softer than reality, known as *hypoacusia.* Modifications of tone and timbre have also been reported in cases of auditory illusions. Localization of sounds in space may be perceived as being more distant or as being closer, as in telescopic illusions, or pelopsia in visual illusions. The localization of lesions remains unclear, but it may involve cortical areas in and around the transverse gyri, as well as the peripheral level of the auditory system.

Illusions and Disturbances of Brain Information Processing

In a manner similar to hallucinations, illusions may be explained by disturbances in the bidirectional system of recognition for objects and movements. It is possible that feature recognition consists of two

191

*Disorders of
Recognition in the
Physical World:
Illusions and
Hallucinations*

levels of processing—high-level processing, in which a list of the proto-types for particular features is connected via bottom-up and top-down processing, and lower-level processing, in which a row assessment of features is performed. In normal conditions, an adaptive resonance is established between these two levels for the assessment of such features as size, shape, and color. In cases of illusions, this adaptive resonance may become tonically hyperactive, bringing to conscious vision the image of an object of increased or diminished size, changed shape, and so forth.

HALLUCINATIONS

A HALLUCINATION IS DEFINED by the *DSM–IV–TR* as "a sensory perception that has the compelling sense of reality of a true perception but that occurs without external stimulation of the relevant sensory organ" (p. 823).

Hallucinations were originally defined by Esquirol (1814) as perceptions without the presence of objects. Jasper (1963) stressed that hallucinations occur simultaneously with perceptions of reality. Vivid mental images differ from hallucinations in that in the first case, vivid images are perceived as coming from an internal source of information, while hallucinations are perceived as being real sensory experiences and are often included in a correctly perceived scene. A patient may see a hallucinatory object included in a real visual scene, for example, or may perhaps hear hallucinatory voices while engaging in conversation with a real individual. In some cases, hallucinations have been reported to occupy entire scenes and may be difficult to differentiate from dreams. Though an individual may recognize and acknowledge that his or her hallucinations are not truly objective, he or she may not be able to voluntarily suppress them.

Hallucinations are categorized according to the sensory modality involved in the false perception—including auditory, visual, somatic, tactile, and gustatory hallucinations—and may be complex, involving two or more modalities. Elementary hallucinations involve primary sensations, such as noises or light flashes, as well as partially or entirely complex hallucinations, involving animals, humans, or perhaps even entire scenes. Hallucinations similar to dreams may develop in the course of falling asleep (hypnagogic hallucinations), or while waking up (hypnopompic hallucinations).

Elementary and complex hallucinations have been described in patients with psychiatric manifestations of various neurological brain diseases and disturbances at the peripheral levels of the sensory system. Visual hallucinations have been reported more frequently, and may

192

LOCALIZATION
OF CLINICAL
SYNDROMES IN
NEUROPSYCHOLOGY
AND NEUROSCIENCE

be accompanied by auditory hallucinations in some cases. Visual and auditory hallucinations are observed especially frequently in patients with epilepsy and are also often reported in patients with brain tumors, infections, and in a few rare cases, strokes. Visual hallucinations, and less frequently auditory hallucinations, have been described in cases of progressive degenerative dementia, such as that suffered during the course of Alzheimer's disease and Huntington's disease. They may also be caused by alcohol withdrawal, various psychomimetic drugs, and medications, as well as by sensory deprivation.

The presence of elementary hallucinations, especially of a verbal nature, is one of the primary symptoms of schizophrenia. These hallucinations have also been noted, though infrequently, in patients with affective psychosis. Schizophrenic patients may perceive these elementary auditory hallucinations as a confirmation of their delusions. Auditory hallucinations of rattling machinery, for example, are considered to be proof that someone is trying to hurt the patient, while a strange noise is thought to be produced by devices that are being used to spy on the patient. The inclusion of elementary and verbal hallucinations in the delusional system is in fact quite common in patients with schizophrenia.

Gustatory and olfactory hallucinations have frequently been observed in patients with brain tumors and in patients with epilepsy, often as an aura before a seizure.

Somatognosic hallucinations may be perceived during simple and complex partial seizures, epileptic auras, or migraine attacks, and are usually short in duration, lasting for only seconds or minutes (Hécaen & Albert, 1978; Kenna & Sedman, 1965). When suffered following a stroke or head injury, or during the course of a brain tumor growth, an infectious illness, or a toxic or metabolic disorder, however, somatognosic hallucinations may persist for hours, days, or even months (Cummings, 1992). Somatic hallucinations such as autoscopy, or the feeling of another presence, may be observed especially frequently in patients with schizophrenia and in some cases of affective psychosis.

AUDITORY HALLUCINATIONS

Clinical Aspects

Two major types of auditory hallucinations have been described thus far—elementary hallucinations and complex, usually verbal, hallucinations.

Elementary auditory hallucinations are described by patients as an unstructured sound, such as a buzzing, a hum, blowing wind, or trickling water. The sounds may have a rhythmic, pulsating nature resembling the rattling of an engine or the ticking of a clock.

193

*Disorders of
Recognition in the
Physical World:
Illusions and
Hallucinations*

Complex auditory hallucinations, on the other hand, include verbal and musical hallucinations. A patient with verbal hallucinations hears single words or sentences that seem to come from one or several voices. These hallucinatory voices were termed *phonemes* by Wernicke in 1900, as cited by Hamilton (1985) and Sims (1988). This term was used for many years in the old German and Continental European psychiatry, but was eventually abandoned due to the use of the same word in linguistics, in which phonemes are considered to be the units of speech sounds that form spoken words.

Verbal hallucinations may consist of orders given directly to the subject, experiences known as imperative hallucinations. A patient suffering from such hallucinations, however, does not often follow the commands given by the voice or voices. The voices are often described as being abusive, accusing the patient of improper behavior. In some cases, the voices are reported as discussing the patient's behavior without directly addressing their comments to the patient. These discussions may be perceived by the patient as overheard conversations. In other cases, the topic of discussion of such voices has reportedly been of a neutral nature.

The voices heard in verbal hallucinations may be clear, located in space, and ascribed to a certain individual. Patients often note, however, that the voices are vague and difficult to describe. A patient may be unable to clearly identify the acoustic features of the voice, such as its timbre, tone, and gender, or the origin and direction from which the voice is coming. Peculiar types of hallucinatory voices have been described in patients suffering from schizophrenia. In such cases, a patient may hear a loud voice, which may seem to originate either internally or externally, and which speaks the patient's own internal thoughts, a phenomenon known as *Gedankenlautwerden* in German, and as *"echo de pensées"* in French (Hamilton, 1985). The appropriate English term would probably be *audible thoughts* (Sims, 1988). Schneider (1930, 1959) included this type of verbal hallucination as one of the major features of the first rank symptoms of schizophrenia.

Musical hallucinations are described by patients as perceived songs or melodies. They may be clearly recognized as the work of a chorus or an orchestra, or perhaps as music from a particular instrument or singer, which is most common.

Anatomical Aspects
Elementary and Verbal Auditory Hallucinations
Primarily elementary auditory hallucinations may be observed in patients with peripheral hearing problems. These hallucinations may manifest as tinnitus and as unstructured sounds of varying pitch and timbre. Progressive bilateral hearing loss may also produce verbal and musical hallucinations.

194

LOCALIZATION
OF CLINICAL
SYNDROMES IN
NEUROPSYCHOLOGY
AND NEUROSCIENCE

Elementary and verbal auditory hallucinations are often experienced by patients with temporal lobe seizures, in many cases representing an ictal event (Hécaen & Albert, 1978; Penfield & Erickson, 1941). Seizures accompanied by auditory hallucinations, elementary and verbal, are most frequently reported in patients with tumors of the temporal lobes (Courville, 1928; Hécaen, 1972; Hécaen & de Ajuriaguerra, 1956). Hécaen and de Ajuriaguerra (1956) observed auditory hallucinations of a paroxysmal type in 8 of 61 patients with temporal lobe tumors, and in only 1 of 80 patients with frontal lobe tumors and 2 of 61 patients with mesencephalic tumors. No clear prevalence of left or right hemisphere lesions has been reported in cases of auditory hallucinations.

The role of the temporal lobe in the development of auditory hallucinations has also been demonstrated in studies of patients with schizophrenia. Barta, Pearlson, Powers, Richards, and Tune (1990) used a quantitative MRI study to measure the volume of different brain regions in 15 young patients with schizophrenia. The brain regions measured in the study included the superior temporal gyrus, the amygdala, the third ventricle, the midbrain area, and the pons. The control group included 15 subjects matched to those of the schizophrenic group by age, race, and education. The subjects in the schizophrenia group were noted as having a smaller left and right superior temporal lobe volume and a smaller left amygdala than the control subjects. In general, the brains of the schizophrenic patients were overall 2% smaller than those of the control subjects, with the right temporal lobe being 10% smaller, and the left temporal lobe being 7% smaller. There was a positive correlation between the percentage difference in the volume of the left temporal lobe and the auditory hallucination severity score as obtained from the Scale for Assessment of Positive Symptoms.

Several studies have demonstrated the role of functional changes, primarily in the superior temporal region, in the development of auditory hallucinations. These studies employed the use of auditory testing accompanied by electrical stimulation, PET scans and fMRI measurements of blood flow.

Electrical stimulation of the anterior transverse gyrus during the course of surgical treatment for epilepsy was shown to produce an auditory sensation (Penfield & Rassmusen, 1950). Patients reported these sensations as "ringing, humming, rushing, chirping, buzzing, knocking, and rumbling" noises. The sounds were often attributed to the opposite ear and were often described not as random, unstructured sounds but as a more structured sound belonging to certain objects, such as wind blowing through a tree, a train passing by on a nearby railroad, or the slamming of a door. Penfield and Perot (1963) described patient S.B. (Case 29), who reported hearing "buzzing" immediately after an electrode was inserted into the anterior transverse gyrus. When the electrode was moved to the cortex of the first temporal gyrus, the patient, apparently experiencing a verbal hallucination, yelled out, "Someone is calling!" In addition to sounds resulting from the stimulation of the anterior transverse gyrus, various sounds could be also produced via the electrical stimulation of the amygdala and hippocampus (Horowitz, Adams, & Rutkin, 1968).

According to Penfield and Perot (1963), the cortical points for the auditory experiential responses, which included a voice, multiple voices, music, or a meaningful sound, were strictly limited to the lateral and superior surface of the first temporal convolution. The authors observed and recorded 48 experiential responses of patients, noting 24 responses in the nondominant hemisphere and 24 responses in the dominant hemisphere of nine patients.

In a study of our own (Bajhin, Wasserman, & Tonkonogy, 1975), thresholds of tone durations of anywhere from 1 to 1000 msec were employed to evaluate the possible involvement of the temporal lobe in the development of auditory hallucinations. We had previously shown that the shortening of a signal to 10 msec, and especially to 1 msec, resulted in a greater increase in the absolute threshold of the tone in the ear contralateral to the lesion in the posterior part of the superior temporal lobe, with the possible involvement of the transverse gyri (Baru, Gershuni, & Tonkonogy, 1964). In a subsequent study, a group of 10 patients, each suffering from paranoid schizophrenia and verbal auditory hallucinations, helped to demonstrate that absolute thresholds of 1000 msec–length tone were symmetrical with differences not exceeding 1.1 db between the right ear and the left ear (Bajhin et al., 1975). A shortening of signal led to significant asymmetry, with thresholds increasing more in the right ear than the left ear. These differences reached 4.6 + 1.6 db ($p < 0.05$) for tone durations of 10 msec, and 8.2 + 2.7 db ($p < 0.01$) for tone durations of 1 msec (see Figure 4.1). The thresholds also increased with the shortening of the signal from 1000 msec to 1 msec both for a group of 12 patients with paranoid schizophrenia, but with an absence of auditory hallucinations, and for a group of 10 normal control subjects. The observed right-left ear differences in absolute thresholds for 1000 msec, 100 msec, 10 msec, and 1 msec were insignificant and did not exceed 0.9 db, even for short duration signals.

Similar asymmetry was found in studies of dichotic listening for fused words in 32 patients with schizophrenia, 65 depressed patients, and 14 normal controls (Bruder et al., 1995). The authors of these studies confirmed the earlier results of Wexler, Giller, and Southwick (1991), who found a decrease in the right ear advantage. This decrease is correlated with positive symptoms in schizophrenia.

An increase in right ear thresholds for tones of short duration in our study pointed to the involvement of the superior part of the left

196

LOCALIZATION
OF CLINICAL
SYNDROMES IN
NEUROPSYCHOLOGY
AND NEUROSCIENCE

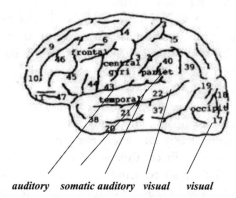

auditory   somatic auditory visual   visual

FIGURE 4.1   Left hemisphere. Localization of lesions in auditory, visual, and somatic hallucinations. Similar sites of lesions may be found in the right hemisphere. The figure shows that the temporal lobe is a predominant lesion site for auditory and visual hallucinations, while the parietal lobe is implicated in somatic hallucinations. Other sites of lesions for visual hallucinations include structures within the deep white matter of the temporal lobe, such as the hippocampus and the amygdala, as well as mesencephalic structures and the upper brain stem for hypnagogic and hypnopompic hallucinations.

temporal lobe contralateral to that ear in the development of auditory verbal hallucinations in patients with paranoid schizophrenia. It is of interest that asymmetry for thresholds of short duration tones was no longer noted in three of our cases in which hallucinations were eventually controlled by medication, pointing to the role of functional changes in the development of hallucinations.

Several studies of auditory hallucinations in schizophrenic patients have been based on the use of MRI scans. Barta et al. (1990) employed the MRI scans to study gyral volumes of the temporal lobe, amygdala, third ventricle, midbrain, and pons in 15 outpatients suffering from schizophrenia, with a mean age of 40.6 ± 4.6 years; a control group consisted of 15 subjects matched for gender, race, and age. According to MRI scans, the schizophrenic patients had smaller superior temporal gyri bilaterally, smaller left amygdalae, and larger third ventricles than the matched control subjects. There was a positive correlation between the size reductions in the superior temporal gyri and the hallucination severity scores on the Scale of Assessment of Positive Symptoms. Similar size reductions of the left superior temporal gyrus and the left anterior hippocampus-amygdala region were reported by Shenton, Kikinis, and Jolesz (1992). These authors used MRI scans for the volumetric study of temporal lobe structures in 15 patients with schizophrenia and 15 matched controls. The volume of the superior frontal gyrus did not differ between patients and controls. Size reductions in the left posterior T1, as evaluated in 13 patients, correlated with scores on the thought-disorder index.

As may be expected, studies commissioning the use of PET and fMRI scans have demonstrated that the areas of increased or decreased blood flow in patients with hallucinations cover many brain regions involved in speech and language processing, as well as other functions. A decrease in blood flow measured via PET scans in patients with auditory hallucinations, however, was observed in auditory and Wernicke's regions by Cleghorn et al. (1992), who also found that relative metabolism was significantly correlated with hallucination scores in the striatal and cingular regions. The authors used PET scans with 18 F-fluorodeoxyglucose to study brain metabolism in 12 patients with schizophrenia, each of whom experienced auditory hallucinations during glucose uptake; the same technique was employed in the study of 10 schizophrenic patients with histories of auditory hallucinations, none of whom experienced hallucinations during the glucose uptake. In patients who experienced hallucinations, lower relative metabolism was found in the primary auditory areas and in the right superior temporal region, while trends toward a higher relative metabolism were revealed in the right hemisphere region homologous to Broca's area. Hallucination scores correlated positively with relative metabolism in the striatal and anterior cingulate regions.

Shergill, Brammer, Williams, Murray, and McGuire (2000) reported fMRI data that showed the activation of blood flow bilaterally in the temporal cortex (with a greater response on the right) in hallucinating patients; other areas of increased activation included the inferior frontal cortex, the insula, the anterior cingular cortex, the right thalamus, the inferior colliculus, the left hippocampus, and the parahippocampal cortex. The study was based on the fMRI recording of six patients with schizophrenia, each of whom experienced hallucinations during the recording, in comparison with brain activation in the same patients during periods of no hallucination. Interpretations of these data include suggestions that the development of hallucinations, in addition to the activation of the right superior and middle temporal gyri, is mediated by an "attentional network" in the anterior cingulate and right thalamus, as well as an "emotional network" in the bilateral insula and the left parahippocampal gyri, as well as in the prefrontal cortex, which is involved with executive function and the impulse control mechanism. Woodruff (2004) also discussed the involvement of various mechanisms based on the different cortical areas in the development of auditory verbal hallucinations, including the effect of attention on cortical sensory responses, emotional responses, memory, volition and verbal self-monitoring, and impulse control. These PET scans and fMRI findings and their interpretations must be analyzed with some degree

198

LOCALIZATION
OF CLINICAL
SYNDROMES IN
NEUROPSYCHOLOGY
AND NEUROSCIENCE

of caution since PET and fMRI scans often produce signs of simultaneous activation in multiple brain areas, while the origin and functional significance of such activation remain unclear and may be related in some cases to the general blood flow changes that are not directly related to brain activation in the targeted areas.

At the same time, a number of fMRI studies have reported significant activation of the right or bilateral STG (superior temporal gyrus) areas during auditory hallucinations, but with brain activation recorded in other areas as well (David, 2001; Lenox & Lowe, 1996). David (2001) examined patients suffering from schizophrenia via the use of fMRI scans during the period of active auditory hallucinations as well as during times in which neuroleptics helped to control the hallucinations. He first studied one patient with schizophrenia and auditory verbal hallucinations, then confirmed the results in a group of seven similar patients. The author observed a reduction in blood flow in the posterior part of the superior temporal gyrus while the patient was listening to the hallucinated speech. The same area became activated when the patient was listening to the hallucinated speech, but with his or her hallucinations disappearing shortly thereafter following treatment with neuroleptics. David (2001) concluded that the pathology underlying the development of hallucinations was functional, and not anatomical.

Musical Hallucinations.   Musical hallucinations may be observed in patients with brain tumors or with an AV malformation involving the left or the right temporal lobe. Fay and Scott (1939) observed a 45-year-old woman who developed a hallucination of "quartets" singing hymns and dance songs, along with episodes of anomia and jargon aphasia; following the removal of the left occipito-temporal meningioma, which had been producing seizures, the woman's hallucinations stopped. Penfield and Erickson (1941) reported musical hallucinations in two patients, each with a meningioma growing from the olfactory groove and suppressing the pole of the left temporal lobe; in one patient, a glioma was infiltrating the second temporal gyrus in the right hemisphere. Keshavan, Brar, and Kahn (1988) reported a 43-year-old man who developed psychotic symptoms with hallucinations of an orchestra playing primarily instrumentally a "monotonous march" in his head; the development of the patient's hallucinations followed the removal of a right frontoparietal meningioma. Keshavan, David, Steingard, and Lishman (1992) reported a 28-year-old woman who developed musical hallucinations along with persecutory delusions following the removal of a right parieto-temporal AV malformation; the reported musical hallucinations consisted of traffic noise and melodies such as "Mary Had a Little Lamb."

199

*Disorders of
Recognition in the
Physical World:
Illusions and
Hallucinations*

Peripheral lesions of the auditory system may also produce musical hallucinations. Such hallucinations in acquired deafness have been described in multiple cases; (Aizenberg, Scwartz, & Modai, 1986; Hammeke, Mcquillen, & Cohen, 1983; Miller & Crosby, 1979; Ross, Jossman, Bell, Sabin, & Geschwind, 1975). In several cases, musical hallucinations developed in patients with partial hearing loss following either a brain stem stroke or a midbrain tumor. Lanska, Lanska, and Mendez (1987) described a 55-year-old patient who, after suffering a stroke, developed slurred speech and right-sided weakness. He complained of hearing low-pitched, slow "musical sounds in both ears." Several days later, the auditory hallucinations became "like people talking" and "like continuous rain falling on a roof." Audiometry revealed bilateral moderate sensorineural hearing loss. Head CT and MRI scans revealed a left-sided pontine hemorrhage involving the caudal half of the pontine tegmentum, including the dorsal and medial acoustic striate. Brain stem auditory hallucinations were also present in three cases described by Cascino and Adams (1986). Hearing loss was present in all three cases. Two patients had suffered from a vascular lesion of the rostral pontine tegmentum; the third patient had a lower midbrain tumor. Hearing loss was also present in cases reported by Murata, Naritomi, and Sawada (1994). One patient developed auditory musical hallucinations lateralized to the right ear following a stroke with a hemorrhage at the right pontine tegmentum. Two years prior to the stroke, the patient had suffered from a mild left-sided hemiparesis secondary to a lacunar infarction in the right internal capsule.

Halgren, Babb, and Crandall (1978) performed a study in which electrical stimulation produced hallucinations of music, which consisted of an orchestra, voices singing, a piano playing, a choir, and a radio theme song. The localization of stimulation points was in the superior temporal convolution on either the lateral or the superior surface in the left or right hemisphere. Hallucinations of music were produced from 17 points in 11 cases.

VISUAL HALLUCINATIONS

Clinical Aspects

Elementary visual hallucinations consist of unformed images of phosphenes, which are flashes of bright lights that appear as lights that flicker and dance, shadows that move up and down, whirling colored balls, radiating gray spots that then become pink and blue, long white marks, colorless or blue stars, circles, spots, and so forth.

Complex visual hallucinations include images of primarily people and animals moving in correctly perceived space and incorporated into that space by the hallucinating subject. "Strange men," for example,

200

LOCALIZATION
OF CLINICAL
SYNDROMES IN
NEUROPSYCHOLOGY
AND NEUROSCIENCE

may be perceived by the patient as sitting around the table in the patient's room or on a deck, or deceased relatives or friends may appear in the patient's room. One of our patients, an immigrant from Russia, who was suffering from Lewy body dementia, told his wife that a Red Army soldier was in the room asking the patient to go with him, then asked his wife to pack his belongings needed for the trip. Another patient, who was in the early stages of Alzheimer's disease, saw "an animal, probably a rat" that would suddenly appear near his legs but then "run out if somebody would enter the room"; the patient also developed persecutory delusions, claiming that the animal was put in the room by a neighbor who was trying to harass the patient. In cases of alcohol withdrawal, the hallucinating patient may see small animals, or perhaps bugs on his clothes or blanket; this may be accompanied by tactile hallucinations of something crawling on the skin.

Palinopsia is a condition of abnormal visual perseveration in which an object image remains in the visual field after that object has been removed. This visual perseveration may spontaneously recur for hours or even days. Palinopsia may develop and then abruptly disappear in patients with brain tumors, head injuries, and strokes. In some cases, however, palinopsia may continue to recur for years (Cummings, Syndulko, Goldberg, & Treiman, 1982).

Visual hallucinations have frequently been observed in the hemianopic field. Patients may sometimes experience *extracampine hallucinations,* a condition in which visual hallucinatory images appear beyond one's visual field, usually in the back of the head. Visual hallucinations may be associated with the emotional affect of terror or fear; pleasant feelings may also accompany visual hallucinations in some cases.

In cases of *scenic hallucinations,* the visual field is completely occupied by a hallucinatory image that consists of a landscape or an event. Scenic hallucinations often represent a vivid memory of events that occurred many years ago in the patient's life. Penfield and Perot (1963) called such images experiential hallucinations in cases of seizure disorders, and experiential responses when they were produced by the electrical stimulation of certain areas of the brain.

Another type of complex visual complex hallucination produces a dreamy or oneiroid state. In this case, patients perceive complex and precise scenes from their past, often seeing themselves as participants in the event (Hécaen & Albert, 1978). This dreamy state was first described by Jackson (1888), who reported the case of a 37-year-old man who had attacks in which he saw "things from boyhood's day." Another patient saw large buildings he had once seen "near a church, close to its wall" and, during another attack, he "could actually see the clock" on the building. In some cases, the scene is ill defined, imprecise, and perceived by the patient as being fantastic. A patient may dream, for

201

*Disorders of
Recognition in the
Physical World:
Illusions and
Hallucinations*

example, of participating in space explorations and collecting peculiar diamonds on the moon, or perhaps of wandering among the dinosaurs during prehistoric times. On a more somber note, other patients may perceive the annihilation of the world, seeing pictures of the death of millions of people, the destruction of cities, and collisions between planets.

In dreamy states, patients may feel somewhat drowsy and confused, perhaps experiencing hallucinated visions that reflect distorted scenes from the external world and perceiving themselves as active participants in such scenes. The hallucinations are reported to be quite vivid and somewhat similar to dreams. They differ from hallucinations in delirium in that images seen in states of delirium are more fantastic in nature. In cases of delirium, images of animals, dead bodies, bugs, and monsters follow each other, but with no apparent connections. Dreamy states are characterized by more systematized, logically connected scenes and fantasies. One of our patients during such attacks would sit in the chair appearing drowsy and unresponsive, but after the episode she reported her participation in the "soap opera with Mel Gibson. . . . I would like to invite Mel and the other participants to my home and get them acquainted with my parents." In some cases, hallucinations can become threatening and can provoke a motor response from the patient.

The recognition of one's surroundings may be changed by feelings of familiarity in previously unknown places, otherwise known as *déjà vu*. A patient may also feel that a well-known situation is completely new and has never been seen or experienced before, a condition known as *jamais vu*.

Hypnagogic and *hypnopompic hallucinations* are other types of primarily scenic hallucinations, which develop either when a subject is about to fall asleep (hypnagogic) or, less frequently, when a subject wakes up during the night (hypnopompic). Though the hallucinations are often visual and/or auditory, somesthetic hallucinations have also been described (Roth, 1980). Somesthetic hallucinations are vivid and often terrifying, but may be pleasant in some cases. The content of a hallucination is sometimes difficult to differentiate from one's own dreams, as insight is often absent during the development of such hallucinations. Later on, however, the patient does usually recognize the alien character of the hallucination.

Pseudo-hallucinations constitute another type of hallucinations that are similar to the dreams and vivid mental images previously mentioned. Like "regular" hallucinations, pseudo-hallucinations are vivid, colored, and persistent and occur in the absence of real objects. They may be visual and auditory, as well as tactile in some cases. The difference lies in the fact that a sufferer from pseudo-hallucinations

202

LOCALIZATION
OF CLINICAL
SYNDROMES IN
NEUROPSYCHOLOGY
AND NEUROSCIENCE

perceives a subject as figurative, "not real," and located in the subjective space being perceived by an inner eye or ear (Sims, 1988). Following their original description by Kandinsky (cited by Sims, 1988), pseudo-hallucinations were analyzed in detail by Jasper (1963), who stressed the presence of gradations between pseudo-hallucinations and vivid imagery. Pseudo-hallucinations have been reported in patients with a wide variety of psychiatric disturbances, including schizophrenia, mood disorders, and histrionic personality disorder, as well as being experienced due to the effects of hallucinogenic drugs and in the course of sensory deprivation. The concept of pseudo-hallucinations and their very existence as a separate form different from "regular" hallucinations has, however, been questioned in the literature (see Hamilton, 1985). The term has not yet been included in previous editions of the *Diagnostic and Statistical Manual,* and *DSM–IV–TR* (2000, p. 823) stresses that "no distinction is made as to whether the source of the voice is perceived as being inside or outside the head."

Anatomical Aspects
Temporal and Occipital Lobes

Brain Tumors. Hécaen and de Ajuriaguerra (1956) observed visual hallucinations in patients with tumors localized in various cerebral regions, primarily in posterior parts of the cerebral hemispheres and the mesodiencephalic region, including 10 of 75 patients (13.3%) with temporal lobe tumors, 6 of 24 patients (24%) with occipital lobe tumors, and 8 of 61 patients (13.11%) with mesodiencephalic tumors. Visual hallucinations were observed in only 5 of 80 patients (6.25%) with frontal lobe tumors, compared to 13–24% of patients with temporal and occipital tumors. Subtentorial tumors led to visual hallucinations in 6 of 85 patients (7.95%), primarily of the elementary types (four of six cases), as may be expected in cases with the involvement of the more peripheral region of the visual pathways.

Hécaen (1972) found that in 13 of 16 cases of auditory hallucinations, the left hemisphere was responsible, including 10 cases of left hemisphere involvement in patients with complex musical and verbal hallucinations. Each hemisphere was involved equally in elementary hallucinations and dreamy states.

The development of both elementary and complex visual hallucinations was also described in cases of patients with tumors in the temporal and occipital lobes (Gibbs, 1932; Tarachow, 1941). Sanford and Bair (1939) studied 211 cases of temporal lobe tumors and 45 cases of occipital lobe tumors. The authors found 22 cases with visual hallucinations, 11 of which were of elementary types out of the cases with temporal lobe tumors, and four cases of visual hallucinations, two of which were of elementary types out of the cases with occipital lobe tumors.

Seizures. Elementary visual hallucinations are usually observed when seizure activity develops in the occipital lobe (Penfield & Erickson, 1941). The visual sensations include moving and spinning lights, colors, and lines. The patient may see the images either in the visual field contralateral to the damaged hemisphere or, as is more often the case, straight ahead in the central visual field. Complex visual hallucinations are rarely noted during occipital lobe seizures.

Complex visual hallucinations in patients with temporal lobe seizures may consist of visual images of animals, humans, and various objects. The images are usually described as possessing the shape, color, and/or size of real objects (Hécaen & Albert, 1978). A patient may be either terrified or pleased, depending on the nature of the hallucinated scene, but his or her insight into the artificial nature of the hallucinations may be either absent or limited in the course of the event. The subject may later describe the hallucinations in full detail, however, and begin to recognize their nonrealistic nature. The localization of lesions may include not only the temporal lobe but other regions as well, including the frontal lobe, the mesodiencephalic region, and even brain stem regions (Hécaen & de Ajuriaguerra, 1956).

Dreamy states have been associated with temporal lobe lesions since the early reports by Jackson (1876), and were described as "uncinate fits" by a series of authors (see review by Hécaen & Albert, 1978). Hécaen and Albert (1978) observed dreamy states in patients with temporal lobe tumors in 5 out of 75 patients, while similar hallucinations were reported in only 1 of 24 patients with occipital lobe tumors. Penfield and his colleagues stressed that this type of hallucination was related to one's memory and the recollection of past events, and recorded such a state during electrical stimulations of the temporal lobe, using the term *experiential responses* to define the nature of such states (Penfield & Erickson, 1941; Penfield & Jasper, 1954; Penfield & Perot, 1963; Penfield & Rasmussen, 1950).

In cases of palinopsia, lesions are localized in the posterior area of the right hemisphere in most cases (Kinsbourne & Warrington, 1963; Meadows & Munro, 1977). Hécaen and Albert (1978) stressed that, according to their literature review, palinopsia is associated with occipital lesions.

Experiential visual hallucinations combined with auditory hallucinations were often described by Penfield and Perot (1963) as part of the seizure experience in 53 out of 520 patients with temporal lobe seizures. No case of an experiential hallucination was found when the focus of the seizure activity was outside the temporal regions in the case histories of 1,132 patients suffering from local seizures who underwent surgery for the treatment of epilepsy. Visual experiential hallucinations were found to occur in 15 nondominant hemisphere cases

204

LOCALIZATION
OF CLINICAL
SYNDROMES IN
NEUROPSYCHOLOGY
AND NEUROSCIENCE

and in six dominant hemisphere cases. Auditory experiential hallu-cinations showed a reverse pattern—four cases with a nondominant hemisphere seizure focus, and eight cases with a seizure focus in the dominant hemisphere.

Electrical Stimulation.   Electrical stimulation in the course of the surgical treatment of epilepsy produced visual and auditory elemen-tary and complex hallucinations, often of experiential response types.

Elementary visual hallucinations were produced by the stimula-tion of the lateral and medial surface of the occipital lobe (Penfield & Rasmussen, 1950). No experiential hallucinations were produced by stimulation of Brodmann's areas 17, 18, and 19. The responses included perceived images of only gross light, shadows, and colors, which were described by patients as "lights flickering, dancing, bright, fawn, or blue, stars, wheels, blue-green and red-colored discs, colored balls whirling, radiating gray spots becoming pink and blue, a long white mark, shadow moving up and down, brown squares, black wheels, colorless stars."

Lee et al. (2000) recently reported results of cortical electrical stim-ulation in 23 patients with epilepsy. In similar fashion to the results reported by Penfield and Rasmussen (1950), Lee et al. (2000) observed elementary visual hallucinations manifesting as very small spots or blobs of flashing lights when electrical stimulation was applied to the occipital lobe, and primarily to the occipital pole, the inferior occipital gyrus, or the striate cortex.

Visual elementary hallucinations of phosphene types may be produced by the electrical stimulation of the striate cortex (Chapanis, Utmatsu, Konigsmark, & Walker, 1972; Marg & Dierssen, 1965) and the parastriate cortex (Dobelle & Mladejovsky, 1974). Adams and Rutkin (1970) reported the development of phosphenes with the stimulation of the visual radiation, while stimulation of the hippocampal forma-tion produced unformed visual sensations, for example, colored balls, flashing lights, and so forth.

Experiential visual responses to electrical stimulation were usu-ally accompanied by auditory responses. According to Penfield and Perot (1963), all types of experiential responses, auditory and visual, fall within the anatomical boundaries of the temporal lobes, especially in the right temporal lobe. Most of the responses were located on the lateral and superior surface of the first temporal convolution. No re-sponse was obtained from the anterior transversal temporal gyrus, but two occurred within the posterior transverse temporal gyri. The few responses were noted from the region near the cortex of the fusiform and hippocampal gyri, which were stimulated much less often than the lateral surface.

The experiential response points were usually located between the anterior temporal gyrus and the occipital cortex. Stimulation of the occipital cortex in Penfield and Perot's patient R.W. (Case 2) produced colored flashes and light, while stimulation applied to the area immediately anterior to the occipital cortex produced the figure of robbers with guns. After an electrode was inserted into the anterior transverse gyrus of patient S.B. (Case 29), the patient immediately reported hearing a "buzzing" sound. When the electrode was moved to the cortex of the first temporal gyrus, the patient exclaimed, "Someone is calling!" (Penfield & Perot, 1963).

In the same study, Penfield and Perot (1963) described visual experiential responses, including reports of a person or group of people, a scene, or a recognizable object, in 19 patients upon the stimulation of 38 points. Nondominant hemisphere stimulation produced responses at all 38 points in all 19 patients, while dominant hemisphere stimulation produced responses at only 10 points in 7 patients. The points were scattered throughout the temporal lobe in the right hemisphere, spreading into the posterior temporal region, covering the speech area in the left hemisphere, and approaching the borders of Brodmann's area 19 in the secondary visual cortex. Most of the points on the left side were situated on the superior surface of the first temporal convolution.

Gloor, Olivier, Quesney, Andermann, and Horowitz (1982) observed experiential responses in 18 of 29 patients with temporal lobe epilepsy and chronic, stereotactically implanted cerebral electrodes. Experiential responses were recorded in most cases both in spontaneous seizures and in response to the electrical stimulation of the amygdala, the hippocampus, or both structures.

Visual hallucinations of faces, people, and objects may be produced by the electrical stimulation of the cortical surface of the anterior temporal lobe, especially with the direct activation of the amygdala and hippocampus (Baldwin, 1960; Halgren et al., 1978; Horowitz et al., 1968; Sem-Jacobsen & Torkildsen, 1960). Lee et al. (2000) noted similar reports, as well as reports of landscapes and scenes from memory, in response to the stimulation of wider areas within the lateral temporal lobe, the lateral occipito-temporal junction areas, and the basal occipito-temporal region.

Stimulation of the right, compared to the left, temporal lobe results in more frequent complex visual hallucinations, while stimulation of the right hippocampus may produce dream-like experiential responses, or *déjà vu* (Halgren et al., 1978). Stimulation of the occipital lobe may also produce complex visual hallucinations. Foerster (1931) described a patient who tried to catch a butterfly that he perceived when Brodmann's area 19 in the occipital lobe was electrically stimulated.

206

LOCALIZATION
OF CLINICAL
SYNDROMES IN
NEUROPSYCHOLOGY
AND NEUROSCIENCE

Stroke. Hallucinations following a stroke may be seen, but they are extremely rare and occur primarily in cases with posterior hemisphere lesions.

Starkstein, Robinson, and Berthier (1992) examined the records of a 10-year period of admission to the stroke unit and found only five patients who developed hallucinations following a stroke. All five patients had suffered from a right hemisphere lesion, with cortical lesions in four of the cases, according to the head CT data. The lesions involved posterior regions of the right hemisphere in all four cases, often with extensions into the two or three adjacent lobes. Extension of the lesion to the frontal operculum was observed in one case, and extension to the frontal region in another case. Posterior lesions included lesions in the occipital cortex in two cases, in temporal areas in two cases, and in the parietal cortex in two cases. A subcortical lesion noted in one case was characterized by the involvement of the head of the caudate, the putamen, and the internal capsule. Seizure disorders developed in three of the five patients after stroke.

Levine and Finkelstein (1982) presented eight cases of the development of hallucinations, delusions, and agitated aggressive behavior following a posterior right hemisphere stroke in seven cases and a head injury with a right temporo-parietal contusion in one case. The stroke lesions included a right occipito-parietal hemorrhage in two cases, a right temporo-parietal hemorrhage in two cases, a right temporo-parietal infarction in one case, a right temporo-parietal-occipital infarction in one case, and a right posterior embolic infarction in one case. Stroke was noted during a 1–8-month time period prior to the onset of hallucinations in six cases, and 11 years prior to the onset of hallucinations in one case. Types of hallucinations and delusions included the following: in Case 1, there was a hallucinatory experience, there were persecutory delusions (e.g., "Everyone is against me. . . . I am doomed here"), and the patient talked to herself; in Case 2, a "soft cloak" was thought to be placed over the patient's left arm and both shoulders, and at night, a broadcaster's voice was heard repeating the same things, classical music interrupted by "Happy Birthday" was heard, loud and insulting voices were perceived, and God was seen as a glorious light that followed her, but she was lucid in the daytime; in Case 3, there were visual hallucinations and illusions of human forms, delusions of being spied upon, and delusions that listening devices had been placed in her house; in Cases 2, 7, and 8, there were pure hallucinations; in other cases, persecutory ideation, agitation, aggressive behavior, fluctuating disorientation, and incoherent thoughts were reported. Seven of the eight patients had seizures—generalized in one patient, and local, leftward turning of the head and eyes and paresthesia, or left-sided twitching, in six cases. No seizure was reported in

207

*Disorders of
Recognition in the
Physical World:
Illusions and
Hallucinations*

Case 3, that is, the patient who had suffered from a right temporo-parietal infarction and experienced hallucinations 11 years after the stroke. There was no reported psychiatric history in any of the cases. An autopsy was performed following the Case 1 patient's death, and head CT scans were employed in Cases 1, 2, and 3. Neurological examinations probably formed the basis of the anatomic diagnoses in the remainder of the cases.

Peroutka, Sohmer, Kumar, Folstein, and Robinson (1982) reported the development of visual and auditory hallucinations in the course of a stroke in a 72-year-old woman. The patient reported seeing and hearing various people sitting at her kitchen table, were discussing her among themselves and making derogatory and vulgar remarks about her. Elementary auditory hallucinations included a loud buzzing noise, which the patient perceived as coming from a large bee. She occasionally experienced tactile hallucinations of having her hair pulled out by her visitors. Head CT scans revealed a small region of hypodensity with rim enhancement at the junction of the temporal, parietal, and occipital regions. An EEG did not show any seizure activity, but on the second day after the onset of the stroke, the patient experienced an episode of uncontrolled movements, which began in the left shoulder and subsequently spread to the entire left upper extremity. The episode lasted for approximately one minute. No similar episode was observed at any other time.

As with the cases involving a single stroke, hallucinations in multi-infarct dementia have been reported in a small number of patients. Cummings, Miller, Hill, and Neshkes (1987) described visual hallucinations in 4 of 15 patients with multi-infarct dementia in the earlier stages of the disease. Three patients were experiencing visual hallucinations, including one patient with a combination of visual and auditory hallucinations. Visual hallucinations were registered in the homonymous field defect in two of the three patients. A marked decrease in vision to 20/800 bilaterally was present in the third case. This may be compared with data from the literature, which relate the development of hallucinations to peripheral sensory losses, or hemianopsia.

In a vascular dementia case of our own, a 79-year-old woman reported seeing several males sitting around the table and "discussing something" on the deck of her house. Head CT scans revealed a large infarction in the cortex and the subcortical white matter of the left occipital lobe.

In summary, visual and auditory hallucinations were observed primarily after stroke with localization of cerebral infarctions or hemorrhages in the posterior parts of the cerebral hemisphere, and more frequently in the right than in the left. Seizures often accompanied the development of hallucinations after stroke.

208

LOCALIZATION
OF CLINICAL
SYNDROMES IN
NEUROPSYCHOLOGY
AND NEUROSCIENCE

The development of a specific type of hypnagogic hallucinations was reported in patients following a stroke in the upper brain stem.

Mesencephalic Region, Upper Brain Stem

Hypnagogic and hypnopompic hallucinations have frequently been observed in patients suffering from narcolepsy. The seizure focus in narcolepsy is probably localized in the mesencephalic region. Visual hallucinations resembling hypnagogic and hypnopompic hallucinations were also described in cases of upper brain stem lesions.

L'Hermitte (1922) described a 72-year-old woman who suffered from a severe vertiginous attack. Several days later she demonstrated a palsy of the sixth cranial nerve, as well as an intentional tremor of the right upper limb. Another few days later, she developed an involvement of the third and fourth cranial nerves, a right hemiparesis with positive Babinski's sign. Two weeks later, the patient reported seeing animals of bizarre appearance, but as soon as she tried to touch them they disappeared through the floor. The patient perceived these images as unreal illusions. She also reported the transformation of the animals into human figures, such as children playing with dolls. The patient also suffered from afternoon somnolence and insomnia at night. The hallucinosis became less frequent following neurological recovery.

L'Hermitte indicated that clinical findings point to an upper mid-brain lesion in this case. He stressed the similarity of the visual hallucinations to dreaming, according to their incoherent nature, the prevalence of mobile and multiple colored images, and visuotactile associations. This type of hallucination was called hypnagogic because of the predilection for appearance during the late evening before falling asleep.

Several years later, Van Bogaert (1924) described a similar case with a pathological verification of an infarction occupying the third nerve nucleus, the inferolateral red nucleus, the superior colliculus, the periaqueductal gray matter, the decussation of the superior cerebellar peduncle, the substantia nigra, and the pulvinar nucleus. He suggested the term "peduncular hallucinosis" (Van Bogaert, 1927). L'Hermitte, Levy, and Trelles (1932) presented pathological findings in another patient with peduncular hallucinosis, in which the researchers found degeneration of the periaqueductal gray matter as well as of the oculomotor nucleus. McKee, Levine, Kowall, Resell, and Richardson (1988) described a case with only bilateral lesions of the substantia nigra, specifically of the pars reticulata.

Peduncular hallucinosis has also been described in cases with lesions in areas other than the upper brain stem. Geller and Bellur (1987) reported "peduncular hallucinosis" in a patient with a cystic craniopharyngioma compressing the brain stem. Posterior thalamic infarc-

209

Disorders of
Recognition in the
Physical World:
Illusions and
Hallucinations

tions were observed in three cases reported by De Morsier (1938), and more recently by Feinberg and Rapscak (1989) in a patient with a right paramedian thalamic infarction.

Cummings (1985) described visual hallucinations in a 78-year-old patient suffering from chromophobe adenoma of hypophysis with complex partial seizures and bilateral EEG abnormalities. The patient had also demonstrated signs of persecutory delusion and delusional jealousy.

Hallucinations Associated With Ophthalmologic Lesions

The Charles Bonnet syndrome is frequently described as a type of visual hallucination observed in elderly individuals with ocular pathology. In 1769, Charles Bonnet, a Swiss naturalist, described complex visual hallucinations accompanied by a loss of vision in his grandfather, an 89-year-old magistrate. The onset of the hallucinations had occurred following bilateral cataract extract surgery. The patient did not show any psychiatric symptoms, and his consciousness and insight were preserved. In spite of his vision loss, the patient continued to see the figures of men, women, birds, carriages, and buildings. Today, Charles Bonnet syndrome is known as a condition that is quite severe and frequently acute and develops in a person with complete or partial blindness. Elementary hallucinations may be observed during the onset of the condition, but complex visual hallucinations are eventually reported. The hallucinations are usually vivid and colorful, with movements on hallucinated scenes (Hécaen & Albert, 1978).

Fitzgerald (1971) reported the development of hallucinations in 15% of his 66 patients within 1 year of becoming blind. Cogan (1973) described visual hallucinations in 11 patients with visual losses of varying degrees. Holroyd et al. (1992) recently reported visual hallucinations in 13 of 100 consecutive patients with vision loss secondary to macular degeneration.

Lesions of optic nerves and of the optic chiasm associated with a loss of vision may also be accompanied by visual hallucinations. These are elementary hallucinations, but they may also appear as fully formed images of objects, people, animals, and scenery (Cummings, 1992). Visual hallucinations are also reported in the hemianopic field defect secondary to occipital lobe damage. Since most of the described cases with Charles Bonnet syndrome were elderly patients, it is unclear whether the development of visual hallucinations in patients with vision loss requires some additional hemispheric lesion.

OLFACTORY HALLUCINATIONS

OLFACTORY HALLUCINATIONS ARE reported as the sudden development of an odor, the smell of which is usually thought of as unpleasant.

210

LOCALIZATION
OF CLINICAL
SYNDROMES IN
NEUROPSYCHOLOGY
AND NEUROSCIENCE

Patients experiencing such hallucinations often refer to the smell of burning rubber, rotten food, and dead animals. Jackson (1876) suggested lesion localization in the uncinate region, and many researchers in the past referred to an olfactory hallucination as a "uncinate crisis." Strobos (1953) reported 62 patients with temporal lobe tumors, 34 with tumors in the right temporal lobe, and 28 with tumors in the left. Olfactory and gustatory hallucinations were present in 18 of the patients.

Hécaen and de Ajuriaguerra (1956) observed olfactory hallucinations in 7 of 75 patients (9.33%) with temporal lobe tumor, in 1 of 80 patients (1.25%) with a frontal lobe tumor (1.25%), and in 1 of 75 patients (1.33%) with a parietal lobe tumor. Penfield and Jasper (1954) noted olfactory hallucinations during the electrical stimulation of both the olfactory bulb and the uncus.

Gustatory Hallucinations

GUSTATORY HALLUCINATIONS ARE usually reported as the perception of a bad taste. They may be experienced either together with olfactory hallucinations or as an isolated symptom in patients with temporal lobe tumors, though the latter rarely occurs (Hécaen & de Ajuriaguerra, 1956). The authors reported gustatory hallucinations in 4 of 75 patients (5.33%) with temporal lobe tumors, and 1 of 75 patients (1.33%) with a parietal lobe tumor. Gibbs (1932) described 1,545 cases of brain tumors, in which he found reports of visual hallucinations in 51 cases, olfactory hallucinations in 74 cases, and gustatory hallucinations in 32 cases. Visual hallucinations developed predominantly in cases with occipital tumors and, to a lesser extent, in tumors of the thalamus and caudate nuclei. Penfield and Jasper (1954) observed gustatory sensations when electrical stimulation was applied to the areas around the insula beneath the Sylvian fissure. Stimulation of the right amygdala produced gustatory sensations.

Conclusion

1. Temporal lobe pathology is observed in most of the neurological cases of elementary, verbal, and musical hallucinations.
2. Data obtained via electrical stimulation in the course of surgical treatment for epilepsy point to the possible role of the anterior transverse gyrus in the development of elementary hallucinations. Verbal hallucinations were reported as a result of electrical stimulation of the first temporal gyrus. No clear differences were observed between the involvement of the left and right hemispheres in the development of auditory hallucinations.

3. Involvement of the peripheral auditory system may lead to the development of auditory hallucinations, most frequently of the elementary type. It is unclear what role other regions play in the development of auditory hallucinations. Further studies are needed in this area.

4. Areas involved in the development of visual hallucinations cover many brain regions, including the cerebral hemispheres, the mesencephalon, the upper brain stem, and the peripheral visual system.

5. Visual hallucinations of elementary and complex types may be most frequently observed in patients with temporal and occipital lobe lesions, in comparison to patients with parietal and frontal lobe pathology. Occipital lobe lesions, as well as manual electrical stimulation, seem to underlie the development of elementary hallucinations in a majority of cases, while experiential hallucinations and responses have usually been observed in relation to temporal lobe seizures and manual electrical stimulation. The areas within the temporal lobe that are usually implicated in the development of visual hallucinations include the first temporal gyrus and, most likely, the posterior transverse gyri.

6. The role of the hippocampal and amygdala regions has also been revealed by some of the studies. Mesencephalic and upper brain stem lesions frequently underlie the development of hypnagogic and hypnopompic hallucinations.

7. Elementary visual hallucinations, and in some cases complex visual hallucinations, have been described in patients with a peripheral loss of vision.

8. The development of olfactory and gustatory hallucinations has been reported in cases with temporal lobe tumors as well as in the course of the electrical stimulation of the olfactory bulb and uncus for the onset of olfactory hallucinations, and the amygdala and insula for the onset of gustatory hallucinations.

9. Anatomical data point to parietal lobe involvement in almost all published cases of various types of somatoagnosia, including somatic illusions and hallucinations. Extensions of lesions, primarily to the adjacent occipital and temporal areas, have been also observed in some cases.

10. Lesions in cases with somatoagnosia are more often seen in the left hemisphere than in the right hemisphere.

11. Involvement of the basal ganglia and hypophysis was reported in some of the cases with autoscopic hallucinations.

12. The development of hallucinations is frequently observed in patients with seizure disorders.

212

LOCALIZATION
OF CLINICAL
SYNDROMES IN
NEUROPSYCHOLOGY
AND NEUROSCIENCE

HALLUCINATIONS IN VARIOUS PSYCHIATRIC AND NEUROLOGICAL DISORDERS

Primary Hallucinations

Hallucinations may be reported in patients with primary psychiatric disorders, especially schizophrenia, as well as in patients with secondary psychiatric disturbances. There is a trend toward more frequent findings of auditory verbal hallucinations in patients with schizophrenia, while visual hallucinations are more frequently noted in patients with psychiatric manifestations of neurological illnesses. These differences, however, are primarily quantitative, since similar types of auditory, visual, and other types of hallucinations may be observed in both groups of patients.

Secondary Hallucinations: Brain Tumors

Hécaen and de Ajuriaguerra (1956) found various types of paroxysmal hallucinations in 58 out of 439 cases of patients with brain tumors. The frequency of hallucinations in patients with other types of tumors was as follows: relatively high in patients with temporal lobe tumors, with hallucinations being experienced by 34 of 75 patients (45%); 8 of 14 patients (33.33%) with occipital lobe tumors; 8.75% of patients with frontal lobe tumors; 12.0% of patients with parietal lobe tumors; 16.39% of patients with mesodiencephalic tumors; and, 9.41% of patients with subtentorial tumors. Specific types of hallucinations were observed more frequently in patients with tumors in particular lobes than others. Auditory, gustative, and olfactory hallucinations, as well as dreamy states, were observed primarily in patients with temporal lobe tumors, while somatognosic hallucinations were present in patients with parietal lobe tumors. Visual hallucinations developed in patients with tumors of a wide variety of localization sites, but most frequently in patients with occipital lobe, temporal lobe, and mesodiencephalic tumors. Hallucinations in patients with brain tumors were also described by Courville (1928), Tarachow (1941), and Strauss and Keschner (1935).

Hallucinations Induced by Drugs

Hallucinations may also be induced by hallucinogens, by commonly used drugs, or during alcohol and sedative withdrawal. The hallucinations experienced in such cases are usually visual. They are vivid and colorful, often including images of objects, people, and/or animals. The hallucinations usually begin with unformed images of lines, circles, and/or stars, then change into more structured objects, such as a lattice or a chessboard, and finally into fully formed images of animals, people, landscapes, and events. Auditory hallucinations are rarely observed and are limited to the perception of noise. Consciousness

213

*Disorders of
Recognition in the
Physical World:
Illusions and
Hallucinations*

may be preserved in such cases, especially in hallucinations produced by hallucinogens. Various degrees of clouding of consciousness may be present in patients with hallucinations induced by commonly used drugs and in patients experiencing hallucinations as a result of alcohol or sedative withdrawal. *Zoopsia,* or visual hallucinations of animals, is a typical occurrence in withdrawal manifestations. Acute intoxication via the use of cocaine, amphetamine, or large quantities of alcohol may produce visual hallucinations of insects, combined with tactile, or haptic, hallucinations, in which the insects are perceived as crawling on the individual's skin.

A list of hallucinogens includes (see review by Cummings, 1992) indoles (including LSD), cocaine, amphetamines, mescaline, psilocine, cannabinols, phencyclidine (PCP), nitrous oxide, and ketamine. Common drugs that may induce hallucinations, often in association with a clouding of consciousness, include numerous medications with a wide variety of chemical structures and pharmacological actions, such as antidepressants, imipramine, maprotiline, almost all known antiparkinsonian medications, hormones, steroids, tyroxin, antibiotics, penicillin, tetracycline, sulfonamide, bromides, phenacetin, digoxin, narcotics, and many others. This points to the role of general toxicity, rather than the specific influence of a particular chemical agent, in the development of hallucinations.

It is possible that the involvement of the hypothalamic and surrounding structures is primarily responsible for the hallucinogenic effects of the toxicity caused by these medications.

Withdrawal syndromes may also be manifested in the development of primarily visual hallucinations that are clinically indistinguishable from drug-induced hallucinations. Hallucinations may be produced by the fast or abrupt discontinuation of the intake of narcotics, such as alcohol, barbiturates, chloral hydrate, opioids, cocaine, or benzodiazepines, especially meprobamate. At the same time, such benzodiazepines as Librium and lorazepam are used to prevent the development of withdrawal symptoms upon the cessation of narcotics intake.

Primary Degenerative Diseases of Older Age
Alzheimer's Disease

Hallucinations are observed less frequently than delusions in cases of Alzheimer's disease, but their occurrence may still reach quite significant numbers. Rubin, Drevets, and Burke (1988) recorded visual or auditory hallucinations in 25% of 110 patients with senile dementia of the Alzheimer's type. Drevets and Rubin (1989) subsequently studied psychotic symptoms via a longitudinal study over the course of the illness and reported that hallucinations were present in 13% of the patients in the middle stages of Alzheimer's disease. Others have reported

214

LOCALIZATION
OF CLINICAL
SYNDROMES IN
NEUROPSYCHOLOGY
AND NEUROSCIENCE

the frequency of hallucinations in Alzheimer's disease as being in the range of 14% to 30% (Berrios & Brook, 1985; Kumar, Koss, & Metzler, 1988; Mendez, Martin, Smyth, & Whitehouse, 1990). Cummings et al. (1987), however, reported hallucinations in only 1 of 30 patients with Alzheimer's disease. The patient experienced auditory hallucinations in the form of voices that belonged to men who intended to harm her. This combination of hallucinations and persecutory delusions is often observed in patients with Alzheimer's disease.

Mendez et al. (1990) undertook a retrospective review of the outpatient medical charts of 217 individuals with probable Alzheimer's disease, and found that 55 of the patients (25%) had apparently experienced hallucinatory episodes. Visual hallucinations were experienced by the vast majority of the patients, in 48 of the 55 cases (87.2%), including six patients who suffered from a combination of visual and auditory hallucinations. Auditory hallucinations alone or in combination with visual hallucinations were observed in only 12 patients (21.8%), and haptic, or tactile, hallucinations were reported in two patients (3.6%). Mendez et al. (1990) also described the phenomenology of hallucinations in Alzheimer's disease. Visual hallucinations were described by patients as colorful, moving, and/or animate. The most frequent feature of a visual hallucination was humans, including both unfamiliar and familiar humans, intruders, and deceased persons (67.3%); animals were also commonly reported during hallucinatory experiences, though to a lesser extent (14%). Other types of reported hallucinations were those of complete scenes, interactions with images, and unformed vague images (21.8%). Auditory hallucinations were predominantly of a verbal type, being frequently reported as voices commenting or arguing about the patient.

Kotrla, Chacko, Harper, Jihnran, and Doody (1995) compared single proton emission computed tomography (SPECT) scans in 10 patients with Alzheimer's disease, all of whom had been experiencing hallucinations, and 36 patients who were not experiencing hallucinatory episodes, including 16 nonpsychotic patients and 20 nonhallucinating delusional patients with Alzheimer's disease. The SPECT scans of the hallucinatory patients revealed hypoperfusion of both parietal lobes; the mean and SD of the hallucinating and nonhallucinating groups were 1.83 ± 0.15 and 1.99 ± 0.18 respectively. The presence of delusions in 20 of the 36 patients in the nonhallucinating group obviously could have influenced the results.

Huntington's Disease

Dewhurst, Oliver, Trick, and McKnight (1969) reported hallucinations in 13 of 102 Huntington's disease (HD) patients, most of whom were inpatients at state mental hospitals. The hallucinations were

215

Disorders of
Recognition in the
Physical World:
Illusions and
Hallucinations

auditory in all 13 cases, and there was one case of a combination of auditory and tactile hallucinations.

Folstein, Folstein, and McHugh (1979) reported hallucinations in 63% of patients with a diagnosis of Huntington's disease, in combination with manic depression and delusions in 45% of the patients and with delusions in 18% of the patients. Folstein (1989) reported auditory, visual, and tactile hallucinations in patients with Huntington's disease. The auditory hallucinations consisted of voices commenting on the patient's behavior.

Parkinson's Disease

Hallucinations in Parkinson's patients are usually the result of either levodopa or other antiparkinsonian medications, including bromocriptine, especially in patients with a previous history of schizophrenia or affective disorders.

The development of hallucinations has also been reported in some patients with Wilson's disease and basal ganglia calcifications, as well as Fridreich's and other hereditary ataxias.

In summary, hallucinations have been described as psychiatric manifestations of various neurological illnesses. They are primarily visual, are often perceived in color, and are frequently vivid and animated. Auditory hallucinations are relatively rare in such patients with neurological illnesses. Haptic and olfactory hallucinations may also be observed in some cases, though less frequently. No significant differences have been observed between types and manifestations of hallucinations in these illnesses. All of these types of hallucinations have also been reported in patients with schizophrenia, though auditory verbal hallucinations are more frequent in schizophrenic patients than in among those with identifiable neurological illnesses, and visual hallucinations are reported more frequently in neurological illnesses with psychiatric manifestations. The origin of these differences remains unclear but may be related to the more frequent site of lesions limited to the superior-posterior part of the temporal lobe, which is involved in the processing of the auditory modality of information, and lesions found in the wide variety of cortical and subcortical areas that are related to the processing of the visual modality of information in patients with neurological manifestations of neurological illnesses.

Brain Information Processing and Hallucinations

Sensory Systems and Hallucinations

According to the anatomical data reviewed in this section, disturbances of brain information processing in hallucinations are related to the pathology localized within the same sensory systems as those that are used to process modality-specific sensory information in the course

216

LOCALIZATION
OF CLINICAL
SYNDROMES IN
NEUROPSYCHOLOGY
AND NEUROSCIENCE

of recognition. The involvement of the temporal lobe, especially the superior-posterior areas and Heschl's gyri, has been reported to be related to auditory hallucinations, while occipito-temporal lesions have been observed in cases of visual hallucinations. The role of peripheral hearing in auditory hallucinations and of vision disturbances in visual hallucinations has also been noted and described. Somatic hallucinations have been connected primarily with parietal lobe lesions.

Agnosia and Hallucinations

At the same time, in spite of the almost identical lesion sites in visual agnosia and visual hallucinations and in auditory agnosia and auditory hallucinations, the hallucinations are usually not accompanied by agnosia; the same is true for somatic agnosia and somatic hallucinations. This points to some preservation of the bottom-up and top-down processing needed for the recognition of real stimuli in patients with hallucinations. The presence of such stimuli may even help to reduce hallucinatory experiences. It may be suggested that bottom-up stimuli, using the adaptive resonance loop, activate the top-down expectation consistent with the bottom-up set of features, in this way suppressing the top-down expectations that are not supported by bottom-up stimuli as they are observed in hallucinations (Grossberg, 1980).

Patients with elementary and complex visual hallucinations often continue to correctly perceive objects and scenes as unchanged, or to hear and comprehend speech with a background of hallucinatory images, often incorporating those images into the real scenes. Usually they do not demonstrate any sign of conventional agnosia. Also, there is no direct evidence supporting the presence of unconventional agnosia in hallucinatory patients.

Similarly, we found that pure tones presented with lengths of 1 msec and 10 msec to the right ear of schizophrenics with auditory hallucinations resulted in higher absolute thresholds compared to those of schizophrenia patients without hallucinations. These differences were not observed for pure tones presented to the left ear (Bajhin et al., 1975). The observed asymmetries point primarily to the involvement of the temporal lobe in the development of auditory hallucinations.

Some indirect link between the mechanisms of unconventional agnosia and hallucinations, however, may be suggested on the basis of findings related to the increase of hallucination severity when sensory input is distorted by noise. Unconventional agnosia may similarly be uncovered by testing one's recognition with the presence of background of noise (Tonkonogy, 1973). But these similarities may be superficial to some extent. It is possible that a broad-range white noise may supply more bottom-up activity to the active component of top-down expectations, thus generating stronger hallucinations (Grossberg, 1980).

217

*Disorders of
Recognition in the
Physical World:
Illusions and
Hallucinations*

In cases of agnosia, on the other hand, the bottom-up activity distorted at the lower level increases the uncertainty and the errors made in choosing the appropriate prototype for further top-down processing. In agnosia, especially of the conventional type, the disturbances probably result primarily from impairments in bottom-up processing, while hallucinations may result from impaired top-down processing. The type of underlying disturbances is also different. Agnosia is usually the result of a relatively large lesion leading to a substantial loss of brain tissue as well as disturbances in bottom-up processing at the hierarchical stages of recognition. Hallucinations may be frequently observed during the course of either seizure or electrical stimulation of certain cortical areas, pointing to the role of excitation, probably of top-down processing, in the development of hallucinations.

Theoretical Models of Bidirectional Sensory Information Processing and Hallucinations

The latest theoretical models of hallucinations use data on the bidirectional system of recognition to explain the mechanism of hallucinations (Grossberg, 1976, 1980). This type of model was proposed earlier in consideration of information processing in normal conditions based on the added weights of selected bottom-up features to form and, later, to activate the corresponding prototypes of real objects or words in stored models or node categories (Grossberg, 1976; Kohonen, 1989; von der Malsburg, 1973). The authors came eventually to the conclusion, however, that such a system will undergo catastrophic forgetting with changes in general input conditions, and Grossberg (1976) introduced the adoptive resonance theory (ART) to demonstrate how to prevent catastrophic forgetting. It was suggested that top-down expectations may help to prevent catastrophic forgetting by selecting and amplifying the activities of cells within the learned prototype of the active category (Grossberg, 1976, 1980).

According to the theory developed by Grossberg (1980), the chosen prototype is considered to be an expectation that is transferred to the lower level for the "testing of the hypothesis" or the "reading out of the prototype" by target cells. The prototype is used for priming and matching against the bottom-up input pattern and for helping to finalize the selection and amplification of cells with the salient combinations of features that are "confirmed" by the "hypothesis." If the prototype is close enough to the input pattern, than a state of resonance develops, producing suprathresholds that excite the target cells and thus lead to conscious vision.

The top-down process on its own cannot lead to the suprathreshold experience usually produced by target cells. In cases of visual imaging, for instance, the inhibitory signals of top-down processing may

218

LOCALIZATION
OF CLINICAL
SYNDROMES IN
NEUROPSYCHOLOGY
AND NEUROSCIENCE

supress the inhibition that prevents the top-down process from activating target cells, thus leading to the generation of volitionally desired images. If this top-down signal becomes "tonically hyperactive" and fires by itself without volitional control, a suprathreshold activation of target cells may develop, and hallucinatory phenomenal perception may be experienced with the lack of bottom-up information.

Other ideas point to the possibility that mental imagery may be related to the central activation of exclusively descending pathways (Farah, 1989), while in the spillover states such as hallucinations and eidetic imagery, this activation involves the ascending pathways that are close to the descending pathways (Pollen, 1999). The phenomenal visual experience requires the activation of at least some minimal resonant loop.

Grossberg's suggestion that "tonically hyperactive" top-down processing results in hallucinations may be compared with the clinical findings of hallucination development both during the course of seizure, especially during the aura, and in response to the electrical stimulation of particular areas of the cortex during surgical treatment of temporal lobe epilepsy. In such cases, the excitation induced by the electrical current may result in the tonic hyperactivity of top-down processing.

It is possible that tonic hyperactivity may develop on different levels within the hierarchical organization of a particular recognition module. Bottom-up processing may include several processing levels. For instance, the complex features level becomes the categories level, and the simple features level, or parts of the objects level, becomes the categories level for the previous complex features level, and so on to the higher levels of abstractions. Bidirectional bottom-up and top-down processing may exist within these sublevels, making it possible for the development of hallucinations and thus reflecting the tonic hyperactivity of top-down expectations at those sublevels. Such a mechanism may underlain the development of either elementary or complex hallucinations, depending on the sublevels involved. This suggestion is somewhat supported by some differences in the sites of pathology described in patients with elementary versus complex hallucinations. Occipital lobe involvement, for example, is frequently observed in cases of elementary visual hallucinations, while temporal lobe pathology is typical for complex visual hallucinations.

Paroxysmal Activity and Hallucinations

There are some similarities between mechanisms of tonic hyperactivity in hallucinations and local paroxysmal activity observed in local partial seizures, or Jacksonian seizures. The excitation develops in the motor cortex in cases of local partial seizures, and involves the sensory, mainly top-down pathways in hallucinations. Some significant

219

*Disorders of
Recognition in the
Physical World:
Illusions and
Hallucinations*

differences should, however, be mentioned. Hallucinations may be transient in the course of an aura, but they often persist for days, months, or even years, while partial local seizures are usually transient and reappear from time to time. Partial local seizures usually respond to treatment with anticonvulsants, while the successful treatment of hallucinations often requires use of neuroleptics, pointing to the role of neurotransmitter abnormalities in the development of hallucinations. Also, the development of paroxysmal activity on EEGs in hallucinating schizophrenics has not yet been reported, and PET scans, as well as fMRI studies, often show a decrease in blood flow (not the "hot spots" typical for paroxysmal seizure activity) in the superior posterior temporal region during auditory hallucinations in patients with schizophrenia (Cleghorn et al., 1992; David, 2001). Further studies are certainly needed in this area.

5

Disturbances in the Recognition of the Social World

SOCIAL AGNOSIA

DISORDERS OF SPEECH, praxis, and gnosis were described under the general term *asymbolia* by Finkelnburg (1870). Jackson (1876) used the term *imperception* to describe disorders of object recognition and actions with objects; aphasia was identified as a separate disturbance. The disorders of object recognition were separated off as an independent syndrome by Munk (1881) who studied the results of an ablation of the occipital lobes in animals, and by Charcot (1883), Wilbrand (1887), and Lissauer (1890) in their clinical studies. Freud (1891) is responsible for actually coining the term agnosia. Liepmann (1900) showed that disorders of motor actions were independent from those of agnosia, and thus suggested the term apraxia to describe such action disorders.

At present, almost a hundred years later, the time has come to clarify and separate the symptoms of recognition and action disorders in the social world, often described under vague and general terms such as social incompetence, disorders of social judgment, and social imperfection. We prefer the use of the term *social cognition,* which has frequently been employed in cognitive neuroscience publications. As a starting point, the terms agnosia and apraxia, implying disturbances of recognition and motor actions in the physical world, may be used to delineate disturbances in the recognition of social situations and socially directed actions or behavior as *social agnosia* and *social apraxia.*

222

LOCALIZATION
OF CLINICAL
SYNDROMES IN
NEUROPSYCHOLOGY
AND NEUROSCIENCE

This may help to bring descriptions of the disorders of social gnosis and actions and their clinico-anatomical specificities in line with more clearly defined terminology, both clinically and anatomically, of disturbances in the recognition of actions in the physical world. We have described social agnosia as a type of recognition disturbance for the social world. Social apraxia is described in chapter 6, section entitled "Social Apraxia."

Agnosia is defined as a disorder of object recognition, while elementary sensations remain relatively intact. Agnosia may be visual, auditory, or tactile depending on the specific disturbed modality employed by the brain for the recognition of objects and their relationships in the *physical* world. Accommodation and adaptation to the *social* structure of the world requires the recognition of persons as participants in social interactions, their emotional and mental states, as well as their positions and roles in the interactions. This helps in anticipating future social actions and in responding appropriately to those actions, for example, by using defensive actions against a perceived threat. Disturbances in the process of social recognition may be called social agnosia.

Social agnosia may also be manifested as a difficulty in the proper positioning of the self in the social world. The patient with social agnosia may overestimate his or her achievements and relative social stature, perhaps causing him or her to insist that he or she is rich, owns the hospital, is a member of a popular profession such as that of a surgeon, especially a neurosurgeon, or is closely connected with God by being his first assistant, and so forth. The terms *grandiosity* and *grandiose delusion* are usually used to delineate this difficulty in social self-assessment. In reality, the patient is unable to correctly recognize his or her position in social space. In other cases, a patient is unable to recognize changes in the dynamics of a social situation and continues to set up and pursue financial, business, or educational plans without recognizing the real pattern of a social situation and the changes that have taken place in this pattern. Social apraxia may be secondary to social agnosia in such circumstances, and it is often difficult to distinguish between the two disturbances. The term social apractognosia may be correct, but is a bit cumbersome. The term *social agnosia and apraxia* are suggested for such disturbances.

AGNOSIA OF PERSON

AGNOSIA OF THE physical world, including various types of object and space agnosia, was described around the turn of the 20th century and has since continued to be studied, while attention began to be paid to the social aspects of agnosia only in the last decades of the 20th cen-

223

Disturbances in the
Recognition of the
Social World

tury. The description of prosopagnosia by Bodamer in 1947 was probably the first attempt to study the disturbances of facial gnosis related to the identification of participants in social activities. Almost 30 years passed before the concept of emotional agnosia was advanced by the studies of Hellman and Ross and their colleagues. Another aspect of agnosia of person is related to the delusional alienation of one's physical appearance from its social meaning, manifesting as a delusional misidentification.

Prosopagnosia, the Disorder of Facial Recognition

The recognition of faces plays an important role in social interactions. Its impairment may lead to significant disturbances in daily social activity as well as in response to various events in social life. A loss in the ability to recognize familiar faces was described as a syndrome independent of visual agnosia by Bodamer (1947), who studied three patients with a "loss of knowledge of faces" but a relatively preserved recognition of objects. Bodamer coined the term prosopagnosia using the Greek word *prosopon,* meaning face. Bodamer related the first clinical report of this disturbance to Quaglino (1867), an ophthalmologist who described a patient who had suffered a loss in the ability to recognize his friends as well as a person with whom he had conversed with for an hour some days before seeing him again. The patient preserved the ability to recognize the person upon hearing his voice, however. The patient also suffered from left hemianopia and achromatopsia. The paper was published in an ophthalmological journal, and then eventually forgotten. Hughlins Jackson (1876), Wernicke (1881), Charcot (1883), and Wilbrand (1887, 1892) described a failure to recognize familiar faces as one of the signs of severe visual agnosia with impairments of various types of visual recognition (for a review, see Grusser & Landis, 1991). Hoff and Pötzl (1937) suggested that a disturbance in facial recognition is a specific form of visual agnosia. They based their suggestion on the description of a case with disturbances in the identification of familiar faces, while the recognition of letters and words, as well as other visual stimuli, was either less impaired or completely preserved.

It was Bodamer (1947) who brought agnosia of familiar faces to the forefront of neurological and neuropsychological interest and established the syndrome as a distinctive clinical entity, which he called prosopagnosia. He presented descriptions of three patients who had suffered from brain injuries during World War II, two of whom were suffering from prosopagnosia. The third patient demonstrated metamorphopsia, or a distortion of facial perception without a failure to recognize familiar faces, while one of the two patients with prosopagnosia also demonstrated transient visual metamorphopsia and was occasionally able to recognize familiar faces. These findings were used by Bodamer to support his suggestion of the clinical independence of agnosia for familiar faces. In spite of an absence of autopsy data in his two cases, Bodamer attributed the development of prosopagnosia to traumatic lesions in both occipital lobes.

Many cases of prosopagnosia have been described in the literature since Bodamer's publication, with the number of reported cases reaching about 50 in 1962 (Hécaen & Angelergues, 1963) and more than 70 in 1967 (Kok, 1967). Many more cases have been published since then (see Farah, 1990; Grusser & Landis, 1991).

Clinical Aspects

Disorders of Conventional Information Processing. Prosopagnosia is defined as a disorder in the recognition of familiar, individual faces with a relative preservation of the recognition of faces as objects. This defines prosopagnosia as a disturbance in the conventional processing of well-known faces. The patient is unable to recognize faces of relatives and other well-known individuals, often including, for example, the patient's husband or wife, daughter, son, and/or physician. The recognition of individual faces of relatives and famous people becomes especially difficult when looking at their photographs. In some difficult cases, a patient may be unable to recognize his own face in the mirror, determine whether it is a male or female face, or assess its age. Recognition usually becomes possible when the patient hears the voices or the typical sounds of the footsteps of his relatives. Recognition of the emotional state of the subjects according their facial characteristics is usually preserved, but may be disturbed in some cases.

Prosopagnosia is often associated with visual spatial agnosia, including disorders of topographical memory, spatial dyslexia, and spatial dyscalculia (Hécaen & Angelergues, 1963). Other associated disturbances include color agnosia, achromatopsia, and, in some cases, loss of visual imagery manifested as an inability to visualize familiar faces. Metamorphopsias with facial distortions may be confused with prosopagnosia, but the recognition of familiar faces is usually preserved in cases of metamorphopsia, unlike prosopagnosia (Bodamer, 1947; Hécaen & Angelergues, 1963). Landis described three such cases and suggested the term *prosopo-metamorphopsia* for such disturbances (Grusser & Landis, 1991). Visual object agnosia may also be present in cases of prosopagnosia, but cases of prosopagnosia have been described with a prominent dissociation between severely impaired object recognition and preserved recognition of faces (Ferro & Santos, 1984; Hécaen, Goldblum, Masure, & Ramier, 1974; McCarthy & Warrington, 1986).

It is reasonable to suggest that, as with visual object agnosia, prosopagnosia may be divided into *apperceptive* and *associative prosopagnosia*. In apperceptive prosopagnosia, the disturbances would be found

225

*Disturbances in the
Recognition of the
Social World*

in the first encoding type of visual processing for individual facial features. Associative agnosia would be related to difficulties in matching the description of individual faces in their storage models with their respective meanings.

Disturbances at the Level of Complex Features Processing: Apperceptive Facial Agnosia. With regard to the first encoding stage, it seems that a patient with apperceptive prosopagnosia has lost his or her ability to use more global, complex features of individual faces, which are needed for the matching of features with the stored models of these faces. The listing and processing of these complex features representing the particular contours and shapes of the individual faces could be predefined in the course of individual experiences. The destruction of such conventional processing requires compensation based on the restructuring of the object using the set of simple features. This may include the use of some of the secondary features of the face that do not form the shape of an individual face and may belong to multiple individuals with various facial shapes. These features include long or short hair, color of hair, and the presence of a beard or mustache, pimples, or scars in particular places on the face. The use of such features to attempt facial recognition, however, is often unsuccessful, since a female with a short, boyish haircut may be recognized as a male, and a well-known person who usually wears glasses cannot be recognized when he or she takes them off. A patient may recognize particular parts of the face, such as the nose, eyebrows, eyes, and ears, but fail to recognize the individual face using its complex gestalt features. As in visual object agnosia, such global features have not yet been clearly identified. One of our patients with prosopagnosia correctly assessed even the peculiar details of the facial features, such as the length of the nose and the height of the forehead, but was unable to recognize the particular familiar faces in their entireties (Levin et al., 1961).

Some researchers have tried to single out the areas of the face that are especially important for facial recognition. These areas include the region around the eyes, the region around the mouth, and the bridge of the nose, termed the occula by Bodamer (1947). These local features are probably used when the ability to recognize global features is lost in patients with prosopagnosia. It was found that matching such facial fragments with an entire unfamiliar face was disturbed in patients with prosopagnosia. Bodamer found that the ability of patients with prosopagnosia to recognize faces is more disturbed if based on the mouth region; Gloning and Quaterner (1966) demonstrated the opposite. De Renzi (1986) reported comparable impairments in the matching of the face as a whole with the facial fragments of the eyes, mouth, and half-face.

The results point to the role of disturbances in the recognition of the salient features of the face in difficulties of compensation for the loss of the ability to recognize global features. The relative role of these salient features remains unclear, but it is important to stress that the recognition of local salient features may be used to compensate for disturbances in the processing of global facial features in less severe cases of prosopagnosia, or in the course of recovery.

The role of perceptual disturbances in prosopagnosia cases is also supported by findings of unconventional disturbances in the recognition of occluded objects in addition to difficulties in the recognition of occluded faces or facial fragments. De Renzi (1999) points to the poor scoring methods of such tests as Ghent's overlapping figures and Gollin and Street's interrupted figures. Patients may also show moderate or mild impairments on a face age discrimination test (De Renzi, 1986) and a face matching test (Benton & Van Allen, 1968). Perceptive disturbances manifested as difficulties and slowness in matching unfamiliar faces have also been reported in more severe cases of prosopagnosia (De Renzi, 1986; Newcombe, 1979; Newcombe, Young, & De Haan, 1989; Whiteley & Warrington, 1977). In our studies of cases with severe prosopagnosia, we found that the recognition of objects in their conventional view was preserved, but prominent disturbances were found in the recognition of overlapping figures and incomplete pictures of the objects (Levin, Povorinsky, & Tonkonogy, 1961).

Disturbances at the Semantic Level: Associative Facial Agnosia. Perceptual disturbances are either less prominent or completely absent in many cases of prosopagnosia. According to studies of face matching, the perceptual stage of visual recognition typical for patients with apperceptive agnosia may be minimal in patients with associative prosopagnosia. It has been observed that patients with impairments in the recognition of familiar faces show a relatively preserved ability to perform in tests of facial matching (Benton & Van Allen, 1972; De Renzi, 1986; Tzavaras, Hécaen, & Le Bras, 1970).

The same-different matching tasks developed by Benton and Van Allen (1972) have often been used in such studies. The subject is asked to match a photograph of an unfamiliar face, viewed from the front, with its identical counterpart, found in one of six photographs of faces taken under different lighting conditions or from different angles. Benton and Van Allen (1972) reported that their patients matched unfamiliar faces at the normal or close to normal level in three of their four cases of prosopagnosia. This relatively preserved facial discrimination in patients with prosopagnosia may be compared with difficulties in facial discrimination tests and the preserved recognition of familiar faces in some of the cases (Benton, 1980; Damasio, 1985), pointing to the relative preservation of perceptual, encoding operations in some cases of prosopagnosia. In such cases, the primary disturbances in prosopagnosia may be related to typical associative agnosia disturbances in the ability to match facial descriptions with their owners' identities, such as those of a relative, parent, doctor, and so forth.

As in patients with visual object agnosia, top-down processing may facilitate the recognition of individual faces by patients with prosopagnosia. This may be achieved by a limitation of the "vocabulary" of the individual faces presented for recognition to include only close or distant relatives, for example, or only the medical staff on the ward. A further restriction of choices could be achieved by the presentation of famous faces, which may then be divided into groups of politicians, actors, athletes, and so on.

Unconventional Information Processing and Disorders of Face Recognition. Disturbances in conventional information processing represent the leading clinical features of prosopagnosia. The visual stimuli used have included familiar faces of relatives or friends and photographs of famous faces. Studies of facial recognition in unconventional conditions have been limited, however, to the direct matching or immediate and/or delayed recall of unfamiliar faces. Each variety of tests used in such studies usually requires the subject to find the identical counterpart of a face presented in a sample photograph among photographs of several other faces.

In addition to the matching of unfamiliar faces (Milner, 1958), unconventional conditions have included different lighting, various degrees of shading, and changes in viewing angles (Benton & Van Allen, 1968; Tzavaras et al., 1970; Warrington & James, 1967; Whiteley & Warrington, 1977). But patients with prosopagnosia have often showed either no or only minor disturbances in these tests, pointing to the relative preservation of the perceptual phase of facial recognition in many cases of prosopagnosia.

Limitation of presentation time to 1 sec for the presentation of faces to be matched reveals prominent perceptual disturbances in patients with prosopagnosia (Grusser & Landis, 1991). Patients with right hemisphere damage and without prosopagnosia showed moderate impairments in face matching in tests with unlimited times of facial presentation. Their performance did not significantly worsen when the time length of face presentation on the screen of a tachistoscope was limited to 1 sec. Patients with prosopagnosia also performed the face matching without difficulty when the time was unlimited, but became unable to correctly match faces when the time of face presentation was reduced to 1 sec. The reported results are similar to our findings of prominent disturbances in object recognition when the

228

LOCALIZATION
OF CLINICAL
SYNDROMES IN
NEUROPSYCHOLOGY
AND NEUROSCIENCE

length of object presentation on the screen of a tachistoscope has been limited.

The matching of unfamiliar faces is certainly a part of the learning process, which is based on the ability to describe the individual features of the face, to temporarily store those features as an individual model in one's operational memory, and to match that model with a presented set of faces. The test is facilitated by the limitation of the number of faces that need to be matched. The process of recognition of familiar faces differs according to the involvement of already existing permanently stored models for many familiar faces, and needs to compare the encoded facial description with the relatively large set of models in storage that have been acquired in the person's individual experience. In the future, it would be worthwhile to study the recognition of familiar faces in unconventional conditions, perhaps including partially occluded familiar faces, as in studies of visual object agnosia. Such tests may help to facilitate the evaluation of mild, unconventional manifestations of prosopagnosia, and to better understand the underlying mechanisms of disorders of the recognition of familiar faces.

Agnosia of Individual Faces and of the Individuality of Living and Nonliving Objects. A series of single cases has been reported in support of the association between disturbances in facial recognition and impaired recognition of particular nonliving objects, such as: different types of chairs (Faust, 1955); a personal pen or mug (Levin et al., 1961); buildings and public monuments (Assal, 1969); particular makes of cars (Boudaresques, Pocet, Cherif, & Balzamo, 1979; Damasio, Damasio, Van Hoesen et al., 1982; L'Hermitte et al., 1972); types of food, articles of clothing (Damasio, Damasio, Rizzo, Varney, & Gersh, 1982); and living objects, including different species of birds (Bornstein, 1963); a specific cow presented to be recognized by its owner (Assal, Faure, & Anderes, 1984); specific racehorses (Newcombe, 1979); and cats (Damasio et al., 1982; Levin et al., 1961). These types of tasks have been related in cognitive psychology to recognition at the subordinate level category, while object recognition as a part of a particular class is attributed to the basic level category (Rosch, Mervis, Gray, Johnson, & Boyes-Braem, 1976).

It seems that the processing of information is quite different in the task of recognizing individual faces and the individuality of objects from the processing of information in the task of recognizing objects that are members of certain conceptual categories, such as faces in general, tables, chairs, plates, dogs, horses, and so forth. The system responsible for the recognition of individual faces and other objects may require model storage for every individual item, while such storage for the recognition of an object as a member of a conceptual category may

229

*Disturbances in the
Recognition of the
Social World*

be limited to one general model, which represents the category of faces or tables, for example, and thus stores various versions of multiple faces and tables. Thus, a very limited number of models of individual faces may be stored and recognized, while a general model of a face provides a memory base for the recognition of many faces as members of that particular category.

Access to later model storage is facilitated by top-down operations and is based on the classification of tables and chairs as furniture, plates and cups as crockery, and so on. The recognition of individual faces or other specific objects cannot rely on such operations, since each individual object needs to be matched with a representation of the same individual object as it is stored in a model.

Similarities in the tasks and operations involved in the recognition of individual faces and of the individuality of other particular objects may explain the frequency of simultaneous disturbances in both types of recognition. Though it seems redundant to have separate systems for the recognition of individuality for each category of objects, it is possible that two separate systems exist for the processing of information related to particular faces and the processing of information related to the individuality of particular living and nonliving objects within the same cognitive category. This may explain reports of some rare cases of patients who suffer from isolated difficulties in the recognition of individual faces without suffering from difficulties in the recognition of particular living or nonliving items. De Renzi (1986) described a patient who experienced prominent difficulties in the recognition of his relatives and close friends but preserved the ability to identify his own personal things, including his own electric razor, wallet, glasses, and neckties. Assal et al. (1984) described a farmer who was suffering from an impairment in the recognition of his cows but was able to recover the ability to recognize faces and celebrities. Bruyer et al. (1983) reported an opposite finding in the case of a patient with a disorder of face recognition and a preserved ability to recognize cows. Due to the rarity of such cases, further studies of similar cases are needed.

It is also of interest that prosopagnosia is often accompanied by disturbances in topographic orientation, which may be interpreted as a common loss of familiarity with previously well-known objects and their topographic orientations. Hécaen and Angelergues (1963) reported a frequent association of prosopagnosia with topographic amnesia—topographic amnesia was recorded in 38% of patients with prosopagnosia, while 77% of the patients with a loss of topographic memory also suffered from prosopagnosia (Hécaen & Angelergues, 1963). Landis et al. (1986) found evidence of prosopagnosia in 7 of 16 patients with a loss of topographic familiarity.

230

LOCALIZATION
OF CLINICAL
SYNDROMES IN
NEUROPSYCHOLOGY
AND NEUROSCIENCE

A patient of our own with severe prosopagnosia demonstrated prominent topographic disorientation (Levin et al., 1961). The patient could not find his room, bed, or toilet on the hospital ward, nor could he draw the plans of his room on the ward and the spatial orientation of the functional rooms on the ward, such as the dining room, the dayroom, and the restrooms. In spite of his ability to visualize the images of faces in general and to recall names and personality features of persons, the patient experienced difficulties in the revisualization of familiar faces.

It is probable that impairments in similar operations underlain disturbances in the recognition of specific and familiar faces, objects, and spatial relationships, as well as in the ability to revisualize a familiar face. The disturbance of a unified module for the processing of individual features is probably responsible for the reported correlations. Another possibility is that the anatomical structures responsible for the processing of individual features are located very close to one another, for example, in the same posterior areas of the right hemisphere. A more extended lesion in the posterior part of the right hemisphere would thus result in the development of associations between various types of recognition disturbances—of individual familiar faces, objects, space locations, and so on.

Anatomical Aspects

Disturbances of Conventional Information Processing: Bilateral Occipito-Temporal Lesions.   As in cases of visual object agnosia, lesions in cases of prosopagnosia are often bilateral, involving both sides of the occipital and temporal lobes. Damasio, Damasio, and Van Hoesen (1982) analyzed 10 previously published postmortem reports of patients with prosopagnosia, as well as 3 new cases, and determined that prosopagnosia resulted from cerebral infarctions in all 3 of the new cases and in 8 of the 10 previously reported cases, and from cerebral tumors in the remaining 2 cases. The occipital lesions were bilateral in all 13 cases and were located predominantly in the inferior parts of the occipital lobe, including the cuneus and the lingual gyri. Lesions involved the temporal lobe, usually the fusiform and parahippocampal gyri, in 10 of the 13 cases, while parietal lobe lesions were reported in only 2 cases. The location of lesions in those 13 cases of prosopagnosia is practically the same as in many cases of visual object agnosia. In fact, visual object agnosia was reported in some of the cases included in the review, including a case described by Wilbrand (1892). Additional cases of prosopagnosia in which CT scans revealed bilateral posterior cerebral lesions were reviewed by De Renzi (1986), Landis et al. (1986), and Michel, Poncet, and Signoret (1989).

Unilateral Right Occipito-Temporal Lesions

Autopsy Data. The similarities of lesion sites bring up the question of the location of lesions that is necessary for the development of different types of visual agnosia. It seems that left occipital and occipito-temporal lesions are sufficient for the development of visual object agnosia (see discussion in the previous paragraph). As to the development of prosopagnosia, some data point to the crucial role of a right hemispheric lesion. To the best of our knowledge, only three cases of prosopagnosia with autopsy-proven unilateral right hemisphere lesions have been published. In a case of prosopagnosia described by Kok (1967), surgery revealed a large arteriovenous malformation (AVM) in the basal area of the right hemispheric occipito-temporal region. The patient died within 2 days after total surgical removal of the AVM. An autopsy revealed atrophy of the basal occipito-temporal area in the right hemisphere. Landis and Regard (1988) published another anatomically verified case of the development of prosopagnosia following a stroke. The patient died 10 days after the stroke from pulmonary embolism, and an autopsy revealed a recent, large infero-medial occipito-temporal infarct, as well as an old frontal infarct in the right hemisphere. A tiny cortical microinfarct in the lateral occipito-parietal area was seen in the left hemisphere. In a third case of prosopagnosia, recently described by Kawamura and Takahashi (1995), an autopsy exhibited a lesion in the right hemisphere alone.

Intraoperative and Brain-Imaging Data. In addition to the rare cases of autopsy confirmation, a series of cases has been reported in which intraoperative and radiological findings have revealed right hemisphere lesions in prosopagnosic patients. These cases were summarized by De Renzi (1986) and Landis et al. (1986).

The development of prosopagnosia followed epilepsy treatment surgery in two cases reported by Hécaen et al. (1956), Hécaen, Angelergues, Bernhardt, and Chiarelli (1957), and Hécaen and Angelergues (1963). The right posterior occipital, temporal, and parietal lobes were removed in one of the cases, and the right occipito-temporal epileptic zone was removed in the other. L'Hermitte and Pillon (1975) presented a patient who had developed prosopagnosia after undergoing a right occipital lobectomy for the treatment of intractable seizures.

CT scans revealed unilateral right hemisphere infarctions in two cases reported by De Renzi (1986) and in three of six cases described by Landis et al. (1986). The infarctions were located in the inferior occipital lobe in all of the cases, including the cuneus, the lingual gyrus, and the lips of the calcarine fissure in De Renzi's patients, and the lingual gyrus and the fibers of the optic radiations in Landis's patients; the infarctions also extended to the posterior-medial temporal lobe, including the parahippocampal and fusiform gyri, in all five cases. The splenium of the corpus callosum was also involved in all five cases.

Right posterior hematoma was reported in four cases of prosopagnosia, the location of which was occipito-parietal in two cases (Assal, 1969; Landis et al., 1986, Case 4), occipital in one case (Whiteley & Warrington, 1977, Case 2), and posterior temporal in one case (Meadows, 1974, Case 4). Hematoma in the posterior occipito-temporal region of the right hemisphere was also demonstrated via CT scan in a case reported by Michel, Perenin, and Sieroff (1986).

Tumors in the posterior region of the right hemisphere were found in three cases of prosopagnosia, including a right occipital astrocytoma in one case (Whiteley & Warrington, 1977, Case 3), a right occipito-temporo-parietal glioblastoma in the second, and a right occipital oligodendroglyoma in the third (Landis et al., 1986).

In summary, unilateral right hemisphere lesions were found in all 19 cases verified by autopsy, intraoperative, or CT scan data. Occipital lesions were found in 16 of the 19 cases, and occipito-temporal involvement was present in 13 of the cases, including all 6 cases with cerebral infarctions. Temporal lobe involvement could be suggested in the remaining 6 cases as the result of mass effect caused by a tumor or hematoma located in either the occipital or occipito-parietal region.

These results demonstrate that a primarily ventral occipito-temporal involvement in the right hemisphere is sufficient for the development of prosopagnosia. A similar lesion in the left hemisphere was observed to be sufficient to produce visual object agnosia.

Also, an extension of mass effect to the opposite hemisphere or a suppression of brain tissue in the left hemisphere cannot be ruled out in some cases of prosopagnosia, especially those with tumors or hematoma. The role of callosal lesions must also be taken into account in cases with infarctions. It is also plausible that head CT may miss some of the small infarctions in the left hemisphere. However, unilateral lesions were found in the posterior right hemisphere in all 19 cases of prosopagnosia, including 6 cases with cerebral infarctions. No cases of prosopagnosia with such unilateral lesions in the left hemisphere have been described in patients with cerebral infarctions in the region of the left posterior cerebral artery (De Renzi, Zambolin, & Crisi, 1987; Landis & Regard, 1988). These findings argue against the suggestion that mass effect from tumors and hematomas in the right hemisphere could reach the opposite left hemisphere, thus facilitating the development of prosopagnosia in such cases.

Disturbances of Unconventional Information Processing:
Role of the Ventral Temporal Cortex

Experimental studies of disturbances in unconventional information processing via the matching or recall of unfamiliar faces have also

233

Disturbances in the
Recognition of the
Social World

confirmed the role of the right hemisphere in the process of facial recognition in unconventional conditions.

More prominent impairments for patients with right versus left
hemispheric lesions have also been shown in tests of the immediate
recall of unfamiliar faces (De Renzi & Spinnler, 1966; Newcombe, 1969;
Warrington & James, 1967), as well as in tests of the direct matching
of unfamiliar faces (Benton & Van Allen, 1968; Tzavaras et al., 1970).
Warrington and James (1967) found that impairments on the delayed-
matching test for unfamiliar faces were more prominent in cases with
right occipito-parietal lesions than in cases with right temporal lesions.
However, there was a significantly higher number of patients with tumors in the group of patients with occipito-parietal lesions than in the
group with temporal lesions. Consequently, an extension of mass effect from the parietal to the temporal lobe cannot be excluded.

No significant correlation was found between impairments in facial recognition in conventional and unconventional conditions using
the matching test for unfamiliar faces and the test for the recognition
of famous individuals (Warrington & James, 1967), pointing to the possibility of differences in the localization of lesions in cases of conventional versus unconventional disturbances of facial recognition.

Data presented by Milner (1968) also support the role of the right
temporal lobe in the development of unconventional prosopagnosia.
The author compared immediate and delayed recall of the photographs
of 12 unfamiliar faces among 25 faces in groups of patients who had
been treated for epilepsy via an ablation of the right frontal lobe and
either the right or left temporal lobe. Milner observed prominent impairments only in patients with an ablation of the right temporal lobe,
especially in cases with an ablation of the hippocampus.

Single-cell recording has been used to study the recognition of faces
in monkeys. The design of these studies specifically involves learning
to discriminate faces, which may fall under the category of unconventional information processing. The recording of single cells showed the
presence of cells in the inferior temporal cortex (IT), which selectively
respond to complete face images (Bruce et al., 1981; Desimone et al.,
1984; Perret et al., 1982; Young & Yamane, 1992). Some cells in the adjacent regions responded only to specific parts of the face (e.g., mouth,
eyes, hair region), and others only to a specific facial orientation (e.g.,
front, profile). Responses to particular faces reflecting personal identity were registered in a small percentage of cell firings. These studies
seem to support the role of the inferior temporal region in the unconventional processing needed for face recognition and, to some extent,
for the recognition of familiar faces in particular.

The role of the ventral temporal lobe in the unconventional information processing of faces was also demonstrated in PET and fMRI
studies of normal control subjects undergoing the face-matching test.

234

LOCALIZATION
OF CLINICAL
SYNDROMES IN
NEUROPSYCHOLOGY
AND NEUROSCIENCE

The changes as recorded via PET scans were compared in the face-matching and dot-location tasks. The face-matching test activated the ventral occipito-temporal cortex, primarily the fusiform gyrus in the right hemisphere, while the dot-location task activated the superior parietal lobe (Haxby et al., 1991, 1993, 1994). This contrasted with data demonstrating bilateral activation, with a dominance of the right hemisphere, of the ventral occipito-temporal cortex during the recognition of non-face objects (Köhler, Kapur, Moscovitch, Vinocur, & Houle, 1995).

Similar fMRI studies by Puce, Allison, Gore, and McCarthy (1995) found that the viewing of faces activated the ventral occipito-temporal cortex bilaterally, primarily within the fusiform gyrus. Bilateral activation of the fusiform gyrus in the course of facial processing was also observed by Gauthier and Tarr (1997), as well as Rossion, Dricot, Devolder, Bodart, and Crommelonck (2000). Kanwisher, Chun, McDermott, and Ledden (1996), however, found that the processing of faces predominantly activated the right fusiform gyrus.

Special attention in the fMRI studies has been given to the role of the fusiform gyrus in the processing of individual faces and objects. Rhodes, Byatt, Michie, and Puce (2004) compared differences in the passive viewing of faces, butterflies, and objects and their matching between trained versus untrained individuals. The authors found that fusiform area activation in response to the viewing of faces was greater than in response to the viewing of butterflies. In fact, little overlap between the fusiform areas was activated by faces or butterflies. This effect was observed in both hemispheres and may support the relative independence of the individuation processes for faces, as discussed in previous paragraphs.

Studies employing the use of single-cell recording and brain imaging in normal control subjects support the pathological findings on the role of the ventral temporal cortex, especially the fusiform gyrus, in unconventional face information processing. A significant discrepancy, however, remains between clinico-anatomical findings and single-cell recording/brain imaging/pathological findings concerning the important role of occipital cortex lesions in disturbances in the recognition of familiar faces in patients with prosopagnosia. It is possible that the conventional processing used in the recognition of well-learned faces is based primarily in the ventral occipital cortex, while more complex unconventional operations needed for the processing of unfamiliar faces are mainly related to the ventral temporal cortex, especially the fusiform gyrus, or the "face area." Another discrepancy is related to the bilateral activation of the fusiform gyrus in the course of facial processing, which differs from the clinico-anatomical data that point to the development of unconventional prosopagnosia occurring

235

Disturbances in the
Recognition of the
Social World

predominantly as a result of right hemispheric lesions. This may be explained via recorded images from PET and fMRI scans that demonstrate changes in local blood flow. These changes are due to the more general mechanisms of blood flow that are not directly related to brain activation in the particular cortical areas, for example, an increase of blood flow in the symmetrical area of the left hemisphere when brain activation is underlined by an increase of blood flow in the right hemisphere, and vice versa. Further studies and comparison with lesion data are certainly needed.

Role of the Inferior-Posterior Prefrontal Cortex

Single-unit recordings in areas of the inferior-posterior prefrontal cortex (PFC) in monkeys show disproportionate activation of neurons in those areas in response to pictures of objects, and almost exclusive activation in response to faces (Goldman-Rakic, Scalaidhe, & Chafee, 2000). The authors stress that in humans, the fMRI and evoked potential studies of the working memory for faces also revealed selective activation of the inferior-posterior prefrontal region. These areas are directly connected to the inferior temporal cortex, which plays a significant role as a ventral pathway for object and face recognition.

It may be suggested that, in similar fashion to its role in object recognition, the PFC receives information about low-frequency properties of individual faces. This information is then used to select a limited number of choices of individual faces for top-down transfer to the inferior temporal areas for further processing. It is also possible that information about individual faces processed in the PFC areas may be transferred to the frontal lobe regions involved in the planning and guiding of social activity.

CONCLUSION

1. Disturbances in the recognition of familiar faces, also known as prosopagnosia, may develop as a result of impairments in the well-learned processing of complex features that helps one describe the unique shape of a particular face (apperceptive face agnosia) and match that description with faces in the stored models (associative face agnosia). Prosopagnosic patients often try to compensate by using the simple features of the face for facial recognition.

2. Visual agnosia for familiar faces may be accompanied by difficulties in the recognition of the individuality of living and nonliving objects. Both disturbances may represent a disorder of individuality recognition for individual faces and objects, or perhaps interconnected disorders in the recognition of individual familiar objects, including a disturbance in both the revisualization of

236

LOCALIZATION
OF CLINICAL
SYNDROMES IN
NEUROPSYCHOLOGY
AND NEUROSCIENCE

familiar faces and the topographic memory. These interconnected disorders are probably related to lesions of the closely anatomically localized operations mediating the recognition of familiarity for different visual tasks. It is conceivable that the recognition of individuality on the subordinate level is mediated by the right hemisphere, while more abstract types of class recognition for objects at the basic, ordinate level, including faces as well as topographic processing, and revisualization are mediated by the left hemisphere.

3. Prosopagnosia, or visual agnosia for the recognition of familiar faces, developed in many cases following bilateral lesions of the ventral occipito-temporal region, in similar fashion to cases of visual object agnosia.

4. Lesions in the occipital or occipito-temporal regions of the right hemisphere are sufficient in many cases for the development of prosopagnosia. Callosal involvement was observed in all cases with prosopagnosia due to right hemisphere infarctions. The role of the cerebral edema and mass effect on the opposite left hemisphere cannot be ruled out in cases with hematoma or tumors located in the right hemisphere. Callosal involvement, edema, and mass effect could produce difficulties in the use of left hemispheric structures for the compensation for prosopagnosia caused by a right hemisphere lesion. It may be suggested that visual object recognition is primarily provided by the ventral pathway in the left hemisphere, while the recognition of individual faces is mainly related to information processing in the ventral pathway of the right hemisphere.

5. Disturbances in unconventional information processing as observed in tests requiring the matching of unfamiliar faces were usually shown to develop following ventral temporal lesions in the right hemisphere. These disturbances may be relatively independent from agnosia for familiar faces. Visual working memory for faces may be provided by the inferior-posterior prefrontal cortex (PFC), which is interconnected with the areas of the ventral pathway in the inferior temporal areas.

6. Delusions of seeing double are more frequently observed in cases with right hemisphere lesions, primarily in the frontotemporal region (Figure 5.1). Unilateral right hemisphere lesions were reported in cases of prosopagnosia with locations in the occipito-temporal region for disturbances in conventional information processing, and in the frontotemporal region for disturbances in unconventional information processing. This stresses the involvement of the right temporal area in the development of both prosopagnosia and delusions of doubles, with lesions extending to the occipital

Right hemisphere   Left hemisphere

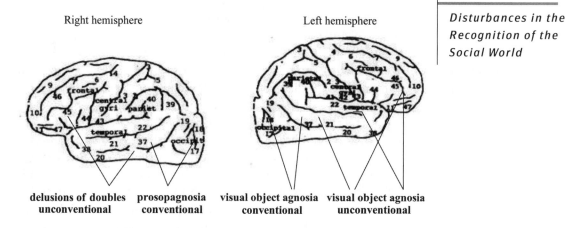

delusions of doubles   prosopagnosia   visual object agnosia   visual object agnosia
   unconventional   conventional   conventional   unconventional

FIGURE 5.1 Similarities of lesion localization in the right hemisphere for prosopagnosia and in the left hemisphere for visual object agnosia. Note also the overlap of lesion localization in prosopagnosia and delusions of doubles, also known as Capgras syndrome. For more details, see section entitled "Delusions."

lobe in conventional prosopagnosia and to the frontal lobe both in delusions of doubles and in unconventional prosopagnosia. Lesions in the frontal area, particularly the PFC, as well as in the temporal area, are thus likely to be instrumental in the development of the delusional quality both of agnosia of person at the semantic level and of unconventional prosopagnosia, while lesions in the occipito-temporal area underlie the onset of conventional prosopagnosia.

Emotional Agnosia and Motor Aprosodia

The term *motor aprosodia* may be useful in describing disturbances in the nonverbal expression of emotions. Emotional agnosia and motor aprosodia may also be considered to be types of communication disorders.

Disturbances of emotion recognition were first described in the 1970s, beginning with a report by Heilman, Scholes, and Watson (1975). The authors described "auditory affective agnosia" in patients with damage to the right hemisphere, suggesting that linguistically neutral sentences differed according to emotional prosody. The patients with damage to the right hemisphere showed marked impairments compared to both normal controls and to patients with damage to the left hemisphere and with resulting mild aphasia. Four years later, Ross and Mesulam (1979) described two patients with an inability to project appropriate emotional prosody in their voices. One of the patients was

238

LOCALIZATION
OF CLINICAL
SYNDROMES IN
NEUROPSYCHOLOGY
AND NEUROSCIENCE

unable to project anger and displeasure, while the second constantly spoke in a "nasty" tone. CT scans revealed suprasylvian anterior lesions in the right hemisphere in both cases.

Based on those and similar cases, Ross (1981) suggested the term *aprosodia* to denote disturbances in the comprehension and expression of emotional prosody. According to this terminology, the term "sensory affective aprosodia" would be used for an impairment in comprehension of the emotional prosody of speech, and the term "motor affective aprosodia" would define difficulties in the expression of emotion by voice. However, disturbances in the recognition of facial expressions, as often seen in cases of sensory affective aprosodia, would be difficult to consider as aprosodia, since the term *prosody* has usually been applied to the nonverbal characteristics of speech, such as intonation, rhythm, pitch, timbre, stress, and accent. Vuilleumier, Ghika-Schmid, Bogousslavsky, Assal, and Regli (1998) used the awkward term "prosopoaffective agnosia" to describe impairments in the recognition of facial expression. Other authors described both disturbances in the recognition of emotional prosody of speech and impairments in the recognition of facial expressions under the term "emotional aprosody" (Starkstein, Federoff, Price, Leiguarda, & Robinson, 1994). It seems that the term *emotional agnosia* would help to bring the various terms under a single heading, with particular terms such as agnosia of emotional prosody or agnosia of face expression used to outline different modalities of disturbances in the recognition of emotion. The introduction of the term agnosia may also be important in bringing the understanding of the agnosia of emotion closer to the well-developed conceptual framework of the studies of object and space agnosia.

Emotional Agnosia
Clinical and Neuropsychological Aspects
Neuropsychological Testing. Agnosia of emotion is usually manifested as disturbances in the recognition of positive and negative emotions. The list of positive emotions is frequently limited to a happy tone of voice and facial expressions. The list of negative emotions, however, varies from at least two emotional states reflected in tone of voice and facial expressions, such as sadness and anger (Darby, 1993; Starkstein et al., 1994), to three or more emotional states that may differ according to particular studies, such as anxiety, sadness, anger, and apathy (Bajhin, Korneva, & Lomachenko, 1980; Balonov & Deglin, 1976; Tonkonogy et al., 1977), or sadness, anger, fearfulness, disinterest, and surprise (Ross, 1981). The recognition of fear and disgust was added in the study of the role of the amygdala in emotional agnosia (Adolphs et al., 1994). Weniger, Irie, Exner, and Ruther (1997) used the 16 pictures of the

239

*Disturbances in the
Recognition of the
Social World*

Ekman series representing the four basic negative emotions—anger, fear, disgust, and grief—and added pictures signifying surprise, lack of emotion, and positive emotions of joy. It must also be stressed that recognition of negative emotions, especially fear, represents a more difficult task than recognition of the positive emotions of happiness and joy. Some researchers have included unemotional faces and neutral voices in the list of tested emotions.

The lower number of negative emotions in the list of emotional states certainly increases the threshold for the diagnosis of emotional agnosia, increasing reliability for more severe cases, while a higher number of emotions in the testing procedure decreases that threshold, helping to uncover the milder cases but increasing the overlap with the normal control subjects. These differences must be taken into account in the comparison of contradictions between various studies, especially in relation to the lesion localization in emotional agnosia, for example, in cases of lesions of the amygdala.

To standardize the evaluation of auditory emotional aprosodia in different patients, it is useful to use a tape recording of the voice of either the examiner or an actor reading the neutral sentences with various emotional intonations. In our own studies, we also tried to bring those emotionally loaded intonations closer to the real-life experience of emotional recognition. In addition to the voice of an actor, we used the recorded voices of psychiatric patients with various emotional conditions such as anxiety, depression, anger, apathy, euphoria, or euthymic mood (Bajhin et al., 1980). Pictures of facial expressions usually include photographs of actors imitating various emotional states.

The testing of emotional agnosia is usually conducted by providing patients with a multiple-choice answer sheet with a verbal list as well as facial drawings of tested emotions. The vocabulary of emotions included in the tests is limited in such designs, facilitating the comparison of the auditory and visual features of emotions with their samples in the stored model.

Emotional agnosia has often been concomitantly tested in auditory and visual modalities. Such an approach helps to differentiate between the roles of modality-related disturbances with multimodal impairments in the recognition of emotion. In most cases, these disturbances are multimodal, with possible differences in the severity of auditory and visual impairments in some patients.

Associative and Apperceptive Emotional Agnosia. Similar to object agnosia, emotional agnosia may include two major types—*associative emotional agnosia* and *apperceptive emotional agnosia*.

Associative emotional agnosia may be considered in cases with multimodal disturbances in the comprehension of emotional prosody

240

LOCALIZATION
OF CLINICAL
SYNDROMES IN
NEUROPSYCHOLOGY
AND NEUROSCIENCE

conveyed by voice intonation and by emotion-laden facial expressions. In such cases, the apperceptive part of the recognition is preserved, since agnosia is multimodal and involves both the auditory and visual modalities. The primary processing of auditory and visual information is thus preserved. This is supported by the absence of prosopagnosia in cases with disturbances in the comprehension of emotion-laden facial expressions; the recognition of facial expression may be preserved in patients with disturbances in either facial identification or prosopagnosia (Bowers, Coslett, Bauer, Speedie, & Heilman, 1987; DeKosky, Heilman, Bowers, & Valenstein, 1980; Tranel, Damasio, & Damasio, 1988). Similarly, either the comprehension of speech is usually preserved or only mild aphasia is observed in patients with disturbances in the recognition of emotional tones of voices (Balonov & Deglin, 1976; Ross, 1981, 1985).

The recognition of more elementary prosodic linguistic characteristics of speech, such as in exclamations, interrogations, questions, and narrations, may also be disturbed in patients with auditory emotional agnosia (Balonov & Deglin, 1976; Heilman, Bowers, Speedie, & Coslett, 1984). This points to the possible role of disturbances at the apperceptive level in such cases. These disturbances may be defined as apperceptive emotional agnosia, especially in cases with an absence of visual emotional agnosia.

Apperceptive Emotional Agnosia. Starkstein et al. (1994) reported cases of apperceptive emotional agnosia in which disturbances in the comprehension of facial emotions were unaccompanied by signs of auditory emotional agnosia in 9 of 32 patients (28%) with emotional agnosia of facial expressions, while the comprehension of facial emotions was preserved in 6 of 29 patients (21%) with auditory emotional aprosody. Apperceptive emotional agnosia could have been considered responsible in these cases. It would be useful to evaluate such unimodal cases for the presence of disturbances in the processing of the more elementary features of visual and auditory emotional expressions.

It may be suggested that the development of associative emotional agnosia results from a lesion at the level concerned with the translation of the auditory and visual signals into a multimodal code compatible with the code that describes positive and negative emotions in the stored model. This storage, or the rule of comparison of the multimodal signal with the code describing emotions, may be destroyed by brain damage, making it impossible to classify information presented for recognition.

Disturbances of Conventional Information Processing. The testing of visual and auditory emotional agnosia is limited to the short list of

241

*Disturbances in the
Recognition of the
Social World*

several basic positive and negative emotions with a well-established set of features typical for *conventional* information processing. The testing procedure is also facilitated by a list of verbal labels for emotions and by drawings of facial expressions, restricting the choice of possible emotions included in the testing. Such a testing procedure reveals the disturbances in conventional information processing, which usually result from local lesions that completely destroy the particular regions of the brain. These lesions may result from a stroke, a tumor, or a traumatic injury, as in cases of visual object agnosia or of conventional prosopagnosia.

Both in patients with schizophrenia and in those with primary degenerative dementia, lesions are often spread over many areas, destroying multiple regions of the brain only partially and manifesting as disturbances of *unconventional* information processing. It may thus be expected that emotional agnosia would not be revealed by the testing of conventional information processing in such patients. Indeed, the results of such testing in patients with primary psychiatric disorders and degenerative dementia did not yield evidence of any significant disturbances in emotional recognition. Also, no correlation was found between mood disorders and emotional sensory agnosia in stroke patients.

Starkstein et al. (1994) studied 59 acute stroke patients, and reported depression in 22% of the patients with severe aprosody and 38% of the patients without aprosody. The authors did not find significant differences in the frequency and severity of depression between the group of patients with either minor or severe aprosody and the group of patients with an absence of sensory emotional aprosody.

On the other hand, Vuilleumier et al. (1998) described a case of hypomania and agnosia of emotionally laden facial expressions, mainly for negative emotions, which developed following an infarction in the right posterolateral thalamus. The authors stressed the possibility that secondary mania in this particular case, as well as sensory aprosodia, probably resulted from diaschisis spreading to the temporal lobe in the right hemisphere. However, the researchers did not discuss the probable direct functional interconnection between mania and sensory aprosodia.

Murphy and Cutting (1990) reported the results of another attempt to study prosodic comprehension and expression in depression and mania in comparison with both schizophrenic and normal subjects. The study included 15 patients in each of three groups with mania, depression, and schizophrenia, as well as 15 normal subjects. While the observed differences between the three groups of patients and the normal subjects were statistically significant, they were inconclusive from our point of view. The mean number of errors for

242

LOCALIZATION
OF CLINICAL
SYNDROMES IN
NEUROPSYCHOLOGY
AND NEUROSCIENCE

emotional comprehension, for example, did not exceed 2 or 3 errors out of 10 answers in the groups of patients, and remained at 1 or 2 errors out of 10 answers in normal subjects. No differences were found between groups of patients with mania, depression, and schizophrenia. Similarly, errors in emotional expressions reached 4–5 in the group of patients with schizophrenia, and 5–6 for the remaining three groups, including the normal subjects.

In the series work conducted in our laboratory (Tonkonogy), either mild disturbances or a complete absence of disturbances of auditory emotional comprehension and emotional facial expression were observed in a group of patients with schizophrenia (Bajhin et al., 1980). It was even observed that some patients with prominent negative symptoms of apathy and loss of interest demonstrated an excellent ability to recognize emotion as conveyed by the tone of voice.

Similarly, inconclusive results in regards to the identification of emotion were reported in patients with Alzheimer's disease. Several authors observed that the accuracy of comprehension of emotional prosody and emotionally laden facial expressions did not differ between patients with Alzheimer's disease and older adult controls (Cadieux & Greve, 1997; Lavenue et al., 1999; Roudier et al., 1998). Ogrocki, Hills, and Strauss (2000) recently published the results of a study that examined the recognition of emotionally laden facial expressions in 17 patients with Alzheimer's disease and 15 healthy older adult controls. The faces were presented for recognition on black-white photographic slides. They expressed five basic emotions, including happiness, sadness, anxiety, anger, and emotional neutrality. The scores on the task were almost identical between the two groups—34.3 + 1.5 for the individuals with Alzheimer's disease, and 34.7 + 1.5 for the control subjects. Some authors, however, have reported differences in emotional recognition between patients with Alzheimer's disease and control subjects (Albert, Cohen, & Koff, 1991; Zandi, Cooper, & Garrison, 1992).

The scores for emotional recognition did not correlate with the severity of the cognitive impairments assessed by Mini-Mental State Examination (MMSE) in the study by Ogrocki et al. (2000). An absence of correlation between the accuracy of emotional recognition and cognitive impairments was also reported by Della Salla et al. (1995). Some authors (Roudier et al., 1998) suggested that scores in emotional recognition are related not to the general cognitive deficit but rather to specific impairments in memory and language. However, statistical control did at least partially eliminate these connections.

Disturbances of Unconventional Information Processing. The evaluation of *unconventional* information processing was included in the test procedure only by a few authors. Bowers et al. (1987) studied the recognition of emotional tone in voices by delivering sentences with either congruent or incongruent semantic content, for example, using a happy intonation while reading a sentence with a seemingly sad semantic content, such as "The woman lay ill and dying." The processing of emotional information in the background of incongruent sentences is required to retain the attentional focus on the emotional intonation, avoiding the contradictory information provided by the content of the sentence. The semantic content of the sentence acts in this case as noise-producing interference at the level of the comparison of emotional descriptions with their stored models. One's attention in such a comparison must be focused on the tone of the voice as it is selected from the background noise caused by the content of the sentence, in a fashion similar to that of the competition between the color of the letters and the verbal label of the color written by the colored letters in Stroop's test. Unconventional information processing involves some additional operations, uncovering cases with agnosia of emotion that are not revealed by conventional forms of testing. Darby (1993), for example, used conventional testing methods to reveal evidence of emotional agnosia in 4 of 43 patients (9.3%) with infarctions of the right (27 patients) and left (16 patients) hemisphere in the territory of the middle cerebral artery (MCA). Starkstein et al. (1994) employed both conventional and unconventional types of testing and observed emotional agnosia in 45% of 59 patients who had suffered an acute stroke.

Further studies of disturbances in unconventional information processing in relation to agnosia of emotion are certainly needed to evaluate the role of the various types of noisy background and incomplete sets of information in the formation of agnosia of emotion. This is especially important for studies of the apperceptive components of emotional agnosia, the comparison with object agnosia and prosopagnosia, and the clarification of localizational aspects of emotional agnosia as they are related to disturbances in unconventional information processing.

Motor Aprosodia

The term affective, or emotional, motor aprosodia refers to disturbances in the ability to bring emotional intonation into verbally neutral sentences in response to a request or repetition task. The condition was first described by Heilman's group in two patients with right parietal lesions (Tucker, Watson, & Heilman, 1977). Ross and Mesulam (1979) reported two patients, one of whom was unable to speak in an angry voice, and the other was unable to speak in a solicitous tone. Both patients suffered from infarctions involving the right anterior suprasylvian region. These publications were followed by studies that stressed the controversies related to the roles of right and left hemispheric

244

LOCALIZATION
OF CLINICAL
SYNDROMES IN
NEUROPSYCHOLOGY
AND NEUROSCIENCE

lesions in the development of emotional motor aprosodia (Ryalls, 1988). Starkstein et al. (1994) also found it practically impossible to distinguish between emotional motor aprosodia and abnormal prosody caused by dysarthria, hypophonia, or even shyness.

Clinical Aspects

According to Ross (1985, 2000), the presence of emotional motor prosody should be recognized via the observation of a patient's spontaneous speech during an interview, especially when the patient is asked emotionally loaded questions about current illnesses or past experiences. Such questions may include, for example, "How you feel about your neurological deficit?" "Have you experienced the loss of a loved one?" or "Have you had any close calls with death or serious injury?" We also asked patients to read neutral sentences and to try to develop and reflect through vocal intonation the emotional modulation of anger, sadness, fearfulness, surprise, happiness, or absence of interest. Similarly, the patient is asked to repeat neutral sentences with the same emotional modulation of voice that was presented either by the examiner or, even better, via previously recorded neutral sentences read by an actor. The emotional modulation of intonation, rather than changes in speech loudness, must be assessed in such cases. The patient may demonstrate disturbances in the emotional coloring of the speech, while linguistic prosody, such as stresses, pauses, exclamations, or questions, may remain preserved. Spontaneous speech characterized by a monotone voice and without clear linguistic intonation may be observed in other cases.

The evaluation of emotional motor aprosodia may be significantly complicated by various types of *dysarthria,* especially during the acute stage of stroke. Dysarthria may differ from emotional motor aprosodia in the slurring of speech, hypophonia, or festination with secondary disturbances of emotional and linguistic intonation. Some flatness or monotone character of voice may be also seen in patients with emotional motor aprosodia, occasionally making it impossible to distinguish emotional motor aprosodia from dysarthria, even for the experienced observer (Starkstein et al., 1994). Studies of emotional motor aprosodia thus require a careful description of abnormalities which are probably related to accompanying dysarthria. The results of these studies must be accepted based after a careful analysis of the original clinical data.

Relation to Language Disturbances

Emotions may be considered as a compact language used for communication with the outside social world. Emotional language is simple, consisting of a limited vocabulary that does not exceed two dozen

245

*Disturbances in the
Recognition of the
Social World*

words. This language may be primarily inherited and is similar, if not identical, for different cultures, resembling some sort of common, innate international language. This may explain attempts to apply the classification of aphasia as a background for the classification of emotional agnosia.

Ross (1985, 2000) compared the comprehension of emotional prosody, its repetition, and its spontaneous production to define various types of aprosodia, including motor, sensory, transcortical, conduction, and global. Ross described transcortical motor aphasia as a disturbance in spontaneous prosody combined with a preservation of the repetition and comprehension abilities of emotional prosody. Transcortical sensory aprosodia includes poor emotional comprehension with a preserved repetition and spontaneous production of emotional prosody. Disorders of conduction aphasia consist of repetition disturbances of emotional prosody, while the comprehension and spontaneous production of emotional prosody remain unimpeded, and so on. According to Ross, differences between different types of aphasia and aprosodia mainly relate to the localization of lesions in the left hemisphere in cases of aphasia, as against the right hemisphere in cases of aprosodia. Ross actually suggested that the sites of lesions in the right hemisphere in various types of aprosodia are similar to the localization of lesions in the left hemisphere in cases with comparable types of aphasia.

Such an approach requires reliable clinico-anatomical confirmation that is difficult to obtain, especially taking into account the difficulties encountered in the assessment of motor emotional aprosody in spontaneous speech and in the course of repetition. Also, despite wide acceptance, the original Wernicke-Lichtheim classification of aphasia has remained controversial since its introduction more than 100 years ago. It must also be stressed that language comprehension is usually disturbed to some extent in cases of Broca's aphasia, and expressive speech is often at least somewhat impaired in cases of Wernicke's aphasia (Tonkonogy, 1986). According to Ross's classification, on the other hand, comprehension is preserved in cases of motor aprosodia, and spontaneous affective prosody remains unimpaired in cases of affective motor aprosodia.

We thus prefer to leave the controversy of aphasia-based classifications of emotional agnosia and motor aprosodia for future studies, and to consider emotional agnosia as a type of agnosia, primarily multimodal associative agnosia.

Anatomical Aspects
   Emotional Agnosia: Right Hemisphere Versus Left Hemisphere and Role of Temporal and Parietal Lobe Lesions.   A series of studies points to the role

of right hemispheric lesions in the development of emotional agnosia. Jackson (1876) suggested that lesions of the right hemisphere lead to disturbances of the emotional aspects of communication, while lesions of the left hemisphere result in impairments of the propositional aspects of communication.

Almost 100 years later, Heilman et al. (1975) published a study of patients with right temporo-parietal lesions that exhibited more prominent impairments in the recognition of the affective component of language than among patients with left temporo-parietal lesions. Ross (1981) studied 10 patients with infarctions of the right hemisphere confirmed by CT scans and found that patients with impaired comprehension of affective prosody tended to have suffered from lesions involving, but not confined to, the right posterior-superior temporal lobe, similar to the left hemispheric lesions commonly observed in patients with Wernicke's aphasia. This conclusion was later supported by a study of 15 patients with right hemispheric infarctions confirmed by MRI scans (Ross, Orbelo, Burgard, & Hansel, 1998).

The role of the involvement of the right hemisphere in the development of auditory emotional aprosodia was also studied during a period of right and left hemispheric inactivation following unilateral electroconvulsive therapy (ECT) in patients with depression (Balonov & Deglin, 1976). The authors studied nine patients after a total of 18 unilateral ECT sessions—9 right-sided ECT sessions and 9 left-sided ECT sessions. The number of correct recognition of emotions was 47 + 4 and 91 + 2 after right-sided and left-sided ECT sessions, respectively.

Darby (1993) subsequently confirmed the role of right temporo-parietal lesions in emotional agnosia in a study of 42 patients with infarctions in the area of either the right (26 patients) or the left (16 patients) middle cerebral artery (MCA). In the first days following the infarction, disturbances in comprehension of the emotional tone of voice and of facial expressions were observed in three out of four patients with infarctions involving the inferior division of the right MCA, and in one patient with an infarction of the left MCA. Disturbances were noted in two patients three weeks after the onset of a stroke that caused a lesion in the inferior division of the MCA, and in one patient in whom a stroke caused a lesion in the superior division of the MCA. These disturbances were not noted in any other cases of left hemispheric lesions.

Starkstein et al. (1994) studied 59 patients with acute stroke lesions using a standardized assessment of the comprehension of emotional intonation and facial expressions. They found evidence of "comprehension emotional aprosody" in 45% of the patients, compared to evidence of the disturbance in only 9.3% of the patients in Darby's study of 43 patients with acute infarctions in the territories of either the right or the left MCA. This may be related to a more difficult second, unconventional task that required the recognition of emotional prosody when the emotional intonation was opposite to the emotional content of the sentence, for example, a happy intonation paired with a sad semantic content. The results yielded by Starkstein et al. (1994) demonstrated that patients with "receptive aprosody" had a higher frequency of right hemispheric lesions, primarily in the temporo-parietal cortex and the basal ganglia.

Similar results were reported by Bowers et al. (1987), who found that patients with lesions of the right hemisphere gave worse responses to sentences in which the semantic content was incongruent with the emotional prosodic content. These sentences, with their contradictory signals, may be considered as unconventional information, as in Stroop's test. The processing of these opposing signals requires the participation of additional cortical and probably subcortical areas, for example, frontal areas for the Stroop test, and may explain why Starkstein et al. (1994) found evidence of lesions in the basal ganglia as well as frontal and diencephalic atrophy in cases of "receptive aprosodia."

Dichotic auditory testing in normal subjects also supported the prevalent role of the right hemisphere in the comprehension of emotional prosody. The tests demonstrated that the emotional tone of a voice is better recognized by the left ear, which is connected by the crossed sensory pathways to the right hemisphere, than by the right ear, which is connected to the left hemisphere (King & Kimura, 1972; Ley & Bryden, 1982). Similarly, the advantages of the left visual field over the right visual field were demonstrated in tests that required subjects to discriminate between emotionally laden facial expressions (Ladavas, Umilta, & Ricci-Bitti, 1980), or to match an emotionally expressive face with a spoken word (Hansch & Pirozzollo, 1980).

In the only case with corresponding autopsy data, Tonkonogy (1986) found evidence of disturbances in recognition of the emotional tone of voice and of facial expressions in patient L.R. These impairments developed following a stroke that involved a large bilateral infarction in the temporal lobe, as well as a partial infarction in the inferior parietal lobe of the right hemisphere. L.R. was a 65-year-old right-handed woman, who was a former teacher and who had a long history of cardiac arrhythmia and several episodes of cerebral emboli, which led to three strokes. After the first stroke, the patient developed mild conduction aphasia with slight difficulties in expressive speech and speech comprehension. The comprehension of emotional prosody was preserved.

The second stroke occurred 8 months later and led to the development of moderate aphasia of word deafness with prominent difficulties in repeating single vowels as well as disturbances in the comprehension of spoken language. L.R.'s expressive speech remained fluent, with no grammatical errors and no evidence of paraphasia. Her

248

LOCALIZATION
OF CLINICAL
SYNDROMES IN
NEUROPSYCHOLOGY
AND NEUROSCIENCE

speech, however, almost completely lost its emotional and linguistic intonation, becoming monotonous and resembling motor aprosodia. The patient's speech differed from dysarthria in that there was an absence of slurring. L.R.'s ability to name objects and actions was preserved. The patient's reading comprehension was much better than her motor prosodia, and the patient was able to read and follow written commands. Sensory amusia was noted, and a moderate auditory agnosia was present.

Agnosia of emotion was noted after the second stroke. Disturbances in the recognition of emotionally laden facial expressions were evaluated by presenting the patient with drawings of smiling, crying, and astonished faces on separate cards. Sometimes the patient was asked to name the emotion associated with the facial expressions, and at other times she was required to choose the card associated with a specific emotion. The patient was unable to understand or discriminate between the different facial expressions and could not tell whether the people in the pictures were smiling, crying, or astonished. At the same time, no sign of prosopagnosia was observed. In spite of language disturbances, the patient could either name or show on the card the names of individual familial faces, as well as the names of celebrities, and could determine which faces were male and which were female.

Evaluation of the comprehension of emotional speech prosody was conducted using a tape recording of two short pseudosentences composed of nonsense words: "An ter fil sol" and "Ak mas sho zu." An actor used various intonations to convey the states of anger, sadness, astonishment, and nervousness as he uttered each sentence. The actor also modulated the expression of the pseudosentence to indicate a declarative, interrogative, or imperative linguistic intonation. After hearing a sentence, L.R. was shown cards with the written words "anger," "sadness," "astonishment," and "nervousness" and was asked to select the card that indicated the correct emotional intonation. The same type of cue was presented for the different linguistic intonations. L.R.'s testing sessions revealed prominent difficulties in the comprehension of emotional and linguistic prosody. The patient was extremely doubtful about the appropriate choice and would often switch from one card to another, trying to find the correct answer.

While these disturbances could be secondary to nonverbal auditory agnosia, the presence of impairments in the recognition of facial expressions supported the significant, if not critical, role of primary emotional agnosia in the development of sensory aprosodia in L.R.

L.R. suffered from a third stroke 3 months after experiencing the second. The patient complained of paresthesia in her right arm and suffered from ptosis of the left eyelid with a right deviation of the left

249

*Disturbances in the
Recognition of the
Social World*

eyeball and an external deviation of the right eyeball. L.R. was able to move her extremities, but unfortunately she contracted pneumonia, which led to her death only 13 days following the onset of the third stroke. An autopsy revealed symmetrical infarctions in the temporal lobes (Figure 5.2).

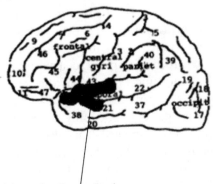

(a) conduction aphasia
(Left hemisphere, lesion after 1st stroke)

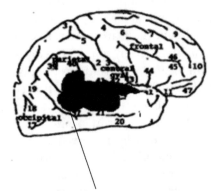

(b) emotional sensory agnosia and motor aprosodia
(Right hemisphere, lesion after 2nd stroke)

FIGURE 5.2 Development of (a) conduction aphasia and (b) emotional agnosia and motor aprosodia. (a) Conduction aphasia developed after the first stroke, which occurred in the left hemisphere. The infarction in the left hemisphere destroyed the anterior two-thirds of the first temporal gyrus, the middle portion of the second temporal gyrus, and the anterior portion of Heschl's gyri. (b) Emotional agnosia and motor aprosodia developed after the second stroke, which occurred in the right hemisphere. The infarction in the right hemisphere completely destroyed Heschl's gyri, the entire first temporal gyrus, the middle and posterior portion of the second temporal gyrus, the posterior part of the supramarginal gyrus, and the portion of the insula at the level of the sensory strip. Smaller, older infarctions were found in the left parahippocampal gyrus and the left cerebellar hemisphere. The most recent infarction was situated in the left thalamus.

After the first stroke, the patient developed mild conduction aphasia, which could be attributed to the left hemisphere infarction in the anterior-middle portion of the first temporal gyrus, and probably to the partially damaged Heschl's gyri as well. The second stroke caused many disturbances related to the right hemisphere, as well as bilateral temporal lesions, including word deafness, sensory amusia, and nonverbal auditory agnosia. Agnosia of emotion also developed after the second stroke and may be attributed to the right hemispheric temporal infarction in the first and second temporal gyri, as well as Heschl's gyri. The most striking and important finding in this case was the development of disturbances in the recognition of facial expression following a lesion largely limited to the superior areas of the temporal lobe in the right hemisphere, with a sparing of the occipital lobe, as well as a sparing of almost the entire parietal lobe; only the posterior portion of the supramarginal gyrus was damaged. This also points to the role of a lesion in that region in the development of an impairment in the comprehension of emotional speech prosody. The auditory emotional agnosia, however, might have been at least partially secondary to the nonverbal auditory agnosia and word deafness that developed after the second stroke.

The findings in this case correspond to data that point to the role of lesions in the right temporo-parietal region in the development of emotional auditory and visual agnosia (Darby, 1993; Ross, 1981; Starkstein et al., 1994). It is still remains unclear, however, what specific part of that region is generally implicated. Our findings underscore the role of a superior temporal lobe lesion. Ross (1985, 2000) stressed that the cortical lesion in such cases involved, but was not confined to, the posterior-superior temporal lobe, a region similar in location to Wernicke's area in the left hemisphere, which is usually destroyed in cases of Wernicke's aphasia. Yet no single case of emotional agnosia with a lesion restricted to that particular area in the right hemisphere has been published.

Disturbances in the comprehension of emotional prosody have also been described in patients with lesions of the left hemisphere. Most of these patients, however, suffered from aphasia with a severe deficit in verbal comprehension (Schlanger, Schlanger, & Gerstmann, 1976). Seron, Van der Kaa, Remitz, and Van der Linden (1979) observed a positive correlation between the severity of emotional aprosody and the comprehension of propositional speech in aphasic patients. This may be related to the development of sensory auditory aprosodia secondary to the disturbances caused by impairments at the apperceptive level of speech comprehension in aphasia. At the same time, auditory emotional agnosia may be observed primarily in patients suffering from a lesion of the right hemisphere but with no sign of aphasia. This lesion would cause a direct impairment of the process involved in the recognition of emotion. It would be useful to compare the recognition of emotionally laden facial expressions in patients with sensory auditory aprosodia and aphasia produced by lesions of the left hemisphere with the recognition of such expressions in patients with such aprosodia and an absence of aphasia but with the presence of lesions of the right hemisphere. This may help to eliminate the role of an apperceptive component in the development of emotional agnosia in patients with lesions of the right and left hemispheres.

Lesions of the Amygdala. Special attention must be given to data concerning the role of a lesion of the amygdala in the development of a disturbance in fear recognition. Damasio's group reported a 30-year-old patient who demonstrated severely impaired recognition of fear following a near complete bilateral destruction of the amygdala caused by Urbach-Wiethe disease (Adolphs et al., 1994). The patient's ability to recognize faces was completely preserved (Adolphs et al., 1994). In their next report, Adolphs et al. (1995) demonstrated that while the processing of fearful facial expressions was impaired in the patient with bilateral amygdala damage, it remained unimpeded in 6 patients with unilateral amygdala damage, as well as in 12 brain-damaged control patients with lesions that did not involve the amygdala. Damage in the unilateral amygdala patients was caused by herpes simplex encephalitis in 2 patients, and by a temporal lobectomy for the treatment of epilepsy in 4 patients.

Calder et al. (1996) subsequently presented two cases with differentially severe impairments of fear recognition following bilateral damage to the amygdala. The damage was caused in one patient by herpes simplex encephalitis, and by neurosurgery for epilepsy treatment in the second patient. The authors reported a high number of errors made in the attempted recognition of six emotional states, those of happiness, sadness, surprise, disgust, anger, and, especially, fear. Scott et al. (1997) noted a particularly impaired recognition of fear and anger in both visual and auditory modalities in a patient following a bilateral amygdalotomy carried out during the course of neurosurgery for the treatment of epilepsy.

These results must be considered with caution, since cases of intact recognition of vocal expression of fear following a bilateral lesion of the amygdala have been described as well (Anderson & Phelps, 1998). The Damasio group also reported unimpeded recognition of facial expressions of emotion in two patients with extensive bilateral damage to the amygdala caused by herpes simplex encephalitis (Hamann et al., 1996). The lesion in one patient extended to the temporal pole and the hippocampal formation. The lesion was more extensive in the second patient and involved several areas outside the amygdaloid complex,

252

LOCALIZATION
OF CLINICAL
SYNDROMES IN
NEUROPSYCHOLOGY
AND NEUROSCIENCE

including the inferior, middle, and superior temporal gyri as well as the hippocampus and the perirhinal, the entorhinal, and the parahippocampal cortices. The authors suggested that the difference between their cases and those of Urbach-Wiethe disease was most likely related to the development of impaired facial emotion recognition, but only if the lesion occurred during early development rather than in adulthood. The noted difference may also be related to differences in the assessment of test results.

The Damasio group (Tranel, Damasio, & Damasio, 1988) also reported a case of impaired fear recognition accompanied by extensive lesions in the ventromedial occipital and inferior parietal regions of the right hemisphere. No damage to the amygdala was found. Rapcsack et al. (2000) subsequently demonstrated that the recognition of negative emotion, especially fear, was a more difficult task than the recognition of positive emotion for 74 control subjects, as well as 80 patients with various localizations of brain damage, including 11 patients who had undergone a unilateral temporal lobectomy, and 2 patients with bilateral amygdala damage caused by herpes simplex encephalitis. A unilateral temporal lobe resection was performed during the course of neurosurgical treatment of epilepsy in 10 patients, and during normal control subjects when differences in overall recognition performance for the other five categories of facial emotion had been adjusted for. The authors concluded that their data did not support a special role for the amygdala in the processing of the facial expressions of fear.

These clinico-anatomical findings seem to contradict the neurophysiological studies in primates and humans that identified cells in the amygdala that would selectively activate in response to facial expressions, including an expression indicating fear (Fried, MacDonald, & Wilson, 1997). As in cases of visual object recognition, however, these responses may not be directly related to the recognition of emotion reflecting other operations, for example, the transfer of information of already classified emotion to the amygdala for further processing related to behavioral responses to perceived fear or other emotions.

Lesions of the Basal Ganglia. Emotional auditory and visual agnosia were also described in single cases either with lesions of the basal ganglia (Cancelliere & Kertesz, 1990) or with infarctions involving the right thalamus and extending into the posterior limb of the internal capsule (Wolfe & Ross, 1987). The presence of additional lesions not detected by head CT scans cannot be completely ruled out in such cases. Further data collection in similar cases with confirmation of lesion anatomy by either MRI or autopsy is needed. The role of the so-called ischemic penumbra, which may involve the cortical areas in the first 6 to 8 weeks after an acute stroke, must also be evaluated. Such a penumbra was implicated in the development of subcortical aphasia, and may exist in a case reported by Wolfe and Ross (1987) in which the patient was evaluated within 10 days and then in 6.5 weeks following stroke.

Motor Aprosodia: Role of Right and Left Hemisphere Lesions and the Role of Frontal Lobe Lesions.   The role of a right hemispheric lesion in the development of motor aprosodia was suggested by authors who originally described that particular type of aprosodia (Ross, 1981; Ross, 1985; Ross & Mesulam, 1979; Ross & Stewart, 1981; Tucker et al., 1977). Ross, Orbelo, Burgard, and Hansel (1998) recently reported 12 cases of emotional aprosodia in spontaneous speech with unilateral ischemic infarctions in the right hemisphere as observed via brain MRI scans. Concerning the more precise localization of lesions in cases of emotional motor aprosodia, Ross et al. (1998) pointed to lesions involving, but not confined to, the posterior-inferior frontal lobe that proved to be similar to the left hemispheric lesions found in patients with Broca's aphasia. He also found an extension of the lesion in that particular area of the right hemisphere in 12 of 15 patients with either pure motor aprosodia (3 patients) or combined motor and sensory aprosodia (9 patients). In the previously mentioned case of patient L.R., combined sensory and motor aprosodia developed following a second stroke with infarctions located in the right superior temporal region and the anterior supramarginal gyrus. The lesion did not extend to the posterior frontal lobe.

Further confirmation of findings related to the clinical features and anatomical aspects of emotional motor aprosodia is certainly needed.

CONCLUSION

1. The clinico-anatomical data points to the primary role of right hemispheric lesions in the development of auditory and visual emotional agnosia. These lesions involve the superior part of the temporal lobe, including the middle and posterior portion of the T1 and T2 areas, as well as Heschl's gyri. This lesion is similar to that observed in the left hemisphere in cases of Wernicke's aphasia. However, no cases of emotional agnosia with an isolated lesion in this particular region of the right hemisphere have been reported.

2. It is important to note that recent studies have revealed the role of this particular region in the visual recognition of movements and actions. Together with data concerning the involvement of the superior temporal areas in the development of visual emotional agnosia, these findings point to the involvement of the upper posterior portion of the temporal lobe in visual information

254

LOCALIZATION
OF CLINICAL
SYNDROMES IN
NEUROPSYCHOLOGY
AND NEUROSCIENCE

processing, especially in the right hemisphere. The roles of parietal and basal ganglia lesions need further exploration, especially in cases of emotional agnosia in which disturbances are limited to unconventional information processing.

3. The development of emotional motor aprosodia may be related to an inferior premotor lesion, primarily in the right hemisphere. A similar lesion in the left hemisphere mediates the development of Broca's aphasia. However, a bilateral temporal lesion was noted in the observed cases. Further studies are needed in this area of research.

AGNOSIA OF SOCIAL ACTIONS

THE RECOGNITION OF social actions plays an important role in social functioning. It helps to navigate the social environment, to choose appropriate responses to the dynamic of the environment, and to plan and anticipate the results of social actions and interactions. The list of social actions includes actions that are aggressive, dangerous, hostile, friendly, deceptive, and so forth.

The existence of special operations to recognize motor actions was demonstrated by studies of so-called mirror neurons, which were activated in the brains of monkeys while the animals were viewing the actions of grasping, manipulating, and placing as performed by another monkey (for more details, see chapter 3, section entitled "Agnosia of Action"). While the monkeys observed others performing the actions of grasping, some neurons fired in response to a particular grip, such as a precision grip or a whole-hand prehension. These particular neurons are located in area F5. Similar neurons were observed in the lower bank of the superior temporal sulcus.

A similar system may provide the ability to recognize the social actions and interactions performed by other individuals in order to allow a proper reaction (Rizzolatti et al., 2000). One of the components of such a system could be an ability to make inferences about the state of mind of individuals involved in particular actions. Disturbances in such an ability have recently been highlighted in a series of studies based on theory of mind tasks.

THEORY OF MIND AND AGNOSIA OF SOCIAL ACTIONS

THE BEHAVIOR OF animals and humans may reflect prediction of others' behavior based on the recognition of emotional states according to clues, such as the emotions present in tone of voice, facial expression,

255

*Disturbances in the
Recognition of the
Social World*

or body posture signaling, for instance, in the case of a threat that requires a defensive response.

We may also recognize the mental states of others using information not provided by emotional expressions. This ability to make inferences about others' mental states and about others' beliefs in the course of social interactions has been termed the *theory of mind* (Premack & Woodruff, 1978; Wellman, 1990).

Testing of the theory of mind usually includes two major tasks—false belief tasks and faux pas tasks (Baron-Cohen, Leslie, & Frith, 1985; Wimmer & Perner, 1983). Both types of tasks depict social interaction between two persons, who, for simplicity's sake, we will call Person 1 and Person 2. In the course of testing (for a review, see Stone, Baron-Cohen, & Knight, 1998), the examiner reads a story about Persons 1 and 2 and presents pictures to the subject. In the false belief tasks, Person 2 changes the location of an object while Person 1 is out of the room, for example, a bottle of Coke is moved from the table to the refrigerator. In the first-order false belief tasks, the tested subject is asked: "When Person 1 comes back in, where will Person 1 think the bottle of Coke is?" The correct false belief answer would be, "on the table." The answer to this question requires a mentalistic inference about the beliefs of Person 1. Several additional questions are asked with the intention of checking the subject's comprehension and memory of actions depicted in the story. These questions may include a reality question, such as "Where is the bottle of Coke?" (correct answer—in the refrigerator), or a memory question, such as "Where was the bottle of Coke originally?" (correct answer—on the table), and so on. These questions require a physical inference rather than a mentalistic inference.

The purpose of second-order false belief tasks is to test the subject's ability to understand what Person 2 thinks about what Person 1 thinks. The beginning of the second story may be identical to that of the first, but when Person 1 leaves the room in the second story, that person may see through the window that the object is moved by Person 2, who remains unaware that Person 1 observed the move. The tested subject is then asked: "When Person 1 comes back in, where will Person 2 expect that Person 1 will think the object is?" The correct answer would be, "in the refrigerator." Control questions are similar to those of the first-order.

The faux pas tasks evaluate one's ability to make inferences about the mental states of Person 1 (the listener) and Person 2 (the speaker). In the stories, Person 2 commits a faux pas by saying something awkward, unintentionally revealing information that was supposed to remain hidden from Person 1. For example, Person 2 may have received a crystal bowl as a wedding gift from Person 1. About a year later, while attending a dinner party in the house of Person 2, Person 1 accidentally

256

LOCALIZATION
OF CLINICAL
SYNDROMES IN
NEUROPSYCHOLOGY
AND NEUROSCIENCE

drops a bottle of wine on the crystal bowl, shattering the bowl. Person 1 apologizes, and Person 2, apparently not remembering that the bowl was a gift from Person 1, responds, "Don't worry. I never liked it anyway. Somebody gave it to me for my wedding." In another story, Person 2 mistakenly reveals to Person 1 that a surprise birthday party has been planned for Person 1.

In each case, the tested subject is asked to confirm the existence of a faux pas, to point to the person who committed it (thus requiring the detection and understanding of faux pas), to explain why Person 2 should not have said what he or she said (requiring an understanding of the mental state of the listener, Person 1), and to explain why Person 2 said it (requiring an understanding of the mental state of the speaker, Person 2). A control question asks the subject to remember details of the story. Various types of theory of mind tests differing in their complexity and general content have been developed in the recent years.

A series of studies demonstrated that children develop the ability to understand the first-order false belief task between the ages of three and four, showing that children are aware that other people may hold mistaken, false beliefs (Johnson & Wellman, 1980). Children between the ages of six and seven begin to understand the second-order false belief task, demonstrating that they are aware that one person can hold a false belief about the mental state of another person depicted in a story, an idea otherwise understood as "belief about belief" (Perner & Wimmer, 1985). Between the ages of 9 and 11, children begin to develop the ability to understand the faux pas task (Baron-Cohen, O'Riordan, Stoen, Jones, & Plaisted, 1997).

Clinical and Neuropsychological Aspects

In general, theory of mind tasks are concentrated on the ability of the tested subject to recognize the state of the mind of a person who develops a false belief as a result of another person's actions. The actions usually include various ways of hiding an object while Person 1 either is not watching or is secretly observing the actions of Person 2. The situation in such stories is underlain by the understanding that while Person 1 relies on his belief in the conventional anticipation that Person 2 will not perform the action of object hiding, Person 2 does not expect himself or herself to be watched while hiding the object. This understanding underlies the development of false belief and is considered to be typical and conventional for the normal healthy subject.

The development of a false belief is based on a predefined conventional model in which the person's state of mind is fixed on the stability of a situation without any expectation or anticipation of normal actions (first-order false belief task) or unusual actions (second-order

257

*Disturbances in the
Recognition of the
Social World*

false belief task) from another person. Those situations are most probably quite simple but do not take into account other possibilities created by the presence and interaction of two persons in the story. Such possibilities could be based on suspicions that the person left in the room may undertake some actions while alone in the room, such as hiding the object, or that the person who left the room will, while remaining undetected, witness the action of the person left in the room. It is expected that the tested subject will consider only the more frequent option. This makes the task quite simple, conventional, and difficult to be disturbed via brain pathology.

A more sophisticated faux pas test requires an understanding of the mental state of the speaker, who has disclosed hidden information that may hurt the feelings of the listener. The state of mind of the speaker and the listener is more difficult to assess in such cases than in false belief tasks, since the speaker has not expected to uncover his deception and to say something awkward. The components of the actions, however, are predefined by the description of "the speaker who says something that he or she should not have said" and "the listener who was hurt by what was said," thus facilitating the ability of the tested subject to correctly predict and assess the thoughts of both the speaker and the listener. This task is certainly more complex than the false belief tasks, and thus may be more vulnerable to brain damage.

Disturbances in the theory of mind tasks were revealed in the majority of a group of children with autism who could not solve first- and second-order false belief tasks (Baron-Cohen et al., 1985; Happé, 1994; Ozonoff, Pennington, & Rogers, 1991; Perner, Leekam, & Wimmer, 1987). One key experiment used a puppet show to reveal impairments in the first-order false belief task (Baron-Cohen, 1995; Leslie, 1990). Each subject in this experiment witnessed the puppet Sally as she placed a marble in a basket and left the room. Another puppet, Ann, then moved the marble to a box in the same room. The tested subject was asked where Sally would look for the marble when she returned. The results of the study showed that children with autism are unable to understand that Sally does not know that the marble has been moved. They cannot distinguish their own knowledge from that of another person. Their usual answer in such tests is that Sally will look for the marble in the box, not in the basket.

The ability to deceive may also be impaired in children with autism due to an inability to understand the beliefs of another person. This can be demonstrated via a deception test in which subjects are asked to hide a penny in one of their hands. A child with autism may hide the penny in a closed fist but leave the other hand open, neglecting to consider what the guesser may think about where a penny may be hidden when he or she sees only one closed fist.

258

LOCALIZATION
OF CLINICAL
SYNDROMES IN
NEUROPSYCHOLOGY
AND NEUROSCIENCE

A subtle theory of mind deficit has also been found in children with Asperger's syndrome, a mild form of autism. These children could pass first- and second-order false belief tasks, but demonstrated disturbances in the faux pas task (Baron-Cohen et al., 1997). Since IQ and language development are often normal in children with Asperger's syndrome, the impairments in theory of mind tasks are considered to be dissociable from other cognitive disturbances, and may be compared with the subtle social deficits in Asperger's syndrome. On the other hand, the ability to pass theory of mind tasks may be preserved, while other cognitive disturbances are found in patients, as in cases of Down syndrome or Williams's syndrome (Karmiloff-Smith, Klima, Bellugi, Grant, & Baron-Cohen, 1995; Ozonoff et al., 1991).

In a study of patients with schizophrenia and persecutory delusions, Corcoran, Mercer, and Frith (1995), Corcoran, Cahill, and Frith (1997), and Frith and Corcoran (1996) found lower performance levels on theory of mind tests compared with the performance levels of control subjects and patients with other diagnoses. The authors suggested that these disturbances were related to a deficit in the theory of mind mechanisms manifesting as an acquired inability to anticipate and assess the intentions of other people. Patients with persecutory delusions, for example, may erroneously interpret the intentions of others as being hostile and aggressive.

Walston, Blennerhassett, and Charlston (2000) employed the use of a limited diagnostic definition of persecutory delusions to include the belief that a specific person or group of persons has hostile intentions toward the patient. This definition excluded delusions of suspiciousness or perplexions, as well as fears with ideas of self-reference, as experienced by more generally paranoid patients. The authors excluded cases with prominent cognitive impairments and instead selected four "pure" cases with "encapsulated" persecutory delusions, a condition in which the patient interprets a specific persecutor as operating with a hostile intent. The authors used in the study the theory of mind tests devised and employed by Frith and Corcoran (1996). All four patients performed at a high level and demonstrated no evidence of disturbances in theory of mind tests. It was thus concluded that persecutory delusions could develop in individuals with preserved theory of mind mechanisms.

According to Damasio (1994), the development of persecutory delusions is explained in such cases by the involvement of a person's own emotional reaction, for example, fear of strangers, in the formation of an inference about a stranger's intention in accordance with the individual's "somatic marker mechanism." According to this interpretation, the theory of mind mechanisms remain intact in patients with persecutory delusions.

259

*Disturbances in the
Recognition of the
Social World*

Anatomical Aspects

Data from functional neuroimaging studies have been presented in support of frontal lobe involvement in the theory of mind task performance (Baron-Cohen et al., 1994; Fletcher et al., 1995; Goel, Grafman, Sadato, & Hallen, 1995). It has also been shown that theory of mind task performance, especially for faux pas tasks, was impaired in five patients with bilateral orbito-frontal lesions caused by head injury; performance was preserved in five other patients with unilateral left dorsal prefrontal lesions caused by strokes (Stone et al., 1998). These findings have been used to support the relative independence of modularity of theory of mind tasks, each with their own mechanisms and structural properties (Stone et al., 1998).

A study employing the use of fMRI scans recently demonstrated that, in addition to the frontal region, two other brain regions—the temporal cortex and the amygdala—are activated in control subjects during theory of mind tests (Baron-Cohen et al., 1999). All three areas are activated to a lesser degree in autistic children. A highly significant hypoperfusion in both temporal lobes, centered in the associative auditory and adjacent multimodal cortex, was also found in 21 autistic children by measuring cerebral flow using PET and voxel-based image analysis (Zilbovicius et al., 2000).

Some negative results have also been reported, such as those noted by Bach, Happe, Fleminger, and Powell (2000), who described an intact ability to perform theory of mind tasks with impaired executive function tests in a patient who suffered bilateral orbito-frontal lesions following a head injury. The author suggested the independence of theory of mind abilities from executive function and pointed to the possibility that a disturbance in theory of mind could be caused by posterior lesions.

The role of the right hemisphere in disturbances in theory of mind task performance was first suggested by Happé, Brownell, and Wimmer (1999). The authors found impairments in performance in 14 patients with a mean age of 64 years, each with a lesion of the right hemisphere CVA, compared to normal performance in five patients with a mean age of 67 years, each with a lesion of the left hemisphere CVA, and normal performance in 19 elderly controls with a mean age of 73 years.

The concept of agnosia of social actions only has only begun to be studied and thus it certainly requires further division into its main components. One such component includes disturbances in the recognition of social actions, manifesting as delusional beliefs in social actions and based on the erroneous recognition of actions and feelings of another person or group of persons in the immediate social environment. Examples include delusions of persecution, delusional jealousy, and erotomania (for more details, see chapter 5, section entitled "Delusions").

260

LOCALIZATION
OF CLINICAL
SYNDROMES IN
NEUROPSYCHOLOGY
AND NEUROSCIENCE

Disturbances of Brain Information Processing

A broad explanation of theory of mind disturbances may be related to the mechanisms of top-down processing in *mind reading* (the prediction and assessment of another's thoughts) and social events recognition. The various types of possible states of mind may be kept in a stored model. In a normal person, mind reading is usually based on the high probability of the simple model, which expects no changes in the social situation depicted by the theory of mind tasks. Other less probable models may include unexpected social actions of another person such as object hiding, or hostile actions. The stored models may also include the more general nonspecific models of suspiciousness and hostility. In some cases, these models may be invoked by impairments in which the theory of mind mechanisms are limited to particular top-down nonspecific choices, for example, a belief in hostility toward the patient manifested as a general paranoid suspiciousness and extending to the interpretation of theory of mind tasks. In other cases, the choice of model may be more concrete and specific, for example, in persecutory delusions with regard to specific hostile persecutors and in delusional jealousy of a beloved person. An emotional state related to the "somatic marker mechanism" may also become involved by invoking one of the specific or nonspecific stored models, for example, fear of a stranger in persecutory delusions. Such a mechanism of delusion formation may be seen more often in patients with mood disorders, mania, or depression than in patients with schizophrenia or similar primary psychiatric illnesses.

Lesions in the temporal and frontal lobes may underlain the development of social delusions as well as social agnosia. A patient with delusions, however, may show a complete preservation of social gnosis outside the realm of false beliefs. Delusions are often directed toward a specific person or group of persons, while other persons and their actions remain excluded from the delusional system. Walston et al. (2000) studied four patients, each of whom suffered from encapsulated persecutory delusions concerning a perceived threat of violence from gangs of strangers. None of the four patients showed any detectable abnormalities in their social interactions; reasoning and affect were also preserved. Theory of mind tests yielded high scores, demonstrating intact theory of mind reasoning ability in all four patients.

Corcoran et al. (1995) studied theory of mind tests in patients with schizophrenia and found that persecutory delusions may certainly be accompanied by a wide range of cognitive problems, including social agnosia and disturbances in theory of mind tests. These findings, however, do not exclude the possibility that persecutory delusions do not have a direct relationship to impairments in the theory of mind, as has been shown in patients with encapsulated delusions (Waltson et al., 2000). On the other hand, delusions may be absent in patients with

261

*Disturbances in the
Recognition of the
Social World*

marked social agnosia, as has been observed in patients with autism, pointing to possible differences in the mechanisms underlying the development of social delusions and social agnosia.

There are no direct correlations between delusions, social agnosia, and dementia. While so-called encapsulated delusions are not accompanied by any clear signs of cognitive decline, mild dementia is a frequent finding in other cases, especially in patients with psychiatric manifestations of neurological illnesses. Delusions and dementia in such cases may be caused by the same pathological process, but the underlying mechanisms are different and will be discussed later. Delusions may become less vigorous and become unsystematized; they may eventually disappear in the course of progression to severe dementia. Prominent disturbances in social gnosis seen in patients with severe dementia do not directly involve the formation of delusions, since such a formation is based on the relatively preserved system of social gnosis. Thus, severe social agnosia in patients with dementia may even prevent the development of delusions, which is probably based on a malfunctioning tonically hyperactive top-down processing system during efforts made in the recognition of social actions described in the following section.

DISTURBANCES OF SELF-IMAGE AND SOCIAL AGNOSIA

SELF-IMAGE IS DEFINED as a virtual self-model that represents a subject in his or her relation to the physical and social worlds. While body image is centered on the physical world in the egocentric and the allocentric space, the self-identity image or self-identity model mediates the interaction of a person with his or her world, primarily with the social world, and assesses the position of the *self* in the social space. The self-identity model contains the awareness of identity, in which a person has an awareness of continuity, of being the same identical person all the time, from past to present. This personal experience "unfolds in a space which is centered on a singular, temporally extended experiential 'self'" (Metzinger, 2000, p. 289). The properties of the social self-model also include the feeling of *my-ness*, for example, *my* volitional act, and the ability to distinguish what is *myself* from the outside world (Metzinger, 2000; Sims, 1988). The self-model may include different submodels in order to be socially adaptive, for example, to process conventional and unconventional social information using different submodels.

The *social self-image* is closely integrated with body image, which is often included in the self-model as described by modern authors (Feinberg, 2001; Grush, 1997; Metzinger, 2000; Ramachandran & Rogers-Ramachandran, 1996; Sims, 1988). The somatic and social self-images,

262

LOCALIZATION
OF CLINICAL
SYNDROMES IN
NEUROPSYCHOLOGY
AND NEUROSCIENCE

however, must be considered as relatively independent models that are involved in the regulation of body image and social world.

Depersonalization and Derealization

Clinical Aspects

In 1873, Krishaber described a syndrome of "cerebro-cardiac neuropathy," which was characterized by a strange and unpleasant alteration either of one's perception of oneself or of one's surroundings, with a "loss of reality of the world." One of Krishaber's patients described the disturbance in this way: "I experience one self that thinks, and another self that acts. . . . At such times, I lose the reality of the world." Dugas and Moutier (1911) introduced the term *depersonalization* to describe such an alteration in the perception of oneself. Mayer-Gross (1935) later suggested the term *derealization* for an altered perception of the environment and of reality, and reserved the term depersonalization for an altered perception of oneself.

According to *DSM–IV–TR* (American Psychiatric Association, 2000), depersonalization is "characterized by a feeling of detachment or estrangement from one's self. . . . There may be a sensation of being an outside observer of one's own mental processes, one's body, or parts of one's body. . . . The individual with Depersonalization Disorder maintains intact reality testing. . . . *Derealization* may also be present and is experienced as the sense that the external world is strange and unreal" (p. 530).

Some characteristic descriptions of depersonalization include the subject's feeling as if he or she is "detached from own body," "observing my body movements from outside," "unreal . . . I can't be quite certain of myself any more," or "like a robot." Derealization often accompanies depersonalization, having been described thus: "I am detached from the environment," "I lose the feeling of reality of the world," "I seem to be walled up in a block of ice," and "There is as a big pane of glass between me and the world." Depersonalization is often accompanied by anxiety, "unpleasant feelings," a fear of "going insane," a loss of ability to experience emotion, and a distortion of one's sense of time.

Depersonalization and derealization have been observed in patients with neurological diseases including infections, brain tumors, degenerative disorders, and epilepsy, in which they have been observed especially frequently. This list may also include patients with primary psychiatric disorders, schizophrenia, depression, mania, and acute stress disorder, as well as patients who have suffered from sensory deprivation exhaustion and sometimes patients who have ingested substances such as marijuana, mescaline, LSD, cannabis and especially tetrahydrocannabinol (THC).

Depersonalization and derealization may appear as an ictal phenomenon and in the interictal period of panic disorder. Personality

263

Disturbances in the
Recognition of the
Social World

disorders, especially avoidant, borderline, and obsessive-compulsive, may coexist with depersonalization and derealization. At the same time, depersonalization and derealization disorders are considered to be a separate clinical entity when they do not occur exclusively during the course of another mental disorder and are not due to the direct physiological effects of a substance (American Psychiatric Association, 2000).

Anatomical Aspects

Few attempts have been made to localize the condition of depersonalization, and they have been published primarily in the epilepsy literature. Devinsky, Putnam, Graftman, Bromfield, and Theodor (1989) studied 71 patients, each with dissociative disorder, and found that depersonalization was most frequently induced by complex partial seizures, mainly with a left-sided focus. The presence of partial complex seizures pointed to a temporal lobe focus in these cases. The role of the temporal lobe in the development of depersonalization was also described by Penfield and Rasmussen (1950). In the course of surgical treatment for epilepsy, an application of electrical current to the superior temporal gyrus produced in one patient a "queer sensation of not being present and floating away," while in another patient the stimulation of the medial temporal gyrus produced feelings of being "far off and out of this world." Penfield and Rasmussen observed "illusions of unfamiliarity, strangeness and remoteness" after cortex stimulation, mainly in the temporal region with probable extension into the adjacent occipital cortex (1950, p. 173).

As may be expected, electrical brain mapping and PET studies have confirmed changes in the temporal lobe in patients with primary depersonalization disorders but have revealed changes in other cortical regions as well. Using an electrical brain-mapping technique in a patient with primary depersonalization disorders, Simeon et al. (2000) conducted a PET study of 8 subjects, all with primary depersonalization disorders, who were compared to 24 subjects in a normal control group. In the group of patients suffering from depersonalization, the authors reported significantly *lower* metabolic activity in Brodmann's areas 22 and 21 of the superior and middle temporal gyri. However, significantly *higher metabolic activity* was also registered in the parietal Brodmann's areas 7B and 39 and in the left occipital Brodmann's area 19.

Disturbances of Self-Identity Image in Relation to Social Space

Multiple Personality Disorders (Dissociative Identity Disorder)

Clinical Aspects. According to *DSM–IV–TR* (American Psychiatric Association, 2000), "the essential feature of Dissociative Identity

Disorder is the presence of two or more distinct identities of personality states" (p. 526). Normally, self-identity image may be adjusted for adaptation to the changing social environment. In some extreme cases, however, these submodels of identity may become independent, manifesting in a clinical syndrome of multiple identities with differences in personality traits, history, and self-image. One primary identity may be quiet, passive, and obedient, while another personality may be unaware or only partly aware of the presence of the first identity and is aggressive, hostile, and controlling.

The alternative subpersonalities may be presented as different in age and in gender, race, and sociocultural background. A particular subpersonality may experience gaps in memory, which are usually related to personal history for lengths of time during which the individual has been occupied by another subpersonality. The transition from one to another subpersonality is often rapid, occurring in a matter of seconds.

According to *DSM–IV–TR* (American Psychiatric Association, 2000), the number of subpersonalities may reach as high as 100 in an individual but reaches 10 or less in half of the reported cases. Females tend to have more identities compared to males, and dissociative identity disorder is diagnosed three to nine times more frequently in females than in males.

Seizure disorders are frequently noted in patients with multiple personality disorders. Actually, an association of multiple personalities and seizure disorders was reported in several publications in the 1800s (Charcot & Marie, 1892; Mitchell, 1817; Von Feuerbach, 1828). More recently, several authors have noted an unexpected frequency of multiple personalities in patients with seizure disorders (Horton & Miller, 1972; Mesulam, 1981; Schenk & Bear, 1981). Benson, Miller, and Signer (1986) described two patients who each experienced shifts from one personality to another following a major seizure. One personality was irritable, hostile, and aggressive with episodes of assault, while the second personality was calm, pleasant, and easy for hospital staff to manage.

At the same time, patients with dissociative identity disorder often have no history of seizures, and an EEG does not show seizure activity. According to *DSM–IV–TR* (American Psychiatric Association, 2000), these patients may frequently exhibit signs of posttraumatic stress disorder. They may also have symptoms that meet the criteria for mood, substance-related, sexual, eating, or sleep disorders. Aggressive behavior, self-mutilation, and suicidal behavior have been observed in some patients, and autosuggestion may be a factor in some of these cases.

Anatomical Aspects. The localization of *multiple personality disorder* may also be related to the involvement of the temporal lobe. Schenk and Bear (1981) observed frequent multiple personalities in interictal periods in 10 out of 53 patients with complex partial seizures, pointing to the probable involvement of the temporal lobe in the development of multiple personality disorder. It is also possible that head injuries involving temporal lobe structures may result in the formation of dissociative identity disorder. Further studies are certainly needed. It is important to stress that both types of identity disorders, depersonalization and multiple personality, have been frequently observed in patients with seizure disorders, pointing to the role of the excitation rather than the destruction of brain tissue in the mechanisms of identity disturbances. Childlike behavior was frequently noted in patients with orbito-frontal localization of lesions, leading to the idea that the role of frontal lobe lesions must also be considered in the development of such disorders.

Disturbances of Self-Identity Image and Amnestic Disorders

Clinical Aspects

The development of self-image is related to memory but is not identical to the detailed memory of one's life events. The interactions of the individual with these events and their positive and negative outcomes are processed and used in the formation of identity image, self-awareness, and its features in interactions with the world. Disturbances of self-image may manifest as a phenomenon independent from memory loss, as in depersonalization and personality changes. In some cases, however, memory problems may either accompany self-image disturbances or manifest themselves as the intrinsic parts of those disturbances. This has been observed in so-called *fugue states, twilight states,* and *generalized psychogenic amnesia.*

In fugue states, called "dissociative fugue" in *DSM–IV–TR* (American Psychiatric Association, 2000, p. 525), disturbances of *self-identity image* may be observed during episodic periods of unrecalled behavior (Cummings, 1985). Such periods are "characterized by sudden, unexpected travel away from home or one's customary place of work, accompanied by an inability to recall one's past and confusion about personality identity or assumption of new personality" (American Psychiatric Association, 2000, p. 519). Such travel may range from hours or days to weeks or months, during which time a person's behavior seems to be coherent, but when under observation such a person may call attention to himself or herself by purposeless behavior, appearing to be drowsy or intoxicated and unaware of his personal identity.

266

LOCALIZATION
OF CLINICAL
SYNDROMES IN
NEUROPSYCHOLOGY
AND NEUROSCIENCE

Fugues are characterized by a tendency to wander away without subsequent memory of the episode, which may last anywhere from hours to days. Delusions, hallucinations, and disturbances of affect are often absent in such cases. A patient may leave his house for a walk to the nearby store, only to find himself later unexpectedly on the other side of the city, unable to understand how he got there. During such travel, the patient crosses the street, rides in public transportation, and responds to simple questions, but leaves the impression of a somewhat perplexed, absent-minded person. The fugue may end as suddenly as it began, and the person may find him- or herself in an unknown situation afterward, with no recollection of the episode. The loss of memory for an episode is usually total (Lishman, 1978).

The essential features of twilight states include an abrupt onset and ending, with an overall duration of anywhere from hours to weeks. The patient demonstrates a prominent disorientation in terms of his or her surroundings but retains the appearance that his or her actions and behavior are preserved and well organized; in fact, he or she often does not seem to be strange when observed from outside. Some patients demonstrate psychomotor retardation with a slowness of reaction. Behavior during twilight states is often guided by perceptual delusions, florid visual hallucinations, and wild affects of terror, fear, and anger. A patient's calm, tranquil state may be suddenly interrupted by sudden outbursts of rage and panic, sometimes accompanied by violent acts of heinous crime with killings of close relatives or bystanders. Everything—humans, animals, and furniture—may be destroyed with unlimited anger and rage. The twilight state usually ends abruptly, often with a subsequent deep sleep. The patient has absolutely no recollection of an experienced twilight state. In some cases, however, recollection of the content of the delusions remains for several minutes after the state ends (so-called retarded amnesia).

Anatomical Aspects

Several EEG studies have been reported of patients suffering twilight states. Lennox (1945) first described a prolonged state of mental confusion in cases with continuous and bilaterally diffuse 1.5 to 4 Hz spikes and wave complexes on an EEG. Similar cases of "spike-wave stupor" or "petit mal status" were described by Schwab (1953), Friedlander and Feinstein (1956), and Niedermayer and Khalifeh (1965). Kroth (1967) and Lugaresi, Pazzaglia, and Tassinari (1971) described a prolonged twilight state in two patients with focal sharp waves and slow waves in the temporal region. Gastaut, Roger, and Roger (1956) and Rennik, Perez-Borja, and Rodin (1969) reported a prolonged twilight state in patients with generalized paroxysmal abnormalities, in some cases with frontotemporal accentuation.

Escueta, Boxley, Stubbs, Waddel, and Wilson (1974) described a 39-year-old patient who had been suffering from generalized tonic-clonic seizures and episodes of confusion since the age of 22. The patient's twilight state was manifested as a general condition of confusion, including an inability to follow simple commands. The patient would turn his eyes toward the direction from which a voice was coming, but failed to respond to his name and to nod his head "yes" or "no" in response to the questions asked; he would simply mumble words with a smile. The patient's behavior appeared to be purposeful; he was able to eat, drink, and go to the bathroom and was able to unbutton his pajamas in preparation for micturition. An EEG performed during such a twilight state revealed polymorphic ½ to 1 Hz slow waves appearing intermittently in the left prefrontal and anterior temporal regions. These same waves rarely appeared in the right medial-anterior temporal region.

The pathological underpinning of fugues remains unclear. In some cases, a clear epileptic history is present. Whitty and Lishman (1996), for example, described a 48-year-old patient who had experienced an episode of wandering from one city to another that lasted for 10 hours. Afterwards, the patient had no recollection of the episode. The patient had a history of infrequent tonic-clonic seizures, and an EEG after the episode of wandering revealed an epileptic focus in the left temporal region. Stengel (1941) found a history of epilepsy in 10% of his cases with episodes of fugues. Berrington, Liddell, and Foulds (1956) revealed a history of severe head injury in 16 of 37 patients with fugue episodes.

In contrast, many authors have stressed a psychogenic origin for the fugues. Schacter, Wang, Tulving, and Freeman (1982) described a patient who developed an episode of fugue while suffering from depression. Other precipitating factors may include severe stress caused by financial problems, marital discord, and especially criminal charges or stress during wartime. It is also stressed that patients with a history of seizures or seizure-like episodes may be more likely to develop fugues of a psychogenic origin.

Fugue states have been more frequently described in patients with seizure disorders, especially in cases of temporal lobe epilepsy. These fugues may be difficult to differentiate from the psychogenic fugues that may develop in patients with mood disorders and in response to psychological stress. The role of seizures or seizure-like electrical activity as recorded via EEG in such cases requires careful clinical attention and further studies.

A loss of memory of one's entire life and personality identity has been also observed in *generalized psychogenic amnesia*. Psychogenic amnesia, known as "dissociative amnesia" in *DSM–IV–TR* (American

268

LOCALIZATION
OF CLINICAL
SYNDROMES IN
NEUROPSYCHOLOGY
AND NEUROSCIENCE

Psychiatric Association, 2000, p. 523), is usually characterized by a sudden onset and an abrupt termination. Psychogenic amnesia differs from amnesia in identifiable neurological disorders by frequent loss of identity (Cummings, 1985). In addition to generalized amnesia, psychogenic amnesia may be selective, with only a partial loss of memory for some of the details of stressful events, or localized, when the loss of memory is limited to relatively brief periods of time, usually several hours after the stressful event. Psychogenic amnesia may be systematized, appearing as a loss of information concerning a particular person, family, or event. Forms of self-aware amnesia do not usually include a loss of identity.

Disturbances of Self-Awareness of Activity in Its Interactions With Social Space

One of the leading characteristics of self-image is the feeling of awareness of activity. Social or physical activity is accompanied by the sense of self-awareness. If there is no such activity, there can be no awareness of the self (Jasper, 1963; Sims, 1988). This highlights the role of self-model activation in the regulation of its interaction with the environment (Metzinger, 2000, p. 290). To regulate such activation, an individual must use the self-model to assess his or her own position and its dynamics in social space. Disturbances in this assessment may result in impairments of social gnosis and social actions.

Disturbances of self-awareness are related to various personality disorders described in detail in psychiatric textbooks and manuals (see American Psychiatric Association, 2000). In this book, attention is given primarily to the disturbances related to identifiable neurological diseases with relatively well-defined localizations of brain lesions. Examples of such disturbances include personality changes and related delusions as the result of lesions of the frontal and temporal lobes.

Clinical and Anatomical Aspects

Overestimation of Self-Image: Role of Orbito-Frontal Lesions. Disturbances in personality may be described as overinflated self-awareness. The patient becomes boastful, overestimates his or her abilities and accomplishments, and/or devises numerous unrealistic plans. He or she dismisses warnings and criticisms from friends and relatives about this overestimation of abilities. This overinflated self-image may be explained by the inability to properly assess the results of one's own actions. It is often accompanied by unconcern about one's own history of failures. Patients with orbito-frontal lesions are often hypomanic, experiencing euphoric episodes that are usually empty, causing one to behave in a fatuous manner without true elation. It seems that an overinflated

269

*Disturbances in the
Recognition of the
Social World*

image is a relatively independent symptom and is only partly related to euphoria.

Another manifestation of orbito-frontal lesions is a loss of social rules or limitations. The patient loses a sense of social distance, often demonstrating overfamiliarity and tactlessness. This loss is also manifested as a preoccupation with inappropriate sexual comments and sexual indiscretion and promiscuity.

In general, orbito-frontal personality changes resemble in some part simple versions of the narcissistic personality disorder of *DSM–IV–TR* (American Psychiatric Association, 2000). They also, however, have some similarities with multiple personality, specifically with the frequent development of childish behavior, such as engaging in prankish joking and punning, described as childish excitement by Jastrovitz (1888) and as *Witzelsucht* by Oppenheim (1889).

Manifestations of overestimated self-awareness may be observed in both patients with mania and with grandiose delusions (for more details, see chapter 11, section entitled "Mood Disorders," and section entitled "Delusions Underlain by Social Agnosia," in the present chapter).

Underactivation of Self-Image: Avolition and Role of Dorsal Frontal Lesions. Lesions localized in the convexital dorsal and parasagittal medial regions of the frontal lobe lead to disturbances in the activation of the mental and physical activity that gives a person the sense of self-awareness. The patient develops apathy and avolition, or a loss of initiative, resulting in a withdrawal from social life. The inner structure of self-awareness, the self-model, may be preserved in such cases, but the activation of the self-model for its interaction with the environment is inhibited and is suppressed secondary to the avolition, in similar fashion to the preservation of the inner structure of language in cases of speech akinesia (for more details, see chapter 10, section entitled "Avolition, Akinesia, and Negative Symptoms").

Underestimation of Self-Image: Role of Temporal Lobe Lesions and Association With Temporal Lobe Seizures. In patients with temporal lobe lesions, primarily with temporal lobe epilepsy, self-awareness in the ability to succeed in a social activity is underestimated. The patient attempts to achieve positive results, often becoming preoccupied with details, circumstantialities, orderliness, and perfectionism, and often losing the major point of the activity. Flexibility, an ability to adjust to the changing environment, is replaced by viscosity and stickiness in actions and thought processes (Bear & Fedio, 1977; Bear, Levin, Blumer, Chetham, & Ryder, 1982; Waxman & Geschwind, 1975). This is also reflected in increased concerns over morality and

270

LOCALIZATION
OF CLINICAL
SYNDROMES IN
NEUROPSYCHOLOGY
AND NEUROSCIENCE

ethical issues, hyperreligiosity, humorlessness, and hyposexuality. Hypergraphia represents another manifestation of these personality changes (Waxman & Geschwind, 1975).

For many decades, the *distinct personality profile* has been considered to be a specific set of personality changes in patients with various types of seizure disorders. Bear and Fedio (1977) devised a special scale to evaluate these personality changes. The authors compared groups of patients with temporal lobe epilepsy, patients with neuromuscular disorders, and normal control subjects and found a distinct personality profile in many patients of the temporal epilepsy group. It was also found that a distinct personality profile includes higher test scores on all tests in patients with temporal lobe epilepsy than in patients with generalized seizures (Bear et al., 1982; Hermann & Riel, 1981; Rodin & Schmaltz, 1984).

Subsequent studies, however, demonstrated these distinct personality changes in patients with generalized seizures as well as in patients with temporal lobe epilepsy (Brandt, Seidman, & Kohl, 1985; Master, Toone, & Scott, 1984; Stark-Adamec, Adamec, Graham, Hicks, & Brun-Meyer, 1985). These personality changes have also been observed in cases with various types of psychiatric disturbances (Hermann & Riel, 1981; Mungas, 1982; Rodin & Schmaltz, 1984).

It remains unclear why these personality changes have been more frequently observed in seizure patients with relatively small lesions, while quite opposite personality changes have been shown to be related to orbito-frontal lesions with neuropathology produced by brain tumors, severe head injuries, or degenerative processes. It is possible that both the localization of lesions and underlying paroxysmal activity play a specific role in the development of the distinct personality disorder in epileptic patients.

Disturbances in Brain Information Processing

Social agnosia develops within the system in the recognition of social subjects and their interactions by a particular person in relation to the self-image of that person. Like recognition in physical space, the system of social information processing has to include two basic levels needed for successful recognition: a lower level for features processing and a higher level that contains the prototypes of social subjects and social actions, consisting of a set of features and their weight for each prototype. The list of object and action prototypes stored at higher levels of the social recognition system, however, differs from the system or module for the recognition of objects and actions in the physical world. The content of this list must include subjects and actions that are socially important for the social self of a particular person, who must recognize the social meanings of persons and their

271

Disturbances in the
Recognition of the
Social World

actions in relation to such categories as danger, deception, and friend-liness, as well as the success or failure of her or his own actions. This system may be disturbed in social agnosia due to general difficulties in the recognition of primary social features, subjects, and actions in the social world.

Various emotions may act in such conditions as a primer, decreasing the thresholds of particular prototypes in the set of social categories: for example, a state of mania increases the probability of overesti-mated self-assessment, while fear increases feelings of suspicion. An underestimation of self-assessment is frequently developed against a background of prominent depression. Emotions may play a significant role in priming, modulating and regulating the social gnosis and self-assessment of the results of a person's actions.

CONCLUSION

1. Localization of lesions in depersonalization and derealization has been reported primarily in patients with temporal lobe lesions (Figure 5.3).
2. Overestimation of self-image seems to be primarily related to orbito-frontal lesions, while underactivation of self-awareness is observed mainly in cases of dorsal frontal lesions.
3. Lesions in the temporal lobe were observed in cases with an un-derestimation of self-image.
4. A primary site of lesions in cases with *somatoagnosia is the pari-etal lobe.* This stresses the relative independence of the self versus body images and their disturbances, at least from the clinico-anatomical point of view.

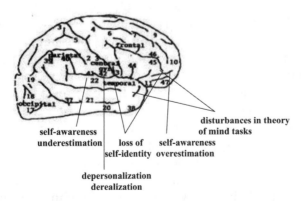

FIGURE 5.3 Right hemisphere. More frequent sites of lesions underlying the development of various types of social agnosia and disturbances of self-image.

272

LOCALIZATION
OF CLINICAL
SYNDROMES IN
NEUROPSYCHOLOGY
AND NEUROSCIENCE

DELUSIONS

A *DELUSION IS DEFINED* as a "false unshakeable idea or belief which is out of keeping with the patient's educational, cultural and social background; it is held with extraordinary conviction
and subjective certainty" (Sims, 1988, p. 82). Delusions are held with
unusual convictions not amenable to the logic of other people of
the same educational and cultural background (Fish, 1967). The overvalued idea may be acceptable and comprehensible but completely
preoccupies the sufferer, becoming so dominant that the patient's
whole life comes to revolve around this one idea (McKenna, 1984).
The condition of suffering from delusions is usually associated with
strong affect.

Primary delusions refer to false beliefs that are not understandable
considering the patient's current conditions and his or her history.
Primary delusions may appear completely out of the blue, with no explanation. Delusions in this sense are referred to as "autochthonous
ideas" (Wernicke, 1906). Primary delusions are often considered to be
bizarre or "absurd," "impossible" from the perspective of one's ordinary life experiences and one's particular culture. "Delusions which
express a loss control over mind and body are generally considered to
be bizarre" (American Psychiatric Association, 2000, p. 299). Examples
of bizarre delusions include disturbances of mind self-image, or beliefs
that one's thoughts have been withdrawn, inserted, or controlled by
outside forces. A patient may feel bizarre changes in body self-image,
for example, that his body has turned into that of a dog or that his
body will wash away if he has a shower (Cutting, 1987), or perhaps that
a stranger has removed her internal organs and replaced them with
somebody else's organs without leaving any scars (American Psychiatric
Association, 2000, p. 324). Such delusions are usually described in patients with schizophrenia.

Secondary delusions are understandable and can be traced from their
origins to the patient's current mood, life circumstances, personality,
and beliefs about his or her peer group (Sims, 1995), but they are characterized by prominent disturbances in reality assessment. They include,
for example, guilt delusions in patients with depression, delusions of
grandiosity in manic states, and delusions of being followed by police
or threatened by a gang.

Delusions are termed *paranoid* when they specifically relate to the
patient or are self-referent, and are often persecutory. The term *paranoid schizophrenia* was originally used in clinical psychiatry to describe
cases with delusions accompanied by hallucinations, while the term
paranoia was used for cases with delusions but with no hallucinations
(Kraepelin, 1905).

The classification of delusions may be based on differences in the content of delusions. They may be called *social delusions* when the content is related to the relations of self to the outside social world. *Somatic delusions* are centered on one's own body. Social delusions include delusions of persecution, control, jealousy, love, grandeur, and guilt, as well as nihilistic delusions and delusional misidentification. Somatic delusions may include delusions of ill health (hypochondriacal delusions), delusions of abnormal, often ugly, body shape (dysmorphophobia), delusions of bad odor emitting from body parts, and delusions of infestation or lycanthropy. Somatic delusions may be considered to be manifestations of disturbances in the somatic self-image. For more details, see chapter 3, section entitled "Somatoagnosia and Disturbances of Somatic Self-Image."

SOCIAL DELUSIONS

SOCIAL DELUSIONS REFLECT the firm, unshakable but false recognition of persons or actions in the social world or its particular components. Two types of social delusions may be distinguished. *The first type* is underlain by the type of social agnosia, in which the social world may be falsely considered as hostile in persecutory delusions, deceptive in delusions of jealousy, and controlling in delusions of control; the outside world may be considered as not existing at all in nihilistic delusions. Delusional misidentification is underlain by a patient's recognition of a relative or friend as an impostor who tries to deceive the patient by presenting an appearance identical to that of his or her relative or friend. *The second type* of social delusion reflects the under- or overestimation of the position of self in the outside world. Patients in such cases may feel delusions of guilt about various social actions that are either minimally or not at all related to them. Delusions of grandeur are opposite to delusions of guilt in that a patient's position of self in relation to the outside world is thought to be on a level of importance, power, and achievement that is either greatly overestimated or completely unrelated to the individual's real position in the social world. Another variety of social delusions is built around disturbances of social self-image, which consist of nihilistic delusions and delusions of control.

DELUSIONS UNDERLAIN BY SOCIAL AGNOSIA

Delusions of Persecution
Clinical Aspects

Delusions of persecution, "in which the central theme is that one (or someone to whom one is close) is being attacked, harassed, cheated, persecuted, or conspired against" (American Psychiatric Association, 2000, p. 822), are the most common types of delusions. They are based on the belief that somebody in the outside world holds hostile feelings and intentions toward the patient. Persecutory delusions, for example, may consist of firmly held false beliefs that someone, perhaps a specific person or group of persons, has tried to kill the patient by poisoning his or her food. A patient may believe that a gang of youngsters is trying to catch and kill him, or that the neighbors are conspiring to damage the his property or "to get rid" of him. A woman may perhaps insist that she is being followed by a man who has the intention of raping and killing her. In other cases, delusions are less encapsulated and the deluded person becomes suspicious and fearful of everybody around him or her, including business colleagues, relatives, neighbors, and doctors who are perceived by the patient as trying to harm him or her, or plotting to steal his or her house.

Persecutory delusions may also be simple and concrete, as in a patient with Alzheimer's disease who accuses his or her son-in-law or daughter-in-law of stealing money or valuables from a locked drawer. In patients with schizophrenia, the delusions may be more abstract, often "high-tech" ideas that manifest as a belief that someone is trying to harm the patient using atomic waves, or perhaps using radio waves from devices hidden inside the wall of the patient's room.

Patients suffering from persecutory delusions often attempt to prove their false beliefs by pointing to some unrelated features, while some of the more demented patients do not bother to look for any form of confirmation of their beliefs. We observed a patient with residual schizophrenia who experienced bizarre delusions, in which she reported, giggling, that her parents, who had both died long ago, were in the cellar where "a machine was cutting their heads."

Persecutory delusions have been described in cases of schizophrenia, and may accompany Schneider's list of first rank symptoms. Delusions of persecution have been described in many infectious and degenerative diseases, as well as in posttraumatic and metabolic encephalopathy. Special attention has been given to the similarity between psychosis in schizophrenia and interictal psychiatric manifestations of epilepsy, especially temporal lobe seizures (Slater, Beard, & Clithero, 1963). These similar manifestations include persecutory delusions in many of the reported cases of schizophrenia and in the interictal periods of temporal lobe epilepsy.

Persecutory delusions are underlined by emotions of fear, emotional states that are driven by fear in response to perceived, but nonexistent, danger. The role of fear may support the suggestion that the temporal lobe and the limbic system are involved in persecutory delusions, since the development of fear has been closely connected with these structures.

Anatomical Aspects

Gal (1958) reported the development of delusions in patients with temporal lobe tumors. White and Cobb (1955) described delusions in a case of a large pituitary adenoma, which was suppressing the adjacent hypothalamic areas.

Malamud (1967) reported the development of a psychiatric disorder in each of 18 patients with intracranial tumors of the limbic system. Delusions were observed in Case 18, with autopsy data of a colloid cyst arising from the roof of the third ventricle. Paranoid delusions developed in two patients with temporal lobe tumors. An autopsy of the patient in Case 1 revealed a ganglioma restricted to the left anterior hippocampal region, largely involving the uncus amygdaloid area. In Case 2, an autopsy revealed a small cystic astrocytoma in the right para-hippocampal gyrus, compressing the hippocampus, but not involving the amygdala; a large, fairly recent hemorrhage was found on the lateral side of the amygdala. Delusions were also reported in Case 10, in which autopsy data revealed a tumor in the right gyrus cinguli in the white matter of the frontoparietal region. All 18 patients described by Malamud suffered from seizure disorders, primarily of the complex-partial, psychomotor type.

The involvement of the temporal lobe and adjacent areas as well as subcortical structures in cases with persecutory delusions has been reported in some patients with cerebrovascular lesions.

Trimble and Cummings (1981) described a 58-year-old male who was experiencing lethargy, a lack of motivation, and persecutory feelings that a plot against him was developing. A CT scan of the patient's brain showed bilateral inferior thalamic infarcts. The patient suffered a loss of voluntary eye movement in the vertical plane, and the authors stressed the role of the involvement of the ventral tegmental area in the midbrain.

Levine and Finkelstein (1982) described the development of delusions, usually persecutory, in six of seven patients with right temporo-parietal (two cases), occipito-parietal (two cases), or temporo-parieto-occipital (two cases) infarctions or hemorrhages. The authors pointed to episodes of seizures in six of the seven patients with delusions and the possible role of these seizures in the development of delusions following stroke.

Peroutka et al. (1982) reported the development of delusions in a case of a right hemisphere infarction in the temporo-parietal-occipital junction.

Persecutory delusions, and in some cases delusions of jealousy, were also reported in patients with late-onset paranoid delusions. MRI data in such cases revealed white matter hyperintensity and cerebral microinfarctions around the lateral ventricles and the centrum semiovale

276

LOCALIZATION
OF CLINICAL
SYNDROMES IN
NEUROPSYCHOLOGY
AND NEUROSCIENCE

(Miller et al., 1989, 1991). These changes were significantly more frequent and prominent in comparison with those of a group of elderly patients with early-onset schizophrenia (Tonkonogy & Geller, 1999), pointing to the role of interruptions of the interhemisphere connections in the development of delusions.

Delusions that are not otherwise specified in *DSM–IV* have been known as *late paraphrenia* in the European literature (International Classification of Disease, [ICD-9]). Delusions experienced in late paraphrenia and in Alzheimer's disease are similar and include beliefs involving having possessions stolen, "phantom boarders," impostors, and jealousy. In addition, delusions of being plotted against and of being harmed are often seen in cases of late paraphrenia. Patients with late paraphrenia are usually characterized by a relative preservation of personality, affect, and intellect. Most researchers have not reported any anatomical or histopathological changes different from similar changes in elderly normal control subjects (Blessed, Tomlinson, & Roth, 1968). A radiological study performed by Naguib and Levy (1982, 1987) showed that ventricular dilatation, as seen on CT scans, was more prominent in 45 cases of late paraphrenia than in age-matched normal controls. The ventricular brain ratio (VBR) was 13.09% in patients but 9.75% in controls. Howard, Almeida, Levy, Graves, and Graves (1994) compared the results of quantitative volumetry measurements of MRI scans in cases of late onset delusional disorders (*n* = 16), patients with paranoid schizophrenia (*n* = 31), and age-matched healthy control subjects (*n* = 35). The volumes of the lateral and third ventricles were significantly larger in patients with delusional disorder of late onset than in control subjects. Enlargement of the lateral ventricles in patients with paranoid schizophrenia compared with controls did not reach statistical significance. The mean age was quite high in all three studied groups—79.83 for the patients in the two experimental groups and 79.48 in the control subjects.

Delusional Jealousy

Clinical Aspects

Morbid jealousy may manifest as an overvalued idea, depressive affect, and anxiety reaching high intensity in, for example, a delusion of infidelity. The spouse is considered as "belonging" to the deluded person, who has "found" various signs that prove the infidelity of the spouse. Such signals may include any "suspicious" spots on the spouse's underclothes or sheets; and even bags under the eyes of the spouse have been considered to be proof of frequent sexual intercourse with someone else.

Delusions of infidelity are frequently associated with chronic alcoholism and other coarse brain diseases, including primary degenerative

277

Disturbances in the
Recognition of the
Social World

dementia during the course of Alzheimer's disease or Pick's disease, Huntington's disease, or Parkinson's disease, and as sequelae of head injury. The delusions may also be observed in affective psychosis, though less frequently, and they are rare in patients with schizophrenia.

Anatomical Aspects

Malloy and Richardson (1994) found only a few cases in the literature with complete neurological workups. The lesions were localized primarily in *the right hemisphere, mainly in the right frontal region.*

Shepherd (1961) reported three cases with delusions of infidelity; an EEG or autopsy in each case revealed dysfunctions or lesions primarily in the right hemisphere or in the right frontal region. Richardson, Malloy, and Grace (1991) described a case of Othello syndrome, which developed shortly after recovery from a large right middle cerebral artery infarction. Silva and Leong (1993) described a 48-year-old patient who had developed delusions of jealousy following a left frontal lobe infarction.

In some cases, delusional jealousy may develop following an infarction involving either the subcortical nuclei or the thalamus. Wong and Meier (1997) reported the development of delusional jealousy in a 72-year-old man following a right cerebral infarction involving the head of the caudate nucleus, the globus pallidus, the putamen, and the internal capsule. Soyka (1998) described a 74-year-old patient with a history of three right hemisphere strokes and lesions in the periventricular areas and the thalamus. The patient developed delusional jealousy following his fourth stroke with a right thalamic infarction.

Erotomania or de Clerambault's Syndrome

Clinical Aspects

A patient suffering from *erotomania* believes that he or she is in love with someone who may not have any knowledge about the patient. A woman, for example, may hold the firm belief that a person, usually older and of high social status, is in love with her, even if that person has never actually spoken to her. The patient may send love letters and perhaps stalk the victim. In one famous case of erotomania, a male patient with schizophrenia developed an unfounded infatuation that involved a celebrity actress. The patient attempted to assassinate a famous politician in an effort to attract the attention of this celebrity.

In addition to being noted in patients suffering from schizophrenia, erotomania has been observed in patients with bipolar disorder, as well as in patients with coarse brain diseases, including head injury, posttraumatic seizures, meningioma, and Alzheimer's disease. For a review, see Malloy and Richardson (1994). No clear neurological data on lesion localizations in cases of erotomania have been described thus far.

278

LOCALIZATION
OF CLINICAL
SYNDROMES IN
NEUROPSYCHOLOGY
AND NEUROSCIENCE

Delusional Misidentification Syndromes

Disturbances in face recognition at the semantic level may manifest as a delusional syndrome when the patient not only alienates the face image from its meaning, as in associative prosopagnosia, but also expresses firm delusional beliefs in his or her own conclusions, suspecting deception and manifesting as a delusion of doubles.

Clinical Aspects

Three basic subtypes of misidentification syndromes are Capgras syndrome (Capgras & Reboul-Lachaux, 1923), Fregoli syndrome (Courbon & Fail, 1927), and the intermetamorphosis syndrome (Courbon & Tusques, 1932). All three syndromes are underlain by the delusion of doubles. These doubles are perceived to be impostors in cases of Capgras syndrome, and familiar persons recognized as strangers in Fregoli delusions. In the intermetamorphosis syndrome, the patient perceives that someone—familiar or unfamiliar—has been transformed into another person with an altered identity and an altered physical appearance. In the syndrome of subjective doubles, the patient believes that a stranger has been physically, but not psychologically, transformed into the patient's own self. Capgras syndrome is also often correlated with paranoid and persecutory delusions (Malloy, Cimino, & Westlake, 1992; Silva & Leong, 1993).

Delusional misidentification syndromes have been described in various nosological entities, but more frequently in cases of schizophrenia (Christodoulou, 1991). The syndromes were also described in cases of bipolar disorder, paraphrenia, cerebral hemorrhage, various forms of encephalitis, temporal lobe epilepsy, metabolic disorders, and Alzheimer's disease. For a review, see Cummings (1985) and Malloy and Richardson (1994).

Anatomical Aspects

Among cases with structural lesions, Alexander, Stuss, and Benson (1979) reported a case of Capgras syndrome resulting from a lesion that had predominantly affected the frontal and temporal lobes of the right hemisphere. Lewis (1987) reported a 19-year-old left-handed female patient who had suffered from complex partial seizures since the age of five. At the age of 19, she developed delusions in which she perceived members of her close family as impostors. An MRI scan revealed bilateral occipito-temporal atrophy, as well as lesser symmetrical atrophy in the frontal lobes.

Weston and Whitlock (1971) described the development of Capgras syndrome following severe head injury with a fracture extending from the left auditory canal upward and backward at an angle of 45° near the parieto-temporal suture. A left carotid angiogram showed a slight

279

*Disturbances in the
Recognition of the
Social World*

elevation of the middle cerebral artery, consistent with a diagnosis of temporal lobe contusion. The patient developed delusions in which he believed that the persons claming to be his parents and siblings were actually impostors who had assumed the appearance of his own family. He referred to his mother, for example, as "that old lady who looks after me." The authors concluded that the patient had some features of a frontal lobe syndrome, together with bilateral temporo-parietal damage. Bilateral atrophy of the frontal and temporal lobes was demonstrated on CT scans of schizophrenic patients with Capgras syndrome (Joseph, O'Leary, & Wheeler, 1990).

Mackie, Ebmeier, and O'Carroll (1994) presented a case of a man in his mid-20s who was experiencing persecutory delusions of being spied upon, followed, and "bugged" by his parents. The patient claimed to hear voices commenting about him and insisted that his parents and relatives would often leave a room, after which almost identical impostors would return. The patient could identify these impostors because, according to him, they were marginally shorter and broader than the real individuals. An MRI scan of the patient's brain showed mild ventricular dilatation. SPECT scans revealed a significantly higher uptake in the left occipital and calcarine regions compared to the right hemisphere indices in the same regions. The latter remained in the normal range without any significant reduction.

Malloy et al. (1992) and Malloy and Richardson (1994) summarized the findings obtained via neuroimaging in 37 cases reported in the literature on Capgras delusions and found that 72% of cases with CT or MRI scans demonstrated right frontal, temporal, and frontotemporal involvement. In some of the cases described, an extension of the frontal or frontotemporal lesion to the parietal and occipital lobes was also observed, but the more frequently noted lesions involving the frontal and temporal lobes in the right hemisphere make this somewhat similar to the localization of lesions in prosopagnosia.

Young, Flude, and Ellis (1991) found only similar data about structural changes in patients with Fregoli syndrome, including a 67-year-old man who developed the syndrome in the *right hemisphere* following stroke. The patient experienced a weakness of the left side with no speech defect. Left visuospatial neglect was noted in cancellation and drawing tasks, pointing to the probable involvement of the right parietal lobe. The patient was visited multiple times by a psychology student, and during one of such visits, the patient misidentified the student as his daughter, asking why she had changed the color of her hair from blonde that morning. The patient became irritated and began to talk about "deception" when the student tried to convince him that she was not his daughter.

280

LOCALIZATION
OF CLINICAL
SYNDROMES IN
NEUROPSYCHOLOGY
AND NEUROSCIENCE

DELUSIONS UNDERLAIN BY DISTURBANCES IN SOCIAL SELF-AWARENESS

Grandiose Delusions

Clinical Aspects

An individual's erroneous beliefs concerning his or her own enormous importance may be defined as a delusion of inflated worth, power, knowledge, identity, or special relationship to a deity or famous person. Some patients with schizophrenia, for example, believe that they have a special relationship to God, perhaps having the responsibility of helping to bring the good dead to humans on earth. One patient may insist on being the king of Egypt, or perhaps a millionaire with an unlimited amount of money in the bank, while another believes he is of blue blood or is a great inventor. One of our patients with schizophrenia insisted she was the queen of Egypt, while another patient, a high school graduate, claimed to be a graduate of several universities, including MIT and Harvard. Still another patient, who was suffering from schizophrenia accompanied by cognitive impairment, proudly described himself as a neurosurgeon, while he was in fact a high school dropout.

Delusions of grandiosity are also manifested in delusions of reference, delusions "whose theme is that events, objects, or other persons in one's immediate environment have a particular and unusual significance" (American Psychiatric Association, 2000, p. 821). A patient suffering from schizophrenia may claim to have a special relationship with God, or claim that a TV anchor transfers special messages to the patient. Grandiose delusions may involve beliefs involving possessing supernatural powers, being an associate or a son of God, or being the president. Multiple personalities may be related to grandiose delusions in some cases. One patient of ours, an African American female who was suffering from schizoaffective disorder, insisted that she was Shirley Temple and insisted that the ward staff call her Shirley. She would not pay attention to questions about the difference in race between herself and the real Shirley Temple, and several hours later she would respond to her real name, showing no recall of her different personality. Grandiose delusions may lead to assumptions of being Christ or a famous political or military figure such as Napoleon Bonaparte.

Grandiose delusions have often been described in patients with schizophrenia or mania, and are often observed in patients with schizophrenia without manifestations of other signs of mania, sometimes with a background of flat affect.

Anatomical Aspects

In some diseases with well-defined brain pathology, for example, general paresis, grandiose delusions are often present and probably

281

*Disturbances in the
Recognition of the
Social World*

related to lesions of the frontal lobe. Only a few researchers have reported the presence of grandiose delusions in patients with Alzheimer's disease (Starkstein et al., 1994).

Delusions of Guilt

Clinical Aspects

Delusions of guilt have often been observed in severely depressed patients. Such a patient may believe, for example, that he or she is a wicked sinner and has ruined his or her family, or that he or she is worthless and deserves to die. A patient may be psychomotorly retarded, repeating in a weak voice self-accusations of responsibility for the problems of a daughter's family, or of living in a stolen house. Delusions of guilt may also develop in some cases of schizophrenia, often reaching bizarre proportions. One of our own patients, a 21-year-old patient with schizophrenia, falsely accused himself of multiple attempts at child molestation. He unfortunately tried to punish himself for such behavior by cutting a small part of the skin on his penis "to prevent the repetition of such terrible behavior."

In patients with neurologically identifiable brain diseases, delusions of guilt have been reported primarily in those with "melancholic depression," which perhaps developed in the course of various infectious, degenerative, neoplastic, and cerebro-vascular diseases.

Anatomical Aspects

Lesions in cases of melancholic depression acquired via brain tumors primarily involve the temporal lobe in either the right or the left hemisphere (Baruk, 1926; Hécaen & de Ajuriaguerra, 1956).

Delusions of Socially Related Self-Image: Nihilistic Delusions, or Cotard's Syndrome

Clinical Aspects

The more pronounced types of depersonalization and derealization are experienced as *nihilistic delusions (délire de négation)*, as described by Cotard (1882). Examples of comments made by individuals experiencing nihilistic delusions include the following: "I am a dead person," "I do not exist," "There is no world anymore," and "Nothing exists any longer." If a patient is asked to name the president of the United States, he or she may answer that there is no president and no government. Patients often insist that they were never born, or that they have no head, no stomach, and no body.

A patient with Cotard's syndrome denies the existence of the world around him and believes that the world has either disappeared completely or is dead (Griesinger, 1845). In the patient's mind, his or her body does not exist. If asked about his age, a patient answers that he

282

LOCALIZATION
OF CLINICAL
SYNDROMES IN
NEUROPSYCHOLOGY
AND NEUROSCIENCE

has no age, as he was never born. Nothing exists any longer, not even himself or herself (Cotard, 1882). One of our patients with paranoid schizophrenia asserted that there is no government. Another schizophrenic patient, who had lived in Boston all her life, answered, "There is no Boston," when asked about places she liked in the city.

While these patients with schizophrenia had no clear signs of depression, nihilistic delusions have been described primarily in patients with severe melancholic depression (Sims, 1988) and sometimes in patients in delirious states (Fish, 1967). Cotard's delusions were also reported in patients following closed head injury, brain tumors, cerebral infarctions, seizure disorders, and prominent brain atrophy of various origins (Malloy & Richardson, 1994).

Anatomical Aspects

Localization of lesions in patients with Cotard's syndrome has been observed primarily in the frontal and temporal regions of the right hemisphere. Drake (1988) reported three patients suffering from Cotard's syndrome, with a right posterior frontal astrocytoma in one patient, right temporal lobe atrophy and right frontal encephalomalacia due to a closed head injury as revealed via CT scans in a second patient, and a right frontal infarct shown in CT and MRI scans in a third patient. Seizure disorders were reported in both the first and third patients, with the disorder having developed during the adult years of the third patient. Joseph (1986) reported two cases of koro, each with a dysfunction of the right temporo-parietal lobe as indicated by EEG and CT scans. Joseph (1986) described a patient with Cotard's in whom CT scans revealed bilateral frontal and temporal atrophy. CT data noting multifocal brain atrophy, though more prominent in the medial frontal region, were also reported in eight patients with Cotard's syndrome (Joseph & O'Leary, 1986). Young et al. (1991) described a young man who, following traumatic brain injury, was convinced that he was dead; a CT scan showed low attenuation over the surfaces of both frontal lobes, suggesting some degree of frontal atrophy, while SPECT scans revealed a reduced tracer uptake in the right temporal lobe and the adjacent parietal region.

Alienation of Thoughts: Delusions of Lost Control Over the Mind

Clinical Aspects

A quite peculiar type of alienation of one's own thought processes has been described in patients with schizophrenia. Schneider (1959) included feelings of passivity of thought in his list of first rank symptoms of schizophrenia. These feelings include *thought withdrawal, thought insertion,* and *thought broadcasting*. Thought withdrawal is characterized

283

*Disturbances in the
Recognition of the
Social World*

by a patient's feeling that his thoughts have been somehow taken out of his head against his will. The feeling is often described by patients as thought blocking, when the train of thoughts is suddenly stopped and the mind goes completely blank (Sims, 1988). Such an individual has the false belief that "his or her thoughts have been taken away by some outside force ('thoughts withdrawal') . . . that alien thoughts have been put in his or her mind ('thought insertion')" (American Psychiatric Association, 2000, p. 299).

Another type of thought withdrawal is *thought broadcasting*. The patient in such cases reports feeling that his thoughts have been withdrawn from his mind and may now be public. This is usually included within the content of a delusion. Sims (1988, p. 123) cited the case of a 21-year-old student, originally described by Mellor in 1970, who said: "As I think, my thoughts leave my head on a type of ticker-tape. Everyone around has only to pass the tape through their mind and they know my thoughts." Thought insertion and thought broadcasting are related to disturbances of social self-image rather than disturbances of body scheme.

Delusions of control have been described in addition to delusions of thought withdrawal and insertion. In such delusions, a person feels "that his or her body and actions are being acted upon or manipulated by some outside force" (American Psychiatric Association, 2000, p. 299). A patient of our own, who suffered from paranoid schizophrenia and resided for many years in a state hospital in Massachusetts, experienced delusions of control and reported that his thoughts were controlled by his elder brother, who lived in California and had not visited the patient for many years. Delusions of control are often observed in patients with schizophrenia. Cutting (1987) compared 74 patients with acute schizophrenia to 74 patients with acute organic psychosis. The author found evidence of delusions of control and thought alienation in 37 patients with schizophrenia but in no patients with organic brain psychosis. These delusions of control were found to be frequently accompanied by persecutory delusions.

Anatomical Aspects

The localization of lesions in patients with delusions of control and of thought alienation remains unclear, but frequent association of these delusions with persecutory delusions may point to the role of temporal lobe involvement.

Social Delusions and Disturbances of Brain Information Processing

In cases of delusions underlain by social agnosia, the development of delusions is usually limited to one particular aspect of social agnosia, such as the misperception of danger, persecution, or deception.

Another scenario for various delusions may be the disturbed social self manifesting as either over- or underestimated self-awareness or as disturbed self-control.

Persecutory delusions may be accompanied by a wide range of cognitive problems, including social agnosia and disturbances in theory of mind tests, an idea originally put forward by Corcoran et al. (1995), who studied theory of mind tests in patients with schizophrenia. These findings do not, however, exclude the possibility that persecutory delusions do not have a direct relationship to theory of mind types of impairments, as has been shown in patients with encapsulated delusions (Walston et al., 2000). Delusions may also be absent in patients with marked social agnosia, as observed in patients with autism, pointing to possible differences in the mechanisms underlying the development of social delusions and social agnosia. Special mechanisms may be suggested as underlying the development of delusions in such cases, an explanation that may be built on the similarities between delusions and hallucinations.

Hallucinations are manifested as a conscious phenomenal vision of objects, animals, and/or humans that are not present in reality. Delusions are similarly characterized by unshakeable false beliefs that are held with conscious certainty but are not supported by social reality. Similarities between delusions and hallucinations also include the absence of agnosia of the physical world in many patients with delusions, and a lack of clear signs of such agnosia in cases with hallucinations. Physical world gnosis in hallucinations and social gnosis in delusions may be preserved outside the areas of hallucinatory visions or delusional beliefs.

Delusions are often accompanied by hallucinations. Persecutory delusions, for example, are often accompanied by auditory hallucinations in patients with schizophrenia. These hallucinations often consist of voices with derogatory comments that are in line with the content of the persecutory delusions. In other cases, while there may be no clearly identifiable hallucinations or delusions, a patient develops a delusional percept when a real percept is being included in the delusional system. A patient with delusional jealousy may, for instance, insist that all the stains on his wife's underclothes are caused by semen (Fish, 1985). Sims (1988) described a patient who believed that the freckles on her arms were actually spots reminiscent of blood injections that were performed at night when she was asleep. One of our patients, a librarian in Oregon with late onset paranoid psychosis, picked up the phone and believed the sounds heard over the phone line to be proof that another librarian from Massachusetts was harassing her using the phone line.

A theoretical model proposed by Grossberg (1980), who attempted to explain the mechanism of hallucinations, may be applied to the explanation of delusions in such cases. In a fashion similar to that of hallucinations, the delusional recognition of a particular category, such as danger or deception, may involve a disturbance during top-down processing, when the features of a corresponding prototype of danger or deception are transferred through the top-down feedback for comparison with the set of features in target cells, thus finalizing the recognition process. These on-center target cells are surrounded by inhibitory, top-down off-surround cells that inhibit the inclusion of weak features in the final set of features in the course of recognition. In cases of delusions, a top-down process inhibits the inhibition surrounding the target cells, activating these cells and producing the conscious, "unshakable" recognition of danger or deception. This recognition is frequently related to a person or group of persons.

Grossberg (1980) suggested that such an inhibition of inhibiting surround cells can become tonically hyperactive without volitional control by an individual, resulting in the development of hallucinations or conscious perceptual experiences with no bottom-up input. A similar process may be responsible for the development of false beliefs without appropriate bottom-up social information.

Various emotions may act in such conditions as primers, lowering the thresholds of particular prototypes in the set of social categories. A state of mania, for example, increases the probability of overestimated self-assessment, while fear increases suspiciousness. Delusions of guilt and nihilistic delusions frequently develop against a background of prominent depression, while grandiose delusions are often observed in manic patients. Fear and suspicions may underlie persecutory delusions, Capgras syndrome, and delusional jealousy. Delusions, however, are absent in the majority of all patients, even in severe cases with depression, mania, or prominent fear and anxiety. Delusions may also be mood incongruent, showing no relation to the emotional state of a patient.

Though emotions may certainly play a significant role in the priming, modulating, and regulating of the social gnosis, as well as in self-assessment of the results of a person's actions, the development of delusions is probably related to some sort of additional mechanism. In addition to the activation of a prototype in the set of social categories, a tonical hyperactivity of top-down processing is needed for the development of delusions. This process may primarily involve prototypes in which thresholds of activation are lowered by particular emotions.

The development of tonical hyperactivity may be related to different hierarchical pairs of low and high layers of the social recognition system. In cases of delusional misidentification syndrome, these pairs of layers disturbed by tonical hyperactivity seem to be related to the levels of social object recognition, particularly the recognition of

286

LOCALIZATION
OF CLINICAL
SYNDROMES IN
NEUROPSYCHOLOGY
AND NEUROSCIENCE

familiar persons. Top-down disturbances at the level of dangerous actions recognition may be related to the development of persecutory delusions.

The pathological mechanisms of tonical hyperactivity remain unclear, but they may be compared in some ways to the frequent observation of hallucinations in patients with seizures. Such connections could be suggested in cases of schizophrenia-like psychosis of epilepsy. Persecutory delusions are often accompanied by temporal lobe epilepsy in patients with stroke and brain tumors. But the delusions included among the first rank symptoms of schizophrenia, such as thought control, insertion, withdrawal, and broadcasting, are not usually accompanied by seizures, including any subclinical seizure activity that may be observed via EEGs. This points to other underlying causes for the onset of delusions, the most likely of which is an imbalance in neurotransmitters. A number of special studies are needed to determine the accuracy of this proposition. It is also possible that these specific neurotransmitter disturbances are underlying findings demonstrating that these types of delusions are usually absent in secondary psychiatric disorders.

Different aspects of brain information processing may be implicated in the development of delusions in both schizophrenia and secondary psychosis. According to Cutting (1987), a deluded organic patient is frequently a helpless onlooker in the enactment of some tragedy or misdeed by others, often in the immediate vicinity. One of our patients with Alzheimer's disease, for example, believes that her son-in-law steals valuables from her drawer. On the other hand, the self-image is intimately involved in patients with schizophrenia. Such delusions include a patient's beliefs that she is "going to have eight children," that his or her brain is rotating, that he or she has "turned into a dog" or "into a different person," and that the "right side of [the] body is empty; personality shifted to the left shoulder." Typical examples of such delusions include the first rank symptoms of thought alienation manifested as thought withdrawal and insertion, as well as delusions of control.

Delusions of self-image are considered to be implausible, absurd, and bizarre, probably because the self-image of mind and body is characterized with a probability of 1.0, which means a full certainty that there exists only one definitive prototype, or model, of mind and body self-image. In cases of delusions related to actions in the outside world, there is at least a possibility that these actions actually happened in reality, but, considering the circumstances outlined in the content of these delusions, the probability is quite low. This points to the idea that possible differences in mechanisms underlie the development of the different types of delusions. In cases of persecutory

287

*Disturbances in the
Recognition of the
Social World*

delusions, for instance, there is a small chance that the individual is being watched by police. Though this idea is rejected via top-down comparison with the results of reality testing in normal conditions, a deluded individual may consider the results of reality testing to be supportive of his or her false beliefs. On the other hand, the probability of thought withdrawal by outside forces is equal to zero in normal conditions and is not included in the preserved conventional and bidirectional process of self-image assessment of one's own mind and body. In cases of delusional thought withdrawal, this zero probability may be changed, making it possible to get involved in the process described.

Chen and Berrious (1998) suggested that established, previously stored patterns may be interrupted by a spurious attractor or pattern (Muller & Reinhardt, 1991) stored in the wide basin of attractions, or prototypes that do not correspond to previously learned patterns in cases of memory overload or certain abnormal conditions in the network. These abnormal network conditions may include reductions in network size or in the number of connections, leading to the development of absurd, bizarre delusions. Those "spurious attractors," however, must be inhibited in normal conditions during the course of learning.

Grossberg (1980) suggested that such an inhibition may be achieved via top-down processing that compares the expectations (attractors) with bottom-up input. An expectation is included in adaptive resonance with low-level processing when the top-down prototype is confirmed by bottom-up input. It is possible in cases of self-image delusions that the formation of adaptive resonance is disturbed, allowing "spurious attractors" with zero probability to be included in the adaptive resonance loops, which process features of my-ness in the self-image. Such disturbances may result from relatively small lesions, leading to the excitation responsible for the development of tonical hyperactivity in top-down processing in patients with schizophrenia. Contrary to the suggestion made by Chen and Berrios (1998), no significant reduction in network neural resources would be required for the development of delusions in such cases.

The site of the lesions responsible for the development of delusions of self-image of mind remains unclear. It has been demonstrated that lesions are often localized in the parietal lobe in cases of body image delusions such as depersonalization. Similar lesion localization may also be suggested in cases with delusions of self-image of mind, but further studies are needed. It is also unclear why delusions of self-image of mind are observed only in patients with schizophrenia, while the self-image of body is more frequently disturbed in patients with psychiatric manifestations of neurological illnesses. The role of neu-

288

LOCALIZATION
OF CLINICAL
SYNDROMES IN
NEUROPSYCHOLOGY
AND NEUROSCIENCE

rotransmitter imbalances, such as high levels of dopamine, may be implicated in cases with schizophrenia, but further studies are certainly needed.

CONCLUSION

1. Lesion localization in various types of delusions primarily involves the temporal and parietal lobes of both hemispheres, though more often in the right hemisphere, as well as the frontal lobe or limbic structures, including the hypothalamic region, in some cases (Figure 5.4).

2. Temporal lobe lesions have been primarily reported in patients with delusions of persecution and of guilt, while frontal and frontotemporal involvement have described in patients with grandiose delusions, Cotard's syndrome, and delusional misidentification syndrome. The development of paranoid delusions has been reported in cases of strokes and brain tumors, with localization in the temporal lobe and limbic structures. Lesions in cases of brain tumors were mainly located in the limbic system, including the anterior-inferior region of the temporal lobe and the hypothalamus.

3. Lesions, primarily of the temporal lobe, were reported in patients with delusions of persecution and of guilt; the involvement of the frontal and frontotemporal areas was described in cases with grandiose delusions, Cotard's syndrome, and delusional misidentification syndrome.

4. Persecutory delusions are frequently accompanied by temporal lobe seizures both in patients with cerebro-vascular lesions and in those with brain tumors. Though lesions were located more often

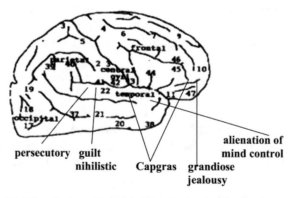

FIGURE 5.4 Right hemisphere. Probable sites of lesion localization in various delusions.

289

*Disturbances in the
Recognition of the
Social World*

in the right hemisphere, lesions of the left hemisphere were also reported.

5. In cases of late onset paranoid psychosis, persecutory delusions were underlined by white matter changes around the lateral ventricles and the centrum semiovale.

DELUSIONS IN PRIMARY AND SECONDARY PSYCHIATRIC DISORDERS

Primary Delusions

Delusions are one of the most important signs of primary psychiatric disorders, especially of schizophrenia. First rank symptoms are observed only in patients with schizophrenia and primarily include delusions of control, thought intrusion, broadcasting, and alien penetration, as well as persecutory delusions in some cases (Cutting, 1987). Disturbances of the self-image, of one's my-ness, are ultimately involved.

Secondary Delusions

Alzheimer's Disease

The frequency of delusions varies from 13% to 33% in patients with Alzheimer's disease (Cummings et al., 1987; Larsson, Sjoegren, & Jacobson, 1963; Mayeux, Stern, & Rosen, 1983; Mendez et al., 1990; Reisberg et al., 1987; Sim & Sussman, 1962; Sulkava, 1982).

Delusions are typical for elderly patients suffering from Alzheimer's disease and may include beliefs that their money or property is being stolen, usually by a relative, or that a spouse is being unfaithful. Capgras syndrome has also been reported in such cases, in which a patient develops beliefs that his or her relative or previously well-known visitor is actually an impostor (Burns, Jacoby, & Levy, 1990; Bylsma et al., 1994; Cummings, 1987; Drevets & Rubin, 1989; Mendez et al., 1990; Rubin, Drevets, & Burke, 1988). Some of the patients believed that imagined people were in the house (phantom boarders) or that the people seen on TV were actually in the room. Perhaps the latter was the manifestation of oneirism. Hypochondriacal delusions and Cotard's syndrome were reported in some cases (Starkstein et al., 1994), as was the misidentification of one's own face in the mirror. The highest frequency of delusions was noted in the moderate stage of the disease's progression.

Delusions in Other Neurologically Identifiable Diseases

Cummings et al. (1987) reported delusions in 7 of 15 (47%) of patients with multi-infarct dementia. The content of these delusions did not differ from that of delusions in Alzheimer's disease and included theft and infidelity. Delusions were also reported in patients with

Huntington's disease (Dewhurst et al., 1969; McHugh & Folstein, 1975), postencephalitic parkinsonism (Bromberg, 1930; Fairweather, 1947), Wilson's disease (Beard, 1959), idiopathic basal ganglia calcification (Cummings, Gosenfeld, Hooulihan, & Mccaffrey, 1983; Frances, 1979) and herpes simplex encephalitis (Rennick et al., 1973).

Hillbom (1960) found a strong correlation between delusions and posttraumatic temporal lobe injuries, with an even stronger association when the injury was in the left temporal lobe. Nasrallah, Fowler, and Judd (1981) reported the case of a 22-year-old college student who lost consciousness after being struck by a car while riding his bicycle. No evidence of psychosis was noted after the patient regained consciousness in the hospital. A carotid angiogram revealed decreased arterial vasculature in the right frontal area with late filling of the right frontal vein, a finding consistent with a contusion of the right frontal lobe. A left carotid angiogram showed an early filling of the deep venous system, which was consistent with either contusion or ischemia of the left basal ganglia. Six months after the injury, the patient visited a mental health clinic complaining of symptoms that included anxiety, irritability, preoccupation with his disability, insomnia, and rumbling speech. Thirteen months after the accident, the patient was admitted to the psychiatric hospital with signs of depression. Two months later, he developed persecutory delusions, believing himself to be considered by others as a "homosexual." The patient believed that his biking accident was part of an "experiment" at the Veterans Administration Hospital. A second admission to the clinic followed an overdose of thioridazine, amitriptyline, and phenytoin, which was explained by the patient as having been an attempt to end the "experiment."

Over the next 5 years, the patient experienced delusions of reference, influence, thought control, and persecution, and his speech and thoughts were disorganized. CT scans revealed that a left lateral ventricle was slightly larger than that of the right. Nasrallah et al. (1981) described the case as a schizophrenia-like illness following head injury. It is quite possible, however, that the authors simply described the onset of schizophrenia in a 22-year-old patient who happened to suffer a closed head injury 6 months before the onset. That injury could have been a trigger for the schizophrenia onset or could have played no role at all in the schizophrenia development.

In summary, no clear differences in the types and manifestations of delusions have been reported in patients with psychiatric manifestations of clearly defined neurological illnesses. Reported delusions mainly tend to involve an individual's misperceptions of social actions in the outside world and their relations to the individual involved. In cases of schizophrenia, delusions are often manifested as disturbances in self-image of mind or, in some cases, as delusions of the body self-image. The latter type of delusions may be frequently manifested as a depersonalization in patients with neurological illnesses.

6

Disturbances of Actions

ACTIONS REPRESENT ONE of the major aspects of brain information processing. While recognition deals with descriptions of both the external and the internal worlds, actions are directed toward achieving certain goals in these worlds. Two major types of action disturbances have been described thus far. The first and more extensively researched type is called *motor apraxia* and represents disturbances of action in the physical world. The second type, related to impairments of action in the social world, is called *social apraxia* and is less clearly defined; it began to be studied in a systematic manner only in recent years.

MOTOR APRAXIA

MOTOR APRAXIA IS defined as a loss of action involving an inability to execute goal-directed, purposive movements, while elementary movements remain preserved or only mildly disturbed. There is no paralysis or paresis, and muscle strength, as demonstrated via active and passive movements in the extremities, is preserved. There are no disturbances of tone, rigidity, dystonia, bradykinesia, chorea, athetosis, or ataxia, but the patient becomes unable to perform both simple and complex actions.

Disorders of actions with objects, disturbances of the symbolic use of signs, and disorders of recognition were described as asymbolia by Finkelnburg (1870) and as imperception by Jackson (1876). Wernicke (1895), who discussed the "loss of the ideas of movements," discriminated between disorders of action and disturbances of recognition. Meynert

(1890) employed the use of the term motor asymbolia to describe disturbances in object manipulation, and sensory asymbolia to describe recognition disorders. The term apraxia was originally introduced by Steinhal (1871), but it was Liepmann who first studied disorders of action in a systematic manner. Liepmann published clinical descriptions, analyses of mechanisms, and pathological data in his paper entitled "The Clinical Picture of Apraxia" (1900) and in subsequent publications (1905, 1908).

In his first report, Liepmann (1900) described the famous case of Imperial Counselor (Regierungsrat) M.T., who suffered from motor apraxia in the right upper and lower extremities, as well as in the head, face, and tongue; praxis was preserved in the patient's left hand. This dissociation helped to prove that apraxia was a primary disorder in such cases, and was not secondary to disturbances of verbal comprehension, visual recognition disorders, or general cognitive decline.

The patient described by Liepmann demonstrated disturbances in the ability to recognize and correctly use a toothbrush, erroneously using it as a writing pen or sticking its handle into his mouth. The patient could not make a fist, shake someone's hand, or point to his nose or ear with his right hand, and was unable to stick out his tongue. When trying to put socks on his feet, the patient would put a sock on his right foot, then hold the other sock down and attempt to put it, again, on his right foot. The patient was also unable to copy simple figures such as squares or circles. Specific disturbances in the patient's writing ability were also noted.

Based on a detailed theoretical analysis, Liepmann (1908) divided these disturbances of action into three major types: *ideational apraxia, ideomotor apraxia, and melokinetic apraxia.*

Ideational apraxia was defined by Liepmann as a disorder of extrakinetic engrams memory, which stores an ideational spatiotemporal plan that determines the path movements will follow, the limbs and parts of the limbs to be used, and the sequence, speed, and rhythm in which the movements will move along the path. This disorder leads to disturbances in complex and novel actions, while simple actions remain preserved. According to Liepmann, a movement formula stored in the extrakinetic memory directs such complex movements using tactile, kinetic, and primarily visual qualities as guides. Damage that impairs the extrakinetic engrams store, or the proper activation of this store, results in gaps and errors in the ideational concept, or in the failure of that concept to emerge at all.

Liepmann considered ideomotor apraxia to be the result of a disconnection between the kinetic engrams store and the extrakinetic store, as well as a disconnection from fresh optic, tactile, and acoustic stimuli, resulting in apraxia of simple, single motor actions. Kinetic limb apraxia, or *melokinetic apraxia,* was defined by Liepmann as a loss of or damage to the kinetic engrams, resulting in an impairment of very simple motor actions, such as skilled, precise movements. Disturbances were usually limited to small muscle groups on one of the extremities, usually contralateral to the side of the cerebral lesion.

Liepmann's analysis and classification of apraxia continue to be accepted in clinical and theoretical considerations. Though some researchers have clarified details or suggested different names for each of the three types of apraxia described by Liepmann, the basic division of apraxia into three types has remained unchallenged. Kleist (1912, 1934) noted and described ideational apraxia and amnestic apraxia. While Kleist described the latter as similar to Liepmann's ideomotor apraxia, he suggested that amnestic apraxia resulted from disturbances of memory for movements. He also gave special attention to "kinetic limb apraxia," which he described as an inability to combine and separate particular innervations, or innervatory apraxia. Foix (1916), Morlaas (1928), and later De Renzi and Lucchelli, 1988 recognized the validity of differentiation between ideational and ideomotor apraxia. This differentiation, however, was suggested not to be between simple and complex motor actions, and ideational apraxia was defined by Morlaas as an "agnosia of object utilization." In more recent publications, ideational and ideomotor apraxia have been described as two different types of apraxia (Hécaen & Albert, 1978; Hécaen & Gimeno, 1960; Heilman, 1973; Heilman, Rothi, & Kertesz, 1983; Rothi, Raade, & Heilman, 1994).

CLINICAL ASPECTS

Ideomotor Apraxia

The disturbances described by Liepmann (1908) under the name ideomotor apraxia have been subsequently divided into relatively independent types of apraxia, each named according to the body parts involved in the particular actions, such as *limb apraxia* or *buccofacial apraxia,* or according to the goal of the actions, including *dressing apraxia, gait apraxia,* and *constructional apraxia.* These types of apraxia may involve disturbances of *conventional* information processing, which are related to simple, well-learned actions using real objects or body parts, as well as disturbances in the processing of *unconventional* information that is novel or unusual.

Disturbances in Conventional Information Processing
  Limb Apraxia: Apraxia of Simple Limb Actions With Real Objects. In cases of apraxia of simple actions with real objects, subjects experience disturbances of single actions using such objects as keys, toothbrushes, combs, and scissors. When asked to comb his hair, for example, a

patient may attempt to do so using the incorrect side of the comb or may move the comb behind one of his ears like a pen. Liepmann (1900) noted a patient who would sometimes attempt to use a toothbrush as if it were a writing pen, or make scooping motions with it as if it were a spoon. When asked to brush off his jacket, the patient moved the brush to the area above his right ear, instead of to the jacket, and performed rhythmic up-down movements with the brush.

Frequent types of incorrect responses in apraxia of simple actions include an alienation of the actual action from its original goal, and the substitution of one requested action by another, which often includes some components of the intended action and may also be called *parapraxia*. Poeck and Lehmkuhl (1980) described a patient who, when asked to open a can of soup with a can opener, attempted to respond to the command by beating the side of the can with the opener. In some cases of spatial apraxia, disturbances are observed when a patient tries to place an object in his or her hand and tries to correctly position his or her hand. A patient may attempt to pick up a spoon and stir his or her coffee, for example, but may have trouble and instead hold the spoon upside down. Action disturbances in such cases seem to be closely related to a loss in the ability to act in egocentric space and resemble disturbances observed in autotopagnosia. The action itself of stirring coffee is performed in allocentric space, and the difficulties experienced are more apraxic than agnostic. The ability to manipulate single objects is usually well learned and conventional, and therefore less vulnerable to brain damage. Apraxia of simple actions with real objects is thus rarely observed.

Though ideomotor apraxia involving actions and real objects is rarely noted, such apraxia is frequently observed in the performance of pantomimic actions and symbolic gestures following verbal command or imitation. In fact, ideomotor apraxia constitutes the majority of cases of apraxia. Liepmann (1908) presented 24 cases of ideomotor apraxia, and the condition was found to be accompanied by ideational apraxia in only 6 of the cases. Hécaen and Gimeno (1960) reported 47 cases of ideomotor apraxia, of which only 7 had accompanying ideational apraxia. Isolated cases of ideational apraxia are quite rare, and some researchers have suggested the possibility that ideational apraxia may represent a more severe stage of ideomotor apraxia (Sittig, 1931).

Dressing Apraxia. Dressing apraxia is the manifestation of a special type of ideomotor apraxia. When attempting to put on a shirt, a patient suffering from dressing apraxia may orient the shirt in the wrong position in respect to his or her own body, turning the shirt upside down or backwards, being unable to lay out the shirt correctly. The patient may begin by attempting to put his or her right arm into the left sleeve, and then switch to an attempt to bring the shirt over the head in a reversed position. Or perhaps, as in the previously mentioned case of Liepmann's patient, while attempting to put a sock on the left foot, a patient turns the sock upside down and begins to put it on the right foot instead (Liepmann, 1900). This type of apraxia was first isolated as a separate syndrome by Brain (1941), who coined the name dressing apraxia. The disorder was subsequently described in detail by Hécaen and de Ajuriaguerra (1942–1945) based on the analysis of 10 cases previously published in the literature as well as five of their own cases.

Apraxia of Symbolic Gestures. The use of gestures with symbolic value is disturbed in those suffering from apraxia of symbolic gestures. Symbolic gestures are performed using parts of the body, especially hands and fingers, instead of real objects. In apraxia of symbolic gestures, the patient is unable to correctly respond to verbal commands or to imitate the threatening movements of another's index finger and hand. The patient instead replaces the correct action with amorphous back and forth movements of the index finger and hand that do not contain the threatening component of the intended gesture. Similar difficulties are observed when a patient tries to blow a kiss, to wave good-bye, to give a military salute, and to perform the "come over here" motion to ask another person to move closer. Such symbolic gestures are not connected to real intent in real life situations and may be considered as unconventional, similar to pantomimic actions. These abilities may be preserved, however, when a patient makes such movements automatically in response to a real situation requiring the use of such gestures.

Apraxia of the Lower Limbs and Axial Body Movements. A patient suffering from apraxia of the lower limbs and axial body movements is characterized by difficulties in placing the lower limbs and trunk in the correct positions to allow the body to walk, to stay, and to sit, in spite of the preservation of lower limb and trunk movements. In cases of less severe disturbances, a patient may experience difficulties in the ability to dance or to bow, or to stand like one about to hit a baseball. Apraxia of gait and trunk movements differs from Parkinson's disease in the absence of rigidity and the presence instead of a shuffling gait. The term *astasia-abasia* has been used to describe disturbances experienced both in this form of apraxia as well as in advanced stages of Parkinson's disease. In some cases, this type of apraxia is limited to disturbances in the ability to walk. Denny-Brown (1958) stressed the "magnetic type" of disturbances in apraxia of gait when a patient is unable to move his or her feet, as they are seemingly attracted by a magnetic force from the

296

LOCALIZATION
OF CLINICAL
SYNDROMES IN
NEUROPSYCHOLOGY
AND NEUROSCIENCE

ground. However, similar difficulties are often observed in patients with Parkinson's disease.

Meyer and Barron (1960) studied less severe types of gait apraxia by asking patients to mimic the kicking of a ball with the feet. Geschwind (1975) asked a patient to stand like a boxer or like a golfer, and found a dissociation between this type of apraxia and upper limb apraxia.

Disturbances of Unconventional Information Processing

Pantomimic Apraxia. Pantomimic apraxia relates to disturbances of descriptive actions of object use without the presence of the object. While there is a full set of components included in the performance of actions with real objects, pantomimic apraxia is observed when a crucial component—the real object—is absent and the set is incomplete. The conditions in cases of pantomimic apraxia are similar to those in cases of visual agnosia of incomplete objects. A regular, well-learned, and simplified set of conventional operations cannot be used in such cases, and a required recognition or action is thus more difficult to perform. The patient with pantomimic apraxia shows disturbances when asked via verbal command or gesture to pretend to stir coffee with a spoon. He or she may place the hand in a clumsy position and begin to move the hand back and forth or move it in slow circles, but is unable to imitate the intended stirring movement. Another patient may stretch out his index finger and try to imitate stirring movements with the finger. Similar difficulties may be observed when a patient pretends to hammer a nail into a block of wood or use a key to lock a door.

Pantomimic actions are more difficult to perform, are less conventional, and are more vulnerable to cerebral damage. As in cases of actions with real objects, pantomimic actions require movements in egocentric space to place the hand in the proper position, and in allocentric space to imitate movements with imagined objects. This type of apraxia may be observed more frequently than apraxia of relatively well-learned, simple, and conventional actions with real objects. In most cases of pantomimic apraxia, simple actions with real objects are usually preserved, while more difficult and complex actions with real objects may be disturbed in some cases.

Buccofacial or Oral Apraxia. Buccofacial apraxia, otherwise known as oral apraxia, is similar to pantomimic apraxia in the preserved ability to perform actions in real situations. The difference between the two disorders lies in the inability of patients suffering from buccofacial apraxia to correctly respond to verbal commands or physical gestures when these actions require the participation of the lips, tongue, facial muscles, pharynx, and larynx. Such disturbances may be observed, for example, when one pretends to chew, purse one's lips, puff out one's cheeks, lick one's lips, suck on a straw, blow out a match, stick out one's tongue, whistle, sniff a flower, or cough. As in pantomimic apraxia, the use of actual objects improves a patient's ability to correctly perform an action such as blowing out a lighted candle, sucking through a straw, or chewing while eating.

Though buccofacial apraxia is often noted in patients with Broca's aphasia, and in some cases with Wernicke's aphasia or conduction aphasia, it may also be observed in patients without aphasia and vice versa. In our own experience, no correlation has been found between the severity of aphasia and the prominence of buccofacial apraxia (Tonkonogy, 1986). The condition may also be present in some cases of apraxia for real objects (de Ajuriaguerra et al., 1960).

Apraxia of Unfamiliar Finger-Hand Positions. Apraxia of unfamiliar finger-hand processing is similar to symbolic apraxia in the common disturbances in finger-hand positions. Patients suffering from apraxia for symbolic gestures, however, experience disturbances in the ability to act in response to verbal commands to imitate previously well-learned gestures with symbolic meanings, while those suffering from apraxia of finger-hand positions have difficulty learning meaningless, unfamiliar gestures. Luria developed special tests to study the integrity of the kinesthetic basis of movements. One such test is designed to study "the optic-kinesthetic organization of a complex movement," in which the patient is asked to imitate the different finger-hand positions produced by the examiner. This becomes even more difficult for the patient when an examiner changes the position of his hand in such a way that the palm is turned down and the appropriate finger sticks out downward (Figure 6.1). In such conditions, a patient may have additional difficulties caused by a need to mentally rotate a finger or hand in order to successfully complete the task. To allow for the study of the kinesthetic component of the test and to exclude the confounding use of visual clues, subjects are asked not to look at their own hand while trying to imitate, for example, the extension of the index and the ring fingers while other fingers are in a flexed position. A patient suffering from apraxia of unfamiliar finger-hand positions may have trouble imitating the positions of the fingers, producing diffuse movements and extending incorrect fingers.

Luria valued the finger-hand position test so much that he often used it to begin the neuropsychological examination of a patient (Tonkonogy, personal observation).

The finger-hand position test was eventually standardized to make possible the scoring of results (De Renzi, Motti, & Nichelli, 1980; Kimura & Archibald, 1974; Pieczuro & Vignolo, 1967). Pieczuro and Vignolo

298

LOCALIZATION
OF CLINICAL
SYNDROMES IN
NEUROPSYCHOLOGY
AND NEUROSCIENCE

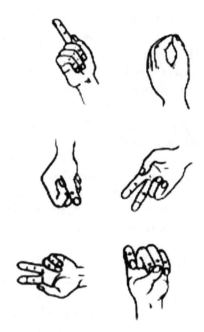

FIGURE 6.1 The finger-hand position test.

(1967), for example, used 10 similar finger-hand positions, asking that each patient copy each position. The results were assessed on a 3-point scale—correct, partially incorrect, and totally incorrect.

Ideational Apraxia

Disturbances of Conventional Information Processing

   Apraxia of Complex Actions With Real Objects.   Complex actions are composed of a series of actions often performed with different objects. Patients suffering from apraxia of complex actions exhibit disturbances in the sequencing of simple actions and often erroneously include elements of other parts of the series in their actions. A patient may produce an incomplete movement, perhaps repeating the first or subsequent action in the series or delaying a transition to the next movement.

   While a patient suffering from apraxia of complex actions may be able to stir coffee in a cup, pour water in a glass, or light a match, disturbances may be observed when the patient has to pour water from a pitcher with a stopper into a glass. Several steps must be performed in such an action sequence: removing the stopper, grasping the pitcher by its neck, bringing the pitcher to the correct place near the glass, tilting the pitcher to an appropriate position, and pouring the water into the glass. A classic task for this type of apraxia is lighting a candle with a match. The patient may be able to remove the match from a box, but he or she may strike the match against the wrong side of the box or bring it to the wick unlighted. The patient may then attempt to strike the candle against the surface of the matchbox. Alternatively, consider, perhaps, that a patient suffering from the disorder is asked to remove sugar from a sugar bowl with a teaspoon, carry the spoonful of sugar to a cup of coffee, drop the sugar into the cup, and stir the coffee with the spoon. The patient may pick up the spoon and attempt to stir the sugar in the sugar bowl with the spoon, or he may carry the empty spoon to the cup of coffee and stir the coffee with the spoon. Patients experiencing apraxia of complex objects tend to omit some of the simpler tasks in sequences of actions, place components in the wrong simple action, and replace the object needed for correct performance with another object included in the complex action.

Ideational apraxia was originally described in patients with senile dementia (Marcuse, 1904; Pick, 1906). According to our own experiences, ideational apraxia may be commonly seen in patients with advanced dementia. It has usually been listed among other manifestations of disturbances in the activity of daily living, a term widely used by rehabilitation and social workers to describe impairments in the everyday functioning of demented patients. It has recently been shown, however, that ideational apraxia may be observed in patients without significant cognitive impairments but with circumscribed lesions in the left hemisphere, a lesion localization similar to that which is often observed in patients with aphasia (De Renzi, Pieczuro, & Vignolo, 1966). Such cases are quite rare, however, and further studies are needed.

Disturbances of Unconventional Information Processing

Apraxia of Unfamiliar Serial Hand and Finger Movements. Several tests were developed by Luria (1966) to study disturbances in sequential series of movements. These tests are widely recognized and are frequently included in various neuropsychological batteries. One such test, the fist-edge-palm test, requires the subject to place his or her hand in three different positions either as verbally commanded or as visually demonstrated by the examiner. Following a short training period, the normal subject performs this test faultlessly. Patients with brain lesions, however, tend either to lose the correct succession of the components in the sequence or continue to repeat the first component, for example, the formation of a fist. To test the flexibility of the organization of motor action, the sequencing may be changed to palm-fist-edge in subsequent trials. Similar difficulties may be observed in the fist-ring test, another version of the serial actions test that requires the patient to thrust his or her hand forward and make a fist, then flex the hand and make a ring with the thumb and the third finger.

300

LOCALIZATION
OF CLINICAL
SYNDROMES IN
NEUROPSYCHOLOGY
AND NEUROSCIENCE

Kimura (1977) subsequently used a special device to test action sequences. The patient is asked to press a button with his or her index finger, pull a handle, and depress a lever with his or her thumb. The results were measured according to learning and action time, as well as the number of correct responses and errors. Kimura classified errors as perseverations, unrelated movements, mistakes in sequencing, incomplete movements, and delays in shifting to another movement in the sequence. Perseverations were found to be the most common error. De Renzi et al. (1980) found that pictorial representations of the required hand position sequencing resulted in a significant improvement in performance, pointing to the role of impairments in the retrieval of patterns of movement from memory in the difficulties of performance for this task. Luria (1966) stressed that additional verbal instructions memorized by the patient, such as "fist," "edge," and "palm," may also greatly improve the performance of such tests.

Kaidanova and Meerson (1964) used a special test, which was actually directed to the study of finger apraxia, to study patients' abilities to learn the serial movements of fingers. Each patient was presented with either visual or kinesthetic cues, and then asked to imitate the serial movements of the fingers. These movements resembled piano playing, for example, a series of finger numbers in the sequence 1–3–2–4, 1–4–2–3, 2–5–3–4, and so on. The number of fingers could also be increased to five, for example, 2–5–4–1–3, or decreased to three, for example, 2–5–3. In cases of disturbances, patients are unable to reproduce the requested succession of the fingers in the series, giving, for example, 1–3–4–2 instead of the correct 1–3–2–4, or repeating the first component of the series, for example, 1–1–1–1, being unable to switch to the subsequent component. Apraxia of the serial movements of fingers is usually bilateral. Though the condition may be secondary to finger agnosia, it has also been observed in cases without finger agnosia.

Kinetic Limb Apraxia

The physical effects of kinetic limb apraxia exclude any effects on the strength and volume of movements. The fingers, however, may lose their delicacy and virtuosity, and may thus become deformed. The patient's movements become rough, angular, and incomplete. Though the coordination of agonists and antagonists remains preserved, patients give the impression of physical sloppiness. The patient may be able to perform simple movements in the course of simple and complex actions, but only the general pattern of actions may be preserved, and simple movements may become so deformed that actions may be difficult to perform properly in some cases. It consequently appears as if a movement loses its goal, its direction becoming apraxic.

This type of disorder has been described as kinetic limb apraxia (Liepmann, 1908), "innervatory apraxia" (Kleist, 1912, 1934), and "melokinetic apraxia" (de Ajuriaguerra & Hécaen, 1960). Luria (1966) incorporated this type of apraxia into the broader syndrome of "kinesthetic, afferent apraxia." The variety of terms reflects differences in the understanding of the psychological and physiological mechanisms underlying the development of this particular type of apraxia. The clinical features of apraxia for single actions, however, remain similar according to these descriptions. In practical terms, apraxia of simple actions may be difficult to distinguish from mild muscle weakness. Some authors thus do not consider apraxia of simple actions to be a true apraxia (Denny-Brown, 1958).

Apraxia and Disturbances of Brain Information Processing

Apraxia and Agnosia

Liepmann (1905, 1908) examined the role of optic, kinetic, and tactile features in motor actions and their disturbances. The role of disturbances of agnosia in the development of apraxia was later discussed by Foix (1916), Schilder (1935), Kroll (1910, 1934), and Semenov (1965). Grunbaum (1930) suggested the term "apractognosia" to stress these connections between apraxia and agnosia. Luria attempted to incorporate agnostic disturbances into the understanding and classification of apraxia (1966).

The Role of Kinesthetic Disturbances. Luria made the distinction between "kinesthetic, afferent apraxia" and "kinetic, efferent apraxia." According to Luria, *kinesthetic apraxia* results from disturbances in the cortical analysis of motor impulses and the kinesthetic synthesis of movement. It differs from spatial apractognosia in that the visual organization of the external spatial coordinates (up, down, right, left) is preserved, while "the ability to select the required kinesthetic impulses that organize the movements" is disturbed (Luria, 1966, p. 206). When a patient attempts to pick up an object, fasten a button, or tie a shoelace, he or she may laboriously search for the required positions of the hand, and will eventually perform the action with the other hand. The effects of kinesthetic apraxia appear in actions with objects and in imitative movements, especially when the object is not present (e.g., when the patient is asked to show how tea is poured into a cup). While kinesthetic apraxia often develops in the hand contralateral to the hemispheric side of a lesion, its bilateral nature may be masked by paralysis of the other hand.

Though Luria did not compare his description of kinesthetic apraxia with Liepmann's classification, kinesthetic apraxia seems to combine the signs of Liepmann's ideomotor apraxia and melokinetic apraxia,

302

LOCALIZATION
OF CLINICAL
SYNDROMES IN
NEUROPSYCHOLOGY
AND NEUROSCIENCE

with some emphasis on the disturbances described in melokinetic apraxia. Luria stressed the similarities of the role of afferent disturbances in kinesthetic apraxia and afferent paresis, which was described by Foerster (1936) as a loss of differentiated hand movements, accompanied by the development of "spade-hand movements" resulting from lesions in the postcentral sensorimotor region. Luria also noted that a series of intermittent disturbances exist between afferent paresis and kinesthetic apraxia.

Kinetic, Efferent Apraxia. *Kinetic apraxia,* also known as efferent apraxia, is the second type of apraxia in Luria's classification and is somewhat similar to Liepmann's ideational apraxia. A key factor in cases of kinetic apraxia is a disturbance in the kinetic organization of motor acts. Series difficulties arise when the patient passes from isolated motor acts to a series of movements of the same type, forming a single skilled movement or kinetic melody (Luria, 1966). The dynamic of the motor act becomes disintegrated, leading to disturbances in the flow of both fast and smooth sequential movements. A loss of complex skilled movements constitutes the central symptom of a motor disturbance (Luria, 1966). The patient with kinetic apraxia is able to perform only single, isolated movements and often continues to repeat these movements, experiencing difficulties switching to new movements. Characteristic examples of such disturbances may be seen when a typist, for example, loses her ability to type at a high speed and begins to laboriously move her finger from key to key. Another example provided by Luria is that of musicians who lose their playing techniques.

In addition to kinesthetic apraxia, Luria considered *spatial apraxia,* also known as *apractognosia,* to be another type of afferent apraxia. The condition is similar, if not identical, to autotopagnosia, and had already been fully described in the literature. Luria named several syndromes as examples of spatial apraxia, including topographic disorientation, Gerstmann's finger agnosia, opticospatial difficulties in constructive apraxia, and agraphia.

The rather important role of visual information processing in motor actions has recently been demonstrated based on single-cell recording techniques in studies of grasping in monkeys. These studies are described in the following paragraph. The authors of these studies consider that motor engrams of actions are limited in their "vocabulary" and are connected with the visual properties of actions. For a review, see Rizzolatti et al. (2000).

Motor Engrams and the Vocabulary of Actions

Special attention must be given to the descriptions of actions stored in the brain, which are also known as motor engrams or motor schemes

(Arbib, 1981). As in recognition, these engrams or schemes require enormous amounts of memory, and thus cannot represent one-to-one descriptions of particular muscle movements needed for specific motor actions. For example, a simple task such as picking up a teaspoon and stirring coffee is not repeated in exactly the same way from day to day: it depends on the initial position of the teaspoon and the location and shape of the cup. Picking up the spoon requires both the proper orientation of the hand relative to the spoon's position, so as to avoid picking up the spoon in the upside-down position, and the shaping of the hand's posture so that its aperture is scaled appropriately to the size of the spoon (Jeannerod, 1984; Soechting & Flanders, 1993). While the spoon is being put into the cup of coffee, the orientation of the spoon in relation to the hand must be changed, and the contact forces of each finger must vary dynamically (Soechting et al., 1996).

Schematic descriptions even of such simple tasks may help to achieve substantial saving in the volume and accessibility of the storage for motor actions. This storage may be organized as the limited numbers of motor schemes, or the vocabulary of motor actions. The term *vocabulary of actions* was first suggested by Rizzolatti in his study of grasping in monkeys (Gentilucci & Rizzolatti, 1990; Rizzolatti & Gentilucci, 1988).

Grasping is characterized by two phases—the initial opening phase and the closure phase (Jeannerod, 1984). During the opening phase, the fingers are shaped according to the size and shape of the object, and the wrist is adapted according to the object's orientation. In the closure phase, the fingers are flexed around the object until they effectively grasp the object. Monkeys most frequently use three major types of grips: the precision grip, the finger prehension grip, and the whole-hand prehension grip. The precision grip, which is based on the opposition of the thumb and the index finger, is used for grasping small objects. The finger prehension grip is used for grasping middle-sized objects and is based on the opposition of the thumb in relation to the other fingers. The whole-hand prehension grip, which is based on the opposition of the fingers in relation to the palm, is used for grasping large objects.

According to Rizzolatti et al. (2000), the motor vocabulary of grasping may contain a limited number of "words" indicating the general goal of one's actions (e.g., grasping), or the execution of these actions (e.g., precision grip or finger prehension). Other words may indicate the temporal segmentation of motor actions, coding the specific phases of the grip, such as hand opening or hand closure, and their sequential order.

Single-cell recording techniques employed during grasping movements helped to demonstrate that separate neurons are activated during the course of each of the three types of grasping. These neurons are localized in area F5 and in the anterior intraparietal sulcus (area AIP).

Area F5 is located anterior to the inferior part of the motor strip, or area F1 in monkeys. There is a high probability that F5 is the monkey homologue of Broca's area, or part of it, and may be compared with Brodmann's area 44 or the *pars opercularis* of the third frontal gyrus (Rizzolatti & Arbib, 1998). Area AIP is located in the rostral half of the lateral bank of the intraparietal sulcus (IPS). Neurons in this area are activated during hand actions (Sakata et al., 1995). Anatomical experiments have demonstrated that areas F5 and AIP are strongly interconnected (Matelli & Luppino, 1997).

The visual and motor properties of F5 neurons were studied in experimental conditions, which were characterized by object fixation followed by grasping and object fixation without grasping (Rizzolatti et al., 2000). In the first condition, half of the tested neurons responded to object fixation, and two-thirds showed selectivity either to a specific object or to a cluster of objects during fixation and grasping. In the second condition, in which object fixation was not followed by grasping, a strong discharge was observed in the neurons, similar to those usually activated by the grasping of the specific object. This was explained in motor vocabulary as the retrieval of specific "wards," which are related to the visual properties of the presented object. The visual properties of the objects were then translated into the potential motor action of grasping.

The third experimental condition required the grasping of objects in the dark with no visual guidance. The monkey learned the characteristics of an object presented in many visually guided trials, and were then shown the object immediately prior to the trial in the dark. In spite of the absence of visual guidance, the neurons were activated in association with grasping.

Two classes of neurons in area AIP—motor dominant neurons and visual and motor dominant neurons—demonstrated activation properties similar to the F5 neurons. The third class of neurons, visual dominant neurons, were strongly activated during object fixation and visually guided grasping, but did not respond when the grasping was executed in darkness (Sakata et al., 1995).

According to a model proposed by Rizzolatti et al. (2000), the AIP-F5 circuit transforms visual information into action. The AIP visually dominant neurons extract specific aspects of object descriptions received from the 3-D object-sensitive neurons in the posterior parietal cortex, caudal area CIPS located posterior to LIP (Shikata, Tanaka, Nakamura, Taira, & Sakata, 1996). The AIP visual neurons decompose the description of an object into the parts important for grasping, for example, the handle of the mug, its body, and so forth. This information is sent to area F5 with suggestions about grasping possibilities. The choice of the grasping schema is made by F5 neurons based on comparisons with the AIP information and concomitant information (purpose of grasping, spatial relationships with other objects, internal drive) received from the prefrontal region. This grasping schema transforms the necessary information to area F1 and to subcortical centers for forming grasping actions, such as hand openings and closures.

This model is based on visually driven motor schemes, or vocabulary of actions, and cannot be considered fully contradictory to the models that reflect the role of tactile and kinesthetic information in motor actions. Gallese, Murata, Kaseda, Niki, and Sakata (1994) studied the effects of AIP inactivation via muscimol injections and demonstrated that grasping with the hand contralateral to the injection side leads to either a complete failure of prehension or an awkward grasping. A successful grasping was achieved in some cases by the use of kinesthetic information obtained by tactile exploration of the object. It can thus be suggested that such kinesthetic information may perhaps participate in the process of the formation of motor schemes, or at least in the process of the transformation of motor schemes into action execution by F1 and subcortical centers.

At the same time, the findings described and analyzed by Rizzolatti et al. (2000) point to the prominent, probably leading role of visual information in the development of motor schemes built as a vocabulary of actions in monkeys. AIP inactivation via muscimol leads to the disruption of hand preshaping and to the posturing of fingers, the effects of which are somewhat similar to the sloppiness of movements in kinetic limb apraxia in humans. Such a disruption of the precision grip in the hand contralateral to the lesion site was also demonstrated following a small injection of muscimol in area F5 (Gallese, Fadiga, Fogassi, Luppino, & Murata, 1997).

Conventional Versus Unconventional Information Processing and Vocabulary of Actions

Conventional Information Processing

Studies of grasping in monkeys point to the existence of a well-defined and limited number of motor schemes or "words" related to the grasping of objects of a specific size and shape. These visual properties of an object elicit the activation of a set of neurons that contain information to allow for the response of a specific type of grasping. Such a structure of information processing may be well suited to conventional information processing when the object being grasped is well known and the set of visual features needed for the selection of grasping type is well defined. Disturbances in this conventional type of information processing are represented in humans by apraxia of actions with well-known real objects, apraxia of dressing, apraxia of well-known gestures, and gait apraxia. It may be suggested that neurons in

306

LOCALIZATION
OF CLINICAL
SYNDROMES IN
NEUROPSYCHOLOGY
AND NEUROSCIENCE

the parietal and, most likely, the frontal areas in humans contain the separate vocabularies of actions and the sets of visual features that are used in the choosing of particular "words" or "instructions" for the selection of specific types of actions. Further studies similar to the studies of grasping in monkeys are needed to describe the types of schemes or the vocabulary of actions stored in the human brain, as well as the mechanisms of their disturbances in various types of apraxia.

The complexity of actions in humans necessitates the existence of a more structurally complicated vocabulary of actions in humans than the vocabulary underlying grasping in monkeys. This may be exemplified by the action of pouring water into a cap from a sealed bottle. This action must be divided into several steps: the bottle is opened; the bottle is grasped and brought to a position that allows the pouring of water into a cup without spilling any; and the water has to be poured into a cup to a certain level. Each step in this sequence of actions requires the use of a different set of "words" in order to adjust to the various visual properties of the objects involved in the action. Objects such as a bottle or a bottle cap may differ in size, shape, and position in space. These differences may require the use of different motor schemas. One schema, for example, may be used to grasp the bottle in one step, while another is used to bring the bottle to the cup, and still another helps to put the bottle in the proper position. Other actions, such as getting dressed, also require several steps, but their types and visual properties may be quite different from the task of pouring water into a cup. It is thus probable that the vocabularies of these different actions may be located in different areas of the brain. The parietal lobe of the left hemisphere may be responsible for allowing one to pour water, while the parietal lobe of the right hemisphere may be employed for the act of getting dressed. These differences in localization are discussed later in this chapter.

Actions may be divided into three levels, in a fashion similar to object classification at the subordinate, the ordinate or basic, and the superordinate levels. The subordinate level describes elementary actions, such as the action of grasping in monkeys. Disturbances at this level may be observed in cases of kinetic limb apraxia. The ordinate level combines elementary actions into simple actions, such as stirring sugar into a coffee cup. Single elements may be represented as a hand posed to pick up a teaspoon, or as a finger adjusted to the texture and size of the spoon, while the combination of a hand's posture and a finger's force represent a combination of single elements involved in a simple motor action. Impairments at this level have been defined as psychomotor apraxia. Action structured at the superordinate level may use combinations of simple actions as invariant kinematic properties and their sequential relationships in time. This type of structure describes the sequential order of actions, leaving their kinematic descriptions to the subordinate and ordinate levels. Disturbances at the superordinate level have been called ideational apraxia.

The classification of actions into subordinate, ordinate, and superordinate levels helps to tune the assessment and use of the visual properties of objects to the selection of types of actions from their vocabulary. It may be suggested that the visual features of an object needed for subordinate actions are different from the features required for ordinate and, especially, superordinate actions. It is possible that superordinate actions need a more general description of an object at the semantic level compared to the importance of some special specific visual features needed for grasping. A general cognitive impairment may thus significantly worsen the condition of ideational apraxia, while not exhibiting any substantial influence on the development of ideomotor apraxia or kinetic limb apraxia.

Unconventional Information Processing

Conventional information processing is an important way to reach saving in operations serving actions. In the course of learning, a conventional description of frequent actions is simplified by an adjustment to the well-known steps included in the actions. Conventional sets of operations become disturbed or destroyed, however, when the conditions of actions are changed and some important elements are missing, as, for example, in pantomimic actions or novel actions.

Pantomimic actions, for example, may be performed using the parts of the relatively automatic, well-learned actions. This may be achieved via a decomposition of the motor schema of action into its parts, followed by the use of some of those parts to imitate the action without the use of objects. The complete schema of stirring sugar into a cup of coffee may be decomposed in such a way that the single action of stirring remains isolated from the preceding and subsequent elements of actions, such as grasping the teaspoon, moving it to the proper position to get sugar from the bowl, and so on. Such a decomposition of the motor schema requires special operations, which are similar to the operations of object decomposition and restructuring in the process of recognition. It has been demonstrated that imitation is an impossible task for a monkey, and so the operations underlying imitation may only exist in the human brain. These operations need special, further exploration.

Another set of operations is needed to learn the new schema of actions in tests of the imitation of finger-hand positions, or in Luria's tests of repeating series of hand positions. Such learning may be based on kinesthetic as well as visual information used in the course of reconstruction of the action and in the sequences of single elements included in the action. A special vocabulary must be constructed to guide

308

LOCALIZATION
OF CLINICAL
SYNDROMES IN
NEUROPSYCHOLOGY
AND NEUROSCIENCE

the proper imitation of the elements composing the action. Since the sets of operations underlying the actions may also differ depending on the type of space in which the actions take place, the role of the body schema in this processing must also be taken into account in future studies. The body schema may be allocentric, with extracorporeal space being relatively independent from the body space, as in the action of pouring water from a bottle into a glass. Other actions may be performed in egocentric space, in which an action is closely connected with one's body image, as in the course of getting dressed, or in the test of finger-hand position. Model storage of these actions may be localized independently from one another, so that the development of apraxia of actions in allocentric space and apraxia of action in egocentric space may each depend on different localizations of brain lesions.

Constructional Apraxia

Constructional apraxia is defined as a disturbance in the drawing or construction of objects and geometric figures either in following a verbal command or in copying another drawing or construction. This type of disturbance was described by Liepmann (1900) as it was experienced by his first apraxic patient as one of the manifestations of ideomotor apraxia, which included an inability to copy simple figures such as a square or a circle. Kleist (1912) isolated disturbances in drawing and construction as an independent syndrome under the name "optic apraxia." Kleist later changed this name to "constructional apraxia," and the syndrome was eventually accepted as a distinctive type of apraxia (Poppelreuter, 1917). Constructional apraxia differs from other types of apraxia in terms of apparent differences in the tasks of disturbed actions. Patients with constructional apraxia show disturbances in the ability to draw an object, either while seeing the object or geometric figure or from memory, while the impaired actions in other types of apraxia are those that require the manipulation of real or imaginable objects and/or body parts.

Clinical Aspects

Constructional apraxia is observed when a patient is asked to replicate a geometric figure or object, either by drawing it or by reconstructing it with sticks or blocks. Disturbances may manifest as difficulties either in the drawing or construction of the general contour or in the configuration of the figure or object. These difficulties are due to underlying disorders in the description of features hierarchies of the decomposed figure or object. Another type of disturbance may reflect difficulties in structural description of the figure, or object invariant properties and their interrelationships. Both disturbances may be present in some cases.

Disorders of Conventional Information Processing

Disturbances in conventional information processing involve a patient's ability to locate the description of a stored model, to evoke that description, and to transfer it to the corresponding actions of drawing or construction. Verbal encoding of the object or figure helps in the search for the appropriate model in storage.

Constructional Apraxia for Geometric Figure and Object Drawings. The patient with constructional apraxia is unable to draw without a sample or to copy geometric figures. In more severe cases, conventional information processing may be disturbed, and he or she may exhibit difficulties in copying such simple figures as circles, squares, and triangles. The drawings of these figures are well learned and verbally encoded. The patient may draw an oval instead of a circle. When verbally asked to draw a triangle or when presented with a picture of a triangle and asked to copy it, a patient draws a triangle with one open angle. The difficulties become more prominent for more complex figures, such as with diamonds or stars. A star may be simplified and drawn as a cross made of two lines, or perhaps as an irregular square. Similar difficulties may be observed when a constructive task requires one to build a square or triangle using sticks of wood.

When verbally asked to draw or when asked to copy a picture of, for example, an animal, a man or a woman, or a face, patients often respond by drawing deformed figures, leaving out important parts and putting some of the parts in the wrong place. When drawing a face, a patient may create an erroneous copy of the face contour, place one eye inside the contour, or draw an eye in the shape of a rectangle (Figure 6.2).

In other cases, the face contour may be correctly drawn, but ears may be placed inside the contour, and the mouth is perhaps missed out completely. Disturbances may also be observed in attempted drawings of a house and its pieces of furniture. A patient may draw an outline contour of the house but may neglect to include windows or doors, or parts of the house are placed in the wrong spatial position. It is especially difficult for such patients to draw a 3-D picture of an object. For example, a patient may draw a table with four legs placed at its four corners, but the 3-D nature of the table is not reflected in the drawing.

Disorders of Unconventional Information Processing

Disturbances of unconventional information processing may be observed when a patient is asked to copy unknown geometric figures that are not represented in stored models, and the patient is thus subjected to the process of structural description and short-term storage

310

LOCALIZATION
OF CLINICAL
SYNDROMES IN
NEUROPSYCHOLOGY
AND NEUROSCIENCE

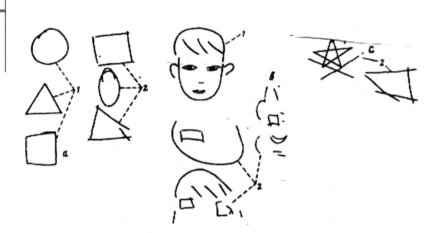

FIGURE 6.2 Copies of the geometric figures and contours of a face as drawn by a patient with constructional apraxia as a result of stroke. (1) Samples. (2) Copies. (a) A circle, triangle, and square are copied with minimal errors, but their spatial relations are altered. (b) Prominent errors are made in the patient's drawings of the face. (c) Drawings of a star are in the shape of an irregular square in one attempt, and in the form of two lines crossing with a "closing-in" sign in another attempt.

as models for drawing or construction. Verbal encoding does not exist for unknown objects or figures and cannot be used in the course of unconventional information processing (Figure 6.3).

It is especially difficult for patients to draw such figures when the sample drawing is removed and the patient is required to recall the image from his or her short-term memory. Unfamiliar figures may also be difficult to construct using sticks of wood in such cases. The Rey-Osterreich Complex Figure Test, which demonstrates special difficulties in the ability to copy and recall figures, has been widely used in neuropsychological testing of constructional apraxia. A patient may be able to draw a figure either by copying the model or from memory and may remember a number of salient details of the figure, but he or she either completely omits the figure's general contour or draws the framework in a piecemeal fashion. In other cases, the framework is set correctly, but details are missed or drawn incorrectly (Kimberg, D'Eposito, & Farah, 1998).

Constructional apraxia is often accompanied by posterior aphasia, spatial agnosia, and/or elements or full experiences of Gerstmann's syndrome (Hécaen & Albert, 1978).

Constructional Apraxia and Disturbances
of Brain Information Processing

Disturbances in the drawing and construction of figures are manifested as a *simplification* of the figures. This simplification leads to the

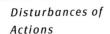

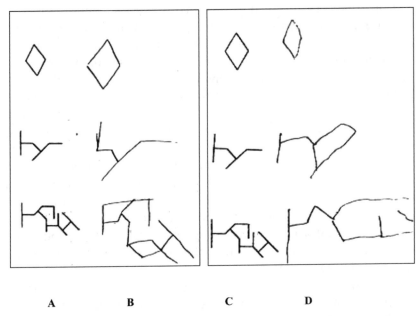

A   B   C   D

FIGURE 6.3 Copies of verbally encoded (upper row) and nonverbally encoded
geometric figures (second and third rows) as drawn by patients with constructional
apraxia. (A) Samples. (B) Drawings by a 61-year-old patient with residual schizophrenia.
(C) Samples. (D) Drawings by a 49–year-old patient with dementia, which had developed
following a suicide attempt via an insulin overdose.

inclusion of fewer details in the figures, with patients omitting or dis-
torting such important details as ears or eyes when trying to copy a face
or draw it from memory (Figure 6.2). In other cases, patients' drawings
have included distortion and fragmentation of the contour outlines of
the figures. Thus, while most of the details are included in the figures,
their spatial relationships are distorted, and the vertical and horizontal
axes of the figure are rotated and disrupted. The correct placement of a
drawing on the page may be also disturbed in such cases, perhaps with
placement being in the upper right or lower left corner of the page. In
some cases, a "closing-in" phenomenon is observed, in which case a patient draws either directly on or very close to the model (Mayer-Gross,
1935, 1936).

   Some researchers have stressed that the simplification and paucity
of drawings may be considered to be deficits in constructional praxis,
while disturbances of spatial relationships in drawings are primarily
of a perceptual nature, and thus perhaps related to some sort of *spatial agnosia* (De Renzi & Faglioni, 1967; Gainotti & Tiacci, 1970; Kirk &
Kertesz, 1989; McFee & Zangwill, 1960; Swindell, Holland, Fromm, &
Greenhouse, 1988). For a review, see Kirk and Kertesz (1994).

Constructional apraxia differs from other types of apraxia in terms of differences in the disturbed main goal of actions. The actions that are disturbed in cases of constructional apraxia are those that are directed toward the drawing of an object, those impaired in cases of limb apraxia, and actions that involve objects, whether real or only reflected in mental images. In this sense, constructional apraxia is closely connected to visual agnosia. The visual properties of an object also play a certain role in other types of motor actions directed toward object manipulation, as shown by studies of grasping actions in monkeys (for more details, see chapter 3, section entitled "Agnosia of Action"). The motor schema, or vocabulary, of an action plays a central role in the execution of such actions. The primary task in constructional apraxia is similar to object recognition, but without the involvement of information processing related to object manipulation. Motor schemas of drawings reflect the visual properties of an object that are important for its recognition. At the same time, a schema may be based on the decomposition of an object into its parts, similar to the process of building motor schemas for object manipulation.

The concrete structure of the motor schemas for drawings remains unclear. This structure may include either the simple features of objects, such as straight lines, curved lines, and line orientations, or the more complex object contours that are built up from these simple features. The drawing of contours may thus be preserved, while the drawing of simple features also remains preserved, as has been observed in many cases of constructional apraxia. It is possible that, as in grasping in monkeys, the operations underlying the act of drawing include motor neurons that contain the motor schemas used in the course of drawing actions, as well as visual neurons that provide motor neurons with information about the visual properties of the object. The main function of visual neurons is to extract from the object description the features needed to invoke the corresponding motor schema for the drawing of the object.

The visual neurons involved in the process of drawing may perform the decomposition of the description of an object or a figure, which is used in the process of the recognition of simple parts or features, such as the straight-line segments needed for a drawing of the object. The line segments may be combined into feature hierarchies, such as corners and vertices. Further combination into a higher-level structure can be used to define shapes such as triangles or rectangles that may form the contour of an object or figure. Damage to these operations may lead to disturbances in the drawing of the general configurations, or contours, of the object or figure.

A second approach is based on the combination of descriptions of invariant properties of the parts of an object or figure and descriptions of interpart relationships. For example, a face may be described according to its simple invariant properties as being composed of two eyes, two ears, and one mouth, while the spatial relationships between these parts and the typical contour of the face may help to define the object as a face. The destruction of this type of object description may manifest as a loss of some invariant properties in the drawing of a face, such as the misplacement of an eye or an ear in relation to the contour of the face. The contour, however, may be drawn correctly, since features hierarchies are preserved.

In both approaches, the disturbances in drawing are primarily related to visual perceptual disturbances, since the main impairment involves the decomposition of object or figure descriptions into parts needed for the selection of the proper motor schema for drawing. The recognition of objects and figures may be preserved, however, since it is based on preserved object or figure descriptions for visual recognition in the stored models, and no sign of visual object agnosia is observed. At the same time, the process of decomposition of an object's description for drawing may be impaired, leading to constructional apraxia caused by visual perceptive disturbances without visual object agnosia.

An absence of visual object agnosia may also be suggested in cases when constructional apraxia is caused by a primary malfunction of motor neurons containing the motor schemas needed for drawing. Single-cell recording used during grasping in monkeys showed, however, that visual and motor neurons are located within the same cortical areas in the parietal lobe. It is thus highly unlikely that a cortical lesion can damage motor neurons but spare the visual neurons in the same area.

In other cases, the damage involves the primary operations used in the description of objects and figures in the process of recognition. This may lead to the development of visual object agnosia accompanied by constructional apraxia, since the visual neurons would be unable to use this impaired description to extract the features needed for the selection of the motor schema needed for drawing. Both constructional impairments and visuoperceptual dysfunctions have therefore been observed in the same patients with brain damage, pointing to the common mechanisms underlying the development of these two kinds of disturbances (Arena & Gainotti, 1978; De Renzi & Faglioni, 1967; Kirk & Kertesz, 1989). This is especially true in patients with apperceptive object agnosia, in which impairments are related to the comparison of object descriptions with stored models. A preserved description may be sufficient in these cases for the extraction of the main features, a process necessary for the drawing of objects. The constructional praxis may thus be either preserved or only mildly impaired.

314

LOCALIZATION
OF CLINICAL
SYNDROMES IN
NEUROPSYCHOLOGY
AND NEUROSCIENCE

Common operations related to the recognition or drawing of a previously unknown object or figure may also include the decomposition and description of the object or figure for short-term storage. An impairment in such operations may result in disturbances either of drawing or of the recognition of new or lesser-known figures or objects. These disturbances are typical for disorders of unconventional information processing. As with well-known objects and figures, the breaking down and the formation of structural descriptions of an unknown object or figure as stored in memory may differ according to whether they are intended for recognition or drawing.

Disturbances in the process of structural description of an object or figure may explain the closing-in phenomenon. A patient suffering from such a disorder is unable to produce or to invoke from model storage a description of an object based on its decomposition into parts, and instead tries to compensate for difficulties in the structural description of an object with one to one, point to point drawings by closing-in the drawing to the sample.

Anatomical Aspects: Upper Limb Apraxia

Left Hemispheric Lesions. The prevalence of left hemispheric lesions in right-handed patients with limb apraxia was first reported by Liepmann (1905), who found evidence of limb apraxia in 20 of 41 right-handed patients with right hemiplegia due to lesions of the left hemisphere, and in none of 42 patients with left hemiplegia due to lesions of the right hemisphere. These findings were supported in a study (Hécaen 1962, 1972) of a large group of patients (415 cases), each with a retrorolandic hemispheric lesion. Ideomotor and ideational apraxia were found only in cases with left hemispheric or bilateral lesions. De Renzi et al. (1980) and Alexander, Baker, Naeser, Kaplan, and Palumbo (1992) stressed the high frequency of apraxia in patients with left hemispheric lesions in contrast to the low frequency in cases with right hemispheric lesions.

The role of left hemispheric lesions in the development of limb apraxia is also supported by the frequent association of limb apraxia with aphasia. De Ajuriaguerra et al. (1960) found evidence of aphasia in 10 of 11 patients with ideational apraxia. Goodglass and Kaplan (1963) administered a battery of quantifiable tests, which included the use of objects and pantomimic and symbolic gestures, to a group of 20 patients with aphasia and a group of 19 nonaphasic brain-damaged patients. Apraxia was found to be more severe in the group of patients with aphasia, but it was also more prominent in nonaphasic patients with left hemispheric lesions than in similar patients with right hemispheric lesions. This points to the role of the left hemispheric lesion in the development of apraxia.

Since cases of apraxia without the presence of aphasia have been described repeatedly by multiple authors, the high frequency of association between apraxia and aphasia cannot be explained by the simple influence of aphasia on the development of apraxia. Kertesz and Ferro (1984) studied 177 cases with left hemispheric stroke and aphasia, and found only 4 cases with severe aphasia and normal scores on tests of voluntary movement. Selnes, Rubens, Risse, and Levy (1982) described the case of a patient who, while continuing to suffer from apraxia, made a rapid recovery from a language disorder. Another localization possibility in the development of apraxia is an extension of left hemispheric lesions, located in the classical language areas around the Sylvian fissure, to adjacent areas in the same region. It is also possible that disturbances in operations of space underlie the development of both apraxia and aphasia. Kimura (1982) stressed that disturbances in a common set of processes may be related to disorders in the ability to organize serial motor actions and language in time. Kimura implicated language disturbances as a leading cause of impairments within the complex system of motor control.

However, the absence of a direct correlation between aphasia and apraxia in a series of cases points to the possibility that common operations underlie some of the aspects of shared space-time control in motor actions and speech. This has been demonstrated in cases with manifestations of so-called semantic aphasia, in which disorders of language operations in space and time were found to be the result of a left parietal lesion (Head, 1926). Some aspects of space-time control operations, however, may be different for motor actions and language, thus leading to the development of either isolated apraxia or isolated aphasia depending on the disturbed aspects of the underlying space-time operations.

Right Hemispheric Lesions. Unilateral right hemispheric lesions were found in cases of dressing apraxia. The lesion localizations in verified cases were parietal and occipital, often at the temporo-parietal-occipital junction (Brain, 1941; Hécaen & Assal, 1970; Hécaen & de Ajuriaguerra, 1942–1945). A lesion of the left hemisphere could be suggested in only 2 out of 15 cases included in a review by Hécaen and de Ajuriaguerra (1942–1945). Lesions of the right hemisphere were also reported in left-handed patients suffering from apraxia.

Left or Right Hemispheric Lesions. Constructional apraxia was first reported in patients with lesions of the left hemisphere (Kleist, 1912). The lesion localization was reported to be in the parietal lobe, primarily in the angular gyrus. Nielsen (1946) paid special attention to a lesion on the border of the angular gyrus and the occipital lobe, pointing

316

LOCALIZATION
OF CLINICAL
SYNDROMES IN
NEUROPSYCHOLOGY
AND NEUROSCIENCE

to the frequent association of constructive apraxia and Gerstmann's syndrome.

Constructional apraxia was later reported in a series of cases with right hemispheric lesions (Hécaen & Assal, 1970; Hécaen, de Ajuriaguerra, David, Rouques, & Dell, 1950; McFie et al., 1950; Paterson & Zangwill, 1944). The role of an extension of the lesion from the right posterior parietal lobe to the adjacent occipital lobe was stressed in these cases. Hécaen et al. (1951), for example, described evidence of constructional apraxia in six cases with occipito-parietal tumors. Differences between the types of constructional apraxia according to the location of the lesion—the right hemisphere versus the left— were stressed following a publication by Paterson and Zangwill (1944). The left hemisphere patients exhibited a tendency to simplify their drawings, preserving the general outlines of the objects and figures. The patients with lesions of the right hemisphere, however, often neglected the left side of the drawing and demonstrated a piecemeal approach, alternating the spatial relationships in the drawing and its position on the paper (De Renzi & Faglioni, 1967; Gainotti & Tiacci, 1970; Kirk & Kertesz, 1989, 1994; Stiles-Davis, Janovsky, Engel, & Nass, 1988; Warrington, James, & Kinsbourne, 1966).

Lesions of the Parietal Lobe and Adjacent Areas of the Temporal Lobe. Following a description of apraxia by Liepmann in 1905, many authors related the development of various types of limb apraxia to a lesion in the parietal lobe of the left hemisphere. The autopsy of Liepmann's government counselor, who suffered from prominent ideomotor apraxia of the right hand, revealed an infarction extending from the supramarginal gyrus to the superior parietal lobe in the left hemisphere (Liepmann, 1905). An additional lesion had destroyed the entire corpus callosum, minus the splenium, which could have been responsible for the development of mild dyspraxia in the left hand. Stauffenberg (1918) and Kroll (1910) each found that an extensive lesion of the supramarginal gyrus in the left hemisphere was often accompanied by severe apraxia in both hands.

Some researchers have stressed the role of lesions in the region around the junction of the parietal and temporal lobes in the development of limb apraxia. According to Foix (1916), ideomotor apraxia resulted from infarctions in the territory of the parietal branch of the angular gyrus artery, while ideational apraxia developed following a lesion in the temporal branch of the same artery. De Ajuriaguerra et al. (1960) connected the development of ideomotor apraxia to parietal and temporal lesions and the development of ideational apraxia to large posterior parietal and temporo-parietal lesions. Heilman (1973) described three patients who exhibited fluent aphasia as well as peculiar types of limb apraxia in response to verbal commands, each with preserved performance in the imitation and use of actual objects with either the right or the left hand. A radioisotope scan performed on one of the patients revealed abnormalities in the angular gyrus. An extension of the lesion to the posterior part of the T1 area may have been responsible, given the presence of fluent aphasia in all three cases.

Following Liepmann's publication on the role of parietal lobe lesions in the development of apraxia, records of an absence of apraxia in cases with similar localizations of lesions began to appear in the literature. Von Monakow (1904), for example, reported a case in which a gunshot wound involved the left supramarginal gyrus, though the lesion was not very large and extended only in front of the interparietal strip, thus partially preserving the supramarginal gyrus. An absence of apraxia was observed 2 years following the injury, and no data concerning an apraxic defect were found in the patient's history, which described his condition immediately following the head injury. In another negative case, a patient was reported as suffering from hereditary epilepsy, and surgery performed to treat this revealed a large area of atrophy in the left parietal lobe, destroying the cortex of the inferior part of the supramarginal gyrus, the largest part of the angular gyrus, and the posterior third of the T1 area. Von Monakow, however, reported evidence of transient apraxia and agraphia immediately following the surgery. The role of developmental compensation of function must also be taken into consideration in this particular case.

In recent decades, the advent of brain imaging has made it possible to study the anatomy of lesions in the large number of cases with lesions of the parietal lobe in the left hemisphere. A number of cases with such localizations of lesions have been reported by several authors. Basso, Luzzatti, and Spinnler (1980) reported the results of ideomotor apraxia testing and CT scans in 123 patients with left hemispheric lesions caused by stroke. The patients were asked to imitate 10 different single gestures with the left hand. The results of each item were quantified— 2 possible points for each item with a maximum score of 20 for all 10 items. The cutoff score for apraxia was 17, and a median score of 12 divided patients suffering from mild versus severe apraxia. The bulk of the lesions observed via the CT scans were located on the junction of the Rolandic gyrus and the Sylvian fissure. The author found that the lesions observed in patients with apraxia included lesions of the anterior, central, and suprasylvian retrolandic areas in the left hemisphere and were consistent with the classical view of apraxia localization. The lesion profiles of patients with ideomotor apraxia (48 patients), however, were similar to those without apraxia (75 patients). This led to the suggestion that the critical factor for the development of apraxia may be the disruption of a portion of the midcollosal connections

318

LOCALIZATION
OF CLINICAL
SYNDROMES IN
NEUROPSYCHOLOGY
AND NEUROSCIENCE

with the right hemisphere due to a lesion, rather than the localization of the bulk of the lesions. The authors recognized the role of the size of the lesions, presenting some evidence in cases with ideomotor apraxia that implicated larger lesions. Indeed, the researchers found that, compared to the lesions in patients without apraxia, the lesions in severely apraxic patients were larger and often involved deep white matter. A comparison of six cases from each group (both groups were composed of patients with small lesions) revealed no differences in the localization of lesions in the left hemisphere. Though the numbers of left- or right-handed patients in each group were not mentioned in the paper, reversed dominance could have been responsible for the absence of apraxia in some of the cases with small lesions.

Kertesz and Ferro (1984) presented a series of 177 stroke patients who had suffered from lesions of the left hemisphere. Though some of the lesions were typical apraxia-causing lesions of the left parietal cortex, none of the patients were suffering from apraxia. The authors used a test battery of 20 items, which included symbolic gestures, pantomimic actions, and actions with single objects. The maximum possible score was 60, with a cutoff score of 49.7 for apraxia. Severe, moderate, and mild impairments were divided by scores of no more than slightly lower than 18, 36 and 49.7, respectively. The researchers found that the severity of apraxia correlated positively with the lesion size. Rather than crediting lesions in the parietal cortex, the authors especially stressed the role of lesions involving the longitudinal white matter tracts (parieto-frontal, occipito-frontal, and anterior callosal fibers) in cases with apraxia. Geschwind (1965, 1975) similarly suggested that lesions of the arcuate fasciculus and supramarginal gyrus should disconnect the portion of Wernicke's area that is important for the comprehension of verbal commands from the motor association cortex in the midfrontal regions responsible for programming movements. Since the imitation of a gesture may not require verbal processing, Geschwind discussed the possibility that the arcuate fasciculus provides visuomotor connections as well.

Different findings were found in studies of anatomical correlation in patients suffering from ideomotor or ideational apraxia. A more anterior localization of the lesion, primarily around the supramarginal gyrus, is often noted in cases of ideomotor apraxia. The development of ideational apraxia is often related either to larger and more posterior lesions around the angular gyrus (de Ajuriaguerra et al., 1960; Foix, 1916; Liepmann, 1920; Morlaas, 1928) or to the more diffuse, unilateral and bilateral cerebral lesions. The latter is often true in cases of bilateral posterior infarcts, tumors, and profound cortical atrophy in patients with Alzheimer's or Pick's diseases (Dejerine, 1914; Denny-Brown, 1958; Ochipa, Rothi, & Heilman, 1992; Pick, 1905; Rothi et al., 1994).

Since the clinical manifestations of ideational apraxia resulting from a lesion of the angular gyrus of the left hemisphere may be enhanced by an extension of the lesion to the other cerebral structures, the primary role of such a lesion cannot be ruled out. The transient nature of apraxia in many cases with circumscribed lesions of the inferior parietal lobe in the left hemisphere supports the idea that this extension may play a decisive role in the severity and persistency of apraxia.

It should also be stressed that apraxia may result from damage to the visual neurons involved in the selection of motor schemas used in actions. Such neurons were revealed via single-cell recording in the parietal area AIP and frontal area F5 in monkeys. It appears that these neurons must be present in humans in the corresponding parietal and frontal areas, especially considering the complexity of motor actions that require quite sophisticated types of visual guidance by humans.

Frontal Lobe Lesions. The role of frontal lobe lesions in the development of limb apraxia was first mentioned by Pick (1905), who described frontal perceveratory apraxia. Wilson (1908) pointed to the possibility of the development of apraxia in patients with frontal lobe lesions. Kleist (1934) described "apraxia of sequential actions" related to lesions in the frontal lobe, specifically of Broadmann's area 10.

Kertesz and Ferro (1984) found severe conditions of apraxia to be caused by subcortical lesions of the frontal lobe in nine cases, and lesions of the parietal lobe in three cases, with an extension to the cortex in two of those cases. The nine frontal lobe patients also suffered from nonfluent aphasia and right hemiplegia. Since the apraxia scores for seven of the nine patients were in the range of 26 to 33, with lower limits of 32 for a mild version of apraxia severity score, it is probable that actions with real objects were not affected in these patients. Thus it is a possibility that lesions localized outside the left parietal lobe may result in primary disturbances of unconventional praxis such as imitation and symbolic gestures, while the development of conventional apraxia may be primarily related to lesions in the left inferior parietal lobe in right-handed individuals. The researchers also examined 16 individuals with large lesions of the left hemisphere and with an absence of apraxia. The inferior parietal lobe was significantly involved in 11 of the 16 patients. Though all of the patients were right-handed, half had a left-handed pattern of skull asymmetry, with larger left frontal and right occipital lobes. In many cases, this absence of apraxia in cases with lesions of the left hemisphere may be related to the reversion of the leading dominant hemisphere to that of the right hemisphere. A more in-depth examination of handedness is certainly needed in such cases.

The role of a frontal lobe lesion in the onset of apraxia was also supported by data presented by De Renzi and Lucchelli (1988), who studied

20 left brain–damaged patients, with sequelae of strokes in 16 cases and brain tumors in four cases. The test for apraxia used by the researchers included the use of single and multiple objects, pantomimic actions, symbolic gestures, and the imitation of static and sequential movements of the hands and arms. No significant correlation was found between disturbances in the test of movement imitation, which are considered to be a manifestation of ideomotor apraxia, and impairments in single and multiple objects tests, which are considered to be indicative of ideational apraxia. CT scans revealed lesions in the parietal lobe in four patients, in the parieto-temporal region in five patients, in the temporal lobe in two patients, and in the occipital lobe in one patient. Lesions outside the classical localization of the parietal lobe and its neighboring regions were revealed in six patients with posterior frontal lobe lesions, the result of a stroke in four patients and of tumors in two patients. The lesions extended to the insula in three cases and to the temporal lobe in one case. Mild impairments were observed in the frontal lobe cases. One patient was found to suffer from hematoma in the right basal ganglia, possibly due to the involvement of the frontal lobe. The CT scan was negative in one patient.

Luria (1966) found premotor frontal lesions to be responsible in cases of learning apraxia for sequential movements of the hand and fingers, and postcentral parietal lesions to be responsible in cases of apraxia for meaningless finger-hand positions. Both of these types of apraxia may be considered unconventional. In a study of apraxia for meaningless finger-hand positions and unfamiliar finger and hand movements, Kimura (1982) found impairments in the test of motor learning both in patients with lesions of the left parietal lobe and in patients with lesions of the left frontal lobe. Kolb and Milner (1981) and De Renzi (1983), however, found a marked deficit in the performance of patients with left parietal lesions in unconstrained sequencing tasks.

Watson and Heilman (1983) reported evidence of bilateral limb apraxia in two right-handed patients with lesions of the frontal lobe in the supplementary motor area. Apraxia was limited to the transitive gestures in both cases. Rothi et al. (1994) discussed the relationship of apraxia in such cases to disturbances in the transcoding of space-time representation into an innervatory pattern, which then allows the individual to adapt himself to changing environmental conditions.

The role of frontal lobe lesions in the development of apraxia is also supported by studies of grasping in monkeys (Rizzolatti et al., 2000). Apraxia of grasping was observed following muscimol injections both to the parietal area AIP and to Area F5 (Gallese et al., 1997). The differences between parietal lobe apraxia and frontal lobe apraxia, however, remain unclear. It seems that frontal lobe apraxia in humans is predominantly related to the unconventional information processing of serial actions, while parietal lobe apraxia primarily involves well-learned actions.

The development of gait apraxia and truncal apraxia has usually been observed in patients with massive frontal lobe lesions. Sittig (1931) described such types of apraxia in a patient with a large tumor of the left frontal lobe, which extended posterior into the parietal region. Denny-Brown (1958) stressed the role of frontal lobe lesions in the development of magnetic apraxia in the lower extremities.

Lesions in the Central Region.   Limb-kinetic apraxia, referred to by Kleist (1934) as innervatory apraxia, is unilateral and develops following superficial and partial lesions in the central gyrus contralateral to the hand with signs of apraxia (Kleist, 1934; Liepmann, 1900, 1906, 1920). More extended and deeper lesions in that area lead to paralysis of the opposite extremities.

Lesions in cases of buccofacial or oral apraxia have usually been localized in the precentral face area (Bay, 1957; Kleist, 1934; Liepmann, 1908; Nathan, 1947) and the adjacent region of the temporo-parietal cortex (Luria, 1966). Frequent associations with Broca's aphasia also point to lesions in the frontal perisylvian region (De Renzi et al., 1966). However, relatively rare cases of comorbidity of oral apraxia and either Wernicke's aphasia or conduction aphasia have supported the possibility that more posterior perisylvian lesions are responsible (Benson et al., 1973; Heilman et al., 1983; Kertesz, 1985). Difficulties in the comprehension of verbal commands, however, may be implicated in such cases. Buccofacial apraxia may also be observed in patients without any sign of aphasia. In some cases, oral apraxia has been noted following a lesion in the right hemisphere (Goldstein, 1909; Hartmann, 1907; Kramer, Delis, & Nakada, 1985; Rapcsak, Rothi, & Heilman, 1987). The possible role of left-handedness must be taken into account in these cases.

Tognola and Vignolo (1980) compared the CT scan findings of two groups of poststroke patients with lesions of the left hemisphere. The first group consisted of 13 patients with oral apraxia, while the second was composed of 8 patients without oral apraxia. A quantitative test of oral apraxia was administered, during which each patient was asked only to imitate simple oral gestures. Verbal commands were excluded from the testing to avoid the influence of comprehensive disturbances on performance. The authors found that the lesions crucial for the development of oral apraxia are located in the following structures of the left hemisphere: the frontal and central (Rolandic) opercula, the adjacent parts of the first temporal gyrus, and the anterior portion of the insula. Though the inferior parietal lobule was involved in only 5 of 13 patients with oral apraxia, it was involved in more than half, 5 of 8, of the patients without oral apraxia. This was considered by the

322

LOCALIZATION
OF CLINICAL
SYNDROMES IN
NEUROPSYCHOLOGY
AND NEUROSCIENCE

authors to be an indication that the parietal operculum and supramarginal gyrus are not as important for the development of oral apraxia as are the anterior operculum and insula. Lesions in patients without oral apraxia were located posterior or, in some cases, anterior to the lesions in patients with oral apraxia. Bilateral lesions sparing the frontal and central opercula and the adjacent insular region did not lead to oral apraxia in the right-handed subjects, supporting the authors' conclusion concerning the role of lesions in the anterior opercular and insular regions in the development of oral apraxia.

Subcortical Lesions. Evidence of apraxia has rarely been reported in cases of *subcortical lesions in the basal ganglia and/or the thalamus* that do not significantly involve the white matter pathways (Agostoni, Coletti, Orlando, & Fredici, 1983; Basso, Luzzatti, & Spinnler, 1980; De Renzi & Luccheli, 1988; Rothi, Kooistra, Heilman, & Mack, 1988). Apraxia in such cases was usually mild, and involvement of the adjacent white matter and cortex by pathological processes must be considered.

Callosal Lesions. Special attention must be given to the localization of lesions involved in unilateral limb apraxia, which may be manifested in the left hand in cases with callosal lesions in right-handed patients. Callosal apraxia was first described by Liepmann and Mass (1907), who observed patients with an inability to imitate pantomimic acts with the left hand and demonstrated clumsiness when manipulating real objects with the right hand. The infarctions in these cases occupied the anterior part of the corpus callosum, sparing the splenium. Geschwind and Kaplan (1962) described a patient with callosal lesions who exhibited an inability to follow verbal commands with the left hand but demonstrated a preserved ability to imitate actions and to correctly use real objects. Graff-Radford, Welsh, and Godersky (1987) observed difficulties in the imitation of actions in response to verbal commands in a patient with the rupture of a left pericallosal aneurism. The aneurism was clipped successfully, and MRI scans performed immediately after the rupture and 4 months later revealed that the hemorrhage damaged the genu and most of the body of the corpus callosum but spared the splenium and the rostrum. A similar pattern of apraxia involving the inability to correctly use the left hand in response to a verbal command was observed in patients who had undergone a comissurotomy for the treatment of intractable seizures (Gazzaniga, Bogen, & Sperry, 1967; Volpe, Sidris, Holtzman, Wilson, & Gazzaniga, 1982; Zaidel & Sperry, 1977). Watson and Heilman (1983) presented a right-handed patient with more severe limb apraxia who was unable to perform actions with his left hand in response to verbal commands as well as to imitate the use of and correctly use objects.

Lesions responsible for the development of apraxia are usually located in the anterior parts of the corpus callosum and in the callosal
genu, with the body of the splenium being spared. It is possible that the
development of apraxia in response to verbal commands with a preservation of motor actions related to visuomotor tasks may be related to
the sparing of the posterior splenium in most of the cases with callosal
apraxia. The information for actions related to visuomotor tasks would
cross from the left to the right hemisphere through the preserved posterior splenium in such cases.

CONCLUSION

1. Lesions in the inferior parietal lobe (Figure 6.4) are often observed
   in patients with limb apraxia of both conventional and unconventional types. More severe lesions that extend from the cortex to
   the underlying deep white matter and interrupt connections with
   the central gyri and the frontal lobe tend to produce more severe
   and persistent forms of limb apraxia.
2. Apraxia of the unconventional, executive type may often be due to
   frontal lobe and subcortical lesions in the left hemisphere.
3. Large lesions in the classical area of the parietal lobe may not
   result in the development of apraxia in some cases. The role of
   left-handedness in the reversal of dominance for limb praxis is
   discussed in such cases. Dressing apraxia usually results from lesions in the inferior parietal lobe of the right hemisphere.
4. Unilateral apraxia in the left hand in response to verbal commands may result from a callosal lesion that damages the anterior
   part of the corpus callosum.

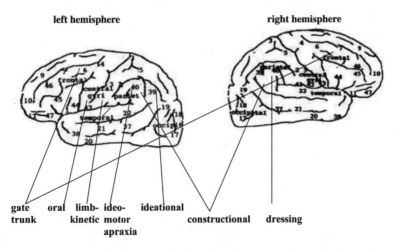

FIGURE 6.4 Frequent localization of lesions in various types of upper limb apraxia.

324

LOCALIZATION
OF CLINICAL
SYNDROMES IN
NEUROPSYCHOLOGY
AND NEUROSCIENCE

5. Constructional apraxia may result from unilateral lesions in the inferior parietal lobe of the left or right hemisphere in right-handed subjects. Some clinical peculiarities are described in relation to the localization of lesions in the right or left hemisphere.

SOCIAL APRAXIA: DISORGANIZATION OF GOAL-DIRECTED BEHAVIOR IN THE SOCIAL WORLD

MOTOR APRAXIA IS defined as a disturbance of goal-directed motor actions in the physical world, while muscle strength and active and passive movements are preserved and paralysis or paresis is either mild or completely absent. The patient is unable to perform actions with objects or to demonstrate pretended actions, such as mimicking how to use a screwdriver or a hammer or how to brush the teeth.

Disturbances of actions in the social world may be described as a disorder of goal-directed behavior related to the planning of social actions, the anticipation of their results, and the execution of social actions. The term social apraxia reflects the similarity between disorders of goal-directed actions in the physical world and behavior in the social world, helping to delineate the clinical content of that disturbance and to describe it in more clearly defined neurological and neuropsychological terms.

Harlow (1868) was probably the first to describe a head injury case that resulted in the changes in social functioning that may be called social apraxia in modern terminology. This case was eventually recognized as a landmark in the history of neuropsychological and neuropsychiatric studies of changes in social functioning and personality caused by a relatively circumscribed frontal lobe lesion.

Phineas Gage sustained a head injury in an accident on September 13, 1848, near Cavendish, Vermont (Harlow, 1868). Twenty-five-year-old Gage was working as the foreman of a railroad construction crew and, on the day of the accident, was using a 3½-foot long and 1-inch thick iron tamping rod to tamp dynamite down into boulders for controlled blasting to level off uneven terrain. Gage did not realize that the explosive powder was not covered by sand, which would have been used to direct the explosion inside the boulder. He inadvertently began tamping on the actual dynamite, triggering a powerful explosion from the boulder toward Gage. The inch thick tamping rod shot right through Gage's head and into the air and landed several yards away. Gage survived the accident and regained relatively good physical health within only a few months.

Prior to the accident, Gage was known and described by others as an honest, amiable, and responsible man. He was praised by his employers as "the most efficient and capable man" of their employees. After the accident, however, Gage underwent a radical transformation, according to his physician, John Harlow. Gage's personality changed drastically. He became ill mannered, profane, irreverent, and capricious, and his social functioning never returned to a level comparable to that prior to the accident. Gage was said to have devised "many plans of future operation, which are no sooner arranged than abandoned in turn for other appearing more feasible.... Previous to his injury, though untrained in the school, he possessed a well-balanced mind, and was looked upon by those who knew him as a shrewd, smart businessman, very energetic and persistent in executing all his plans of operation. In this regard his mind was radically changed, so decidedly that his friends and acquaintances said he was 'no longer Gage'" (Harlow, 1868). Gage lost any sense of responsibility and could no longer be trusted. He became unable to continue his work as a foreman and was dismissed from his job. Interestingly enough, however, Gage suffered no apparent decline in intelligence, memory, speech, or ability to learn new things in comparison with his preaccident levels.

Following the dismissal from his job, Gage began a new life of wandering, trying to profit from his story by displaying himself and the fateful temping rod in backwoods carnival sideshows (Burns & Burns, 1998). He worked as a hostler at a stable in 1851, and as a stagecoach driver in Chile in 1852. His failing health forced Gage to return home in 1860, and he lived under the custody and supervision of his family in San Francisco until his death on May 20, 1861, more than 12 years after the accident. Though no autopsy was performed, Gage's mother granted permission in 1866 to Dr. John M. Harlow to have the body exhumed so that the skull could be recovered and kept as a medical record. Both Gage's skull and the tamping rod eventually arrived in the Warren Anatomical Museum at Harvard University, where they are still held and preserved. An examination performed following the exhumation of the body revealed that the tamping rod was blown upward, entering the skull through the left maxilla and exiting just to the left of the midline of the frontal skull. This report demonstrated the severe injury caused to the frontal lobe.

Based on Gage's case, it was suggested that a frontal lobe lesion may play a specific role in the development of personality and social behavior changes. The absence of an autopsy, however, made it easy to dismiss the conclusion that the frontal lobe serves a role as a specific center of the social faculty (for more details, see the review by Damasio, Grabovski, Frank, Galaburda, & Damasio, 1994). A recent study by Damasio's research team (Damasio et al., 1994), however, made

326

LOCALIZATION
OF CLINICAL
SYNDROMES IN
NEUROPSYCHOLOGY
AND NEUROSCIENCE

suggestions concerning the localization and extent of frontal lobe lesions that made the case more clear and reliable. Employing the use
of both measurements from Gage's skull and modern neuroimaging
techniques, the authors developed a model of probable lesion localization in Gage's brain. In the left hemisphere, the lesion involved the
anterior half of the orbital frontal cortex, the polar and mesial frontal
cortices, and the anterior-most section of the superior cingular gyrus.
The lesion spared both the supplementary motor area and the frontal
operculum. In the right hemisphere, the lesion involved part of the anterior and mesial orbital region, the mesial and polar frontal cortices,
and the anterior segment of the anterior cingular gyrus. There was no
damage to any area outside the frontal lobes. The lesion thus favored
the ventromedial regions of both frontal lobes and sparing the dorsolateral areas.

Interest in the disturbances of social functioning was subsequently
rekindled by studies of patients who sustained frontal lobe head injuries
resulting from gunshot wounds in World War I and World War II (Faust,
1960; Feuchtwanger, 1923; Kleist, 1934; Kretchmer, 1949; Lishman, 1966,
1968). In addition to patients with head injuries, changes in social functioning were also reported in cases of frontal lobe tumors (Ackerley, 1937;
Brickner, 1936; Hebb & Penfield, 1940; Hécaen, 1964; Penfield & Evans,
1935). The clinical description of the disorganization of social actions,
however, was mainly described as secondary to the personality changes
frequently observed in patients with frontal lobe lesions. Primary disturbances in the disorganization of social functioning have begun to be
outlined only recently, primarily by Antonio Damasio and his cowork-
ers (Damasio, Tranel, & Damasio, 1991; Eslinger & Damasio, 1985).

CLINICAL ASPECTS

DISTURBANCES OF FUNCTIONING and of actions in the social environment may be manifested as impairments in conventional information processing, usually defined as disturbances in the activity of daily
living. Disturbances of unconventional information processing, on
the other hand, are usually manifested in the various areas of higher
levels of social functioning, including more complex occupations, education, and relationships with family and friends.

Disturbances in Conventional Information Processing

In advanced stages of underlying disease, for example, tumor growth,
degenerative dementia, or certain types of schizophrenia processes,
the person's everyday life becomes disorganized. The social aspects of
the activity of daily living become disrupted. The individual fails to
adhere to the daily schedule of social life at home and at work, requires

assistance to get up on time and to adhere to his or her work schedule, is unable to properly keep up his or her social relations, and frequently forgets to carry out his or her daily washing, grooming, and other personal hygiene requirements. The individual thus becomes dysfunctional, requiring daily assistance to meet basic personal needs.

Disturbances in Unconventional Information Processing

Disturbances in unconventional social functioning have been primarily described in patients with frontal lobe syndrome, which is caused by relatively circumscribed lesions as a result of brain tumors and head injury. The primary features of such disturbances include the disorganization of more complicated social actions, a loss in forethought and execution of plans, an inability to set and pursue realistic goals in one's career, education, finances, and job performance, and an inability to adjust to a complex, frequently changing social environment.

Some authors used specific terms to define disturbances of actions in the social world. Ackerly and Benton (1948) described what they called a primary social defect in a patient with bilateral frontal lobe damage. Eslinger and Damasio (1985) reported the results of a detailed clinical, neuropsychological, and neuroanatomical study of patient E.V.R., who suffered from a general impairment of "the automatic solving of social problems." In some sense, these disorganized actions in social space are similar to ideational motor apraxia, in which simple actions are preserved while a series of actions lose their order and become disconnected and disorganized. This disorganization of social actions may be defined as social apraxia.

A student suffering from social apraxia, for example, would become unable to hold to the standard requirements of learning activity, would lack the ability to complete his or her usual studies in a timely fashion, and would develop difficulties in both short- and long-term planning of educational activity, perhaps eventually dropping out of school or college.

The person with social apraxia experiences difficulties or becomes unable to perform his or her occupational duty at the previous level, especially in more complicated and challenging professional jobs, for example, in the job of a construction foreman (Harlow, 1868, Gage Case), a stockbroker (Brickner, 1936, Case A), or an accountant (Eslinger & Damasio, 1985, E.V.R. Case). Following the removal of a large orbitofrontal meningioma that was compressing both frontal lobes, patient E.V.R. became involved in a home-building venture with a former coworker of questionable reputation, despite warnings from family and friends (Eslinger & Damasio, 1985). The business eventually had to declare bankruptcy, and the patient lost all of his personal investment.

Patient E.V.R. tried to resort to simpler jobs, such as those of a building manager or a warehouse laborer, but was fired because of disorganization and tardiness. The patient's basic skills, manners, and temper, however, were appropriate and unaffected.

The patient with social apraxia becomes unable to hold gainful employment and is often fired because of an inability to uphold reliable standards or complete his or her usual expected workload, and because of repeated tardiness and an overall lack of productivity. The individual experiences difficulties in both short- and long-term planning, and is unable to anticipate the probable consequences of his or her planned actions.

This picture may stand in stark contrast to the relatively preserved general cognition. The person with a loss of occupational and academic functioning demonstrates a preservation of recent and remote memory, including knowledge about major social and autobiographical events (Brickner, 1936, Case A). Patient E.V.R. exhibited "knowledge and comprehension of complex social issues, the economy, industry, and financial matters" (Eslinger & Damasio, 1985, p. 1732). Neuropsychological testing results demonstrated a verbal IQ of 125, and a Wechsler memory quotient of 143. Normal scores were also attained by patient E.V.R. in both the Wisconsin Card Sorting Test and the Trail Making Test, both of which are more complicated tests currently used for the testing of executive function.

A patient would be able to verbally explain the plan of his or her intended actions but would fail in the real-life situation and in the execution of the plan. Penfield and Evans (1935) reported that, following the bilateral removal of a convexital meningioma depressing both frontal lobes, their patient (Case 1) was able to verbally outline a plan to prepare a dinner for invited guests but failed to prepare the dinner in a timely manner, becoming confused with the sequences and timing of the required actions. Patient E.V.R. (Eslinger & Damasio, 1985) regularly needed approximately 2 hours to get ready for work in the morning, or to decide which restaurant to choose for dinner.

The patient often develops marital difficulties, many times resulting in divorce, and is often unable to successfully continue a new marriage. The individual becomes dependent on family members in many, if not all, daily activities, and relationships with friends become weaker and emptier.

This independence of social apraxia from other manifestations of a frontal lobe syndrome is supported by an absence of significant personality changes in some patients with social apraxia (Ackerley, 1937; Eslinger & Damasio, 1985, E.V.R. Case; Penfield & Evans, 1935, Cases 1 and 2). The disorganization of social activity may be enhanced in other cases by personality changes manifesting as disturbances of the self, which are often observed in patients with frontal lobe syndrome.

Disorganization of Social Actions and Brain Information Processing

Similarities To Motor Apraxia

Social actions and their disturbances may be defined in comparison with motor actions and motor apraxia. Disturbances of goal-directed behavior in physical space or social space are similarly related to an impairment in the ability to select a goal, to plan the steps needed to attain the goal, to anticipate the results, and to execute the series of actions to reach the chosen goal. These similarities may be discussed using the recent studies of grasping in monkeys, in which single-cell recording was used to note neuronal activity (Jeannerod, 1984; Rizzolatti & Gentilucci, 1988). For more details, see "Motor Apraxia" earlier in this chapter.

It has been demonstrated that area F5, located anterior to the inferior portion of the motor strip in monkeys and in the anterior interparietal sulcus (area AIP), contains neurons that become active during motor acts such as grasping, holding, and tearing but are not activated during individual movements. The hierarchical structure of motor actions coded by the neurons of the F5-AIP circuit may be described by a "motor vocabulary" that contains a limited number of "words" that indicate the particular operations by a group of neurons in the course of a particular motor act.

These words may indicate the general goals of the actions, such as grasping, holding, or tearing. Other words help to adjust the motor act to the size of the object targeted for grasping. These words specify the manner of execution of the particular action depending on the size of the object. The grasping of middle-sized objects is executed using finger prehension based on the opposition of the thumb to the other fingers. A precision grip is used to grasp smaller objects, however, and is based on the opposition of the thumb to the index finger. Other words deal with the temporal order of the actions, coding the specific phase of the grip and each part of the sequential order, for example, hand opening, hand closing. Disturbances of hand preshaping and precision grip similar to those in kinetic limb apraxia may be caused by the inactivation of either area F5 or AIP via muscimol injections in these areas.

The vocabulary of motor actions in humans may certainly have a more complicated structure for both simple and, especially, complex actions. Their disturbances may manifest as ideomotor apraxia for a simple action and as ideational apraxia for a series of actions. A special vocabulary may exist for such actions, including motor schemes for

330

LOCALIZATION
OF CLINICAL
SYNDROMES IN
NEUROPSYCHOLOGY
AND NEUROSCIENCE

conventional and unconventional information processing (for more details, see "Motor Apraxia," p. 324). Similarly, disturbances of social actions could result from the disorganization of a vocabulary of actions that is based on a quite different set of words or instructions. Such a vocabulary includes goals, planning, anticipation of results, and ways of executing social actions. The system based on the specific words and vocabulary of social actions must be organized in a separate module to function properly and may be located separately from the system guiding the motor actions.

As with motor actions, the social module must include the processing of gnostic information that is anticipated or received in the course of social actions. This gnostic information is needed for proper adjustment to the specifics of the social environment, such as schedules, tasks, instructions, mental state, and the emotions and actions of other participants in social actions. As in various types of visual or auditory agnosia, disturbances of social gnosis or social agnosia may be observed independently from disorganization of social actions. These disturbances could manifest as emotional agnosia or prosopagnosia or as an impairment in the correct perception of another's thoughts or emotions (for more details, see chapter 5, section entitled "Social Agnosia"). The perceptual component, however, may also play an important role in the planning, anticipation, and execution of actions.

A module of social actions seems to be built on operations that are somewhat automatic and are not fully reflected verbally, as in motor praxis. It is naturally difficult to learn to ride a bicycle, or even to perform a simple motor action such as hammering a nail, following only verbal instructions. These actions are often disturbed in motor apraxia, while their verbal description remains relatively preserved. Similarly, patients with frontal lobe lesions may demonstrate a preservation of verbal planning and anticipation and description of planned social actions, but their execution in real life is markedly disturbed (Eslinger & Damasio, 1985, E.V.R. Case; Penfield & Evans, 1935, Case 1). In other cases, personality changes lead patients to become boastful, devise plans of returning to work, and verbally spell out numerous plans, but they often end up getting involved in questionable business ventures and losing their investments. Patients are then unable to implement even realistic plans in real-life situations (Brickner, 1936, Case A; Eslinger & Damasio, 1985, E.V.R. Case).

Disturbances in Conventional and Unconventional Information Processing

The operations involved in the information processing of social actions may be reflected in the vocabulary of "words," instructions that are well learned, predetermined and used as building blocks for social actions with well-defined sequences of simple actions, for example, elementary jobs or the basic activities necessary for regular daily living. In more severe cases of frontal lobe lesions, this well-automatized conventional information processing may be disorganized and segmented into simple, not properly connected, components of complex actions.

In less severe cases, disturbances primarily involve unconventional information processing. A patient in such cases becomes unable to continue his or her professional, sophisticated work as a business manager, stockbroker, or lawyer, for example, but may be employed in a less-challenging job assignment based on conventional information processing. One 24-year-old patient, for example, underwent a left frontal lobectomy for the treatment of a seizure that developed at the age of 16 following a head injury. The patient was employed as a workman helping his father, a groundsman at McGill University. According to his father, however, the patient never had a job that his father did not get for him at the university (Penfield & Evans, 1935, Case 2).

Operations involved in the processing of social unconventional information require the recognition of more complicated, more dynamic social situations, which are often presented with an incomplete set of features and are not based on well-defined vocabulary in which "words" outline the appropriate sequence of actions. The planning, anticipation, and execution of actions may require the development of flexible responses tuned to the specifics of new or often vague social conditions. A preset vocabulary of actions does not work in these situations, and the use of a large and often newly developed set of words underlies the actions instead.

Anatomical Aspects

The relatively circumscribed lesions of frontal lobes caused by tumors or head injuries are usually reported in cases with social agnosia (Figure 6.5). One such case, reported by Eslinger and Damasio (1985), was patient E.V.R. The patient was examined following the removal of a large orbitofrontal meningioma arising from the cribiform plate and compressing both frontal lobes. He developed a general impairment of automatic solving of . . . social problems, as described above. Head CT and MRI scans showed a low-density area in both frontal lobes, merging with the ventricular system and corresponding to the extensive surgical resections of the entire orbital area on the right side and part of the orbital cortex on the left. The large area of low density found in the right hemisphere involved the orbital cortex and extended to the adjacent dorsolateral prefrontal and premotor cortices with underlying white matter. The area of low density found in the left hemisphere was more restricted, involving white matter of the orbital area but sparing a portion of its cortices. Other cerebral areas were entirely preserved.

332

LOCALIZATION
OF CLINICAL
SYNDROMES IN
NEUROPSYCHOLOGY
AND NEUROSCIENCE

We observed evidence of social apraxia in a 19-year-old patient who had sustained a closed head injury in a car accident when he was 14 years old. The patient had experienced a loss of consciousness for approximately 24 hours. Following the accident, the patient's behavior changed dramatically. He dropped out of school, was unable to hold a job for more than 1–2 months, and became sexually promiscuous. He was brought to the hospital for forensic evaluation after an attempted sexual assault with a diagnosis of "conduct disorder." On his way to the hospital, the patient attempted to rape a nurse who was escorting him in the ambulance. The patient became calm and pleasant following admission to the hospital and demonstrated a preservation of formal cognitive levels. Head CT scans revealed two scars—one in the left orbitofrontal region and another in the white matter close to the first scar. These findings point to the role of the left orbitofrontal lesion in the development of social apraxia.

Stroke sequelae manifested as social apraxia are quite rare, since CVAs do not usually involve the territory of the anterior cerebral artery (ACA) in the frontal lobe, due to the circulatory interconnections between the right and left ACA. Lesions that are more extended and less circumscribed may lead to manifestations of social apraxia in patients with primary degenerative dementia, especially in patients with frontotemporal dementia characterized by a progressive atrophy of the frontal and temporal lobes. The development of social apraxia may be seen among negative symptoms in patients with schizophrenia. In fact, social apraxia becomes the leading syndrome in some cases of schizophrenia. This condition was previously described under the name simple schizophrenia, and more recently as "simple deteriorative disorder" (American Psychiatric Association, 2000, p. 769).

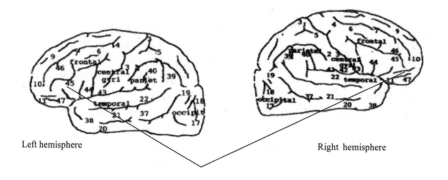

Social apraxia

FIGURE 6.5 Probable localization of lesions in social apraxia.

Lesions of the same region have been also implicated in the development of orbitofrontal changes in self-image that often underlie or possibly accompany disturbances of social functioning of the social apraxia type. Eslinger and Damasio (1985) stressed the intactness of intellect on the Wisconsin Card Sorting Test, which was probably a reflection of either the preservation of the superior dorsolateral frontal lobe, especially on the left side, or the preservation of the mesial frontal regions. Lesions of the latter regions may be responsible for the development of avolition, apathy, loss of initiative, and loss of interest.

We are certainly only beginning to uncover and understand the set of operations involved in information processing in the course of social actions and their disturbances, and lesion localization in cases of these disturbances.

7

Communication Disorders

THE INDIVIDUAL'S COMMUNICATION with the outside world is achieved primarily through language, which plays an important role in the externalization of experiences and feelings, communication with the outer world, and reception of information from the outer world about others' internal and external experiences. In this sense, language plays an important role both in social activity and interactions and in the recognition of actions in the physical world. Other types of communication include gestures and emotional expressions, which may also be considered types of language important for communication in the social world. One specific form of communication is provided by music, which may be considered an expression of emotion.

In addition to disturbances of spoken language, this chapter will also discuss disturbances of the use of emotion as a short, probably genetically installed international language, as well as the various types of amusia. Disturbances in gestures are described in chapter 6, section entitled "Motor Apraxia."

APHASIA SYNDROMES AND OTHER LANGUAGE DISORDERS

ATTENTION WAS CALLED to the significance of the faculty of language in brain information processing in the course of interaction with the outside world in studies of speech and language disorders as a manifestation of brain pathology beginning in the late 17th century. For a review, see Benton and Joynt (1960) and Tonkonogy (1968a).

At the beginning of the 19th century, Gall tried to localize various abilities in the human brain, suggesting that the ability to speak is localized in the frontal regions of the brain (Gall & Spurzheim, 1810–1819). Bouillaud (1825) supported Gall's suggestion about localization of the ability to speak in the anterior parts of the brain. However, as was the case with Gall, he did not possess any reliable data in support of his theory.

Dax (1865) then presented to a medical congress in Montpelier a report of speech disturbances as observed in 125 patients with right hemiplegia. Dax connected speech disturbances with lesions in the left cerebral hemisphere. The study became widely known, however, only after it was replicated by Dax's son in 1865.

The history of systematic studies of aphasia must be dated to 1861, when Broca presented the brain of his patient, Leborgne, at a meeting of the anthropological society in Paris. A second patient, Lelong, was presented in November 1861.

Leborgne, Broca's first patient, had suffered from epileptiform spells since his teenage years. He lost the ability to speak at the age of 30, at which time he was admitted to the Bicêtre Hospital. The patient was able to understand spoken language, but said only the word "tan" in response to all questions. When a listener was unable to understand, the patient would become irritated and swear. Ten years after his initial admission, the patient developed a weakness followed by paralysis of the right hand with a subsequent progressive development of weakness in the lower right extremity. At the age of 44, the patient was unable to stand or to walk, and was confined to his bed. Extended cellulites began to develop on the patient's lower right extremities, and he was transferred to the surgical ward on April 11, 1861, where Broca worked as the attending physician. Broca passed on information about the patient to Aubertin, Bouillaud's son-in-law, who was a fierce supporter of the principles of functional localization in the brain. The case was accepted as a control case, since Aubertin considered the peculiar speech disorders observed in the patient as corresponding to previously recorded cases of speech disorders related to a lesion in the anterior regions of the brain.

The patient died on April 17, 1861. Broca presented the patient's brain the following day (Figure 7.1) at the meeting of the Paris Anthropological Society in support of Bouillaud's suggestion concerning the role of the anterior brain in speech. As the brain had not yet been dissected, Broca gave a verbal description of the brain based on external observations. A large cyst in the left hemisphere replaced the posterior part of the F3 area, extending to the adjacent parts of the posterior F2 area and spreading to the lower parts of the central gyri, the insula, the T1 area, and parts of the T2 area. A softening was seen in the corpus callosum

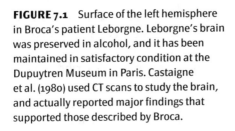 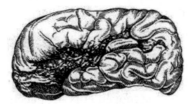

FIGURE 7.1 Surface of the left hemisphere in Broca's patient Leborgne. Leborgne's brain was preserved in alcohol, and it has been maintained in satisfactory condition at the Dupuytren Museum in Paris. Castaigne et al. (1980) used CT scans to study the brain, and actually reported major findings that supported those described by Broca.

through a window in the ventricle made by Broca. The lenticular nucleus was entirely destroyed, and atrophy was noted in both the F1 area and the orbital gyri.

Lelong, Broca's second noteworthy patient, was an 84-year-old gardener who had resided at the Bicêtre Hospital since 1853 and had been diagnosed with senile dementia. In April 1860, at 83 years of age, the patient fell and lost consciousness. When the patient awoke, he was able to say only a few words and demonstrated difficulties in word articulation. The patient understood almost everything that he heard, however, and seemed to experience no weakness in the extremities. On October 27, 1861, the patient fell again and suffered a fracture of the left hip. He was transferred to Broca's care. At that time, the patient's speech was almost completely absent, and the patient was able to say only "oui" (yes), "non" (no), "toisu," "toujours" (instead of "bonjour"), and "Lelo" (instead of "Lelong"). The patient was not able to write. Comprehension of spoken language was almost completely preserved, and no sign of weakness in the extremities was noted. Lelong died less than 2 weeks after the hip fracture incident, on November 8, 1961. The brain was described based on external observation. Fifteen millimeters of the F3 area in the posterior half of the left hemisphere were destroyed. The lesion was connected to the Sylvian fissure on the level of the insula and extended from the other side to the F2 area, which remained preserved as a 2-millimeter slice of tissue. The F1 area and the central gyri were completely preserved. Broca considered the lesions in the posterior F3 area and the F2 area to be the result of cerebral hemorrhage, since the patient had developed a sudden loss of speech in April 1860 following a brief period of unconsciousness.

Broca concluded that the loss of speech in each of his two cases resulted from a lesion in the posterior F3 area of the left hemisphere. Right-sided hemiplegia, as well as other disturbances, developed because of other lesions found in the patients. The second case seemed to fit more convincingly with Broca's conclusion, since the lesion was primarily limited to the posterior F3 area, with an extension to the posterior F2 area. More extended lesions may be suggested, however, since the patient had suffered for many years from senile dementia, and atrophy of the adjacent and other cortical areas was probably present.

Broca (1861a, 1861b) considered the speech disorders described above to be of a central origin, which included two types—aphemia and verbal amnesia. Aphemia was related to disturbances in the ability to connect the movements of speech organs into words. Verbal amnesia was described as the result of a disconnection between an idea and its corresponding word.

Soon after Broca's (1861a,b) publication, Trousseau (1864) pointed to the negative connotation of the word *infamy* in the modern Greek language and suggested that the term aphemia should be replaced by the term aphasia. In spite of Broca's opposition, Trousseau's suggestion was accepted by many authors, and the term aphasia gained long-standing recognition in the literature. Some authors later tried a more limited use of the term aphemia to denote more peripheral language disturbances of articulation (Albert, Goodglass, Helm, Rubens, & Alexander, 1981; Bastian, 1897) or speech akinesia (Petit-Dutaillis, Guiot, Meising, & Bourdillon, 1954). These suggestions, however, did not gain significant recognition from other researchers in the field.

Thirteen years after Broca's famous publication, Wernicke (1874) published a small book with descriptions of 10 patients who suffered from disturbances in the comprehension of spoken language. The patients also suffered from impairments of naming, expressive speech, writing, and reading. Three of the patients had died, and an autopsy revealed a diffuse lesion in two cases, and a lesion in the left posterior T1 area and the adjacent T2 area in one case. Wernicke noted that none of his patients could understand or correct his or her own speech, and concluded that a lesion of the auditory speech center in the posterior T1 area may result in the development of sensory aphasia with disturbances of speech comprehension and secondary impairments of expressive speech.

Wernicke suggested that the processing of sensory images of words takes place in the posterior T1 area, while motor images are processed in the motor speech center, which was described by Broca as being found in the posterior F3 area. An interruption of connections between these two centers resulted, according to Wernicke, in the development of conduction aphasia with disturbances in the repetition of words and sentences, while expressive speech and comprehension remained relatively intact.

These ideas were further developed by Lichtheim (1884), who suggested a scheme that explained the development of some of the clinical types of aphasia as a disruption of connections between cortical speech centers and concept centers. This approach formed the basis for the introduction of a classification of aphasia known as the Wernicke-Lichtheim model, which was not considered of any importance until recently.

THE CLASSIFICATIONS OF APHASIA

ACCORDING TO THE Wernicke-Lichtheim model, the differentiation of various types of aphasia must be based on disturbances of expressive speech, comprehension, repetition, reading, and writing. A disorder of expressive speech or of comprehension with disturbances of repetition, reading, and writing is manifested in two different syndromes—cortical motor aphasia, resulting from a lesion of the cortical motor speech center, and cortical sensory aphasia, resulting from a lesion of the cortical sensory speech center. An interruption of connections between the center of concepts and the cortical motor speech center leads to transcortical motor aphasia, with a disorder of expressive speech and a preservation of repetition. Similarly, an interruption of connections between the center of concepts and the cortical sensory speech center results in transcortical sensory aphasia, with disturbances in comprehension and a preservation of repetition. Mild disturbances of reading and writing are typically noted in cases of transcortical aphasia. Repetition is not impaired in these cases, since the pathway between cortical motor and sensory centers is preserved. Repetition disturbances are, however, the leading symptoms in cases of conduction aphasia. Expressive speech, comprehension, reading, and writing are relatively speaking spared in cases of conduction aphasia, which result from a disruption of connections between the cortical motor and sensory speech centers. Subcortical motor aphasia, which is a relatively isolated disorder of expressive speech, is the result of an interruption of connections between the cortical motor speech center and deep brain structures. In the same way, subcortical sensory aphasia, which is an isolated disorder of comprehension, is caused by an interruption of connections between the cortical sensory speech center and deep brain structures (Figure 7.2).

Through decades of aphasia studies, a number of classifications of aphasia have been suggested. Kleist (1934) described types of aphasia according to the primary language disturbances prevalent in particular types, such as impairments of articulation in "sound muteness," of word production in "word muteness," of sentence production in "sentence muteness," and of naming in "naming muteness." These types of aphasia are similar, if not identical, to the subcortical, cortical, and transcortical motor aphasia of the Wernicke-Lichtheim model. Kleist also included in his classification the "deafness of speech sounds," "deafness of words," and "deafness of naming," which corresponded

340

LOCALIZATION
OF CLINICAL
SYNDROMES IN
NEUROPSYCHOLOGY
AND NEUROSCIENCE

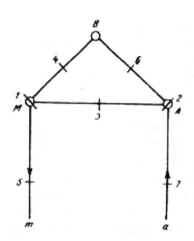

FIGURE 7.2 Localization scheme of aphasia syndromes, according to Lichtheim. Lesions resulting in the development of various types of aphasia.

A: Auditory center of words. M: Motor center of words. B: Concept center. a: Connection from subcortical auditory center to A. m: Connection from M to subcortical center of movements.

to subcortical, cortical, and transcortical sensory aphasia, respectively. Conduction aphasia was considered as a stage of recovery from "word deafness."

Another classification frequently cited in literature was suggested by Luria (1966, 1970), who considered the role of the motor and sensory aspects of speech disorders in the formation of different types of aphasia. Luria divided motor aphasia into three types: kinetic (efferent) aphasia, kinesthetic (afferent) aphasia, and dynamic aphasia. In kinetic aphasia, a patient loses his or her ability to pronounce a series of speech sounds or words in what would be considered easy consecutive order as a result of disturbances in the formation of the kinetic system of skilled movements. Kinesthetic aphasia develops because of an impairment of the kinesthetic basis of speech articulation. Dynamic aphasia is characterized by difficulties in the ekphorization of the entire expression, a disturbance of speech initiative, and an inability to compose the scheme of an expression. Kinetic aphasia is similar to cortical motor aphasia in the Wernicke-Lichtheim model, while kinesthetic aphasia may be compared with subcortical motor aphasia. Dynamic aphasia is considered a type of transcortical motor aphasia.

Luria described only two types of sensory aphasia; sensory aphasia as a type of acoustic agnosia of speech sounds, with an impairment primarily in phonemic hearing; and acoustic-mnestic aphasia, similar to transcortical sensory aphasia. Word deafness, known as subcortical sensory aphasia in the Wernicke-Lichtheim model, was included as agnosia of speech sounds in the description of sensory aphasia. Conduction aphasia, on the other hand, was considered to be a stage in recovery from sensory aphasia. Disturbances at the phonological and semantic levels were primarily analyzed as being secondary to the primary disturbances of the kinetic and kinesthetic systems of speech in motor aphasia, and the auditory agnosia of speech in sensory aphasia.

In summary, the description of particular types of aphasia has been significantly enriched and altered through the years. Seven major types of aphasia from the Wernicke's-Lichtheim schema, however, have continued to be included in the various subsequent classifications of aphasia syndromes. While most of the terms defining these syndromes have been changed, some continue to be used, including *transcortical motor aphasia, transcortical sensory aphasia,* and *conduction aphasia.* The terms cortical motor aphasia and cortical sensory aphasia were eventually replaced with *Broca's aphasia* and *Wernicke's aphasia,* respectively, to avoid the controversy arising from findings of sensory and comprehension deficits in *motor aphasia* and prominent expressive speech disorders in *sensory aphasia.* The term subcortical sensory aphasia was replaced by the term *pure word deafness* early in the history of the study of aphasia, and the term subcortical motor aphasia has been described as *aphemia, phonetic disintegration syndrome, motor dysprosody,* and *articulation aphasia.*

In this textbook, we describe two major types of aphasia syndromes: anterior aphasia, with underlying lesions in the anterior regions of the left cerebral hemisphere; and, posterior aphasia, which develops secondary to lesions in the posterior regions of the left hemisphere. Special attention is given to Broca's aphasia in cases of anterior aphasia, and to Wernicke's aphasia in cases of posterior aphasia. While these syndromes present patients with disturbances at many levels of language processing, primarily at the semantic, phonological, and grammatical levels, they are markedly different in terms of disturbances at those levels, as reflected in their clinical features and in the anatomical localization of underlying lesions. We also describe remaining special types of aphasia syndromes, specifically those with disturbances primarily limited to one of the stages in language processing. These syndromes include transcortical motor aphasia and transcortical sensory aphasia as disturbances at the central semantic levels of language processing, and conduction aphasia as disturbances at the phonological level. Two main syndromes at the peripheral levels of language processing are articulation aphasia, which occurs at the level of motor output, and word deafness, also known as phonetic-sensory aphasia, which occurs at the auditory input level. Mixed types of anterior-posterior aphasia are also described.

CLINICAL ASPECTS

Anterior Aphasia: Broca's Aphasia
Disturbances of Expressive Speech

Clinical symptoms reflect disturbances on several levels of speech production, including the semantic/phonological and syntactic levels, the articulation level, and speech prosody and activation of speech.

Semantic level disturbances are manifested as impairments in word finding, production, and *verbal paraphasia*. This is compounded, however, by phonological disturbances manifested as *literal paraphasia*. Disturbances of syntax are exhibited via motor agrammatism, with a prevalence of nouns in expressive speech. Motor dysprosodia manifests as nonfluent, laborious, expressive speech characterized by a distortion of its rhythmico-melodic structure and a decrease in activation in speech production. Articulation production is less disturbed for single phonemes, but may be frequently observed in articulation sequences involved in word production. *Motor agrammatism* is present in almost every case of moderate Broca's aphasia. This disorder of the motor aspect of language production is accompanied by disturbances in reading and writing, as well as by a comprehension deficit, which is usually less prominent than observed in cases of Wernicke's aphasia.

These multilevel disturbances are usually underlain by relatively extensive lesions involving several adjacent language areas in the cortical and subcortical structure of the hemisphere dominant for speech, which is the left cerebral hemisphere in most individuals.

Disturbances of Conversational Speech

Disturbances at the Semantic Level: Word-Finding Disturbances and Decrease of Speech Output. An individual suffering from Broca's aphasia experiences an inability to recall words that are identical in meaning at the semantic level. A patient with severe Broca's aphasia suffers from an almost complete loss of word finding, often manifested in markedly limited speech output combined with a loss of articulation, especially in sequences. The most severe manifestation of speech disturbances is the restriction of speech output to three or four stereotyped series of words or syllables, such as "pa-pa-pa," "ma-ma-ma," "a-tu-tu," or "yes-yes-yes." The stereotypical series "tan-tan-tan" was first observed in patient Leborgne, the first of two famous cases described by Broca in 1861 (1861a). This has also been known as verbal stereotyping or *embolophasia*. A patient with embolophasia often tries to communicate by applying various intonations to the same word or syllable to stress a negative or positive emotion. Sometimes the word may be nonstereotypic, but it typically represents the echolalic repetition of the last word of the question. For example, the question, "Do you have pain?" may elicit a response of "pain . . . pain . . . pain," in such a patient.

In some cases, usually in the acute stage of stroke, Broca's aphasia begins with mutism manifested as aphonia, a complete loss of voice. A patient does not produce any sound and may rarely make any attempt to vocalize. The patient may occasionally move his lips or tongue or open and close his mouth, but is unable to make his tongue protrude from his mouth, and the tongue moves slowly and feebly in the mouth. Swallowing is generally preserved, however, pointing to a limitation of disturbances to the speech-producing system: more a dynamic disorder of initiation than a primary paresis of voice-production muscles. Vocalization thus often occurs during an involuntary cough or groan or in the course of an examination of the larynx, when the patient is asked to say "ah . . . ah . . . ah" and his attention is focused on the examination rather than on the vocalization. These particular types of mutism, or aphonia, usually last 2–3 days following the onset of stroke. Though vocalization generally returns in subsequent days, prominent Broca's aphasia emerges in many cases with typical signs of embolophasia. No sign of aphonia or mutism is observed in patients with Wernicke's aphasia in the acute stage of stroke. A fluent and unrestricted flow of indistinguishable sounds is usually observed in patients with severe Wernicke's aphasia in the acute stage of stroke.

In patients suffering from moderate Broca's aphasia, conventional conversational speech becomes possible, but is disturbed by prominent word-finding difficulties manifested in diminished speech output. This diminished speech output is impoverished, simplified, and probably constrained either by the absence of anosognosia or by a preserved insight of language impairment. This is different from the word-finding problems observed in cases of Wernicke's aphasia. It is similar, however, to Broca's aphasics in the difficulties they experience in finding the word that appropriately matches the intended meaning. Speech output is markedly increased in these patients via either an excessive number of wrong words or verbal paraphasia, which is less constrained by insight since prominent anosognosia of speech disorder is often observed in patients with Wernicke's aphasia. The articulation of single phonemes and their sequences is usually preserved in patients suffering from Wernicke's aphasia.

Sentences created by patients with Broca's aphasia include primarily high-frequency words, usually 1–3 in number. This relative preservation of high frequency words and sentences is especially apparent in automatized speech. A patient with a prominent loss of speech output usually has few difficulties in producing sequences of the weekdays (Monday, Tuesday . . .), months (January, February . . .), and especially single digits (one, two . . .), in reciting correct words while singing the melody of a very popular song and in reciting a common prayer.

Disturbances at the Semantic Level: Naming Disturbances. The expression word-finding disturbances is usually applied to impairments in the ability to find a word in the course of conversational speech. Another type of word-finding problem may be experienced when a

344

LOCALIZATION
OF CLINICAL
SYNDROMES IN
NEUROPSYCHOLOGY
AND NEUROSCIENCE

subject is required to identify isolated objects or actions as they are presented via auditory, visual, or tactile modalities. The terms *anomia, anomic aphasia,* and *amnestic aphasia* have been applied to identify this disorder of naming. Anomia seems to be the term most frequently used in recent literature.

A clinical examination of naming capabilities would consist of having the examiner point to objects around the patient, for example, a pillow, the floor, or a window, and to body parts, for example, an elbow, a knee, an eyebrow, or an eyelash, and ask the patient to name each of the presented objects. Special sets of 80–100 pictures of objects and actions have been developed for the testing of naming in aphasia test batteries. The number of items that a patient is unable to name roughly demonstrates the degree of the naming disorder.

Prompting by the examiner, giving the first phonemes of the correct word, usually helps a patient to make a correct identification, pointing to the possibility that the retrieval of words from the individual's vocabulary may be facilitated by a catalogue based on the phonological properties of words, known as the lexical module.

Anomia is usually observed in patients with Broca's aphasia and other types of anterior aphasia but may be seen more frequently in patients with posterior aphasia, especially in cases of transcortical sensory aphasia. Cueing based on the use of the phonemic directory of lexicon storage is often less helpful for correct naming in cases of anterior aphasia than it is in cases of posterior aphasia. Patients with Broca's aphasia generally require a clue consisting of two or three syllables from three- or four-syllable words, respectively. A prompt of one or two phonemes often leads to correct naming in patients with posterior aphasia.

In recent decades, naming disturbances have been studied in relation to different variables. For a review, see McCarthy and Warrington (1990). It has been found that naming may be disturbed for low-frequency words, the naming of specific categories such as body parts, color naming, letter naming, and the naming of shapes, numbers, objects, and actions (Goodglass, Klein, Carey, & Jones, 1966), as well as proper names (Semenza & Zettin, 1988), pointing to disturbances of specific sites in the directory that provide access to the stored lexicon. Modality-specific impairments of naming include both *optic aphasia* (Beauvois, 1982; Freund, 1889) and *tactile aphasia* (Beauvois, Saillant, Meninger, & L'Hermitte, 1978; Raymond & Egger, 1906).

Disturbances at the Semantic and Phonological Levels: Literal and Verbal Paraphasia. After finding the word that corresponds to its meaning at the semantic level, a patient with Broca's aphasia often experiences difficulties at the phonological level both in the production of the correct sequence of phonemes in the word and in successfully transferring these phonemes to the corresponding articulation sequences. He or she may skip over an articulem or replace it with an incorrect articulem, producing literal paraphasia. These replacement articulems often follow a certain pattern, for example, *p* often replaces *b*, *c* replaces *z*, *d* replaces *t*, and *m* replaces *n*. The omission of articulems or syllables from the word may also be observed, so that *window* may sound like *wind*. It should be emphasized that the severity of articulem replacement in conventional speech often does not correspond to the degree of disturbance in formal phonological analysis in the same patient pointing to the role of disturbances in translation from a phonologically correct word to its corresponding articulation sequences.

Literal and verbal paraphasia are characterized in Broca's aphasia by a relative stability of replaced articulems and words, that is, *standard paraphasia*, which may be related to the decrease in language-processing activity at the phonological level. This is distinguished from *labile paraphasia* in cases of Wernicke's aphasia, in which language-processing activity is markedly increased and less constrained. A patient with standard paraphasia quite regularly changes *v* to *f*, *z* to *g*, *table* to *cable*, *house* to *home*, and so on. Replacement in labile paraphasia, on the other hand, tends to be unstable and unpredictable: for example, *v* may be replaced by *f*, then by *s*, then to *b*, and so on.

As in severe cases of Broca's aphasia, a patient with moderate Broca's aphasia may sometimes avoid the difficulties in finding the appropriate articulem sequences or word via the perseveration of an articulem, syllable, or word. The result is that the patient continuously repeats a syllable, for example, *be-be-be* or *a-a-a*, or a word during conversational speech.

Phonological disturbances in Broca's aphasia, as discussed in the following paragraphs, may generally be secondary to the impairment of sequences in articulation patterns transferred from lexical stores for further transfer from a more general to a more detailed description at the level of articulation production. These impairments may be persistent and nonlinguistic, and may lead to standard literal paraphasia, omissions of phonemes, perseverations, or errors in the mapping of corresponding phonemes at phonological levels.

Disturbances in word finding may be manifested at the semantic level as verbal paraphasia, characterized by the replacement of a correct word with another word. Cases of verbal paraphasia, however, are relatively infrequent compared to those of literal paraphasia. The substitute word often belongs to the same semantic field as the replaced word: for example, *light* may be used instead of *lamp*, *wash* instead of

346

LOCALIZATION
OF CLINICAL
SYNDROMES IN
NEUROPSYCHOLOGY
AND NEUROSCIENCE

sink, or *table* instead of *desk.* Though the replacing word occasionally seems to be chosen in an accidental manner, a primarily semantic connection can usually be found.

Motor Agrammatism or Telegraphic Style. Agrammatism in Broca's aphasia is characterized by a marked decrease in sentence length. The usual phrase consists of either one or two nouns or one noun and one verb, and small functional words such as articles, connective words, and auxiliaries are often omitted. When verbs are present in the sentences, their inflectional forms tend to be missed. This preponderance of declarative grammatical forms, often accompanied by uninflected nouns and verbs and the omission of small functional words, has been termed telegraphic style. A telegram, for instance, is usually written on the assumption that the receiver of the telegram is well informed about the topic of the message and needs only several key words, primarily nouns and some uninflected and declarative verbs, to understand the message. This style decreases the number of necessary words in the telegram, helping to reduce the word count in the message and thus the cost of the telegram. Such a decrease in verbage in a patient with Broca's aphasia is caused by word-finding disturbances, mainly those involving the use of small functional words.

Disturbances at the Level of Single Articulation Production: Disturbances of Articulation. Disturbances of articulation are usually observed in patients suffering from severe cases of Broca's aphasia. Articulation production in these cases may be lost almost entirely, and the patient is unable to produce any articulation requested for repetition or needed for conversational speech. Though the patient opens his or her mouth and moves the lips and tongue, he or she produces standard embolophasic words or syllables, such as *yes-yes-yes, pa-pa-pa, ta-ta-ta,* or *ma-ma-ma* in response to every question. While spontaneous speech may be possible in less severe cases of Broca's aphasia, vowels and consonants are often distorted, and their differential features are easily missed. One of the most frequently distorted features is voicing, so that a patient utters a distorted sound resembling *p* instead of *b, s* instead of *z,* or *ch* instead of *sh,* for example. Studies have shown that two phonetic features, voicing and nasality, represent significant deficits in patients with anterior aphasia (Blumstein, 1995; Blumstein, Baker, & Goodglass, 1977; Gandour & Danderananda, 1984). These deficits are considered to be the result of a nonlinguistic impairment in particular maneuvers relating to the timing of articulators, rather than an impairment in the articulatory implementation of phonetic features (Blumstein, 1995).

In some patients, articulation production disorder becomes a key manifestation of aphasia. The term articulation aphasia is thus used in such cases. While a patient suffering from articulation production disorder is able to correctly identify the needed phoneme, the sound is distorted and deformed. In literal paraphasia, the phoneme is replaced by another, which is often similar in articulation but without the deformation seen in patients with single articulation production disturbances. Disorders of articulation production may be seen in cases of Broca's aphasia, but are usually either absent or exist only on a subclinical level in cases of Wernicke's aphasia (Blumstein, 1995).

Motor Dysprosody.   Nonfluent dysprosodic speech represents one of the most prominent features of Broca's aphasia. It is characterized by a distorted rhythmical-melodic structure of speech. A free flow of speech or melodic line is interrupted, and speech becomes characterized by effort, tension, prolonged pauses, and arrests filled with a laborious effort to find the next word in a sentence or to start a new sentence between words and while pronouncing a word. The intonation changes sharply from low to high pitch and back to low pitch, so that the normal melodic line of fluctuation between low and high pitches is disrupted.

Disturbances of Oral Movements: Buccofacial Apraxia
Buccofacial apraxia, also known as oral apraxia, is characterized by an inability to carry out the required complex facial and tongue movements in response to verbal instruction or in attempts to imitate such movements as requested by an examiner. At the same time, while no paralysis or weakness of buccofacial or tongue movements is typically observed in cases of oral apraxia, patients are unable to respond to a command or to imitate the act of blowing out a match, sipping through a straw, coughing, licking the lips, whistling, sniffing, or clicking the tongue. These same movements, however, may often be carried out involuntarily in real-life situations.

Buccofacial apraxia is seen in almost every patient with Broca's aphasia, probably contributing to the disturbances at the level of articulation. Buccofacial praxis is preserved in most patients with Wernicke's aphasia.

Disturbances at the Phonological Level: Disturbances of Repetition, Reading, and Writing
The phonetic description of a word based on its acoustical features is transferred to the nonspecific modality for phonological descriptions and is built on sequences of phonemes. The description of a particular phoneme in these sequences differs from the phonetic description,

348

LOCALIZATION
OF CLINICAL
SYNDROMES IN
NEUROPSYCHOLOGY
AND NEUROSCIENCE

since it depends on the phonemes before and after the particular phoneme in the sequences. The description may also be based on combining the simpler features of particular phonemes in the sequences into more complex features, thus describing the whole word, especially for high-frequency words used in the conventional processing of lexical information.

Disturbances of Repetition. The presence of phonological disturbances may be suspected in cases of Broca's aphasia when a patient demonstrates difficulties in the repetition of words. Numerous literal paraphasic errors, or the omission of phonemes, are noted even in the attempted repetition of one- and two-syllable words, such as *cat, table, chair,* and *window.* The number of errors increases when the patient is asked to repeat a long, multisyllabic word such as *industrialization,* a nonword such as *zelrun* or *danseez,* or an irregular word. To minimize the role of articulatory components in repetition disturbances, the patient is asked to raise his or her hand if the two auditorally presented words are the same (*table-table*), and not to raise his or her hand if the two words are different (*table-gamble*). Some improvement of word comprehension may be noted in patients with Broca's aphasia during the course of this test.

Formal phonological analyses, such as the spelling of words, are usually impaired in patients with either severe or moderate Broca's aphasia, as well as in patients with Wernicke's aphasia. Such a patient is unable to estimate the number of phonemes and syllables in a given word, especially if the word consists of three or more syllables. Many mistakes are also made when such a patient is asked if a certain phoneme is present or absent in a word. For example, a patient is asked to raise his or her hand if the phoneme *b* is present in an auditorally presented word, and not to raise his or her hand when the phoneme *b* is absent, as in *table, chair, bread, cat.*

Disturbances of Reading and Writing. These disturbances represent another finding, both in patients with Broca's aphasia and in those with Wernicke's aphasia, that supports the role of the nonspecific modality disturbances at the phonological level in such patients. Though reading seems to be impossible in a patient with severe Broca's aphasia, he or she may be able to use global reading to match cards with the correct name and picture of an object if the choices are limited, perhaps by using a set of cards with the names and pictures of three or four objects. Global reading may also be preserved for ideographs or words that may be well known to the patient, such as "U.S.A.," "Washington," or part of his or her name. Writing is also severely disturbed in these patients. A patient is usually able to write only very familiar words, such as his or her first and last names, or to slowly copy letters, syllables, and short words, though the patient often omits letters in such cases, producing many examples of literal paralexia that reflect disturbances in phonological analysis. In some cases, copying is actually slavish imitation, performed very slowly. Reading is much better than conversational speech in cases of moderate Broca's aphasia. While a patient may be able to read a series of two or three words, literal paralexia and the omission of phonemes are prominent, especially in longer words and phrases. A disorder in dictated and spontaneous writing is much more striking than a disorder in reading. Most patients can write only a handful of phonemes, syllables, and short, high-frequency words in response to dictation. This points to the role of disturbances in phonological analysis in the translation of sequences of phonemes into graphemes and written words. Copying is usually preserved in such cases, although some patients only slowly draw a slavish copy of the presented word.

It must be emphasized that repetition, reading, and writing in response to dictation may be processed on a semantic level, bypassing the phonological level. In such a case, a visual or auditory pattern of the entire word is used to retrieve the corresponding word from lexicon storage via the semantic directory for further processing by the motor output. The latter route may also be partially used in the course of spontaneous writing. Damage to this pathway may lead to the development of disturbances in repetition, reading, and writing in cases of a preserved phonological route.

Comprehension Disturbances

Comprehension of Conversational Speech. The comprehension of *conventional* conversational speech concerning familiar subjects is usually adequate in patients with both moderate and severe Broca's aphasia but is disturbed in patients with Wernicke's aphasia. Early aphasia studies led to the description of Broca's and Wernicke's aphasia as motor and sensory aphasia, respectively.

An examination of conversational speech comprehension usually includes questions about the patient's family, work, and illness. Disturbances in the comprehension of *unconventional* speech, however, may be revealed when a patient with Broca's aphasia attempts to understand the content of a telephone call, a radio broadcast, or a conversation between other persons.

Disturbances at the Semantic Level: Disorders of Word Comprehension and Alienation of Word Meaning. A patient suffering from a disorder of word comprehension experiences difficulties in the identification of word meaning, while his or her phonological or primary acoustical

350

LOCALIZATION
OF CLINICAL
SYNDROMES IN
NEUROPSYCHOLOGY
AND NEUROSCIENCE

recognition capabilities may be preserved. The patient may be able to follow a command, demonstrating a preservation of phonological and phonetic images of the word, but may have trouble when asked to point to an object in response to a command. The condition may also be called an alienation of word meaning (Luria, 1966; Tonkonogy, 1973).

In order to test the semantic aspects of conventional word comprehension, a patient is asked to repeat a simple command, then to follow that command. The command requires the patient to point to an object or a part of the body, such as to a table, a window, a door, a lamp, an elbow, a knee, an eye, or a nose. Patients with Broca's aphasia tend to perform very well on this test, often either committing no errors or having only minor difficulties, while a moderate or prominent alienation of word meaning may be present in patients with Wernicke's aphasia.

Unconventional word comprehension is tested by repeatedly asking a patient to point to the same three objects or body parts, but presented in a different order, for example, "ear–nose–ear–nose–eye–ear–eye." This test is called the ear–eye–nose test with one component. Since a subject in the conventional condition expects to be confronted with different objects, the probability of the repetition of the same object is low, and a subject does not expect the repetition to make comprehension more difficult. This test reveals alienation of word meaning not only in patients with Wernicke's aphasia but also in patients with Broca's aphasia. The addition of a sequential aspect to the test makes performance especially difficult for a patient, for example, when the patient is asked to "point to the ear, then to the eye," or "to the nose, then to the ear," and so forth. This version of the test is called the ear–eye–nose test with two components. Alienation of word meaning may also be observed when the probability of the next item is altered by switching to another semantic field, such as from objects in the room to body parts.

Alienation of word meaning is, in a sense, a mirror image of naming disturbances. A patient with anomia is unable to find the word that corresponds correctly to the meaning of the object presented for naming. In alienation of word meaning, an object cannot be matched with the meaning of the word presented. This is described in further detail in the section entitled "Wernicke's Aphasia."

Disturbances at the Level of Nonlanguage Auditory Gnosis

Disturbances at the level of nonlanguage auditory gnosis are usually absent in patients with Broca's aphasia, while mild and moderate degrees of such disturbances are observed in patients with Wernicke's aphasia, especially in experimental studies of tone pitch differentiation.

Associated Neurological Symptoms. Severe or moderate right-sided hemiplegia or hemiparesis is observed in most cases with Broca's aphasia. The patient walks slowly, with circumduction and other signs typical of spastic hemiparetic movement. Most patients demonstrate right-sided hemihypesthesia in response to pinpricks, as well as some disturbances in the sense of position. Visual field defects are usually absent in patients with Broca's aphasia.

Transcortical Motor Aphasia

Patients with transcortical motor aphasia (TCMA) have a combination of semantic level disturbances, manifesting as impoverishment and simplification of speech output, decreased speech activation and preserved repetition. Speech comprehension and naming, as well as reading and writing, are either completely preserved or only mildly disturbed in such cases. Two major types of TCMA have been described—the *classical variant* and *dynamic aphasia*. These two types differ primarily in the disturbances of expressive speech.

Classical variant is characterized by spontaneous speech, as in Broca's aphasia. The disorder begins with mutism at the onset of stroke, with the subsequent development of nonfluent verbal output. The patient's speech contains short phrases or simple words typical for Broca's aphasia, and the patient has to make laborious, effortful attempts to find the appropriate word and to produce even short sentences. This is combined with the perseveration and echolalic repetition of the last words of posed questions. A loss of initiation may be observed in some patients. The patient's speech differs from that of a patient experiencing Broca's aphasia only by minimal numbers of examples of verbal and literal paraphasia.

Dynamic aphasia is described as being almost identical to transcortical motor aphasia. As recently noted by Alexander (2002), dynamic aphasia is the core of transcortical motor aphasia, stripped of mild agrammatism and articulation impairment.

Disturbances of speech activation are one of the major signs of dynamic aphasia. The patient lacks the starting impulse to initiate speech and is unable to engage in free conversation, needing repeated stimulation to answer questions. When asked to describe his or her own biographical data, the patient frequently stops after one or two short sentences and has to be repeatedly encouraged to continue. When describing the story of a train crash that was prevented, as depicted in a series of pictures, the patient needs to be stimulated by additional questions such as, "Who stopped the train from crashing?" and "How did the train engineer become aware of the broken rails ahead of the train?"

352

LOCALIZATION
OF CLINICAL
SYNDROMES IN
NEUROPSYCHOLOGY
AND NEUROSCIENCE

Disturbances of speech activation in dynamic aphasia are manifested as frequent arrests of speech after one or two short sentences. This laborious effort to continue to talk is not a condition that is commonly experienced in patients with either Broca's aphasia or classical TCMA. Speech is usually fluent in such patients, and no sign of motor dysprosody is generally noted.

Disturbances of complex sentence production are seen in both types of TCMA. A patient's answers to questions are short, often consisting of small, 2–3 word simple sentences that are usually grammatically correct. The patient's speech is impoverished, with an absence of auxiliary verbs and complex sentences. While describing a series of pictures, the patient often prefers to use either short sentences or idiomatic expressions, for example, "Train not crashed. . . . that's it, what I can say," when asked to describe a series of pictures showing children preventing a train crash. The patient tries to replace an active full-scale answer with a short, abbreviated answer, perhaps with an echolalic passive repetition of the last word of the question. It appears that the ability to produce grammatically correct conventional types of simple sentences, such as those used in everyday life, may be preserved, especially in cases of dynamic aphasia. The ability to construct unconventional, complex sentences is disturbed, however, and these types of sentences are absent in the speech of these patients. In some cases, motor agrammatism is manifested as a partial loss of small functional words and a tendency to use substantive, uninflected words.

Patients suffering from TCMA and/or dynamic aphasia experience either mild disturbances or no disturbances at all in phonological analysis, articulation, repetition, comprehension, naming, reading, and writing.

Associated neurological signs include a mild right-sided hemiparesis, in some cases with a prevalence of weakness in the lower extremities. Right-sided hemihypesthesia in response to a pinprick is infrequently noted, and the patient's sense of position is usually preserved. Visual fields remain in the normal range.

Articulation Aphasia

Expressive speech is characterized by the deformation and distortion of articulems, while simple oral movements remain preserved and no sign of slurring dysarthria is usually noted. The disorder of expressive speech is different from other types of aphasia in that it involves only mild disturbances at the semantic and phonological levels, with almost complete preservation of word and sentence production. While comprehension and reading are either preserved or only mildly disturbed in such cases, prominent disturbances in writing are often noted.

Lichtheim (1885) believed there was an interruption of the white-matter pathway from the preserved Broca's area to the corresponding subcortical motor centers, and thus termed this disorder subcortical motor aphasia. The differences between this and other common types of aphasia were emphasized in the names given to this type of aphasia by later authors. These names included aphemia (Albert et al., 1981; Bastian, 1897), anarthria (Marie, 1906b), pure motor aphasia (Dejerine, 1914), mutism of speech sound (Kleist, 1934), phonetic disintegration syndrome (Alajouanine, Ombredane, & Durand, 1939; LeCours & L'Hermitte, 1976), and afferent motor aphasia (Luria, 1966, 1970).

Monrad-Krohn (1947) also added a new term to the mix, dysprosody, stressing the disorder of melodic line, rhythm, and accent in speech. Though the author's patient, a native Norwegian speaker, had never traveled outside Norway in her entire life, she developed a German accent after a stroke. She demonstrated dysprosody in her pronunciation of short sentences with an emphasis on the final pronoun and a raised pitch of voice rather than a lowered one, both of which are highly unusual in spoken Norwegian. In subsequent studies of similar cases of patients speaking with foreign accents, the role of the distortion and deformation of articulemes was stressed primarily in articulation aphasia, while motor dysprosody was determined to be a sign of Broca's aphasia.

Expressive Speech, Conversational Speech

Articulation disturbances are characterized by the deformation of articulems, often caused by the omission of the distinctive features of the sounds in speech (Trubetzkoy, 1939/1969; see also Jackendoff, 1992), giving rise to what are often considered foreign or childish accents. The missing voicing in the articulems may lead to the development of a Scandinavian accent, for example, if the individual's native language is Russian. The patient softens the sound *ch* to *sh*, *b* to *p*, and *d* to *t*. Since the new articulem is distorted and does not completely replace the previous one, this is not a case of literal paraphasia, which results from the replacement of one articuleme by another. The unvoiced articulem preserves some resemblance to the original one, such as when a patient changes the sound *t* to *b*, or *sh* to *ch*, pointing to the preservation of phonological analysis.

Literal paraphasia with normal pronunciation of a new articulem seldom occurs in patients with articulation aphasia. In cases of the development of a German accent in a native English speaker or in a native speaker in one of the Scandinavian languages, the replacement may move in the opposite way, with the unvoiced consonants being replaced by the voiced. We observed a patient who was a native

354

LOCALIZATION
OF CLINICAL
SYNDROMES IN
NEUROPSYCHOLOGY
AND NEUROSCIENCE

Russian speaker and who, following a stroke, developed a French accent, stressing the nasal features in the pronunciation of corresponding articulations. Articulation impairments may also be related to the relative complexity of articulems. These impairments are manifested as the replacement of difficult to pronounce consonants with easier ones, underlying the development of a so-called childish accent, as when *l* replaces *r*, and *c* is used instead of *ch*. We observed such a childish accent in some patients who were suffering from Broca's aphasia accompanied by prominent articulation disturbances.

Motor dysprosody was first observed by Monrad-Krohn (1947) in his case of the development of a German accent in a native Norwegian woman. The melody of the patient's speech was completely changed becoming typical of German speech, with a slight accentuation of the final pronoun in the phrase and a raised pitch of voice rather than a lowered one. We observed opposite changes in melody of speech in our cases of Russian speakers who developed Scandinavian accents following stroke. The accentuation of the final pronoun and the raising of voice pitch, in a manner typical of the Russian language, changes in such cases to the more melodic features of the Scandinavian language, with a characteristic lowering of voice pitch at the end of each phrase. Changes in speech melody were also observed in our cases of patients who acquired a childish accent. The melody resembled childish speech, in which a relatively equal application of accentuation is applied to the beginning of a phrase, regardless of the content of the phrase.

The changes of motor prosody described in cases of articulation aphasia are different from the motor dysprosody in Broca's aphasia, which is characterized by the rapid rising or falling of the voice pitch and is marked by obvious effort and tension.

Word finding, word production, and sentence production remain preserved in patients with articulation aphasia. Recitation and automatized speech show some pattern of acquisition of a foreign or childish accent, but not as noticeably as in conversational speech. Though naming is completely preserved, the distorted accent remains unchanged. Repetition of a single phoneme or syllable improves articulation, and most of the deformation disappears, but the distortion may be revealed again when the patient is asked to switch from the phoneme *p* to the phoneme *b*, from *t* to *d*, from *ar* to *ra*, and from *el* to *le*, and so forth.

Though buccofacial apraxia is often observed in patients with articulatory aphasia, the two disturbances do not necessitate the concurrent presence of one another.

The comprehension of conversational speech, single words, and phrases is preserved in these patients. Only a mild alienation of word meaning occurs following the commands in the eye–ear–nose test, Head's test, and the test for verbal reflection of space and time relations.

Phonological analysis and silent reading are preserved or only slightly disturbed. Reading aloud, however, reveals all of the distortion and deformation of articulemes observed in spontaneous speech, which also demonstrates a striking increase in the number of examples of literal paralexia in comparison to the few true examples of literal paraphasia in speech. In spite of preserved phonological analysis, writing is often more disturbed than would be expected in cases with only a slight disorder of phonological analysis, reading word production, and speech comprehension. Patients with articulation aphasia are often unable to write even single phonemes and well-known ideographs in response to dictation. Copying remains either preserved or only slightly disturbed by literal paragraphia and the omissions of phonemes, especially in longer, grammatically complicated words and phrases. Some patients with prominent articulation aphasia demonstrate preserved writing capabilities.

Associated neurological signs are characterized by a mild right-sided weakness of movement in the lower and especially upper extremities. In most cases, movement of the extremities is completely preserved, which is reflected in the term motor aphasia without hemiplegia, which was used to denote such cases in the old literature.

Posterior Aphasia: Wernicke's Aphasia

Clinical signs represent a combination of a comprehension disorder with prominent disturbances of word comprehension, which are usually more severe than observed in patients with Broca's aphasia, fluent expressive speech characterized by an overabundance of small functional words, verbal paraphasia, literal paraphasia to a lesser extent, logorrhea, and disturbances of reading and writing.

Comprehension Disturbances

The main feature of a comprehension disorder in Wernicke's aphasia is a disturbance in the recognition of words on both phonological and semantic levels. While the differentiation of isolated phonemes as single speech sounds may remain intact, the recognition of phonemes and their sequences as they constitute a word and the recognition of a word as a whole are disturbed. A disturbance in the recognition of words manifests as alienation of word meaning, while sensory agrammatism is often experienced by patients with Wernicke's aphasia as difficulties in the comprehension of a more complicated grammatical structure.

356

LOCALIZATION
OF CLINICAL
SYNDROMES IN
NEUROPSYCHOLOGY
AND NEUROSCIENCE

Comprehension of Conversational Speech. The comprehension of conversational speech is significantly disturbed in many patients with Wernicke's aphasia and involves various frequently used aspects of comprehension at the phonological, syntactic, and semantic levels. Disturbances may extend in some cases to comprehension at the phonetic level, which consists of acoustic sounds of the isolated speech sounds or of auditory patterns of words as a whole.

The patient is often unable to understand simple questions about his or her feelings or family problems, and is unable to understand simple words or to follow elementary commands. Sometimes a patient will not pay attention to the examiner's question and begins to listen only after being repeatedly touched on the shoulder. The patient's comprehension of gestures may also be disturbed. In less severe cases, the patient may demonstrate an understanding of simple questions about his or her health problems, but is unable to understand speech over the phone or to comprehend a conversation between two persons in which the content is not directed toward the patient.

Disturbances at the Semantic Level: Alienation of Word Meaning. In normal speech and comprehension, the acoustical, phonological, and/ or whole word descriptions must be semantically matched with a corresponding word in the word vocabulary. A disturbance in this process is called alienation of word meaning (Luria, 1966; Tonkonogy, 1973). A patient suffering from this type of disturbance may be able to repeat a command to point to an object or body part, demonstrating a preservation of word comprehension at the phonetic and phonological levels. The patient cannot, however, carry out a correct response to such commands and is unable to point to the target. A verbal command for a patient to point to his or her own knee, for example, may elicit a response such as, "knee . . . knee . . . knee . . . what is that?" In this type of comprehension testing, the examiner must be careful not to accidentally provide a clue to the patient, such as by subconsciously looking at the corresponding object or body part, for example, looking at the patient's knee when asking the patient to point to his or her knee.

A complete inability to follow any simple command is seldom observed in these patients. The first command is usually comprehended fairly well, and the patient closes his eyes in accordance with the examiner's instructions. The next command, for example, "Raise your hand," often cannot be carried out, however, and the patient continues to close and open his eyes and is unable to switch to another semantic field. This switch may eliminate the facilitation of the task provided by a limitation of choice to the same semantic field. But in a normal situation, the listener does not expect to be asked to point repeatedly to the same object, and alienation of word meaning may develop when the patient is required to repeatedly point to the three body parts or objects within the same semantic field, for example, "point to the eye . . . ear . . . eye . . . nose . . . ear . . . eye." This test is known as the eye–ear–nose test with one component.

Alienation of word meaning may be related to an inability to compare the correct general pattern of the word with its meaning due to damage to the semantic directory, which guides the search for the corresponding word meaning. The patient in this case may exhibit more prominent disturbances in the comprehension of specific categories of words, such as living things compared to man-made objects (McCarthy & Warrington, 1988). Another possibility is the destruction of word model storage, which may be the cause of alienation of word meaning in some cases, especially those with extended brain damage.

Disturbances of Word Comprehension at the Phonological Level. A patient with a relatively moderate version of Wernicke's aphasia shows a relative preservation of comprehension at the phonetic level of acoustic analysis of word sound. The patient becomes able to repeat isolated phonemes and to perform well on a simple test, for example, "Raise your hand when I say *a,* and do not raise your hand when I say *o.*" Sequences of two or three vowels, for example, *aou* and *auo* or *aou* and *oau,* cannot be differentiated correctly, and the patient continues to raise his or her hand, indicating a belief that the sequence is the same when the order of vowels has been changed in the series. The ability to find out if a certain phoneme is present in the word may also be disturbed. A patient is asked to raise her hand if the requested phoneme is present in the word pronounced by the examiner, and not to raise her hand when it is absent, as in, "Raise your hand if the phoneme *t* is found in the words *cat, cross, table,* and *crack.* It is especially difficult for such patients to differentiate between words that differ by one phoneme, such as *dot* and *pot* or *bat* and *pat.* This may be related to the changes in the auditory features of phonemes when they are included in a sequence of phonemes, as, for example, when syllables become dependent on the preceding or subsequent phoneme and not to the auditory features of the isolated phonemes. A disturbance in phonological analysis is also apparent when a patient shows an inability to estimate correctly the number of phonemes and syllables in a word. Low levels of education certainly worsen the results of phonological tests when a subject is asked to analyze the phonemic structure of sequences. The differentiation of sequences, however, does not require such a formal analysis and may be performed at a level based on the features that describe the entire auditory pattern of the sequence or its phonemic structure, which would not be reflected in the lack of formal knowledge in an illiterate individual.

358

LOCALIZATION
OF CLINICAL
SYNDROMES IN
NEUROPSYCHOLOGY
AND NEUROSCIENCE

Disturbances of comprehension at the phonological level may also be responsible for disturbances in the repetition of isolated words and sentences. While the repetition of isolated phonemes is usually preserved in less severe cases of Wernicke's aphasia, disturbances of repetition appear when a patient is asked to repeat single words or syllables. It is especially difficult for the patient to repeat nonwords and words of two to three or more syllables, such as *industry* or *prescription*.

It is important to stress that disturbances at the phonological level are not limited to the auditory modalities of the phoneme sequences. While trying to read or write words or sentences, the patient often produces only some single, isolated letters, demonstrating an inability to understand simple written commands. The ability to copy written letters or words is also impaired, but is better for a limited number of letters, and sometimes for short words. Dictated writing is severely disturbed in the patient.

These disturbances of visual and auditory phonological analysis point to the existence of a special modality-independent type of phonological analysis and its malfunctioning across the various modalities in patients with various types of anterior and posterior aphasia, in this case in patients with Wernicke's aphasia. Patients with word deafness, a more peripheral form of posterior aphasia also known as acoustic-sensory aphasia, experience disturbances at the phonetic level. These disturbances are limited to the auditory modality, and no disorder of reading and writing is generally present in such cases. It is possible that a modality-independent phonological analysis is provided by a special "inner language," which has the ability to transfer the auditory and visual features of the "communication language" into the vocabulary of the modality-independent unitary language to effectively connect the results of the recognition with their semantic meanings.

At the same time, disturbances at the phonological level may be only partially responsible for difficulties in auditory language comprehension in Wernicke's aphasia. Research has shown that there is no direct correlation between auditory language comprehension and the ability to conduct a phonological analysis of speech (Basso, Casati, & Vignolo, 1977; Blumstein et al., 1977). Since these impairments in the reading and writing of phoneme sequences constituting a word or syllable are usually more prominent than phonological disturbances in the comprehension of acoustically presented syllables and words, disturbances of such analyses may play a more significant role in reading and writing impairments in patients with aphasia. This may be related to the unique role of formal phonological analysis in learning to read and to write.

Disturbances of Word Comprehension at the Auditory Verbal Level. The role of accompanying disturbances at the auditory verbal level must also be taken into account. While such disturbances may not reach the level of severity seen in word deafness, they may become an important factor in combination with disturbances at the phonetic level related to impairments in the processing of primary features of acoustic signals. The patient experiences difficulties at the initial stages of auditory word comprehension, and has trouble recognizing single vowels or consonants, often replacing *e* with *o, b* with *k,* or *t* with *j.* The patient also makes many errors when asked to raise his hand if both single speech sounds are either the same, such as *a-a* or *o-o,* or different, such as *a-o, t-k.* The comprehension of words is noticeably disturbed in such cases, and the term word deafness has been used to indicate the primary clinical feature of this disorder of word comprehension. At the same time, reading, writing, and expressive speech are preserved in patients with word deafness, stressing the nonphonological nature of this disorder.

Disturbances at the Level of Nonverbal Auditory Gnosis. At the clinical level, the existence of disturbances at the level of nonverbal auditory gnosis is supported by the impression that a patient with Wernicke's aphasia suffers from some hearing-related problems, and it is often difficult to bring the patient's attention to the speech directed toward him or her. Auditory gnosis for nonverbal sounds remains preserved in many cases with Wernicke's aphasia, and a patient may be able to recognize the sounds of wind or a train, the clinking of keys, and the voices of common animals, such as cows, cats, dogs, and so on. Auditory agnosia, however, may be observed in some patients with Wernicke's aphasia. Prominent disturbances in the discrimination of simple auditory features, such as a tone pitch or a series of tone pitches, have been observed in experimental studies in which the nonverbal auditory working memory of patients with Wernicke's aphasia is challenged. (For more details, see below.)

Disturbances of Comprehension at the Syntactic Level. Object relations in time and space may be reflected by simple and complex syntactic rules.

Simple syntactic rules. The comprehension of sentences constructed according to the simple conventional syntactic rules is usually preserved in cases of both Broca's and Wernicke's aphasia. Such simple sentences include instructions such as "Point to the window," "Raise your hand," "Close your eyes," or "Touch the door." Another example includes so-called active sentences, when the logical order of an action is reflected by the order of the words identifying the agent and subject of the action, as in, "The wolf killed the fox," "The boy hit the girl," or "The man touched the woman." These simple sentences usually constitute conventional conversational speech and are easy to comprehend.

360

LOCALIZATION
OF CLINICAL
SYNDROMES IN
NEUROPSYCHOLOGY
AND NEUROSCIENCE

The number of such sentences may be limited to reflect the small number of typical actions represented in stored models of sentences describing these actions.

The use of more complicated syntactic rules in the structure of sentences may be considered unconventional information processing, requiring additional operations and being more vulnerable to the sequelae of brain damage in language-processing areas than sentences built on simple syntactic rules.

Complex syntactic rules. Disturbances at this stage of language comprehension may be revealed by testing the comprehension of sentences that exemplify various complex syntactic rules. Pierre Marie (1906a, 1906b) was most likely the first author to introduce special tests for the examination of sentence comprehension and noted disturbances of unconventional speech comprehension in patients with Broca's aphasia. Marie created the three pieces of paper test, in which the patient was given the following instructions: "Here on this table are three pieces of paper of different size; give me the largest one, crumple the middle-sized paper and throw it on the floor, and put the smallest one in your pocket." Based on the difficulties that patients with sensory as well as motor aphasia experienced in performing this test, Marie concluded that every type of aphasia is really a form of Wernicke's aphasia either with or without an expressive speech disorder, the presence of which depended on the existence of an additional lesion in the anterior lenticular speech zone. Though Marie's theory has not been supported in more recent studies of aphasia, the testing of unconventional comprehension that Marie initiated has been further explored by many authors and plays a valuable role in the examination of patients suspected of suffering from aphasia. A recent example of the use of Marie's test in language examination is the inclusion of the modified version of the test in the popular Mini-Mental State Examination, or MMSE (Folstein, Folstein, & McHugh, 1975).

An actual challenge of Marie's test may be related to the task of sentence comprehension, which requires the patient to connect and to memorize three types of actions with three pieces of paper, each different from the others in size. This sentence structure may be compared with the semantically reversible sentences used by Caramazza and Zurif (1976) in their sentence-picture matching test. Consider, for example, the following sentence: "The horse that the bear is kicking is brown." The adjective "brown" in this sentence could connect with either of the two nouns, "the horse" or "the bear." Patients with Broca's aphasia scored at chance level for the comprehension of reversible sentences. Marie's test is apparently similar, though more difficult since it requires that three types of actions each be connected with one of three objects.

These difficulties in sentence comprehension requiring a *spatial connection* of agent and object are also observed in the hand–ear–eye test suggested by Head (1926). The patient is asked to follow the oral commands of an examiner, which may include "Point to your right ear with the index finger of your left hand"; "Point to the left eye with the index finger of your left hand"; "Point to my right shoulder with the index finger of your right hand"; and, "Point to my left shoulder with the index finger of your right hand." For more details, see Tonkonogy (1997). Alienation of word meaning is manifested in this as pointing to the ear instead of the eye, or to the right ear instead of the left ear. To avoid the influence of right-left orientation disturbances, the patients are checked before the start of the test by asking each patient either to raise his or her right or left hand. This test is very sensitive and reveals disturbances of language comprehension not only in patients with posterior aphasia but also in the majority of patients with anterior aphasia.

Another type of the syntactic rules used for unconventional information processing includes the comprehension of passive sentences. The logical sequence of any given sentence does not usually correspond to the sequential order of the words in the sentence, and the sentence may be better understood by using prepositions such as "after," "before," and "with" that make it possible to invert the passive agent-subject order in the passive sentences. The comprehension of relationships in time as they are described by prepositions such as "after" and "before" may be tested by sentences such as, "I ate lunch after I called my friend. What did I do first?" or "Do you put your shoes on before your socks?" The use of the preposition "with" may point to the order of actions tested in the passive sentence, such as "Touch the pencil with the key," or "Touch the key with the pencil" or an active sentence, such as "With the key touch the pencil." Similarly, in the Token Test (De Renzi & Vignolo, 1962), which is popular in aphasia studies, the simple sentence construction includes active sentences such as "Pick up the blue circle" or "Pick up the red triangle." More complex sentence constructions consist of sentences such as "Touch the red triangle with the blue circle." Comprehension of passive sentences is disturbed in patients with various types of Broca's and Wernicke's aphasia. The passive subject-object order is also tested by sentences in which inversion is created by using the small functional word "was." Examples of such sentences include, "A fox was killed by a wolf: Which animal is dead?" and "The girl was hit by the boy: Who is hurt, the boy or the girl?"

A difficult to comprehend structure may also be created by sentences that describe the spatial relationship between two objects, as

362

LOCALIZATION
OF CLINICAL
SYNDROMES IN
NEUROPSYCHOLOGY
AND NEUROSCIENCE

expressed by terms such as "to the right of," "to the left of," "behind," "under," or "above." Examples of such sentences include "Put the paper clip under the pencil, but above the key" or "Put the key to the right of the pencil but to the left of the paper clip."

Most patients with Wernicke's aphasia, as well as those with Broca's aphasia, demonstrate impairments in comprehension for all of the types of complicated sentences just described, while the comprehension of sentences with identical logical and grammatical sequencing may be preserved.

Disturbances of Expressive Speech

In patients both with moderate and, especially, severe Wernicke's aphasia, expressive speech is characterized by a constant flow of often unintelligible speech sounds and words, with an overabundance of small functional words, verbal paraphasia, and jargonaphasia. Fluency and the prosodic structure of speech are generally preserved in such cases. Disturbances of expressive speech are usually combined with a severe comprehension disorder.

Expressive speech in patients with Wernicke's aphasia is fluent, presenting a picture opposite to that of the nonfluent, dysprosodic *speech* of patients with Broca's aphasia, for whom characteristically laborious efforts are needed to find the required word or sentence.

Disturbances of Conversational Speech

Disturbances at the Semantic Level: Word-Finding Difficulties Manifesting as Verbal Paraphasia and Jargonaphasia. While the conversational speech of patients with Wernicke's aphasia is characterized by word-finding problems, there is no decrease in speech output, as is observed in cases of Broca's aphasia. The flow of speech is free and fluent, without the effort and tension typical of dysprosody in patients with Broca's aphasia. Speech activity is actually increased and becomes almost completely incomprehensible, especially in severe cases of Wernicke's aphasia, and consists of a fluent flow of undistinguishable sound pronounced loudly, but without a slurring dysarthria. Though these sounds resemble speech sounds, it is impossible to recognize what phoneme has been pronounced, and single vowels such as *a* or *o* sometimes emerge from the unintelligible flow of sounds. In less severe cases, the patient tries to compensate for the loss of key words by using circumlocution and committing numerous verbal as well as literal paraphasic errors, though to a lesser extent, thus producing a mixture of senseless words commonly known as "word salad" or jargonaphasia. This word salad is almost pathognomonic in severe cases of Wernicke's aphasia. Word salad in Wernicke's aphasia must be differentiated from phonemic jargon (Brown, 1979), otherwise known as "undifferentiated jargon" (Alajouanine & L'Hermitte, 1964; Alajouanine, Sabouraud, & DeRibaucourt, 1952), which consists of strings of phonemes without either meaning or morphological or grammatical organization. This type of jargon is primarily observed and described in patients with conduction aphasia.

The free flow of senseless words is enhanced by an almost complete anosogonosia of speech disorder in patients with severe Wernicke's aphasia. These word salad patients are often unaware that they have a language disorder and tend to become angry and agitated when someone fails to understand them.

Increased speech production, characterized by a nonstop flow of words of hyperactive speech, may occur with seemingly no external stimulation, making it appropriate to use the term logorrhea in such cases. Augmentation is a term used to define the tendency of the patient with Wernicke's aphasia to add an extra two or three syllables or words when asked to repeat something or in an attempt to overcome his naming difficulties: "pa-ba" will be repeated as "pa-ba-da-ta," or "table-house" will become "table house-chair-dog."

Disturbances at the Semantic Level: Naming Disturbances. The naming of objects, parts of the body, or actions is markedly disturbed in patients with both moderate and severe Wernicke's aphasia. Naming attempts typically result in increased speech activation, with striking mispronunciations of words caused by prominent literal paraphasia, or by the replacement of the correct word with a series of incorrect words caused by verbal paraphasia. Patients with Broca's aphasia, on the other hand, exhibit a characteristic slowing down of speech activation accompanied by long pauses filled with effortful, laborious attempts to find the needed word. Prompting by providing the first one or two syllables of the name or word sometimes helps the Broca's or Wernicke's patient to find the appropriate word.

Disturbances at the Semantic and Phonological Levels: Verbal and Literal Paraphasia. Literal paraphasia reflecting disturbances at the phonological level is less prominent than verbal paraphasia in expressive speech, which is related to disturbances at the semantic level in patients with Wernicke's aphasia. This may be noticed as an augmentation of syllables when a patient repeats syllables, as when a series of two syllables, "pa-ba," is repeated as "pa-ba-da-ta." When engaging in spontaneous speech, patients with Wernicke's aphasia may produce neologisms, such as "verter" or "krossy stuff," in response to the question, "What is your favorite food?" (Butterworth, 1979). The formation of neologisms in Wernicke's aphasia seems to be facilitated by increased and unrestrained speech production, labile literal

364

LOCALIZATION
OF CLINICAL
SYNDROMES IN
NEUROPSYCHOLOGY
AND NEUROSCIENCE

paraphasia, and augmentation. This stresses important differences in the phonological disturbances of expressive speech in Wernicke's versus Broca's aphasia. While literal paraphasia is usually standard in cases of Broca's aphasia, it does not change in the course of spontaneous speech and reflects the decreases and the constraints of speech output; the examples of paraphasia become labile in cases of Wernicke's aphasia, frequently changing in the framework of increased speech production.

The correlation between phonological disturbances of expressive speech and impairments in phonological comprehension was not noted by Gainotti, Caltagirone, and Ibba (1975), but was reported by Basso et al. (1977) and Blumstein et al. (1977), who used synthetic sounds to find the correlation between identification deficits and phoneme production. However, taking into account phonological differences in conversational speech between Broca's and Wernicke's aphasia and more prominent comprehension disturbances in Wernicke's aphasia, it may be suggested that the phonological stage of language processing may consist of two well-connected but relatively independent components, one related to expressive speech and another to speech comprehension.

Disturbances at the Syntactic Level: Posterior Motor Agrammatism. In severe cases of Wernicke's aphasia, most substantial words, predominantly nouns and verbs, are either missed or are replaced via verbal paraphasia, and speech consists of small functional words. This mixture of words is known as jargonaphasia, or word salad. Though jargonaphasia is often either nonexistent or not noticeable in less severe cases, a reduced number of content nouns and a preponderance of small functional words may be noted. At the same time, the syntactical structure of conversational speech in Broca's aphasia represents some mirror image of that speech in Wernicke's aphasia. Speech is characterized by telegraphic style, with a preponderance of nouns, and to a lesser extent verbs, without typical inflections and often with an absence of small functional words.

Agents and subjects of actions seem to be relatively well reflected by the use of nouns in the conversational speech of Broca's aphasics, while descriptions of actions are better represented by small functional words in Wernicke's aphasics. In normal conditions, therefore, the Broca's region provides the transfer of descriptions of actions from the semantic level to the phonological level of expressive speech. The Wernicke's region participates in the transfer of the meaning of objects and actions to the same phonological level of expressive speech. These two parts become united at the phonological level for further translation to expressive communication speech describing the agent, the subjects, and their actions.

Articulation, Motor Prosody, and Buccofacial Praxis

While disturbances of this type are usually absent in patients with Wernicke's aphasia, some degrees of disturbance are observed in patients with Broca's aphasia. Some subclinical phonetic impairments in the speech production of Wernicke's patients have been observed. These impairments include an increased variability in phonetic parameters, such as vowel formant frequencies and vowel durations (Ryalls, 1986; Tuller, 1984).

This variability, however, may reflect the general tendency of variability in speech output typical for cases of posterior aphasia.

Associated Neurological Signs

Movements and sensations are generally preserved. Transient right-sided hemiparesis, which occurs within the first 24–48 hours following stroke, completely disappears. Mild weakness of movements in the right hand, however, may be seen in rare cases. While right-sided hemihypesthesia in response to a pinprick is seldom noted, right upper quadrant hemianopia occurs in approximately 20%–25% of cases.

Transcortical Sensory Aphasia (Anomic-Sensory Aphasia)

Patients with transcortical sensory aphasia (TCSA) have moderate disturbances of speech comprehension at the semantic level, while conversational speech, repetition, reading, and writing are relatively preserved. A prominent disorder of naming is especially noticeable, making the clinically descriptive term *anomic-sensory aphasia* useful in stressing the severity of anomia against the background of signs typical for mild to moderate sensory aphasia.

Disturbances of Comprehension

Conversational Speech.   While the comprehension of conversational speech is usually preserved, some mild difficulties may be noted in the comprehension of conversation over the telephone, or while the patient tries to understand the content of a conversation in a crowded and noisy room. These difficulties are less prominent than in patients with Wernicke's aphasia.

Disturbances at the Semantic Level: Alienation of Word Meaning.   The patient may experience difficulties in following commands to point to objects in a room, or in pointing to an object among 10–12 other

366

LOCALIZATION
OF CLINICAL
SYNDROMES IN
NEUROPSYCHOLOGY
AND NEUROSCIENCE

objects in a drawing. Severe alienation is often noted in the ear–nose–eye test with one component, and especially in the version of the test with two components, as in, "Point to your ear, then to your nose" or "Point to your nose, then to your eye."

Disturbances at the Syntactic Level.   The patient is unable to follow complicated commands related to the time and space relationships between objects and sequences, especially when these sequences are presented in reverse order, for example, "Point to the pencil with the pen" or "Point to your right ear with your left hand." Frequent errors are also made when a patient is asked to explain an action described in a series of passive sentences, such as "The tiger was killed by the lion. . . . Who was dead?" Reading, writing on dictation, and volitional phonological analysis writing usually reveal mild literal paralexia, paragraphia, verbal paralexia, or moderate slowness in preserved reading and writing. Repetition may be disturbed only for series of 3–4 words, syllables, or vowels.

Disturbances at the Level of Nonverbal Auditory Gnosis.   Experimental studies of differentiation of tone pitches in a condition challenging the nonverbal auditory working memory demonstrated that such disturbances tend to be absent in most patients with transcortical sensory aphasia. Minimal to mild disturbances may be found only in some patients, especially in learning to differentiate between tone differences not exceeding 5–10 Hz via corresponding motor reactions. No sign of verbal agnosia for nonverbal sounds such as wind, a car, a train, various animals, and so forth has been described in such patients.

Expressive Speech
Conversational speech is fluent, and prosody and articulation capabilities are preserved, though some impoverishment of speech, notably simplification of grammatical structure, may be noted. This impoverishment is similar to that of mild dynamic aphasia, though without arrests or decreases in speech activity. A mild prevalence of simple functional words and verbs may be noted, accompanied by a decrease in numbers of nouns. Literal and verbal paraphasia, primarily of the semantic type, have been reported, though infrequently.

Speech activation may be mildly increased, manifesting as augmentation with literal and verbal paraphasia in the course of a repetition of syllables and words, and, in some cases, during spontaneous speech.

Naming is prominently disturbed, markedly exceeding the degrees of disturbances of comprehension in most cases. A patient is unable to correctly name anywhere from 40%–50% to 70%–80% of presented objects, body parts, or actions. Relatively low-frequency words, such as eyelash, handle, knuckle, eardrum, and fingernail, are particularly difficult for a patient. In trying to find a proper name, the patient demonstrates an increase in word activation, producing a series of examples of literal aphasia, as well as verbal paraphasia with some acoustical or semantic relation to the word he or she is seeking. The patient is sometimes able to demonstrate the correct use of the presented object, such as a comb or a pencil, but is still unable to recall its proper name. A prompting consisting of the first two or three phonemes of the word usually helps the patient correctly name the presented object.

Buccofacial apraxia has not been described in patients with transcortical aphasia. Mild right-sided hemiparesis may be noted in the first days following stroke. A slight weakness in the right hand persists through the chronic stage in some cases. Right-sided hemihypesthesia in both the acute and chronic stages of stroke occurs in only a few cases. Persistent complete right hemianopia, or a defect in the right upper quadrants of the visual field, is noted in many cases.

Primary disturbances involved in transcortical sensory aphasia have been observed at the semantic level of word comprehension, accompanied by primarily unconventional impairments of syntax comprehension and a strikingly prominent disorder of naming. Phonological analysis, repetition, writing, and reading remain only relatively mildly impaired. No significant impairment is noted at the level of nonverbal auditory processing.

Conduction Aphasia

Conduction aphasia is characterized by disturbances at the phonological level and manifested as a disorder in the repetition of words and phrases, with a relative preservation of expressive speech and comprehension. Other prominent signs of disturbances at the phonological level include literal paraphasia. Some disturbances at the semantic level are manifested as anomia.

Wernicke (1874) was the first to point out that an interrupted connection between the acoustical and motor centers of speech may lead to aphasia with a predominant disorder of repetition. The very idea that this type of aphasia exists has long been controversial, with some authors denying it exists at all and others staunchly supporting it. Liepmann and Pappenheim (1914), Kleist (1934), and Hopf (1957) attributed this type of aphasia to a stage in the regression of Wernicke's aphasia, while Luria (1966, 1970) did not mention this type of aphasia at all. Goldstein (1948), on the other hand considered it a type of central aphasia with inner speech disturbances. Hécaen and Albert (1978) even reported that 12% of all aphasia patients seen via a large aphasia service suffered from this specific type of aphasia. Though we have encountered only six patients with the specific syndrome of conduction

368

LOCALIZATION
OF CLINICAL
SYNDROMES IN
NEUROPSYCHOLOGY
AND NEUROSCIENCE

aphasia out of the hundreds of aphasia patients we have examined, the clinical and anatomical differences between central aphasia and both Wernicke's and Broca's aphasia are apparent, supporting the independent nature of this syndrome.

Conversational speech in conduction aphasia is fluent and bears some resemblance to Wernicke's aphasia in its tendency toward augmentation, reflecting an increase in speech activation as well as a diminished number of nouns. Prominent literal paraphasia may be noted against the background of mild disturbances of expressive speech, especially when the patient tries to tell a story. Albert et al. (1981) presented an excellent example of such paraphasia compounded by prominent augmentation. The patient, while intending to say "Nelson Rockefeller," instead said, "Nelson Nockenfellen, I mean Relso Rickenfollow, I mean Felso Knockerfelson."

Naming disturbances are also characterized by prominent literal paraphasia and augmentation, as when a patient tries to find the correct word. One patient with conduction aphasia, for example, attempted to say the word "flower" and instead said, "flowing . . . flying . . . tower . . . flushing."

Repetition. The patient with conduction aphasia experiences prominent difficulties in the repetition of words, phrases, and series of syllables, while the repetition of single phonemes is usually preserved. While repetition in conduction aphasia is significantly more disturbed than expressive speech and comprehension, the severity of repetition impairments usually corresponds to some extent to the severity of expressive speech and comprehension disturbances in other types of anterior and posterior aphasia.

Comprehension disturbances are mild and may be noted in only some of Head's hand–ear–eye test and in tests with complex syntactical structures. Alienation of word meaning is infrequent, however, even in the ear–eye–nose test with two components.

Phonological analysis is only slightly disturbed in these cases. Patients experience difficulties in assessing the number of syllables in words consisting of four or five syllables. Reading is usually preserved in these patients. Difficulties in writing in response to dictation and in volitional writing are characterized by a distortion of words via literal paragraphia. It is, however, easy to understand most of the words written by patients with conduction aphasia.

Associated neurological signs. Movements in the extremities in patients with conduction aphasia are intact. Right hemihypesthesia and, more often, right-sided hemianopia are observed in these patients.

Word Deafness (Phonetic-Sensory Aphasia)

While patients with phonetic-sensory aphasia are unable to understand spoken language, their expressive speech, reading, and writing are almost completely preserved. Phonetic-sensory aphasia was first described by Kussmaul (1877) as *reinen Worttaubheit,* or pure word deafness, 3 years after Wernicke's famous description of sensory aphasia. Many authors doubted the existence of this aphasia syndrome from the beginning. Some investigators, including Wernicke and Friedlander (1893), attributed the difficulties to incomplete sensory aphasia. Luria (1966) more recently excluded pure word deafness from his classification of aphasia. He described Wernicke's sensory aphasia as acoustic-sensory aphasia with primary difficulties in auditory phonological analysis, or the phonemic hearing of words, thus combining both types of aphasia into one syndrome.

Freud (1891) and Freund (1889), on the other hand, stressed the role of peripheral hearing loss in the development of word deafness. More recently, Jerger (1964), Albert and Bear (1974), and Auerbach, Allard, Naeser, Alexander, and Albert (1982) demonstrated a more complicated auditory processing disorder in patients with pure word deafness. These authors stressed the role of central auditory nonverbal processing in the mechanism of pure word deafness, recognizing the syndrome as an independent clinical entity.

Comprehension Disorders

Conversational Speech. Patients with word deafness differ from those with Wernicke's aphasia, in that the former reveal a more noticeable disorder of comprehension of conversational speech. When asked about well-known everyday events, a patient with phonetic-sensory aphasia looks at the examiner with a puzzled expression on his or her face, trying to listen carefully to the voice of the examiner, just as a deaf person does. The term *word deaf* seems to be appropriate in such cases.

Auditory Agnosia of Speech Sounds. Further examination reveals that the patient's actual disturbance is a severe disorder in the auditory gnosis of speech sounds. The patient is unable to repeat even single phonemes, and has difficulties with consonants especially. Patients with moderate aphasia, however, are often able to repeat some vowels. The patient experiences difficulties in differentiation between two individual phonemes. Especially troublesome for the patient are voicing differences between phonemes, such as, *p-b, d-t,* and so on. These disturbances in the auditory gnosis of speech sounds may be responsible for difficulties in repeating and recognizing syllables, words, and phrases. The patient with word-deafness often complains that spoken

370

LOCALIZATION
OF CLINICAL
SYNDROMES IN
NEUROPSYCHOLOGY
AND NEUROSCIENCE

language sounds like an unknown foreign language, or in more severe cases like mumbling or indistinguishable noise. The patient is able to recognize words and phrases, however, if he or she can correctly repeat them. No sign of alienation of word meaning is noted in such cases.

Disturbances at the Nonverbal Auditory Level. Though auditory agnosia for nonverbal sounds may accompany phonetic-sensory aphasia in some cases, agnosia is absent in many patients with phonetic-sensory aphasia, and vice versa. Sensory aprosodia is frequently present, manifesting as difficulties in the recognition of intonations, melodic structures, and emotional characteristics typical of anxiety, fear, anger, depression, surprise, and happiness. (For more details, see chapter 3, section entitled "Auditory Agnosia.") Prominent sensory amusia is also noted in some cases with word deafness.

Severe disturbances in the differentiation of the primary features of nonverbal acoustic signals are frequently noted in cases of word deafness, both with and without signs of nonverbal auditory agnosia. One of our patients with word deafness was asked via a written request to raise her hand when she heard a pitch frequency of 200 Hz (Tonkonogy, 1986). After a rehearsal of 20 trials, different pitch frequencies, including 205 Hz, 210 Hz, 300 Hz, and 350 Hz, were presented along with a written command: "Do not raise your hand." The patient could reliably distinguish only tones 200 Hz from 400 Hz or 500 Hz. The differentiation threshold for pitch-frequency retention was thus approximately 200 Hz, which is in contrast to that of 10–20 Hz in patients with Wernicke's aphasia. Such significant disturbances may certainly underlie the difficulties in the differentiation and recognition of phonemes.

Albert and Bear (1974) observed disturbances of temporal acuity in a patient with word deafness. The patient had an increased intersignal threshold for detecting when a pair of successive clicks was presented. For more details, see review by McCarthy and Warrington (1990).

Expressive Speech

Conversational speech is fluent and grammatically sound in such patients, and there is typically no evidence of logorrhea or augmentation. Literal and verbal paraphasia, as well as occasional difficulties in word finding in conversational speech and in confrontation naming, are sometimes noted.

Some degree of motor aprosody may be observed in patients with phonetic-sensory aphasia. In more severe cases, motor aprosody may manifest as an almost complete loss of intonation and fluctuation in expressive speech. The typical patient speaks in a loud but expressionless voice, and with an indistinguishable emotional tone. Buccofacial and general apraxia are absent.

Phonological analysis is preserved, as it is noted in expressive speech, reading, and writing.

Associated neurological symptoms. Transient right- or left-sided hemiparesis may be noted in only some cases during the first hours following the onset of stroke. Hemihypesthesia, whether left- or right-sided, may persist longer, especially affecting the patient's vision in the upper quadrants of the visual fields.

Word deafness and anomic-sensory aphasia are thus characterized by primary disturbances in auditory recognition and in the processing of the auditory features of verbal sounds. Either no disturbances or only minimal impairments may be observed in expressive speech; naming, nonauditory phonological analysis, reading, and writing. Word deafness is often accompanied by auditory agnosia for nonverbal sounds as well as sensory amusia and motor and sensory aprosody.

Semantic Aphasia and Semantic Dementia
Head (1926) was probably the first to try to describe an unusual type of aphasia, which he called *semantic aphasia*. He described disturbances in this type of aphasia as a failure to recognize the full meaning of words and phrases independent from their immediate verbal meaning. The patient is unable to understand the final goals and tasks of an action that is either initiated spontaneously or suggested by someone else. The patient cannot precisely formulate for him- or herself and others the general concepts that he or she speaks about, reads about, or sees in a picture, in spite of a preserved ability to correctly outline most of the details. Disturbances extend to the construction of simple spatial plans, orientation, and planning of actions, leading to difficulties in everyday functioning and often making the patient unable to continue his ordinary work. Memory and general intellect remain largely preserved.

Head developed a special test battery for the evaluation of semantic aphasia. The battery includes a series of tests intended to study language performance with regard to spatial orientation, including body image, spatial orientation in the surrounding space and in the concept of space, mathematical operations, drawing, and the retelling of complex stories that also require a description of a spatial relationship. He considered that a semantic defect in language function underlies disturbances in semantic aphasia. One of Head's tests was directed toward an examination of the ability to point with the hand to particular parts of the face in response to either an oral command or an equivalent

372

LOCALIZATION
OF CLINICAL
SYNDROMES IN
NEUROPSYCHOLOGY
AND NEUROSCIENCE

picture. This particular test was frequently used in subsequent studies of speech comprehension in aphasia.

Luria helped to focus attention of researchers on semantic aphasia as a special aphasic syndrome. The second volume of his doctoral thesis was devoted to the study of semantic aphasia, which he considered a manifestation of language disturbance in the area of complex spatial orientation and synthesis. Luria developed a series of tests for this disturbance, including logicogrammatical structures, to examine the spatial relationship between single objects or figures. Another test asked patients to compare the semantic sequences of inverted phrases and sentences, such as passive sentences (Luria, 1966). Luria included anomic aphasia as a subcategory of semantic aphasia. Luria's logico-grammatical structures, along with Head's hand–body parts test, eventually became major instruments in the study of speech comprehension in aphasia. The term semantic aphasia, however, has never been fully accepted in aphasiology and has been largely abandoned. This may be due to the vague and imprecise description of semantic aphasia, which lacks a clear clinical picture and is somewhat similar to transcortical sensory aphasia.

Interest in semantic aphasia has recently increased due to a description of *semantic dementia* in slowly progressive fluent aphasia. For a review, see Della Sala and Spinnler (1999). The clinical picture of semantic dementia in cases of slowly progressive aphasia primarily includes anomia and semantic paraphasia. Taylor and Warrington (1971) and Warrington (1975) described patients who were able to reconstruct 3-D representations of objects but were unable to name or to comprehend the names of objects presented either acoustically or in written form. Each of the patients demonstrated normal performance on an intelligence test. Patient A.B., for example, had an IQ of 122.

The description of semantic dementia is similar to the original suggestions of Liepmann (1908), who observed patients with senile dementia who also exhibited disturbances in accessing the concept or meaning of an object, manifesting as a disturbance in verbal categorization and nonverbal performance. The matching of perception of outer words and crystallized engrams, however, remained preserved. Liepmann called these disturbances *ideatorische,* or disjunctive. It seems that these disturbances may be observed at the supra-ordinate level of the semantic network, while their sub-ordinate patterns are either not impaired or only mildly disturbed.

The addition of anomia also makes Head's description of semantic aphasia a perfect example of semantic dementia, in which disturbances at the semantic level of space orientation and categorization are primarily related to language performance. The similarity between semantic aphasia and semantic dementia is also reflected in the term Gogi aphasia, or aphasia for meaning (Tanabe et al., 1992; Tanabe et al., 1994). Further studies and clarification of the terms semantic aphasia and semantic dementia, as well as their clinical patterns, are certainly needed.

Mixed Anterior-Posterior Aphasia

An aphasia syndrome often results from a lesion involving both the anterior and posterior parts of the language zone. A typical example is *global aphasia,* which is a combination of severe Wernicke's aphasia and Broca's aphasia caused by an extensive lesion of the anterior and posterior language zones. Another example is *mixed transcortical aphasia,* which combines symptoms of transcortical motor aphasia and transcortical sensory aphasia.

Global Aphasia

Global aphasia is characterized by an almost complete loss of expressive speech, combined with a noticeable disorder of comprehension, often including gesture comprehension. Severe disturbances in reading and writing are also noted. Expressive speech is similar to severe Broca's aphasia in its restriction to the pronunciation of only one or two words or syllables, known as speech embolus, or emobolophasia. Patients often answer every question with only "yes" or "no," or "ta-ta," "tu-tu-tu-tu," "a-la-la," and so forth. The intonation of words or syllables often reveals their emotional meaning.

Repetition, naming, and automatized speech are greatly disturbed in these cases. Patients produce a speech embolus in almost every attempt to do any of the following: repeat a speech sound, syllable, or word; name a presented object; or recite a series of numbers, the days of the week, or the months of the year. Some patients may repeat single vowels, isolated short syllables (e.g., *ma, pa,* or *la*), or short words (e.g., *cat, dog,* or *house*), but often with literal labile paraphasia, in this way exhibiting a similarity to patients with Wernicke's aphasia.

Comprehension of conversational speech is significantly disturbed in all patients with global aphasia, as in cases of severe Wernicke's aphasia. Some cases are also characterized by a prominent disorder of gesture comprehension. Patients are often unable to understand such simple questions as "Do you have children," "What is your profession," and so on.

Alienation of word meaning. Patients have difficulty following most simple commands. Though a patient may be able to respond correctly to the first command in a series, such as "Close your eyes," subsequent commands reveal severe alienation of word meaning. The patient continues to close and reopen his or her eyes in response to all later commands, or to point to his or her ear instead of to the window, for example.

374

LOCALIZATION
OF CLINICAL
SYNDROMES IN
NEUROPSYCHOLOGY
AND NEUROSCIENCE

Phonological analysis, reading, and writing are prominently impaired. These impairments are even more severe than those that have been observed both in patients with severe Broca's aphasia and in those with Wernicke's aphasia. The typical patient cannot recognize his or her own last name in print and is unable to match printed words with corresponding pictures. When verbally asked to write something, the patient will often draw a figure somewhat resembling the corresponding letter, or will sometimes print the same letter embolus, such as "A," "B," or "P" in response to every task. The patient is also unable to write well-known ideographs, such as "U.S.A." An occasional patient, however, is able to copy letters in a slavish imitation manner.

Buccofacial apraxia is noticeable in all patients. This disturbance is recognizable when a patient is verbally asked, for example, to put his tongue inside his cheek, to put his tongue between his upper lips and his teeth, to whistle, to cough, to blow out a match, or to suck through a straw, and is unable to do so.

The associated neurological signs are quite prominent, including right-sided spastic hemiplegia and right-sided hemihypesthesia. In a few cases, however, movements may be completely preserved. Right hemianopia, predominantly for the upper quadrant, may be revealed in some patients if their comprehension is substantial enough to understand the test.

While global aphasia in general manifests as a combination of signs of severe Broca's and Wernicke's aphasia, the degrees of disturbances in expressive speech, and especially in comprehension, writing, and reading, are more prominent in global aphasia compared to those "purer" types of anterior and posterior aphasia.

Mixed Transcortical Aphasia

Mixed transcortical aphasia is characterized by prominent disturbances of spontaneous speech and severely disturbed comprehension, while repetition capabilities remain strikingly preserved. Embolophasia is not observed, though conversational speech may be completely absent. Patients have a tendency toward echolalic responses of single words from the posed question or toward the repetition of entire questions, though at times adding another appropriate word. The question, "How are you feeling," for example, may elicit a response of "Feeling good" from a patient. The answer is usually produced fluently, with no sign of the motor dysprosody typical for Broca's aphasia. The patient often remains mute, even when asked to tell his or her first and last name, thus demonstrating the decrease in speech initiation usually seen in cases of dynamic aphasia. The patient's ability to recite automatized sequences is also severely disturbed. Often he or she is able to count only to 10, and is unable to recite the days of the week or months of the year in the correct order.

Naming is impossible for these patients. Though the patient may be able to name an object when prompted by a phonemic clue consisting of the first one or two syllables of the word, correct naming is often distorted by literal paraphasia.

The comprehension of conversational speech is prominently disturbed in such cases. A patient may be able to follow commands and to point to some objects in the room, but he or she often demonstrates alienation of word meaning and points to the wrong objects. Severe alienation of word meaning is observed in Head's hand–ear–eye test, and in the comprehension of complex syntactical sentences.

Repetition capabilities are significantly better in these cases. Patients often correctly repeat single phonemes, syllables, and words, including four- and five-syllable words, as well as short simple phrases, in similar fashion to patients with TCMA and TCSA. Literal paraphasia and omissions of phonemes are exhibited only in the repetition of uncommon, multisyllabic, and low-frequency words, series of three vowels or words, oppositional phonemes, such as "pa-ba" or "da-ta," and longer, more complicated sentences.

Phonological analysis, reading, and writing are noticeably disturbed in most cases. A patient may be able to read only two or three well-known ideograms, such as "U.S." or "N.Y.," and to read and write only his or her own last name. Some patients can copy short words, but only with slavish imitation, in which one is able to draw letters but not to rewrite them.

Associated neurological signs. Right-sided hemiparesis varies from mild to severe. Right-sided hemianopia may be demonstrated in some cases.

In summary, while the clinical picture here is similar to that of global aphasia, disorders of expressive speech and comprehension are not as total as in global aphasia, and the remarkable sparing of repetition capabilities defines the clinical picture typical for transcortical aphasia. The disturbances of expressive speech in MTCA, which include a marked decrease in speech initiation combined with elements of Broca's aphasia, are somewhat similar to those observed in cases of severe transcortical motor aphasia and dynamic aphasia. Impairments in comprehension accompanied by severe anomia, on the other hand, resemble transcortical sensory aphasia with elements of Wernicke's aphasia. While these elements of Broca's and Wernicke's aphasia may be responsible for writing and reading disturbances, the latter may be related to other mechanisms, taking into account the remarkable preservation of repetition capabilities.

Aphasia in Dementing Illnesses

Both early and more recent studies of aphasia have been based primarily on analyses of aphasic syndromes in patients with circumscribed,

376

LOCALIZATION
OF CLINICAL
SYNDROMES IN
NEUROPSYCHOLOGY
AND NEUROSCIENCE

focal cortical and subcortical lesions caused by tumors, head injury and, especially, chronic stages of stroke, all of which helped to minimize the role of edema and other more generalized pathological factors in the development of aphasia.

Early writers seem to have mentioned aphasia in cases of generalized cerebral pathology relatively infrequently. Among these authors was Alzheimer, who described the development of aphasia as one of the early symptoms in his cases of presenile dementia (Alzheimer, 1906). Aphasia was also reported by Pick in a case that was later considered an example of Pick's disease, known as frontotemporal dementia in current terminology (Pick, 1892). Irigaray (1973) later began a movement in which language disturbances in dementia were subjected to systematic studies.

Aphasia is reportedly observed in the majority of cases with Alzheimer's disease, reaching a prevalence rate of 80% in cases with histopathological confirmation (Price et al., 1993). The clinical profile of aphasia in Alzheimer's disease more frequently resembles that of transcortical sensory aphasia (Cummings, Benson, & Hill, 1985; Rapcsak & Rubens, 1994) in the following symptoms and side effects: fluent but impoverished speech; frequent verbal paraphasia, predominantly of the semantic type; disturbances in speech comprehension, especially for syntactically complex sentences: and prominent naming disturbances. Repetition is usually remarkably preserved in such cases, even in those in the more advanced stages of dementia, pointing to the predominance of language disturbances at the lexical-semantic level. One of our patients was in the moderate-severe stage of Alzheimer's disease and was exhibiting prominent TCSA, and was able to repeat flawlessly not only well-known short words but also more complicated and lengthy words, such as "industrialization" and "civilization," as well as series of syllables, such as "da-ta" and "pa-ba." In most cases, however, repetition begins to deteriorate with advances to moderate or, especially, severe manifestations of Alzheimer's disease (Appel et al., 1982; Bayles, Tomoeda, & Rein, 1996; Glosser, Kohn, Friedman, Sands, & Grugan, 1997).

The preservation of repetition in patients with Alzheimer's disease may be related to the sparing of the primary and secondary association areas around the Sylvian fissure, while cortical atrophy in the association areas at the temporo-parietal-occipital junction may lead to the development of the lexical-semantic disturbances typical for TCSA (Chui, 1989).

Progressive aphasia may develop as a single early sign of degenerative disease, and while the patient may subsequently develop cognitive problems, signs of significant cognitive decline may be completely absent in the first 2 years of aphasia progression (Mesulam, 1982;

Wechsler, 1977; Weintraub, Rubin, & Mesulam, 1990). This progression of cognitive decline is thus similar to that in typical cases of degenerative disease. Neuropathology in such cases reveals neurofibrillary tangles and senile plaques, which are usually found in Alzheimer's disease, as well as a non-Alzheimer's type of pathology typically noted in Pick's disease (Kirshner, Webb, Kelly, & Wells, 1984; Lippa, Cohen, Smith, & Drachman, 1991). For a review, see Kertesz (1994).

The speech of patients with Pick's disease is often characterized by the stereotypic repetition of brief words and phrases accompanied by periods of mutism. According to our experience, speech in Pick's disease often resembles dynamic aphasia in the decrease in speech initiation, as well as the impoverishment of speech production against the background of general apathy, which is typical for frontotemporal dementia. One patient of ours, patient M.S., suffered from Pick's disease and demonstrated a pronounced lack of initial impulse to talk. (For more details, see chapter 11, section entitled "Anxiety Disorder," and section entitled "Obsessive-Compulsive Disorder" [OCD].) Patient M.S. had to be encouraged and prodded to answer questions, and eventually developed complete mutism with aphonia. Her comprehension became prominently disturbed at this stage, and she could understand only simple gestures. A head CT scan at that time revealed bifrontal cortical and bilateral caudate atrophy, with additional involvement of both anterior temporal regions. A subsequent autopsy showed lobar atrophy in these regions (Tonkonogy, Smith, & Barreira, 1994).

Language Disturbances in Schizophrenia

Language disorders are also observed in some patients with schizophrenia. These disorders were originally called *schizophasia* in the psychiatric literature and were defined by Kraepelin as alienation of speech from the relatively less disrupted thought process (Bleuler, 1951). Expressive speech in such cases is similar to the jargonaphasia, or word salad, typical for patients with Wernicke's aphasia and characterized by a constant stream of words with verbal and literal paraphasia, disturbances of the grammatical structure of sentences, and a prevalence of verbs and auxiliary words. Comprehension, including that of more complex syntactical structures, is preserved in these cases. Schizophasia is in this way different from cases of Wernicke's aphasia.

We conducted a study in which 20 patients with schizophasia and 15 patients with positive formal thought disorders, originally known as *ataxic thinking* in psychiatric literature, and found that patients with schizophasia show disturbances in the grammatical structure of sentences, manifesting as incomplete sentences, and an absence of grammatical connections between primary and auxiliary sentences in the passage. The ratio of nouns to verbs had a mean of 1.0 in schizophasia

378

LOCALIZATION
OF CLINICAL
SYNDROMES IN
NEUROPSYCHOLOGY
AND NEUROSCIENCE

patients and 2.8 in patients with ataxic thinking, and reached 13.0 in some patients whose speech consisted almost entirely of nouns. These differences were especially prominent in the writings of patients with schizophasia and ataxic thinking (Ryabova, Sluchevskiy, & Tonkonogy, 1964), pointing to the probability of posterior temporal lobe pathology in schizophasia, and a more anterior location, possibly in the frontal lobe, in patients with ataxic thinking. These findings also stress a relative independence of expressive speech and comprehension disturbances in Wernicke's aphasia, since jargonaphasia without any significant comprehension is observed in patients with schizophasia. Further studies, however, are certainly needed.

It must be stressed that negative thought disorders somewhat resemble the speech akinesia in patients with circumscribed lesions in the posterior F3 and cingulum areas. Conversely, these negative thought disorders in patients with schizophrenia may be secondary to negative signs such as general akinesia, apathy, and abulia, which are all probably caused by pathology related to the same cortical areas, as well as some subcortical structures.

Disturbances in Primary Psychiatric Illnesses:
Formal Thought Disorders and Language

Communication disturbances may manifest as a formal thought disorder, reflecting impairments in the thought process itself. Thinking may be considered a type of language that is directed primarily to "myself" and is concentrated on the description of the outer world in its dynamics, as well as on the planning and performance of actions. In this sense, thinking represents a form of internal communication. Disturbances in this process may be reflected in the individual's language, demonstrating a so-called formal thought disorder, which is manifested as a loss of association between parts of the train of thought, while the grammatical and phonological structures of thoughts remain preserved.

According to Andreasen (1979a, 1979b), thought disorder may be conceptualized as consisting of two basic types—positive and negative. Positive thought disorders are reflected in speech as incoherence, illogicality, a loss of goals, tangentiality, derailment, and pressure of speech. Negative thought disorders are manifested as poverty of speech and poverty of content of speech. Andreasen compared 18 subtypes and severity of thought disorders in 113 patients, including 45 schizophrenics, 32 manics, and 36 depressive patients, and found an almost equal frequency of tangentiality, derailment, incoherence, and illogicality in both mania and schizophrenia. Some of the subtypes were observed more frequently in mania: these included pressure of speech, circumstantialities, and distractibility.

Other differential signs stressed by previous clinical studies include the sliding of speech from one topic to another closely related topic in cases of mania, while the content of speech tends to be disjointed and disrupted by an absence of any apparent logical connection in cases of schizophrenia. Prevalence of abstract words and abstract topics is also typical for schizophrenia. The tendency to make long speeches lacking both a clear content and a connection to reality may also be observed in some schizophrenics.

Andreasen also demonstrated that a substantial number of schizophrenics exhibited a negative type of thought disorder manifested as poverty of speech and poverty of content of speech. The negative type of thought disorder was observed in depressed patients only occasionally. Speech blocking was observed in only some of the schizophrenics, and rarely in cases of patients with mania.

Aphasia and Disturbances of Brain Information Processing

Disturbances at the Phonological Level

Broca's aphasia, Wernicke's aphasia, and conduction aphasia differ from other types of aphasia with regard to disturbances at the intermediate stage of language processing, known as the phonological level. As in the process of visual object recognition (see chapter 2, section entitled "Visual Object Agnosia"), the phonological level is involved in part decomposition, as well as in the structural description of words. These structural descriptions are based on the assumption that each word may be described as a sequence of invariant primary parts or components, defined as phonemes in modern linguistic studies. Though there are predefined sets of particular phonemes that are similar, identical, or different in various languages of the world, the number of phonemes remains around 30 or 40 in each specific language. The phonemes may be grouped in many thousands of different sequences and thus may be used to form various words using only the limited number of primary parts in the course of word production and recognition.

Phonemes may be further broken down into distinctive phonological features (Jackendoff, 1992; Trubetzkoy, 1939/1969), which describe the variations between speech sounds and define the composition of particular phonemes. These phonological features include: voiced *b, d, g, z* sounds versus unvoiced *p, t, k, s* sounds; nasal *m, n* sounds versus nonnasal *b, k, s* sounds; constricted lips used to make the sounds *w, p, m* versus unconstricted lips to make the sounds *k, e, n, i*; consonants versus vowels, and so on. These features may be used in the process of word decomposition to recognize or to produce the phonemes in the sequences that comprise a particular word.

380

LOCALIZATION
OF CLINICAL
SYNDROMES IN
NEUROPSYCHOLOGY
AND NEUROSCIENCE

In cases of Broca's aphasia, Wernicke's aphasia, and conduction aphasia with disturbances at the phonological level, the process of word production and recognition may be destroyed by a malfunction of the phonological system based on the decomposition of the word into phonemes or syllables. The patient becomes either completely unable to use this system to produce, to recognize, or to repeat a word, or retains only a limited ability to do so. This may manifest as literal paraphasia, an omission of phonemes and syllables in expressive speech, disturbances of repetition, or impairments of word comprehension. Since this system may be modality independent, similar difficulties often appear in reading and writing.

The phonological disturbances in the production and comprehension of speech seem to be identical in patients with Broca's aphasia, Wernicke's aphasia and conduction aphasia, leading to the conclusion, advanced in modern neurolinguistic studies, that the neuroanatomical sites of phonological analysis cannot be strictly localized and are instead distributed over the large perisylvian region in the left hemisphere. For a review, see Blumstein (1995).

The role of local components in phonological disturbances requires further investigation. It is possible that the primary phonological disturbances in Broca's aphasia are concentrated around the process of the translation of the phonemic sequences needed for word production to sequences of corresponding articulatory movements. At the same time, this process of translation to articulatory level is mainly preserved in cases of Wernicke's aphasia, and disturbances are mainly related to the transportation of the auditory patterns of words and phonemes to the phonological level for further processing. The major type of information processing disturbances at the phonological level may thus be defined in cases of Broca's aphasia (type I) as impairments in the translation of phoneme sequences into articulatory sequences in the course of word production. In cases of Wernicke's aphasia, these disturbances (type II) are manifested as interruptions in the translation of auditory patterns of phonemes and their sequences to the modality-independent phonological level.

The role of type I phonological disturbances is supported by data that show no evidence of a disorder affecting the articulatory production of feature voicing in anterior aphasics, pointing to the preservation of the use of voicing, which represents the distinctive phonetic feature at the phonological level. While the patient is able to maintain the distinction between voiced and voiceless stops on the basis of the duration of a preceding vowel, he or she still suffers from disturbances in particular articulatory maneuvers, such as timing or the integration of the movements of two independent articulators (Baum, Blumstein, Naeser, & Palumbo, 1990; Blumstein, 1995; Tuller, 1984). This data demonstrate that translation from the phonological level to the articulatory level is not directly related to the translation of voicing, one of the distinctive features of phonemes, but is instead more complicated and probably involves another set of distinctive features specific to articulatory sequences.

Type II phonological disturbances may be expected in patients with Wernicke's aphasia. Some of the data, however, show that while the labeling of phonemes is disturbed in cases of both Wernicke's aphasia and Broca's aphasia, the ability to recognize and to differentiate between acoustic patterns of phonemes is preserved (Blumstein, 1995). This seems to contradict Luria's view that the basic disturbances in cases of Wernicke's aphasia are impairments of phonetic hearing (Luria, 1966). Furthermore, simple testing of the discrimination between acoustic patterns of phonemes may not reveal more complex conditions in speech comprehension. These complex conditions include the use of the auditory working memory to store the auditory patterns of speech sounds for the processing of their sequences in the course of word comprehension. Disturbances of this short-term storage may lead to impairments in the translation of the auditory patterns of phonemes and words to the phonological level for further processing. The role of such disturbances is supported by a marked increase in thresholds of tone pitch differentiation when the interpair intervals between two tones are increased from 1 sec to either 5 or 10 sec, as well as when differentiated tones are presented as a part of a series of tones (see below).

Phonological disturbances may thus be observed in both types of aphasia. The types of disturbances, however, differ according to whether the patient is suffering from Wernicke's aphasia or Broca's aphasia. Patients suffering from Broca's aphasia find it difficult to translate the phonological pattern of the word to the articulation program, and those suffering from Wernicke's aphasia have difficulties translating the acoustical pattern of speech sounds to the phonological level.

The auditory processing of words in cases of Wernicke's aphasia may not be very elaborate and may thus produce auditory patterns that may be easily translated into phonemes at the modality-independent phonological level. The auditory image of a word may also be processed as an entire object, then transferred either to the phonological level for further processing or directly to the semantic system for comparison with the acoustic images of words preserved in lexical storage. The auditory pattern of the entire word may thus be translated into modality-independent language at the phonological level without a description of the word's phonemic structure. Disturbances in these translations may also be related to the translation of entire visual images of the

382

LOCALIZATION
OF CLINICAL
SYNDROMES IN
NEUROPSYCHOLOGY
AND NEUROSCIENCE

written words, leading to the development of reading disturbances in patients with Wernicke's aphasia.

Speech comprehension in such cases may be less impaired than phonological analysis if the acoustical images of the entire word can be directly compared with words at the semantic level. This suggestion is supported by the identification of prominent phonological disorders in patients with Broca's aphasia, though the relation of these disorders to disturbances of comprehension remains weak, as the comprehension of conventional conversational speech is largely preserved in such patients.

The use of the acoustical pattern of a word in the process of comprehension may be compared with the suggestion, made by Luria (1966), that disturbances of comprehension in sensory aphasia are underlined by impairments in phonemic hearing. This suggestion correctly points to the role of disturbances in auditory processing in the development of comprehension disorders in Wernicke's aphasia, but relies on the suggestion that speech comprehension impairments are primarily related to phonological disturbances. The phonological system using structural descriptions based on word decomposition into phonemes and their distinctive features does, however, seem to be quite complicated in light of the fast and reliable recognition and production of words in conventional speech and comprehension. Such a system requires the processing of the huge number of possible combinations of phonemes that compose the thousands of words. Such a system may underlie the development of language based on its phonemic description, but the recognition and production of conventional speech require a faster and less complicated system based on the processing of a limited amount of information. Like visual object recognition, such a system for processing speech sounds may be based on invariant features that describe the auditory pattern of the entire word, while simple phonetic recognition is preserved and recognition is processed predominantly at the semantic level.

Disturbances at the Semantic Level

The pattern of the entire word may represent a less complex feature than the pattern built up as a sequence of phonemes. Such a pattern offers advantages for processing in the course of recognition. Instead of being processed as a sequence of phonemes, the word is described as a whole image that must be processed on the semantic level to be matched with its corresponding word in the stored vocabulary. This mode of processing is much faster in that the phoneme-by-phoneme stage of phonological analysis of the word is avoided, and one moves instead directly to the assessment of the entire word and, subsequently, to the stage of semantically driven comparison. This manner of processing also helps to reduce the time needed for comparison, since it does not require phonological analysis of the words held in the stored vocabulary. Use of the pattern of the entire word is especially helpful in the conventional information processing of frequently used words. The recognition of both new and low-frequency words, however, may require phonological analysis, since the general patterns of these words do not exist in the stored vocabulary.

Disturbances of recognition using the entire pattern of the word may be compared to attempts by patients with visual agnosia to differentiate between two figures through a slow process of sequential comparison of simple features, while they are not able to use general shape descriptions as contours. (For more details, see chapter 2, section entitled "Visual Object Agnosia.") These disturbances may also be compared to spelling dyslexia, a condition in which a patient is unable to read a word as a whole and tries to compensate for these disturbances by reading the word letter by letter. It remains unclear how such an assessment may be performed. In studies of object recognition, various types of features were proposed as global invariant features sufficient to describe the entire object. In recognition devices, invariant properties may be based on the measurement of area elongation, perimeter length and shape moments (Bolles & Cain, 1982), on the total number of given parts. A square, for example, has four equal straight lines, four vertices, and no free line terminator, while a triangle consists of three vertices and three lines terminated by pairs of lines at those vertices (Ullman, 1996). Similarly, the entire word may be described using some global features that are based on the use of sound frequencies, such as constant frequency, noise-burst, and frequency-modulated components representing the sonograms of animal and speech sounds. These or similar features participate in the formation of phonemes, though their use may likely bypass the phonemic level, composing a pattern for the recognition of the entire word. An example of such a bypass at the peripheral level is presented by hieroglyphic writing and reading. Another example involves disturbances in differentiating between tones in a series of pitches. (For more details, see chapter 3, section entitled "Auditory Agnosia.") While a patient with either Wernicke's aphasia or transcortical sensory aphasia may be able to differentiate between single tone pitches presented in succession at 1 sec intervals, he or she demonstrates prominent difficulties when presented with a series of tones that vary by a sequence of tone pitches, for example, 200 Hz–1000 Hz–2000 Hz versus 200 Hz–2000 Hz–1000 Hz (Meerson, 1986; Tonkonogy, 1973; Traugott & Kaidanova, 1975). Further studies are certainly needed concerning the existence and types of such global features in spoken and written language at the peripheral and phonological levels.

LOCALIZATION
OF CLINICAL
SYNDROMES IN
NEUROPSYCHOLOGY
AND NEUROSCIENCE

Disturbances of Working Memory

We observed striking disturbances in auditory working memory in patients with conduction aphasia. Repetition disturbances as noted in cases of conduction aphasia differ by some peculiar features related to prominent disturbances of verbal working memory. Repetition in patients with Broca's or Wernicke's aphasia is usually possible, though often incorrect and characterized by literal and verbal paraphasia, word omissions, phonemes, and distortions of the structures of phrases. The repetition disturbances in cases of conduction aphasia are often quite different, reflecting an inability to recall any portion of a recently heard series of syllables or of a single multisyllabic word. One of our patients who was suffering from moderate conduction aphasia was able to repeat single vowels, consonants, and well-known words consisting of one or two syllables with no difficulty. However, when the patient was asked to repeat the syllables "da-ta," or the word "industry," she responded, "flied out" or "disappeared," and was unable to recall a single phoneme from the items originally presented for repetition. In another case, a patient was occasionally able to recall the second syllable of a two syllable series, but not the first. When the patient was asked to repeat "pa-ba," for example, he responded, "a-a . . . remainder flew out." After the second presentation, the patient responded, "ba-ba-ba . . . but the first disappeared."

The retention of the word span and repetition capabilities of the patient is limited to only one or two items, so that the patient can repeat only single phonemes, syllables, and short words. Series of phonemes, syllables, and short and long phrases, however, are quite difficult to repeat, and in such attempts, the patient produces numerous instances of paraphasia, primarily literal, demonstrating a significant inclination toward augmentation. An impairment of auditory working memory for speech sounds is thus likely to be a basic disturbance underlying the formation of a typical pattern of repetition disorder as a major clinical sign of conduction aphasia. Verbal working memory is also limited in other types of aphasia, and the limits in word span retention are usually three or four items for most types of aphasia. These limits increase to five or six items in cases of articulation aphasia and transcortical aphasias.

Disturbances in Auditory Nonverbal Processing
in Cases of Posterior Aphasia

Disturbances in the formation of the general auditory and phonological pattern of a word may be partially underlain in patients with Wernicke's aphasia by more peripheral impairments in nonverbal auditory gnosis. These nonverbal impairments are related to the processing of pure tone and tone pitch sequences in the auditory working memory and were apparent in experimental comparative studies of tone pitch differentiation in groups of 13 patients with Wernicke's aphasia, 9 patients with transcortical sensory aphasia, and 19 patients with Broca's aphasia (Dorofeeva & Kaidanova, 1969; Tonkonogy, 1973; Traugott & Kaidanova, 1975). (For more details, see chapter 3, section entitled "Auditory Agnosia.") The conventional examination of absolute and differential thresholds for low tone pitches within 200–300 Hz was within normal limits in all three groups of patients.

An experimental study was directed toward the evaluation of auditory working memory in the process of the differentiation of tone pitches. In the first series, the patient was instructed to push a button in response to a basic pitch frequency of 200 Hz, and not to push the button in response to other tones, for example, 205 Hz, 210 Hz, 220 Hz, and 300 Hz. The patient was thus required to keep the basic tone of 200 Hz in his or her auditory working memory all through the testing in this series. The second series of tests was designed to study directly the role of immediate working memory, without requiring the patient to keep the basic tone pitch in his or her auditory working memory all through the testing. A pair of signals, which consisted of a basic tone of 200 Hz and either an identical tone of 200 Hz or a tone from somewhere between 205 Hz and 300 Hz, was presented with intersignal intervals of either 1 sec or 10 sec. In the third series, the role of proactive and retroactive auditory inhibition was examined via the repetition of the first testing series, and patients were required to differentiate between two unrelated tones of 100 Hz each, followed by a tone of 2000 Hz one second later. Training began with a series of 2–10 repetitions during which the subject was required to push a button when a tone of 200 Hz was presented, and not to push the button when a tone of 300 Hz was presented. The next series of training exercises required the subject to push the button when two consecutive, identical tones were presented, and not to push the button when the two successive tones were different from one another.

The results of this study indicated that patients in both the Broca's aphasia group and the transcortical sensory aphasia group were able to differentiate between pitches of 200 Hz and 300 Hz, as well as between pairs of 200 Hz–200 Hz and 200 Hz–300 Hz after two or three repetitions. Patients with Wernicke's aphasia required between 5 and 10 repetitions, and 7 of the 13 patients were unable to successfully differentiate between pitch tones in the first series of repetitions following a set of 15 repetitions.

Patients with Wernicke's aphasia demonstrated prominent disturbances in auditory working memory for tone pitches, especially when they were expected to keep the tone pitch in memory for the entire set

386

LOCALIZATION
OF CLINICAL
SYNDROMES IN
NEUROPSYCHOLOGY
AND NEUROSCIENCE

of testing, as was required in the first and third series. In the first series, the numbers of Wernicke's aphasia patients able to reach the steady state of single tone differentiation for tones of 205 Hz, 210 Hz, and 220 Hz were only one, two, and four patients, respectively. These numbers were even lower for the third series with proactive and retroactive noise, with only two patients being able to differentiate between tones of 200 Hz and 220 Hz, and no patients being able to differentiate between tones of 200 Hz and 205 Hz. Similar testing in nine patients with transcortical sensory aphasia yielded much better results. All of the patients reached regular patterns of successful differentiation for tones of 220 Hz in the first and third series, while eight patients regularly differentiated tones of 210 Hz. Only five of the patients in the first series and four of the patients in the third series reached regular patterns of differentiation for tones of 205 Hz. Successful differentiation patterns were reached by all 19 patients with Broca's aphasia both for the differentiation of tones at 220 Hz in the first and third series and between tones of 210 Hz and 220 Hz. Only 3 of the 19 patients in the first series, and 4 in the third series, were unable to reach these successful differentiations.

Immediate working memory, which was tested in the second series, was found to be disturbed primarily for the differentiation between tone pairs of 200 Hz–200 Hz and 200 Hz–205 Hz both in patients with Wernicke's aphasia and in those with transcortical sensory aphasia. Four out of 13 patients (31%) with Wernicke's aphasia, as well as 4 out of 9 patients (44%) with transcortical sensory aphasia, demonstrated patterns of correct tone differentiation. Nine of the 13 patients with Wernicke's aphasia were able to repeatedly differentiate between tones of 210 Hz and 220 Hz. All 19 of the patients with Broca's aphasia demonstrated a steady pattern of differentiation for all tested tone frequencies in the second series.

Tests of visual signals, which were similar in format to those of the first, second, and third series, such as differentiations between angles of different degrees, yielded performances at the normal level. (For more details, see chapter 2, section entitled "Visual Agnosia.")

Disturbances of auditory working memory for nonverbal stimuli are thus prominent in patients with Wernicke's aphasia, and to a lesser extent in patients with transcortical sensory aphasia. The majority of patients with Broca's aphasia, however, demonstrate a complete preservation of auditory working memory for nonverbal stimuli. For those who do have problems, these disturbances are manifested primarily as difficulties in the ability to learn and to memorize sounds and tones for a length of time, as when differentiating between tones with a boundary of a 200 Hz frequency and tones with differences of 5–20 Hz, for example, differentiating 200 Hz from 205 Hz, 210 Hz, or 220 Hz.

The boundaries of the memorized 200 Hz frequencies seem to be sufficient to allow the differentiation of 100 Hz differences between tones of 200 Hz and 300 Hz. This may be explained by differences in the reliability of auditory working memory for both narrower and wider boundaries of particular frequencies.

The relationship of disturbances in nonverbal auditory working memory and the clinical signs of transcortical sensory aphasia, especially Wernicke's aphasia, require individual and specialized studies. It is apparent, however, that prominent impairments in the processing of nonverbal auditory features may be found frequently in patients with Wernicke's aphasia, infrequently in patients with transcortical sensory aphasia, and virtually never in patients with Broca's aphasia. Inferences may be made concerning the role of such disturbances in the recognition of the general auditory pattern of an entire word and its phonological structure when a task requires the participation of working memory, as in the frequency assessment that is important for the auditory pattern of speech sounds.

This conclusion seems to contradict previously presented evidence of categorical perception both in patients with anterior aphasia and in those with posterior aphasia. Two phonetic dimensions have been examined—voicing and place of articulation in stop-consonants (Basso et al., 1977; Blumstein et al., 1977). For a review, see Blumstein (1995). Our results showed that even in aphasic patients, who were able only to discriminate between stimuli and lacked the ability to label the stimuli correctly, the discrimination functions and the locus of phonetic boundary were comparable to those of normal subjects. These results lead to the conclusion that aphasic patients with comprehension disturbances preserve the ability to extract the specific spectral patterns corresponding to the specific phonetic categories of speech.

It is possible, however, that while the extraction of a specific spectral pattern is preserved in tested patients, their labeling is disrupted because of disturbances in the auditory working memory of those patterns required for the process of stimulus labeling and typically created by the phonological system. This explanation is supported in part by our testing of the discrimination between two simple vowels, *a* and *o*, by patients with Broca's aphasia. While the patients were able to discriminate between vowels presented as *a-a* and *a-o*, prominent difficulties arose when vowels were presented with interpair intervals of 2 sec, and even more so when the intervals were increased to 15 sec. The auditory working memory for single tones was preserved in our patients, pointing to specific impairments of the verbal working memory. It may be also suggested that the categorical discrimination of specific spectral patterns may be disturbed in some patients with more severe cases of Wernicke's aphasia characterized by prominent

388

LOCALIZATION
OF CLINICAL
SYNDROMES IN
NEUROPSYCHOLOGY
AND NEUROSCIENCE

comprehension disturbances, as well as in patients with the word deaf-ness type of aphasia.

Working Memory and Disturbances in Complex Syntax Processing

Disturbances in the recognition of complex sentences may be related to impairments in some additional operations needed in the course of syntactic processing. One such operation is the use of working memory in the comprehension of sentences, since parts of sentences must be held in the memory while the person tries to integrate the different parts. In Head's hand–ear–eye test, for example, the subject is required to store words and their meanings in order to form appropriate connections in the working memory between the words *left, hand, right,* and *ear* for the planning of appropriate actions. Similarly, several words had to be stored for the operations required in Marie's three pieces of paper test, as well as for the operations needed to comprehend both passive sentences and spatial relations between objects. Our own observations (Tonkonogy, 1986) confirmed that the word span for working memory does not exceed two to three words in patients with Broca's aphasia and patients with Wernicke's aphasia. It may be suggested that impairments of working memory are primary disturbances leading to the secondary problems often noted in various types of unconventional information processing in both posterior aphasia and anterior aphasia, and especially in cases of both Broca's aphasia and Wernicke's aphasia.

An understanding of role of working memory in the complex syntax process has recently been advanced by a series of publications. Some of the authors believe that working memory is specialized for the processing of syntactically complex sentences (Caplan & Waters, 1999; Gordon, Hendrick, & Levine, 2002; Lewis, 1996), while other authors hold the opinion that the processing of complex syntax sets and the memorizing of a list of words may be related to the same area of working memory (Just & Carpenter, 1992; Just, Carpenter, & Keller, 1996). Our data point to the possibility that working memory for various examples complex syntax processing may be related to the site that is responsible for the short-term storing of the list of words, since prominent limitation of word span retention was usually observed in patients with Broca's and Wernicke's aphasia characterized by prominent impairments in complex syntax comprehension.

Disturbances of working memory may explain differences in the localization of syntactic impairments in patients with Broca's aphasia as against the localization of similar impairments in patients with Wernicke's aphasia. It is possible that the structure of working memory at the syntactic level of speech processing includes both auditory and articulatory components. The first is destroyed in patients with

Wernicke's aphasia, and the second is impaired in Broca's aphasia, and this leads to the similar clinical manifestations of complex syntax processing.

The primary disturbances of these complex unconventional operations are also important, for example, disturbances of spatial orientation in the body, as demonstrated in Head's hand–ear–eye test, in relation to other objects, and in the relationship of the space and time of two different objects, as demonstrated in tests that employ the words *beyond, above, behind, below, before,* or *after.* Primary disturbances may also be responsible for disturbances in the comprehension of passive sentences, in which the logical order of words and the grammatical structure of the sentence are reversed: for example, "The cat was hit by the dog." This may be especially important in cases with lesion extensions to the lower parietal lobules, which are known to play a role in the orientation of space and time. Such isolated cases of verbally mediated primary disturbances in the orientation of space and time have been described as semantic aphasia in patients with left parietal lobe lesions, primarily of the supramarginal gyrus (Head, 1926; Luria, 1970; Tonkonogy, 1973, 1986).

In cases of other widely accepted types of aphasia, however, the presence of comprehension disturbances in many types of complex sentences strongly points to the possibility of secondary disturbances, which are underlain by a decrease in word span retention. No primary disorder of verbally mediated orientation in space and time is noted in such cases.

ANATOMICAL ASPECTS

Anterior Aphasia: Broca's Aphasia

Large Cortico-Subcortical Lesion.   In most cases in which Broca's aphasia is caused by stroke, a large infarcted area is found in the inferior-posterior portion of the frontal lobe in the left hemisphere of right-handed subjects, primarily in the posterior F3 area, the operculum, and the insula. The lesion usually extends to the corona radiata, the internal capsule, and the striatum (Kertesz, 1979; Mazzocchi & Vignolo, 1979; Mohr et al., 1978; Tonkonogy, 1986).

A similarly localized large lesion was present in the brain of Leborgne, the first of two famous cases of aphasia reported by Broca (1861a, 1861b). Broca paid attention only to the lesion in the posterior part of the third frontal gyrus in the left hemisphere, which was later named Broca's area in his honor. The lesion, however, actually extended from the posterior F3 area, through the lower part of the central gyri, to the anterior part of the first temporal gyrus. Leborgne's brain was preserved in alcohol by Broca and, since Broca's death, has been maintained in satisfactory

390

LOCALIZATION
OF CLINICAL
SYNDROMES IN
NEUROPSYCHOLOGY
AND NEUROSCIENCE

condition at the Dupuytren Museum in Paris. Castaigne et al. (1980) and Signoret, Van Eeckhout, Poncet, and Castaigne (1987) studied the brain using CT scans and found that the lesion of the posterior F3 area, the lower parts of the central gyri, and the anterior T1 described by Broca actually extended through the insula to the lenticular nuclei and the ventricular system in the left hemisphere.

Posterior F3 Area (Brodmann's Area 44).   The large cortico-subcortical lesion may explain the development of various disturbances at the different levels of language processing—semantic, phonological, rhythmical-melodical, and articulatory. In the early studies of aphasia, on the other hand, it was believed that various types of aphasia developed because of an isolated lesion in a specific region of the cerebral cortex. Broca suggested that a lesion of the posterior F3 area, specifically the pars opercularis of the third frontal gyrus, leads to the development of aphasia by the destruction of the motor memory of speech. However, further studies showed that isolated lesions in the posterior F3 area of the dominant for speech hemisphere may cause only transient aphasia or no aphasia at all, while instances of Broca's aphasia were reported in cases in which the F3 area was spared (Marie, 1906a; Moutier, 1908; Tonkonogy & Goodglass, 1981). For a review, see Tonkonogy (1986). Persistent aphasia was not manifested in cases with bilateral lesions of the posterior F3 area (Moutier, 1908; Tonkonogy & Goodglass, 1981).

However, speech changes were noted during electrical stimulation of the left posterior F3 area (Penfield & Roberts, 1959). Also, an isolated lesion of the left posterior F3 area was often found to produce a mild, transient form of Broca's aphasia, mainly characterized by disorders of word finding and word production, with the preservation of articulation abilities, according to our data and data from the literature.

Subcortical Lesions.   Other areas within this large cortico-subcortical zone were suggested as crucial lesion sites for the development of Broca's aphasia. Special attention within these areas was given to the role of lesions in subcortical structures in the development of Broca's aphasia. Subcortical lesions were originally related to the development of subcortical motor aphasia with expressive speech disturbances, similar to cortical motor aphasia, but differing in the preservation of speech comprehension, reading, and writing, resulting from a lesion separating the cortex of the posterior F3 area from the brainstem (Wernicke, 1874).

The important role of a subcortical lesion in the development of aphasia was later stressed by Marie (1906b). Along with his colleague, Moutier (1908), Marie collected most of the cases of aphasia that had been studied anatomically and had been described in the literature at that time, including the two famous cases of Broca's aphasia, and added some of their own cases to demonstrate the role of subcortical lesions in the development of a peculiar type of aphasia syndrome. This peculiar syndrome was named anarthria by Marie and bore a clinical resemblance to the subcortical motor aphasia described by Wernicke. Marie attributed the development of anarthria to a lesion of the lenticular zone, which included, according to Marie, the caudate nucleus, the putamen, the globus pallidus, the internal and external capsule, the insula, the Rolandic operculum, and the supramarginal gyrus on the inner side of the Sylvian fissure (Figure 7.3). According to Marie, "true" aphasia includes a disorder of comprehension, which is accompanied by "anarthria" in cases of motor aphasia. This comprehension disorder may be noted only if there is an additional lesion in Wernicke's area. However, Wernicke's area was found to be spared in many cases of Broca's aphasia with disorders of speech comprehension (Tonkonogy, 1986), and no single case of pure subcortical infarction accompanied by anarthria was presented in the Marie-Moutier collection of aphasia cases, each of which was anatomically verified.

More recent studies have shown a revived interest in the role of isolated subcortical lesions in the development of aphasia. Several researchers used CT scan data to promote the new concept of putaminal aphasia. Naeser et al. (1982) described eight clinical cases of aphasia in which CT scans showed predominantly subcortical lesion sites. The authors attributed the development of an aphasia syndrome, which was similar to Broca's aphasia, to the more anterior capsular-putaminal infarction, while Wernicke's aphasia was considered to be the result of a more posterior capsular-putaminal infarction. Damasio et al. (1982) published 11 cases of various types of what the researchers considered to be atypical aphasia. CT scans of the patients showed relatively small and deep subcortical infarctions, with no sign of cortical involvement in the left hemisphere. Levin and Sweet (1983) presented a case of severe Broca's aphasia, which had developed following an infarction and was, according to the head CT data, limited to a deep lesion in the lenticular zone extending upward into the corona radiata.

Involvement of the cortical areas, however, is sometimes overlooked by CT scans, and thus cannot be ruled out in such cases. DeWitt et al. (1984) reported cases of aphasia in which MRI scans found cortical lesions, while CT scans detected only purely subcortical lesions. Both transient cortical dysfunction, since many cases of "ubcortical aphasia demonstrate a relatively good recovery of language function, and additional pathology related to cerebral subcortical infarctions may play important roles. Metter et al. (1987) reported cortical metabolic changes in addition to subcortical hypometabolism in a PET study of three patients with both a subcortical lesion and aphasia. Cortical involvement

392

LOCALIZATION
OF CLINICAL
SYNDROMES IN
NEUROPSYCHOLOGY
AND NEUROSCIENCE

may result in such cases from an ischemic penumbra spreading from subcortical infarcted areas to the cortex.

At the same time, an extension of the lesion from cortical to subcortical structures has been reported in many autopsies and CT scan studies of patients with Broca's aphasia (Kertesz, 1979; Mohr et al., 1978; Tonkonogy, 1986). The absence of such an extension is observed only infrequently, and primarily in patients with either transient or mild Broca's aphasia (Tonkonogy, 1986). In spite of the data showing lesions of the subcortical structures in patients with Broca's aphasia, however, authors continue to describe various types of aphasia as accompanying lesions of a primarily cortical nature.

The Insula (Area 13 and Area 14). Lesions of the insula have been observed in many cases of aphasia (Brown, 1979; Henschen, 1920–1922; Mohr et al., 1978; Moutier, 1908). The insula was also noted as having been destroyed in four of our own patients with severe Broca's aphasia, as verified by autopsy (Tonkonogy, 1986). Some researchers have considered the anterior insula to be either part of Broca's area or part of a wider speech area that encompasses the posterior F3 area (Dejerine, 1914; Mazzocchi & Vignolo, 1979). To the best of our knowledge, however, there is no reliable, anatomically verified case of either persistent or transient aphasia due to an isolated insula lesion. While electrical stimulation of the insula was not shown to cause speech changes or speech arrests (Penfield & Roberts, 1959), Ojeman and Whitaker (1978) reported the development of dysphasia during stimulation of the left anterior insula.

The Rolandic Operculum (Area 43). The Rolandic operculum area occupies the lower portions of the precentral and postcentral gyri and is often destroyed in patients with Broca's aphasia. Marie (1906a) included the area as an upper part of the lenticular zone (quadrilateral space) and considered a lesion here to be crucial for the development of anarthria, which Marie said corresponded to the subcortical motor aphasia of Wernicke-Lichtheim.

Lesions involving the Rolandic operculum have been described in many cases of Broca's aphasia (Hécaen & Consoli, 1973; Henschen, 1920–1922; Mohr et al., 1978; Nielsen, 1946). Trojanowski, Green, and Levine (1980) described a case of severe, lasting Broca's aphasia in which a postmortem examination showed an infarction limited to the cortex and the subcortical white matter of the precentral gyrus. Electrical stimulation of this area has been shown to induce vocalization (Penfield & Roberts, 1959). However, this area may be spared in some cases. In our own research, a lesion of this area was noted in only two of four autopsy-verified cases with severe Broca's aphasia (Tonkonogy, 1986). It

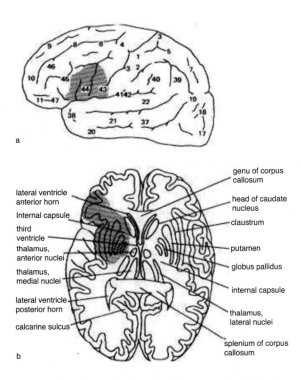

a

genu of corpus
callosum

lateral ventricle
anterior horn

head of caudate
nucleus

Internal capsule

claustrum

third
ventricle

thalamus,
anterior nuclei

putamen

thalamus,
medial nuclei

globus pallidus

internal capsule

lateral ventricle
posterior horn

thalamus,
lateral nuclei

calcarine sulcus

b

splenium of corpus
callosum

FIGURE 7.3 Broca's aphasia. Localization of the large cerebral infarctions in the cortical and subcortical structures of the left hemisphere. (a) Diagram of the cortical infarction with destruction of the posterior part of the third frontal gyrus and the lower parts of the motor and sensory strips. (b) Diagram of the horizontal section. Lesion spreads from the cortex to the striatum. The damaged areas probably mediate several levels of language processing. Limited lesions in the single areas within this large language zone seem to result in only mild and transient language disturbances. It may be suggested that language processing conducted by a damaged single speech area is probably overtaken in such cases by the spared language areas within the large anterior and posterior language zones.

seems that isolated lesions in this area may be at least to some extent responsible for the development of articulation aphasia (see below).

In summary, large lesions involving several areas of the anterior language zone are usually observed in cases of lasting Broca's aphasia. The lesions usually affect any of the following areas: the lower end of the motor and sensory strip; the Rolandic operculum and adjacent areas, including the posterior F3 area; the insula; and subcortical structures such as the putamen and the globus pallidus (Figure 7.3).

Articulation Aphasia

Several studies have emphasized the importance of specific areas in the development of articulation aphasia. Niessl Von Meyendorf (1930) stressed the importance of a lesion in the Rolandic operculum in the

394

LOCALIZATION
OF CLINICAL
SYNDROMES IN
NEUROPSYCHOLOGY
AND NEUROSCIENCE

development of an articulation disorder in his reported case of glo-bal aphasia with a large infarction in the anterior and posterior lan-guage zones in the left hemisphere. One of the areas destroyed was the Rolandic operculum; Broca's area was intact. Kleist (1934) also sug-gested a lesion in the Rolandic operculum as a factor in what he termed aphasic dysarthria. Finally, Luria (1966) suggested the role of a lesion in the lower part of the sensory strip and the adjacent area of the supra-marginal gyrus in cases of what he called afferent motor aphasia with a predominant disorder of articulation.

LeCours and L'Hermitte (1976) and Tonkonogy and Goodglass (1981) reported the localization of an isolated lesion in the Rolandic opercu-lum as verified via autopsy in cases of articulation aphasia. LeCours and L'Hermitte (1976) described a patient with a phonetic disintegra-tion syndrome who suffered from characteristic poor control of pitch in speech sounds. An anatomo-histo-pathological examination in this case revealed an infarction in the cortex that had destroyed the middle and lower parts of the left motor strip, as well as the immediate subcor-tex, including U-fibers to and from the second and third frontal gyri. The infarction extended to the insular cortex. A microscopic examina-tion verified that the posterior part of the F3 area had been spared. Tonkonogy and Goodglass (1981) reported the case of a patient whose speech was characterized by a degree of deformation of articulation and motor dysprosody. Speech sounds were distorted by the omission of some of their distinctive features, predominantly correct voicing. A postmortem examination revealed an ischemic necrotic lesion in the lower part of the left motor strip, as well as a lesion of the anterior part of the Rolandic operculum (Figure 7.4). In both cases, the speech disor-ders were transient, just as in patients with an isolated lesion of Broca's area. Articulation disturbances were primarily associated with lesions of the operculum, however, while transient word-finding difficulties were reported in cases with posterior F3 lesions.

The frequent development of prominent agraphia with relatively pre-served reading and phonological analysis in patients with articulation aphasia may be explained by an extension of the lesion from the motor

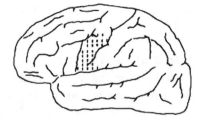

FIGURE 7.4 Articulation aphasia. An infarction in the left hemisphere involves the lower part of the motor strip and the operculum, sparing the posterior F3 area.

strip to the posterior F2 area, which represents the site previously known as Excner's writing center. LeCours and L'Hermitte (1976) noted such an extension to the subcortical white matter of the F2 area in their patient. Agraphia, as well as alexia, may result from the general disorders of phonological analysis in cases of Broca's aphasia. A lesion of the posterior F2 area certainly increases agraphia in such cases of Broca's aphasia.

Transcortical Motor Aphasia

Transcortical motor aphasia (TCMA) was originally described by Lichtheim (1885), who reported a patient with reduced expressive speech accompanied by preserved comprehension and repetition. He suggested that the syndrome resulted from an interruption of the pathway connecting the "center of motor images" and the "center of concept" caused by a lesion of white matter at the base of the third F3.

Subsequent research has shown that lesions in cases of TCMA are localized in the dominant frontal lobe, either above or anterior to the posterior F3 area. Lesions primarily involve the dorsolateral convexity in the prefrontal and premotor regions both anterior and superior to Broca's area. Luria (1966, 1970) referred to such cases as *frontal dynamic aphasia*. On the contrary, the lesions tend to spread to and involve areas beyond the frontal lobe, including the lower end of the central gyri, the insula, and subcortical structures in cases of Broca's aphasia. Most authors agree that lesions in cases of TCMA tend to spare Broca's area in the posterior F3 area. In some cases, however, a transient form of TCMA may be noted with small lesions involving Broca's area and the underlying white matter. For a review, see Rapcsak and Rubens (1994). Cases of TCMA with disturbances primarily of speech initiation have recently been reported in patients with lesions in the mesial aspects of the dorsolateral convexity involving the supplementary motor area.

Dorsolateral Frontal Region (Area 9)

Marie and Foix (1917) found lesions in cases of TCMA to be located both anterior and superior to Broca's area. Kleist (1934) reported similar findings in cases with adynamia of speech. Luria (1970) presented eight cases in which frontal dynamic aphasia developed following a head injury during World War II, and found that dynamic aphasia resulted in these cases from lesions in both the upper and middle parts of the premotor region of the left hemisphere, as well as anterior to Broca's area. Dynamic aphasia has been found to become more prominent when the lesion is located close to the pars opercularis of the posterior F3 area.

Goldstein (1948) determined two subtypes of TCMA. The first subtype was attributed to a mild partial lesion of Broca's area, which had been observed in some cases of TCMA during the process of recovery from a perisylvian lesion (Alexander, 2002; Kertesz, 1979). The second subtype was attributed to a predominantly subcortical lesion and included an area that spread from the deep white matter of the frontal operculum down to the paraventricular white matter anterior to the left frontal horn (Freedman et al., 1984).

Supplementary Motor Area and Adjacent Left Mesial and Superior Frontal Regions (Area 6)

The role of lesions in the area in the development of TCMA has been actively discussed in recent years, especially since Penfield and Rasmussen (1950) reported a supplementary motor area at the mesial surface of the hemisphere directly anterior to the lower area of the motor strip. Electrical stimulation of this area in either the right or left hemisphere produced, in addition to peculiar movements of the extremities, either speech arrest or persistent vocalization. Stimulation of the area in the left hemisphere produced an aphasic response that was often manifested as the perseveration of the word that a patient had begun to say at the moment of stimulation. An aphasic type of response was also elicited via stimulation of the classic aphasia areas, posterior F3 and posterior T1, in the left hemisphere.

These experiments increased interest in clinical studies of speech disorders in patients with lesions of the supplementary motor area. Patients were described as having lesions in the upper-posterior part of the frontal lobe in the left hemisphere, which produced marked impairment in speech initiation as well as decreased speech activity (Alexander & Schmitt, 1980; Masdeu et al., 1978; Petit-Dutaillis et al., 1954; Rubens, 1975; Tonkonogy & Ageeva, 1961). Most of the authors classified these speech disorders as a form of TCMA, called dynamic aphasia, since the morphological and syntactic structures of speech were usually preserved in such cases (Alexander, 2002; Freedman et al., 1984; Goldberg, 1985; Rapcsak & Rubens, 1994; Stuss & Benson, 1986).

Signs of decreased speech activity are often noted in patients with Broca's and global aphasia, especially in the acute stage of stroke. Nonetheless, we found the extension of a cerebral infarction to the caudal part of the first frontal gyri to exist in only 1 of 11 anatomically studied cases with global aphasia, and 2 of 4 anatomically studied cases with Broca's aphasia (Tonkonogy, 1986). In cases with TCMA, however, lesions of the posterior F1 area may be present in many cases, thus underlying the decrease of speech initiation and activity as well as the disturbances in the production of complex sentences.

In summary, both TCMA and its core syndrome, dynamic aphasia, have been described in cases with lesions of the frontal lobe structures in the middle and upper posterior parts of the frontal cortex both superior and anterior to Broca's area. Lesions often spread deep to the periventricular white matter anterior to the left frontal horn. Involvement of Broca's area was also reported in some cases of transient TCMA (Figure 7.5).

TCMA may be considered to be a type of frontal lobe aphasia, since lesions in this type of aphasia are concentrated in frontal lobe areas. In cases of Broca's aphasia, however, the frontal portion of the posterior F3 area represents only the anterior part of the lesion, which extends posterior to the Rolandic operculum, the insula, and subcortical structures (Figure 7.5). This was first understood by Luria, who described frontal dynamic aphasia in his book *Traumatic Aphasia* (1970) and used the term in subsequent publications (Luria, 1966). TCMA, or dynamic aphasia, represents an important and yet often overlooked part of frontal lobe syndrome, especially in cases with frontal abulic syndrome related to lesions in the dorsolateral and mesial parts of the frontal lobe.

Posterior Aphasia: Wernicke's Aphasia

Posterior T1 Area (Area 22). Lesions in patients with Wernicke's aphasia have traditionally been attributed to the posterior T1 area in the dominant hemisphere of the individual. Wernicke (1874) was the first to describe sensory aphasia, and did so by reporting 10 cases with lesions of the posterior T1 area in the left hemisphere. Three of the 10 cases were studied via autopsy and were found to have had an area of lesion in the left posterior T1 area. In these three cases, just as in documented cases of Broca's aphasia, the lesion was not confined to the single T1 area and extended to the adjacent part of the posterior T2 area in one case. A diffuse cerebral lesion was noted in the two

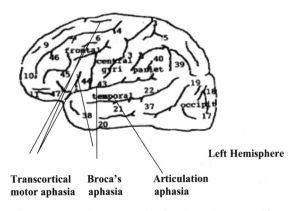

Left Hemisphere

**Transcortical   Broca's   Articulation
motor aphasia   aphasia   aphasia**

FIGURE 7.5 Primary localization of cortical lesions in various types of anterior aphasia.

398

LOCALIZATION
OF CLINICAL
SYNDROMES IN
NEUROPSYCHOLOGY
AND NEUROSCIENCE

remaining cases. Such an extension of lesion to the adjacent T2 areas, the supramarginal gyrus, and Heschl's gyri was reported in a number of subsequent publications.

Hopf (1957) presented a detailed serial anatomical and histopathological study of various types of posterior aphasia. In four cases with Wernicke's aphasia, lesions were found to extend from the posterior T1 area in the left hemisphere to the caudal part of the T2 area and Heschl's gyri. Kertesz (1983) described anatomical findings in 10 cases with severe Wernicke's aphasia—5 autopsied cases and 5 cases in which lesions were localized via isotope scans and angiography. The lesions were large, involving the posterior T1 area and extending to the temporal lobe, the supramarginal gyrus, the temporal and parietal operculi, and the underlying white matter. Temporal involvement was minimal in some cases. In our own research, an extension of the lesion from the posterior T1 area to the inferior parietal lobule was recorded via postmortem examination of two cases with severe Wernicke's aphasia (Tonkonogy, 1986). We observed only one case of Wernicke's aphasia with a small area of infarction confined to the posterior T1 area in the left hemisphere. Wernicke's aphasia was transient in that particular case and lasted several hours following a stroke. Expressive speech and comprehension improved remarkably on the second day, and a diagnosis of moderate transcortical sensory aphasia was made.

However, to the best of our knowledge, Wernicke's aphasia has not been described in cases without the accompanying presence of a lesion of the posterior T1 area, and no evidence of lasting Wernicke's aphasia has been reported in cases with lesions completely sparing Wernicke's area at the posterior T1. This may be the reason why no researchers have seriously challenged the role of the posterior T1 lesion in the development of Wernicke's aphasia, as has been done with Broca's area and Broca's aphasia.

Word Deafness

Cases of word deafness have been found to be quite rare, and no systematic studies of such cases have been conducted thus far. Most lesions in the cases that have been published are bilateral and involve Heschl's gyri, auditory radiation, and the superior-medial part of the temporal lobe (Brain, 1965; Henschen, 1920–1922; Kleist, 1934). Heschl's gyri are primary projection areas of the auditory pathway to the temporal cortex and occupy the inner surface of the temporal lobes deep in the Sylvian fissure. Though a bilateral lesion of Heschl's gyri does not produce any noticeable changes in elementary auditory function (Lemoyne & Mahoudeau, 1959; Tonkonogy, 1973), the recognition of single phonemes and syllables may be markedly disturbed. As previously mentioned, word deafness, otherwise known as *auditory-phonetic agnosia,* has often been described in such cases.

An isolated unilateral lesion of the left Heschl's gyri does not usually produce a persistent, severe syndrome of auditory-phonetic agnosia. In cases of severe Wernicke's aphasia, however, an extension of the lesion in the left hemisphere from the posterior to the middle T1 area and to Heschl's gyri often results in a striking disorder of recognition and of repetition of single phonemes and syllables. The same is true in cases with auditory-phonetic agnosia, or word deafness.

Conduction Aphasia

The localization of lesions in cases of conduction aphasia remains controversial. Wernicke (1874) first suggested that a lesion in the insula may be responsible for the development of conduction aphasia. Lichtheim supported Wernicke's suggestion by describing a case of conduction aphasia in which an autopsy allowed for the localization of the main lesion in the insula. Similar cases were described by Goldstein (1948). The absence of a lesion in the insula, however, has been described in subsequent cases of conduction aphasia (Benson et al., 1973; Liepmann & Pappenheim, 1914).

Geschwind (1965) attributed the development of conduction aphasia to a lesion of the arcuate fasciculus in the deep white matter of the inferior parietal lobule, which interrupts the auditory-motor speech pathway, leading to disturbances of repetition. The role of the arcuate fasciculus lesion was also supported by Damasio and Damasio (1983), who stressed that a lesion of the supramarginal gyrus, in which the arcuate fasciculus is compromised, leads to conduction aphasia. Other lesion sites responsible for the development of conduction aphasia include both auditory and insular cortices, as well as the underlying white matter.

The role of lesions in the auditory cortices was considered by Kleist (1934), who suggested that a lesion of the middle temporal gyrus anterior to Wernicke's area leads to the development of conduction aphasia. Hopf (1957), on the other hand, considered the role of partial damage to the caudal half of the T1 area and of Heschl's gyri.

However, as observed in other types of aphasia, the lesions underlying the development of lasting conduction aphasia have usually been found to be rather large, covering several brain areas. Green and Howes (1977) reviewed 25 cases of conduction aphasia with either postmortem examination or surgical confirmation of the localization of lesions. The lesion affected the supramarginal gyrus in 22 out of 25 cases, extended to the posterior T1 are in 13 cases, and was restricted to the superior temporal gyrus in the remaining 3 cases. Benson et al. (1973) presented three cases of conduction aphasia. Autopsy data revealed lesions in the supramarginal gyrus in Cases 1 and 3, though neither the insula nor Wernicke's area was affected. Data from Case 2, however, showed evidence of lesions in both the insula and the auditory cortex, while the supramarginal gyrus was spared. Damasio and Damasio (1980) reported five cases of conduction aphasia, which persisted in all five cases. All patients underwent head CT scans, which revealed thrombotic infarctions in four cases, and hemorrhagic infarction in one case, all were in the individual's dominant hemisphere. In four cases, lesions involved the superior temporal region, extending to the inferior parietal region. The insular region was compromised and the white matter underlying the cortical lesions was involved in all five cases. No involvement of the angular gyrus, the posterior T2 and T3 areas, or Broca's area was observed in any of the patients.

In summary, the development of conduction aphasia is usually underlined by relatively large lesions in the dominant hemisphere, involving the cortex and white matter of the anterior, and especially the middle parts of the superior temporal lobe and adjacent areas of the inferior parietal lobule in the supramarginal lobule. Lesions may compromise the insula and/or a portion of the posterior T1 area in some cases.

Transcortical Sensory Aphasia

Transcortical sensory aphasia (TCSA) was originally described by Lichtheim (1885), who reported a patient who exhibited fluent paraphasic speech and a severe disorder of comprehension, but whose condition differed from the sensory aphasia of Wernicke in that the patient's ability to repeat words and sentences preserved. Lichtheim believed that the syndrome was caused by the interruption of connections between the concept center and the intact center of auditory images, which is usually damaged in sensory aphasia, as described by Wernicke. Lichtheim suggested that the lesion responsible for the development of this syndrome involved the white matter association pathway at the base of the posterior T1 area, thus interrupting pathways to the concept center. This localization of lesion permits repetition, since language information may be forwarded from the sensory speech center in the T1 area to the motor speech center in the F3 area.

Though the clinical term transcortical sensory aphasia has been used and refined in numerous subsequent publications and clinical practice, the underlying mechanisms and localization of lesions have been questioned by many researchers. Some authors have pointed to lesions of the posterior T2 and T3 areas (Hopf, 1957), and others have suggested the middle T3 area (Kleist, 1934). Partial involvement of a lesion at the posterior T1 area has also been suggested (Bastian, 1897; Goldstein, 1948).

Special attention must be given to the role of occipito-temporal lesions in cases of TCSA. Vix (1910) found TCSA to be accompanied by a lesion involving the posterior temporal regions and the junction of the temporal and occipital lobes. Luria (1970) later observed acoustic-mnestic aphasia, a condition that is clinically similar to TCSA, in cases with lesions in the inferior-posterior portion of the left temporal lobe in the area bordering the occipital lobe. He presented a summary of lesion localization in nine cases of open head injury acquired during World War II. The lesions involved the left temporal lobe in all nine cases, and extended to the occipital lobe in five cases and to the parietal lobe in one case. Luria did not discuss the role of the occipital lesion in these cases. Damasio (1981) reported a series of patients with TCSA, in whom lesions were found to be in the posterior T2 area, with an extension to the occipital cortex in some of the patients and to either the posterior T1 area or the angular gyrus in other patients. The role of the posterior temporo-parietal lesion has been stressed by other researchers as well (Berthier, Leiguarda, Starkstein, Sevlever, & Taratuto, 1991; Kertesz, 1979). We observed a case of TCSA in which a postmortem examination showed a large infarction occupying the white matter of the posterior T1 and T2 areas and extending to the cortex of the angular gyrus (Tonkonogy, 1986, Case 15). In some cases, Wernicke's aphasia observed in the acute stage of stroke has been found to change to TCSA in the course of recovery. A patient observed by our own research team (Tonkonogy, 1986, Case 9) developed TCSA during a stage of recovery from Wernicke's aphasia. The patient died on the 42nd day after the onset of stroke, and a postmortem examination revealed a small infarction in the cortex of the left posterior T1 area bordering the angular gyrus.

Special attention must be given to the role of generalized cortical atrophy in the development of TCSA. While nontranscortical types of aphasia are usually observed in cases of circumscribed local lesions, transcortical sensory aphasia has been observed relatively frequently in patients with generalized cortical atrophy (Dejerine, 1914; Henschen, 1920–1922). TCSA was noted in patients with late onset Alzheimer's disease characterized by generalized cortical atrophy (Appel, Kertesz, & Fishman, 1982; Cummings et al., 1985; Rapcsak & Rubens, 1994). It is possible that a local accentuation of atrophy is responsible for the development of TCSA in such cases.

In summary, according to the data in the literature, lesions in cases of TCSA are usually relatively large, occupying two or more parts of the posterior language zone, and are typically centered in the posterior T2 and T3 areas, with extensions to the occipital lobe. Lesions may also involve the inferior parietal lobe, primarily the angular gyrus, and the posterior T1 area in some cases. TCSA may also be observed in cases of

402

LOCALIZATION
OF CLINICAL
SYNDROMES IN
NEUROPSYCHOLOGY
AND NEUROSCIENCE

generalized cortical atrophy, probably with local accentuation at the posterior language zone (Figure 7.6).

Global Aphasia

An extensive cerebral infarction in the left hemisphere is noted in cases of global aphasia. This infarction occupies the cortex as well as the underlying white matter around the Sylvian fissure in the left hemisphere, destroying the anterior and posterior language zone and extending from Broca's area, the Rolandic operculum, and the insula through the supramarginal gyrus and the anterior and middle parts of the first temporal gyrus to the angular gyrus. The infarction usually extends deep into the caudate nucleus, the putamen, and the internal capsule.

An involvement of Broca's and Wernicke's areas is usually noted in global aphasia, though one of these areas may be preserved in some cases. In a case of our own (Tonkonogy, 1986, Case 10), severe Wernicke's aphasia developed after a first stroke, and global aphasia developed following a subsequent stroke. The patient died from cardiac arrest 7 months after the second stroke. An autopsy revealed old cysts that had developed following infarcts in the gray and white matter of the left hemisphere. The largest cyst extended from the posterior T1 area and the angular gyrus to the supramarginal gyrus and the posterior lower third of the sensory strip. The cyst had apparently underlain the development of Wernicke's aphasia after the onset of the first stroke. Three additional smaller cysts were found in the middle part of the motor strip, in the posterior parts of the F1 and F2 areas, and in the lenticular nuclei. Broca's area at the posterior F1 was spared.

In case 17 (Tonkonogy, 1986) with global aphasia, Wernicke's area in the posterior T1 was preserved, while an infarction destroyed Broca's

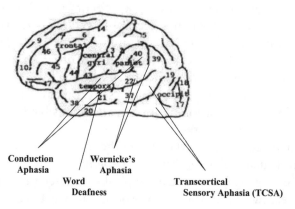

FIGURE 7.6   Main localizations of lesions in the left hemisphere in various forms of posterior aphasia.

area, the Rolandic operculum, the insula, the posterior F1 area, the inferior parietal lobule, and the anterior T1 area. The preserved areas of the posterior language zone included, in addition to the posterior T1 area, the middle portion of the T1 area and Heschl's gyri, in spite of a severe disorder of speech and gesture comprehension in this case. No lesion of subcortical structures was found in a performed autopsy. The role of edema involving these preserved areas may be ruled out, since the patient died 18 months after the stroke led to the development of global aphasia.

Mixed Transcortical Aphasia

The localization of lesions in cases of mixed transcortical aphasia (MTCA) remains unclear. This type of mixed aphasia has been described mainly in patients either with multifocal and diffuse brain pathology accompanied by degenerative dementia (Appel et al., 1982; Mehler, 1988; Whitaker, 1976) or with hypoxic encephalopathy in carbon monoxide poisoning. Rapcsak and Rubens (1994) found that pathology in these cases primarily affects the parietal and frontal association area, but spares the perisylvian language zone, which may explain the preservation of repetition in such cases.

MTCA is relatively rare and is usually experienced as a stage of recovery from global aphasia following a stroke (Rapscak, Krupp, Rubens, & Reim, 1990; Tonkonogy, 1986). MTCA has usually been described in cases with a left interior carotid occlusion leading to infarctions in the upper posterior part of the frontal lobe and in the watershed areas between the anterior, middle, and posterior cerebral arteries. Bogousslavsky, Regli, and Assal (1988a) presented a case of acute MTCA with an occlusion of the left internal carotid artery, which led to the simultaneous development of two infarctions, in the anterior precentral-central sulcus and in the posterior watershed area. Ross (1980) described the development of MTCA in a patient with an extensive mesial frontoparietal infarction. Previous studies have shown infarctions in the anterior area to be located superior to Broca's area, while infarctions in the posterior area are found above and posterior to Wernicke's area. Since the anterior localization of lesions is typical for cases of TCMA, and the posterior site is usually seen in cases of TCSA, it may be suggested that the development of mixed transcortical aphasia in these cases results from a combination of TCMA and TCSA.

The perisylvian region is usually spared in such cases, though the perisylvian language zone may be severely damaged by infarctions in cases of MTCA (Berthier et al., 1991; Stengel, 1947). It is thus possible that the preserved right hemisphere mediates repetition, at least in some patients (Rapscak & Rubens, 1994).

404

LOCALIZATION
OF CLINICAL
SYNDROMES IN
NEUROPSYCHOLOGY
AND NEUROSCIENCE

Cerebral Dominance and Localization in Aphasia

Various aphasia syndromes result from a lesion of the left hemisphere in all right-handed persons (Boller, 1973; Boller, Kim, & Mack, 1977), which points to the dominance of the left hemisphere for language and movement in right-handed individuals (Sperry, 1981). In left-handed people, cerebral dominance for language and movements is often located in the right hemisphere, so that lesions of the right hemisphere lead to the development of an aphasia syndrome. Lesions of the left hemisphere however, result in aphasia in more than 50% of left-handed persons with aphasia (Albert & Obler, 1978; Goodglass & Quadfasel, 1954; Hécaen & Albert, 1978; Luria, 1966). On the other hand, aphasia due to a unilateral lesion of the right hemisphere is rarely noted in right-handed patients.

These discrepancies are usually explained by a frequent dissociation of movement and language dominance in more than 50% of left-handed persons, as well as possible language ambidexterity in some left-handers. This language ambidexterity may underlie the more frequent development of a milder, transient aphasia in left-handed persons than in right-handed persons.

Conclusion

Language disturbances in Broca's and Wernicke's aphasia are manifested as an extensive involvement of the multiple levels of speech production and comprehension at the central and peripheral levels. Central level disturbances include the production and comprehension of words and sentences at the semantic, syntactic, and phonological levels. Impairments at the peripheral levels involve articulation disturbances and motor dysprosody, as well as buccofacial apraxia at the motor output level in Broca's aphasia. Auditory phonetic and verbal comprehension disturbances and auditory agnosia for nonlanguage sounds at the auditory input level are noted in cases of Wernicke's aphasia. Speech activation is decreased in cases of Broca's aphasia and increased in cases of Wernicke's aphasia. Disturbances in speech comprehension are prominent in cases of Wernicke's aphasia, as well as in mild cases of Broca's aphasia, primarily on the level of complex syntax processing. Disturbances in repetition, reading, and writing are similar, though prominent impairments in cases of Broca's aphasia tend to affect writing capabilities.

The role of more peripheral disturbances in the production of articulation, and especially of articulation sequences, in cases of Broca's aphasia are reflected in the localization of lesions in the areas in and around the lower ends of the central gyri and the Rolandic operculum. These areas are related to the central control of the oral and larynx movements involved in articulation production. The areas damaged in cases of Broca's aphasia include the posterior F3 area, the insula, and the Rolandic operculum in the left hemisphere, which is the hemisphere dominant for speech. An extension of lesion to the striatum, as seen in many cases of lasting Broca's aphasia, probably partially mediates the development of motor dysprosody. In addition to lesions in cortical areas, lesions in the subcortical region may mediate the decrease in speech production activity. It seems that central level word-finding and sentence production disturbances are also underlain by a lesion around the Rolandic operculum, probably in Broca's area.

In cases of Wernicke's aphasia, a prominent auditory component in speech comprehension disturbances is underlain by left hemisphere lesions in or around Heschl's gyri, with involvement of the posterior T1 and surrounding areas of the lower parietal lobules. This lesion must be responsible for word-finding disturbances, which are manifested in expressive speech, primarily by the loss of noun production, accompanied by a marked increase in speech activity. The similarity of phonological and syntax disturbances in Broca's and Wernicke's aphasia has generated significant controversy in modern neurolinguistic literature. Similarities in complex syntax processing, however, may be explained as a result of secondary disturbances caused by working memory impairments related to auditory processing in Wernicke's aphasia, and to articulatory problems in Broca's aphasia. The nature of phonological disturbances in cases of Broca's aphasia may also be different, and may perhaps be based on the translation of modality-independent descriptions of words phoneme by phoneme into their articulatory counterparts. In Wernicke's aphasia, the disturbances involve the opposite method of translation, from the acoustical pattern of a word to its phonological modality-independent representation.

Disturbances may be limited to the one or two levels of speech production and comprehension in other types of aphasia. Impairments are limited to the peripheral levels of articulation in cases of articulation aphasia, and to auditory phonetic comprehension in cases of word deafness, or acoustic-sensory aphasia. Lesions in cases of articulatory aphasia lesion are primarily localized in the Rolandic operculum, the center of a region that is damaged in cases of Broca's aphasia. Word deafness is caused by bilateral lesions of Heschl's gyri in the region, which is damaged in the left hemisphere in patients with Wernicke's aphasia. More extended lesions in these areas would result in Broca's and Wernicke's aphasia, respectively.

Disturbances of repetition with prominent literal paraphasia represent the primary feature of conduction aphasia, the development of which is usually underlain by disturbances of auditory working memory for speech sounds. Lesions in such cases are localized in the central

406

LOCALIZATION
OF CLINICAL
SYNDROMES IN
NEUROPSYCHOLOGY
AND NEUROSCIENCE

portion of the T1 area, often extending to the supramarginal gyrus. A role in auditory verbal working memory may thus be suggested for this area.

Semantic and syntactic levels may be impaired in cases of transcortical aphasia, while phonological and peripheral levels are preserved. Speech production is disturbed mainly at the semantic and syntactic levels in cases of transcortical motor aphasia (TCMA), combined with a general decrease in speech activation. The lesions involve primarily the posterior F1 and F2 areas, as well as the area anterior to the posterior F3 region in the left hemisphere. This may point to the role of these areas in speech production at the semantic and syntactic levels, as well as in speech initiation and speech activity.

Speech comprehension is impaired at the semantic and syntactic levels in combination with prominent anomia in cases of transcortical sensory aphasia (TCSA). The localization of lesions seems to be primarily at the temporo-occipital-parietal junction beyond Wernicke's area at the posterior T1 area in the left hemisphere. Prominent anomia points to the role of optic aphasia in such cases, with an extension of lesions to the occipital convex.

The localization of lesion in cases of mixed transcortical aphasia (MTCA) usually reflects the involvement of the anterior posterior-superior frontal areas, which are damaged in cases of TCMA, as well as the posterior temporo-parietal area on the border of the occipital lobe, which is damaged in cases of TCSA. Lesions in some cases of TMCA may extend to the perisylvian areas, including the posterior T1 or Wernicke's areas, without the onset of the symptoms of phonological and auditory disturbances that are typical for Wernicke's aphasia. A preserved right hemisphere is considered to be responsible for this preservation in such cases, though another explanation may also be valid.

ALEXIA AND AGRAPHIA

DISTURBANCES OF READING and writing are commonly known as *alexia* and *agraphia,* respectively. Such conditions are usually observed in patients with central types of aphasia resulting from disturbances at the phonological and semantic levels of verbal information processing. Yet they may also be manifested as disturbances of either reading or writing independent from aphasia. As impairments of verbal information processing, however, the particular types of alexia and agraphia are similar to the types of aphasia in the manifestations of disturbances at either the peripheral or the central levels of verbal information processing.

Alexia and agraphia were originally described in cases with relatively severe disturbances of reading or writing of conventional, well-learned words. Special attention was subsequently given to impairments in the reading or writing of unconventional words at the phonological and lexico-semantic levels, including nonwords in *deep dyslexia* or agraphia, and irregular, exceptional words in *surface dyslexia* or agraphia.

ALEXIA

Clinical Aspects
Peripheral Alexia
Pure Alexia, or Pure Word Blindness. The main symptoms in cases of pure alexia, or *pure word blindness,* include disturbances in the recognition of single letters, and to a lesser extent words, while both spontaneous writing and writing in response to dictation are preserved. The condition resembles word-deafness, also known as phonetic-sensory aphasia, in its primary impairments of peripheral mechanisms of reading single letters based on visual gnosis, which are similar to the disturbances of peripheral mechanisms of auditory gnosis of speech sounds in cases of word-deafness.

Patients suffering from literal alexia frequently confuse letters that are similar in their visual shapes, such as "O" and either "D" or "C," or "P" and either "R" or "B." They have difficulties in matching identical letters that are written in different types of print or in both upper case and lower case. Errors are noted in the naming of letters, a condition known as amnestic alexia. A patient may even recognize, for example, that the letter "A" is placed at the beginning of the alphabet, but is unable to name the letter. In some cases, a patient's ability to read print is better than the ability to read his or her own handwriting.

The reading of words is also disturbed in these cases, especially for multisyllabic and low-frequency words. A patient may be able to read the individual letters that compose the word, but the reading is characterized by delays during transitions from one letter to another, and is performed in a very slow manner, with the patient making frequent omissions and substitutions of letters (also known as spelling dyslexia).

The copying of letters and words becomes disturbed not only for the transcoding of print to handwriting but also for the drawing and, in effect, copying of letters or words. At the same time, processing at the phonological and lexical-semantic levels remains intact, and a patient with literal alexia is able to write in response to dictation and to engage in spontaneous writing. The patient remains, however, unable to read his or her own writing.

Peripheral alexia is often accompanied by disturbances in the reading of musical notes, while the reading of numbers usually remains

408

LOCALIZATION
OF CLINICAL
SYNDROMES IN
NEUROPSYCHOLOGY
AND NEUROSCIENCE

preserved. A reverse pattern may be seen in some cases in which prominent alexia for numbers is accompanied by relatively mild literal alexia.

Peripheral alexia is quite often accompanied by color agnosia. Visual object agnosia is seen less frequently, pointing to the relative independence of literal alexia as a visual gnostic disturbance. Right-sided homonymous hemianopsia is often observed in patients with peripheral alexia.

Attentional Alexia

Attentional alexia is characterized by disturbances of reading when more than one letter or word is in view (Shallice & Warrington, 1977). This type of peripheral dyslexia may be related to impairments in the filtration of a signal from background noise in the course of reading (see chapter 2, section entitled "Visual Object Agnosia").

Attentional alexia may also be manifested as spatial alexia, which is characterized by difficulties in the ability to keep one's gaze on a line, to transfer one's gaze from one line to another, or to find a particular line or word. The patient may try to compensate for these difficulties by using his or her index finger in an attempt to fixate oneself on the line, especially when moving from one line to the next. Though these difficulties are reminiscent of optic ataxia in cases of Balint's syndrome, optic ataxia in attentional alexia is relatively independent from other disturbances of gaze fixation and may be primarily limited to reading tasks (Tonkonogy, 1973).

Neglect dyslexia is another type of attentional dyslexia and is characterized by visual errors made at either the beginnings or ends of words. The most frequent type of error is failure to read the side of the area contralateral to the damaged hemisphere. For a review, see McCarthy and Warrington (1990), and Black and Behrmann (1994). In cases of right hemispheric lesions, errors may be made in reading the beginnings of words, or words found on the left side of an open book. Neglect alexia may be observed in individuals with a seemingly intact visual field and with no signs of either hemianopia or hemispatial neglect (Patterson & Wilson, 1990; Riddoch, Humphreys, Cleton, & Fery, 1990).

Disturbances of Conventional Information Processing: Central Alexia

Agraphic Alexia. In the older literature, disorders of reading were observed in combination with disturbances of writing or agraphia, and were known as cases of *agraphic alexia*. A patient with central alexia is impaired primarily in the reading of both well-learned, conventional words and less frequently used words. The reading of individual letters is significantly less disturbed in these cases than in those of peripheral alexia. Verbal and literal paralexia are frequent, and there are seemingly no attempts by patients to compensate for disturbances of word reading with letter-by-letter reading.

Classic descriptions note that one of the major differences that distinguishes central alexia from peripheral alexia is disturbances of writing, in which patients with central alexia are unable to write letters or words. Attempts to write letters involve the drawing of straight and curved lines, with only some elements of the desired letter. In more severe cases, writing abilities are destroyed, and patients are able to draw only several simple lines. Writing in response to dictation is preserved for well-learned and simple words in less severe cases, but disturbances reappear when patients correctly writes one or two letters from other words.

Copying abilities in cases of agraphic alexia are impaired to a lesser degree than are the abilities to write spontaneously or in response to dictation. An opposite pattern is typical for cases of peripheral alexia. Patients with agraphic alexia are often able to transcode printed letters into handwriting.

Agraphic alexia is often accompanied by anomia, acalculia, various types of apraxia, and space disorientation. Right-sided hemianopia is frequently present as well.

Disturbances of Unconventional Information Processing

Surface and Deep Dyslexia. Surface dyslexia and deep dyslexia, which are subtypes of central alexia, have been described relatively recently. Alexia for the reading of conventional, well-learned words is relatively mild. Impairments mainly involve unconventional types of reading materials, including nonwords, in cases of deep dyslexia, and involve the reading of irregular words in cases of surface dyslexia. Marshall and Newcombe (1966, 1973) were probably the first to study patients with these two somewhat contrasting types of reading disorders.

Disturbances at the Phonological Level: Deep Dyslexia. Deep dyslexia is characterized by disturbances in the translation of the orthography of an entire word, or its decomposition from sequences of orthographic segments to articulation sequences. The primary manifestation of deep dyslexia is *phonological dyslexia* (Beauvois & Dérouesné, 1979), which is also described as an impairment in print-to-sound correspondence. For a review, see McCarthy and Warrington (1990).

Marshall and Newcombe (1973) described patient G.B., who suffered from deep dyslexia accompanied by both semantic paralexia and phonological dyslexia, which is a selective difficulty in the ability to read a meaningless series of letters, for example, nonwords. Shallice and Warrington (1980) noted evidence of phonological dyslexia in C.R.N., one of their patients. Though the patient was significantly impaired in the ability to read nonsense words, C.R.N. was able to read many real words, most likely by comprehending the word meanings through the semantic channel. Another patient, known as W.B., demonstrated a complete inability to read nonwords but was able to read correctly almost 90% of single, real words (Funnel, 1983).

Some of the authors suggest that, in addition to phonological dyslexia, a deficit in the semantic route is also present in deep dyslexia, leading to the semantic errors often observed in cases of deep dyslexia. These deficits were noted in patient G.B. as described by Marshall and Newcombe (1973). Semantic errors are absent in cases of pure phonological dyslexia. For a review, see Denes, Cipolotti, and Zorgi (1999). The patient suffering from deep dyslexia may demonstrate particular difficulties in attempts to read functional words, such as *if, and, for, to,* and *by,* and may exhibit a more efficient reading of nouns than verbs and function words, as well as a more efficient reading of concrete words than abstract words.

Deep dyslexia is frequently associated with severe cases of Broca's aphasia (Kertesz, 1982), pointing to the possibility that deep dyslexia, similar to Broca's aphasia, is a multicomponent syndrome involving a deficit in both the phonological route and the lexical-semantic route (Newcombe & Marshall, 1980; Shallice & Warrington, 1980).

Disturbances at the Semantic Level: Surface Dyslexia. Surface dyslexia is characterized by a loss in the ability to utilize semantically mediated reading of words, as well as in the ability to read an entire word, from the direct translation to the articulation sequences. At the same time, the phonologically based translation of the orthographic description of a word to its pronunciation remains preserved in such cases (Caplan, 1996). Reading in patients with surface dyslexia remains unimpeded for individual letters, regular words, and nonwords. The patient often tries to compensate for his or her difficulties in reading by utilizing this phonologically based reading. This type of reading includes the set of common pronunciation rules of language, which may be used as a substitute for the disrupted semantic route. When given a word that does not correspond to the common pronunciation rule, such as a so-called irregular word, a patient with surface dyslexia will try to read the word according to the common rules, making errors in reading due to so-called regularization. For a review, see McCarthy and Warrington (1990). Marshall and Newcombe (1973) described two patients, J.C. and S.T., who made such errors. Warrington (1975) studied two patients who exhibited difficulties in reading such irregular words as *nephew,* but who were better able to read regular words such as *classification.* The examples of irregular words provided by McCarthy and Warrington (1990) include *yacht, busy, debt, sew, ache,* and *quay;* regular words included *boat, time, cash, hike,* and *tree.* Researchers have stressed that reading according to rules may be applied to words that are meaningless and perhaps unusual for the reader but are nonetheless classified as regular words. Such words may include *shibboleth, chitterling,* and *herpetology.* A patient suffering from surface dyslexia may also be able to read nonwords without difficulty, whereas a patient suffering from deep dyslexia would be unable to do so. In some cases of surface dyslexia, disturbances in the reading of irregular words may be especially prominent, involving common irregular words. McCarthy and Warrington (1990) reported patient K.T., who read and pronounced *have* and *love* as "hayve" and "lowve," respectively. Surface dyslexia is frequently associated with both Wernicke's aphasia and agraphia.

In spite of preserved abilities in reading regular words and nonwords, the comprehension of read and spoken words may be prominently impaired in patients with surface dyslexia, pointing to a lesion involving the semantic system. Patterson and Hodges (1992) stressed a frequent association of surface dyslexia in patients with semantic dementia and impaired reading comprehension. However, abilities in reading regular words, nonwords, and irregular words were noted to be intact and unperturbed in some cases of semantic dementia with disturbances of the comprehension of written and spoken words (Cipolotti & Warrington, 1995; Schwartz, Saffran, & Marin, 1980).

Surface dyslexia may be detected relatively easily in patients speaking languages that have many examples of irregularities in correspondence between spelling and sound, for example, English or French. It may be more difficult to detect in patients using languages with shallow orthographies and with spelling-to-sound conversion rules that may be applied to almost all words, for example, Russian or Italian. Some of the irregularities in such languages may be found in the suprasegmental level, as in stress assignment (Miceli & Caramazza, 1993).

In our opinion, it is possible that the primary symptom of surface dyslexia in such languages is a disturbance in accessing the meaning of the words that a patient can read, either aloud or silently, a disturbance known as word meaning blindness, or alienation of read word meaning. Disturbances in the reading of irregular words may thus be the additional symptom related to the mechanism of compensation for impairments in the semantic routes of reading that is primarily observed in non-shallow languages such as English. Surface dyslexia may be compared in such cases with the alienation of spoken word meaning in cases of transcortical sensory aphasia, while deep dyslexia resembles the phonologically based repetition disturbances experienced in cases of Broca's and Wernicke's aphasia. Some types of peripheral alexia, such as pure word blindness, may be compared with repetition

412

LOCALIZATION
OF CLINICAL
SYNDROMES IN
NEUROPSYCHOLOGY
AND NEUROSCIENCE

disturbances in cases of pure word deafness. Further studies of both deep and surface dyslexia are certainly needed, especially in patients who speak shallow languages.

Ideographic Alexia

Alexia in Japanese patients represents a special interest, since the Japanese learn to read and write in a phonetic alphabet, known as the *Kana,* and to create ideographic signs, known as *Kajii.* A low number of reported cases of alexia in Japanese patients points to the development of pure alexia for Kana and Kajii in cases with left occipital infarctions (Kurachi, Yamaguchi, Inasaka, & Torii, 1979). In cases of alexia for phonetic Kana reading accompanied by a relative preservation for ideographic Kajii reading, the localization of lesions was reported to be more anterior (Soma, Sugishita, Kitamura, Maruyama, & Imanaga, 1989; Varney, 1984). Based on an analysis of the literature, other authors have come to the same conclusion (Benson, 1979; Greenblatt, 1983). It has been suggested that ideographic Kajii reading is processed by the direct lexical route, while phonetic Kana reading is processed by both lexical and nonlexical phonological letter-to-sound reading (Black & Behrmann, 1994). The role of the right hemisphere in lexical Kanjii reading has also been discussed. Selective Kanjii alexia has not been reported in cases with right hemisphere lesions.

Anatomical Aspects

Peripheral Alexia

Pure Word Blindness. Déjerine (1914) described a patient who suffered from a stroke, which resulted in the development of pure word blindness, with no apparent evidence of either agraphia or aphasia. The patient was able to read only his own signature and single numbers. A right homonimous hemianopia was noted. Four years later, the patient had another stroke, which was accompanied by an additional development of agraphia and aphasia. An autopsy revealed two lesions—an earlier lesion and a later lesion. The earlier lesion was found to be localized in the left occipital lobe and occupied the base of the lingual gyrus, as well as the calcarine gyrus, with an extension to both the fusiform gyrus and the splenium of the corpus callosum. The second and later lesion was localized in the angular gyrus, as well as adjacent areas of the parietal and temporal lobes of the left hemisphere.

Subsequent publications generally confirmed the localization of lesions in cases of alexia without agraphia, as was reported by Déjerine (1914). These cases were summarized by Benson and Geschwind (1969), who reviewed 17 well-studied clinico-anatomical cases of pure word blindness, which were reported in the literature from the end of the 19th century through 1966. Greenblatt (1983) added 10 cases, which had been published from 1967 to 1981. According to Greenblatt, the lesions in most of these 27 cases were almost identical with the lesion noted in the case described by Déjerine (1914) and included the lingual and the fusiform gyri, the calcarine cortex, the occipital white matter, and the splenium of the corpus callosum. Lesions in the hippocampus, the parahippocampal gyrus, and the posterior thalamus were observed in some of the cases, but the author stressed that those lesions were generally not associated with the development of alexia.

Cloning, Cloning, and Hoff (1968) described 27 patients with pure alexia who had been selected from a consecutive series of 708 patients with cerebral lesions of varying etiology, including stroke, tumor, trauma, and abscess. Lesions of the occipital lobe were found in 24 of the 27 cases with pure alexia, including 17 cases with lesions involving the occipito-temporal region, and 7 cases with an extension from the occipital lobe to the parietal lobe. The lesions were located in the left hemisphere in 25 patients, including 6 patients with bilateral left-right hemispheric lesions. Two of the 25 patients were left-handed. Unilateral right hemisphere lesions were noted in 2 cases, one of whom was a left-handed patient. Many subjects with pure alexia also suffered from color agnosia.

Damasio and Damasio (1983) studied 16 patients who suffered from alexia not accompanied by agraphia using both standardized reading tests and other neuropsychological tests. The authors compared the results of the tests with findings from head CT scans. They found that the lesions involved the inferior and superior medial occipital cortex but concluded that paraventricular white matter damage in these areas had caused a disconnection for signals moving from the occipital association areas in the left and right hemispheres to the left temporo-parietal language area, which had been critical for the development of pure alexia. An extension of the lesion to the association occipital cortex and the splenium of the corpus callosum was sometimes present but was not essential for the onset of the disorder. For a review, see Black and Berman (1994).

Some of the data point to the role of a callosal lesion in the development of pure alexia. It was suggested that destruction of the splenium leads to the disruption of the flow of visual lexic information from the calcarine cortex in the right hemisphere to the left hemisphere, resulting in alexia (see Greenblatt, 1983, for a review). The role of callosal lesions is especially important for the development of *hemialexia* in the left visual field. Hemialexia has been described in cases of surgical callosal sections for the approach to a colloid cyst and tumor (Trescher & Ford, 1937) or for the treatment of seizures (Gazzaniga, Bogen, & Sperry, 1962). The lesion may be limited to the splenium of the corpus callosum in such cases (Gazzaniga & Freedman, 1973), and hemialexia is completely absent when the splenium is either not involved or only partially cut (Greenblatt, 1983; Greenblatt, Saunders, Culver, & Bogdanowicz, 1980).

Attentional Alexia. Shallice and Warrington (1977) reported two cases of attentional alexia, both of which were associated with tumors found in the white matter of the left parietal lobe. A parietal localization of lesion seems to be the common lesion site in cases of neglect alexia. Behrmann, Moscovitch, Black, and Mozer (1990) reported several cases of neglect alexia with lesions extending from the parietal cortex to the basal ganglia and the centrum semiovale.

Central Alexia

Alexia With Agraphia. The localization of lesions was relatively well studied in agraphic alexia, and probably represents various combinations of deep and surface alexias. Déjerine (1914) was the first to describe the postmortem data of a patient with agraphic alexia, which revealed an infarction in the left angular gyrus with an extension to the occipital horns. In a second case, Déjerine (1892) reported the development of agraphic alexia related to an infarction in the left angular gyrus and adjacent temporal and parietal areas. This and similar cases led to the conclusion that alexia with agraphia results from a lesion in the left angular gyrus, and may also be called angular alexia. Another conclusion is that pure alexia develops following an occipital lesion, which is reflected in the term occipital alexia.

Based on three of our own cases and 17 other cases from the literature, Nielsen (1939) stressed the role of a lesion of the angular gyrus in the development of alexia with agraphia. Nielsen also noted, however, that comprehension of the visual word extends from Wernicke's area to the angular gyrus. Many authors later stressed the involvement of the angular gyrus in cases of alexia with agraphia (Albert, 1979; Benson & Geschwind, 1969; Kertesz, 1979). For a review, see Greenblatt (1983).

Surface Dyslexia. For a review, see Black and Behrmann (1994). Based on a study of six patients with surface dyslexia, Roeltgen (1983) found that a common area of lesions was the posterior T1 area. Patterson, Marshall, and Coltheart (1985) studied the localization of lesions in cases of surface dyslexia via the slice-by-slice anatomical description of several well-documented cases. The authors concluded that the common area involved in these cases was the posterior superior T1 area, as well as the T2 area, with underlying white matter.

Deep Dyslexia. Large lesions involving the perisylvian language region are usually reported in cases of deep dyslexia. For a review, see

Black and Behrmann (1994). Such extended lesions were revealed by CT scans in five patients with deep dyslexia (Marin, 1980). The lesions in these cases involved the inferior frontal, inferior parietal, and superior temporal regions, as well as subcortical white matter and the basal ganglia. Deep dyslexia, however, was often described in patients with Broca's aphasia without any lesion extension to the posterior temporo-parietal region (Kertesz, 1982), while surface dyslexia was observed in patients with Wernicke's aphasia, or other types of posterior aphasia, with a primary localization of lesions in the posterior T1 area. Further studies of deep and surface dyslexia in various forms of aphasia may well help to highlight the localization of lesions in these types of alexia. Agraphic alexia characterized by the typical involvement of the left angular gyrus also deserves consideration in its relation to the popular concept of surface and deep dyslexia.

Another topic of interest is the role of residual reading capacity in patients with deep dyslexia, which may be based on the preserved visual language ability in the right hemisphere. This hypothesis continues to be a topic of debate and requires further study.

Agraphia

Clinical Aspects
Peripheral Agraphia

Apraxic Agraphia. The patient with *apraxic agraphia* is often unable to hold a pen or pencil in the correct position while writing. When he or she is in fact able to do so, the writing of isolated letters is disturbed by a deformation of the general pattern of the letter and its elements, which is accompanied by a loss of some of the elements, a distortion of the spatial relationships between those elements, or mirror writing of letters. In more severe cases, a patient is able to draw only some short lines and arcs that cross each other and only vaguely resemble the patterns of the particular graphemes.

Disturbances involve writing in response to dictation, spontaneous writing, and copying. It is impossible for a patient to switch tasks during the course of copying a print into handwriting, even if only to produce a slavish drawing. Apraxic agraphia may be observed in both hands or may be limited to the right hand.

Apraxic agraphia may appear as a relatively isolated type of apraxia, with no signs of aphasia. The condition may be observed in association with ideomotor apraxia (Hécaen & Albert, 1978).

Spatial Agraphia. The spatial organization of writing is distorted in patients suffering from *spatial agraphia* (Hécaen, 1972). Such patients are able to create graphemes well, but the line of their writing is either

416

LOCALIZATION
OF CLINICAL
SYNDROMES IN
NEUROPSYCHOLOGY
AND NEUROSCIENCE

not horizontal, with a tendency to undulate, or appears in a stepwise manner, with the left side of the paper often being neglected, so that the writing occupies the right side of the page. Other signs of spatial alexia include large gaps between the letters of a word, and a tendency to produce extra strokes in such letters as *m, n,* and *u.* Spatial agraphia is frequently associated with both spatial alexia and spatial acalculia.

Disturbances of Conventional Information Processing: Central Agraphia

Spelling Agraphia. This type of central agraphia has been described as pure agraphia, isolated agraphia, and more recently as a disorder of spelling assembly (McCarthy & Warrington, 1990). Patients suffering from *spelling agraphia* experience disturbances of writing in response to dictation and in the spontaneous writing of well-learned, conventional words, while copying capabilities remain relatively preserved. Spelling agraphia is manifested as a difficulty in the ability to retain the correct order of letters in words, characterized by frequent substitution errors (literal paragraphia) and by the omission of letters. A typical reported disturbance involves a failure to find the grapheme that correctly corresponds to a particular phoneme, a condition also known as amnestic agraphia. When asked to write a certain letter of the alphabet in response to dictation, the patient sometimes tries to find the correct grapheme, but may eventually write another, incorrect grapheme. Disturbances are especially prominent in the writing of words and sentences, manifesting as literal paragraphia, with both letters and words being substituted. Some grammatical difficulties may be observed, including the misspelling of word endings and an absence of punctuation. Similar difficulties may also be seen in the composition of words from letters printed on individual cards. At the same time, copying is much easier and errors relatively rare in patients with spelling agraphia.

Disturbances in the spelling of written words may be observed in some cases with preserved oral spelling (Kinsbourne & Rosenfeld, 1974). A converse dissociation was described in a patient who was able to write without spelling difficulties but made numerous errors when spelling words orally (Kinsbourne & Warrington, 1965).

Spelling agraphia is often accompanied by finger agnosia, acalculia, and disturbances of left-right orientation, and constitutes one of the primary components of Gerstmann's syndrome.

Disturbances of Unconventional Information Processing

As with patients suffering from surface and deep dyslexia, patients with relatively preserved writing of conventional words may demonstrate the two major types of impairments involving the writing of unconventional words—nonwords in cases of *deep agraphia,* and exceptional words in cases of *surface agraphia.*

Phonological Agraphia and Deep Agraphia

In *phonological agraphia,* disturbances of spelling are relatively selective, primarily involving nonwords. The spelling of most real words may remain preserved in such cases. Disturbances in the spelling of nonwords are also more prominent in spelling dyslexia, but the discrepancy between the preserved writing of regular words and impairments in the writing of nonwords is remarkably more pronounced in phonological alexia. Phonological agraphia was first described by Shallice (1981) in patient P.R., who experienced disproportionate disturbances in the writing both of nonwords and of isolated graphemes corresponding to particular sounds, while the writing both of real, familiar words and of irregular words was preserved at an above-average level. A number of similar cases was subsequently reported (Baxter & Warrington, 1985; Nolan & Caramazza, 1982; Roeltgen, Sevuch, & Heilman, 1983). Agraphia was more prominent and included semantic errors in some cases that were similar to deep alexia (Assal, Buttet, & Jolivet, 1981; Bub & Kertesz, 1982; Kremin, 1987). The term *deep agraphia* was suggested for such cases.

Disturbances at the Semantic Level: Surface or Lexical Agraphia

As with surface alexia, disturbances of writing through the lexico-semantic channel in cases of surface agraphia, also known as lexical agraphia, are compensated for via phonological phoneme-grapheme conversion, which leads to the regularization of exception words. Beauvois and Dérouesné (1979) described evidence of lexical agraphia, or orthographic agraphia, in a French-speaking patient, who erroneously wrote the French word *monsieur* as *messieu.* Similarly, the word *answer* may be written as *anser* by a lexical agraphia patient. A list of similar regularization errors described by McCarthy and Warrington (1990) includes the word *mighty* written as *mite, build* as *bild, door* as *dor,* etc. Special difficulties may also be observed in the spelling of words with a high level of orthographic ambiguity, such as *team.*

Anatomical Aspects

Apraxic Agraphia. Exner (1881) suggested the existence of an isolated writing center at the foot of the second frontal gyrus in the left hemisphere. Henschen (1920–1922) suggested the existence of a motor graphic center in Exner's area, and a sensory graphic center in the angular gyrus. In addition to the lesions in the posterior F2 area, posterior

418

LOCALIZATION
OF CLINICAL
SYNDROMES IN
NEUROPSYCHOLOGY
AND NEUROSCIENCE

parietal lesions may be implicated in some cases of apraxic agraphia (Auerbach & Alexander, 1981; Baxter & Warrington, 1986; Brain, 1965; Crary & Heilman, 1988; Russel & Espir, 1961).

Spatial Agraphia. Hécaen et al. (1956) stressed the role of lesions of the right hemisphere in the development of spatial agraphia, calling it the nondominant-hemisphere syndrome, which is usually marked by damage to the right parieto-temporo-occipital junction. In some cases, spatial agraphia was limited to right-sided neglect resulting from a left frontoparietal lesion. Neglect of the left side of words was found to be the result of a left-sided parietal lesion in two patients with right hemispheric language lateralization (Baxter & Warrington, 1983; see also McCarthy & Warrington, 1990).

Spelling Agraphia. Gerstmann (1927) pointed to lesions in the left parietal lobe as being critical for the development of spelling agraphia. Miceli, Silvery, and Caramazza (1985) reported evidence of spelling agraphia in a patient with a lesion in the superior parietal lobule, with a possible extension to the upper portion of the angular gyrus.

Phonological and Deep Agraphia. Roeltgen et al. (1983) reported four patients with phonological agraphia. Head CT scans found evidence of lesions that overlapped portions of the anterior-inferior part of the left supramarginal gyrus. Roeltgen et al. (1983) noted a patient with phonological agraphia with a lesion that was relatively isolated at the insula. Other patients with lesions in the same region have been reported by Shallice (1981), and Baxter and Warrington (1985). An extension of the parietal lesion to the temporal lobe has been reported in cases of deep agraphia (Baxter & Warrington, 1983; Bub & Kertesz, 1982; Kremin, 1987).

Surface Lexical Agraphia. Roeltgen and Heilman (1984) found that an overlap of the lesion in four patients with lexical agraphia included the left posterior angular gyrus and the occipito-parietal lobule. A similar lesion localization was also found in cases described by Baxter-Versi (1987) and Alexander, Friedman, LoVerso, and Fischer (1990).

In conclusion, further collection of clinico-anatomical data may help to clarify the anatomical basis for clinical differences between conventional and unconventional disturbances of reading or writing. It is possible that surface and deep alexia and agraphia differ from other types of central alexia or agraphia in underlying lesion localization.

AMUSIA

THE RECOGNITION AND production of musical sounds and melodies represents a specific type of communication with high emotional content. In some sense, disturbances of this type of communication may be considered as a form of emotional agnosia and motor aprosodia.

Two major types of amusia have been described—*motor amusia* and *sensory amusia*. Motor amusia is characterized by disturbances of singing and playing on musical instruments. *Sensory amusia* is manifested as a disorder in the recognition of musical sounds and melodies. Amusia, or a disorder of musical skills, is a relatively isolated disturbance. Language disorders and forms of aphasia are either completely absent or only minimally present in many cases of amusia.

Proust (1872) was probably the first to describe amusia. He presented two patients who were suffering from motor amusia, one of whom was a musician. Both patients were unable to hum a tune but were still able to recognize melodies. The musician was able to play, read, and compose music, in spite of a severe form of aphasia. Oppenheim (1889) described 16 cases of aphasia with musical disturbances. Knoblauth (1888) proposed the first classification of amusia, which included motor and sensory amusia. Motor amusia included avocalia, instrumental amusia, and musical agraphia. Sensory amusia consisted of musical deafness with paramusia, amnestic amusia, musical blindness, and musical alexia.

Musical abilities are often preserved in aphasic patients and may be disturbed in patients without aphasia or agnosia for environmental sounds. In a review of all published cases of amusia up to that time, Henschen (1920–1922) found evidence of sensory amusia in only 20 out of 65 cases with word deafness. More recently, Sacks (1985) described a case of amusia and a preserved understanding of speech and recognition of environmental sounds. On the other hand, mild signs of amusia or an absence of amusia was described in a large number of cases of Wernicke's aphasia (Assal, 1973; Assal & Buttet, 1983; Basso & Capitani, 1985; Signoret et al., 1987; for a review, see Basso, 1993). One of the most striking cases of this type was that of Shebalin, a Russian composer and the director of the Moscow Conservatory. Shebalin suffered from a stroke in the left hemisphere at the age of 57, followed by sensory aphasia and right-sided hemiparesis. Luria et al. (1965) examined the composer 6 months after the stroke, and found evidence of a prominent comprehension disorder and paraphasic errors in his speech, which persisted until the patient's death 3 years later. His ability to compose music, however, remained preserved until his death, and he

420

LOCALIZATION
OF CLINICAL
SYNDROMES IN
NEUROPSYCHOLOGY
AND NEUROSCIENCE

was able to compose his Fifth Symphony in C flat, which was praised by another famous composer as a brilliant creative work.

Preserved musical abilities are often seen not only in patients with Wernicke's aphasia but also in patients with Broca's aphasia. These patients are often able to sing familiar melodies accompanied by fluent strings of corresponding words. Interestingly, patients with Broca's aphasia are unable to produce these words in expressive speech without singing. Yamadory, Osumi, Masuhara, and Okubo (1977) studied singing in 24 patients with Broca's aphasia. The singing was considered excellent in 6 patients, and satisfactory in 15 patients, including 6 patients who were unable to produce words otherwise. This phenomenon has been successfully used for language rehabilitation in patients with Broca's aphasia.

Certainly, disorders of musical abilities may be primarily observed in patients who have previously demonstrated musical skills. Amusia has thus been more frequently described in professional musicians. At the same time, some aspects of musical skills, for example, singing and the recognition of popular melodies, are well developed in individuals without special musical education, and musical disturbances may be observed in this population in the course of brain disease as well as in musicians. In addition to the two types of amusia, motor and sensory, musical alexia and musical agraphia may be observed in some cases.

Motor Amusia

Clinical Aspects

Patients suffering from motor amusia are unable to sing, a condition known as *avocalia*, or to play musical instruments, a condition known as *instrumental amusia*. Patients with avocalia demonstrate a lost ability to sing popular melodies. Melodies are presented incorrectly, and their melodic contour and rhythm are often destroyed. Singing correct succession of the musical tones becomes impossible for these patients, and tones are often replaced with incorrect tones that often differ by anywhere from a half to a whole tone from the correct tone, in a manner similar to paraphasia in language disorders. This erroneous substitution of tones may be called *melodic paratonia*. The patient suffering from avocalia does not usually demonstrate dysprosodia, and the melodic and intonational structure of speech is generally preserved.

Instrumental amusia is manifested as a disturbance in the ability of both professional and amateur musicians to play a musical instrument. The patient experiences difficulties in playing the instrument, reading the notes, and playing well-learned melodies or compositions. The patient becomes unable to find the correct succession of musical tones and to produce the correct rhythmic pattern. It becomes especially difficult to play the correct harmonic pattern of a new, un-known melody, or to reproduce correctly the intervals between tones and the rhythmic patterns of the melody.

SENSORY AMUSIA

PATIENTS SUFFERING FROM sensory amusia demonstrate distur-bances in the ability to recognize melodies that were once well known to the patient. As with visual object agnosia, two types of musical agnosia may be distinguished—*associative musical agnosia* or amnestic musical agnosia, and *apperceptive musical agnosia* or acoustic musical agnosia.

Associative Musical Agnosia
The patient is unable to identify well-known melodies, losing the abil-ity to match the melody with its sample in the individual's stored mem-ory, while the abilities to detect incorrect notes, to recognize whether various musical instruments are in tune, and to recognize the rhythm of a song are either completely preserved or only mildly disturbed.

Bonvicini (1905) described one such patient, who was unable to rec-ognize well-known popular melodies, including the national anthem. The patient's sense of rhythm and his ability to detect incorrect notes were preserved. Similarly, Lamy (1907) observed a patient who was able to transcribe the national anthem correctly but was unable to recog-nize that the melody was familiar to him.

Apperceptive Musical Agnosia
Difficulties in melody recognition are related to difficulties in the per-ception of basic features of melodies, such as sequential variations in pitch, duration of tones, and tempo. Wertheim and Botez (1961) de-scribed a patient with musical agnosia who suffered from disturbances in the identification of measures and the reproduction of rhythms. The patient also lost absolute pitch. In more severe cases (for a review, see Hécaen & Albert, 1978), the musical quality of sound becomes com-pletely lost (Shuster & Taterka, 1926), and the patient may claim to hear a "screeching car" (Foerster, 1936), the sound of hammering on a metal sheet (Quensel & Pfeiffer, 1923), or a "strident, dissonant, and piercing quality" to the music (Pötzl, 1937).

In some cases, the recognition of melodies is disturbed, while rhythm discrimination remains preserved, or vice versa. Sacks (1985) described a patient who was unable to discriminate between the melodies of hymns and had to rely on the words or the rhythm for correct recognition. Fries and Swihart (1990) described a similar case in which an amateur musi-cian developed a dissociation between impaired melody processing and

422

LOCALIZATION
OF CLINICAL
SYNDROMES IN
NEUROPSYCHOLOGY
AND NEUROSCIENCE

preserved rhythm discrimination. An opposite pattern was observed by Mavlov (1980) in a 61-year-old professional musician following an infarction of the left hemisphere. The patient developed severe difficulties in the recognition and production of rhythms, whereas he was able to produce and to recognize tones and tone sequences. This dissociation between recognition of melodies and recognition of rhythms was experimentally studied by Peretz (1990), who asked patients to compare musical stimuli that were altered in one dimension, either melody or rhythm. Two patients exhibited impairments in the use of melody as a discriminating cue, while two other patients were found to be impaired when the cue was rhythmic.

A similar dissociation between melody and rhythm may be seen in cases of motor amusia. Singing may be characterized by a loss of melody with a preservation of rhythmic organization (Mann, 1888), or vice versa (Brust, 1980; Mavlov, 1980).

These data point to the possibility of a relatively independent processing of musical features, such as melodies and rhythms, similar to the processing of shape, color, and motion in visual object recognition. A further division of musical features may be related to the processing of the melody contour as ascending and descending pathways and the processing of specific tone intervals within the melodic contour.

In general, it is difficult to find a case in which either isolated associative or isolated apperceptive musical agnosia is present, as various degrees of both types of sensory amusia are present in the majority of cases.

Musical Alexia and Agraphia

Musical alexia for note reading and musical agraphia for note writing may accompany motor and sensory amusia or may be observed in cases without amusia. They may be observed together with alexia and agraphia for language, as in two professional musicians described by Brust (1980). One case was that of a 22-year-old student who underwent an anterior lobectomy and the removal of a meningioma in the left temporal lobe. After the surgery, the patient developed severe transcortical aphasia. Eighteen months later, the patient was suffering from only mild anomia and comprehension difficulties but was still unable to sight-read simple melodies and made frequent errors when attempting to copy intervals. His reading and writing language capabilities were more prominently disturbed. No sign of motor or sensory amusia was observed. In the second patient described by Brust (1980), alexia and agraphia for language and music developed after the rupture of a cerebral infarction. CT scans showed infarctions in the left posterior temporal lobe and the left inferior parietal lobe. In this case, the reading and writing of music was more severely disturbed than were the reading and writing of language.

Anatomical Aspects

Motor Amusia

Motor amusia is usually observed in cases with frontal lobe lesions in the right hemisphere. Mann (1888) described a case of motor amusia without the accompanying presence of aphasia. An autopsy of the patient revealed a cyst in the second frontal gyrus of the right hemisphere. Henschen (1920–1922) analyzed all previously published anatomical cases of amusia and concluded that a lesion of the second frontal gyrus of the left hemisphere was the most typical lesion site in instrumental amusia, while the development of avocalia is primarily related to lesions of the triangular portion in front of Broca's area in the same hemisphere. Botez and Wertheim (1959) and McFarland and Fortin (1982) described right hemispheric lesions and instrumental amusia in two patients, including one case with avocalia.

Experimental studies of motor amusia have been primarily limited to singing. Gordon and Bogen (1974) found evidence of a loss of melody with a relatively less-impaired rhythm during the course of a test in which amital sodium was injected into the right side of the brain in eight patients. The test investigated patients in preparation for either a temporal or a frontal lobectomy in cases of seizure disorders. Melodic contour and rhythm were preserved, but not perfect, following left-sided injections in five patients. Patients with anterior lesions performed worse than those with posterior lesions, regardless of the side of the injection. Similar data were reported by Borchgrevink (1980). Following a right-sided injection, the patients lost the melodic line but not the rhythm. A gradual loss of rhythm was observed in one patient following a left-sided injection of amital sodium.

Sensory Amusia

Henschen (1920–1922) stressed the role of the left temporal pole in cases of sensory amusia but also considered the possibility that hemispheric dominance for music is not as rigid as for language. This was an attempt to explain the development of amusia without aphasia in cases of right hemispheric lesions (Henschen, 1920–1922). Feuchtwanger (1930) discussed amusia in a special monograph, during which he concluded that the posterior part of the first temporal gyri in both hemispheres represents a special auditory area for the integration of noise, music, and speech. Wertheim and Botez (1961) observed receptive amusia in a patient with mild Wernicke's aphasia, pointing to a lesion of the left hemisphere in the posterior part of the first temporal gyrus.

424

LOCALIZATION
OF CLINICAL
SYNDROMES IN
NEUROPSYCHOLOGY
AND NEUROSCIENCE

Lately, an absence of clear hemispheric dominance in sensory amusia has been investigated in a series of experimental studies in patients with unilateral brain lesions caused by temporal lobectomy for the treatment of either intractable seizures or stroke. A predominance of the right hemispheric lesions was noted in disturbances in the processing of music in most of the studies, though disturbances were also found in patients with left hemispheric lesions.

Milner (1962) used the Seashore test for musical talent to measure discrimination of pitch, loudness, rhythm, duration, timbre, and melodic memory both before and after a temporal lobectomy. No impairment was found in any test prior to surgery. Some degree of impairment was noted in all of the studied types of auditory perception following the temporal lobectomy, regardless of the side of the surgical procedure. More prominent disturbances, however, were recorded for the discrimination of two short musical sequences and for the perception of timbre after a right temporal lobectomy than after a left temporal lobectomy. The inclusion of Heschl's gyri in the surgery yielded similar results.

A dichotic melody test also showed a predominance of the right hemisphere for music processing in patients following either a right or left temporal lobectomy (Schankweiler, 1966), as well as in patients with right hemispheric stroke compared to normal control subjects (Schulhoff & Goodglass, 1969). Left hemispheric patients showed better detection of errors in familiar songs than did right hemispheric patients (Shapiro, Grossman, & Gardner, 1981). However, the ability to identify familiar melodies may be more pronounced in left hemispheric patients, for whom the words of the song may help the subject choose the correct song, while right hemispheric patients exhibit a more impaired recognition of melodies without words (Gardner, Siverman, Denes, Semenza, & Rosentiel, 1977). This points to the possibility that words are closely associated with melodies, and that the development of sensory amusia may be explained by an impairment of word processing in cases with lesions of the left hemisphere.

Differences between music information processing in the right versus the left hemisphere have also been stressed by studies derived from the two-component model of melody stored in memory. One component contains information about the overall contour of the melody, while the second characterizes the specific intervals between individual tones. It has been suggested that the first component is processed by the right hemisphere, while the second is typically processed in the left hemisphere.

Bever and Chiarello (1974) used dichotic listening techniques to compare the recognition of melodies in nonmusicians, who supposedly relied on the contour-based component of melodies, and musicians, who learned to utilize an interval-based recognition of melodies. In accordance with the hypothesis, musicians exhibited right-ear advantage (left hemisphere superiority) in tasks of melody recognition, while nonmusicians demonstrated left-ear advantage (right hemisphere superiority) in the same task. Peretz (1990) subsequently tested vascular patients with unilateral strokes of either the right or left hemisphere. The test required each subject to compare two melodies, which could be the same or could differ in terms of a violation of contour or in changes of the exact interval size between two adjacent tones while their direction (ascending or descending) was preserved. A lesion in the left hemisphere was found to impair the ability to use an interval-based approach, whereas the contour-based approach was preserved. Right hemisphere patients showed impairments in both contour-based and interval-based approaches, perhaps pointing to the possibility that the use of interval-based approaches somehow relates to the preservation of contour-based information processing. Though further studies are certainly needed, these findings stress the role of both hemispheres in the processing of musical information, with some major role of the right hemisphere, which is generally contralateral to the effective language functioning of the left hemisphere.

Musical Alexia as an Agraphia

Few anatomical of isolated disturbances of musical reading and writing have been published. Musical alexia and agraphia are often accompanied by sensory amusia. Brust (1980) recently described evidence of both musical alexia and agraphia in two patients with lesions of the left hemisphere. A less prominent disturbance of alexia and agraphia for language was also observed in both cases.

8

Memory Disorders: Disturbances of the Major Supportive System of Brain Information Processing

MEMORY IS THE general term used to describe the ability of a living system to retain and to utilize acquired information and knowledge (Tulving, 1995). This ability helps to encode, store, and retrieve information in the course of recognition and action. To avoid overloading the memory with an enormous volume of point-by-point descriptions of information used by the brain processing systems, it is organized in a way that selects and compresses incoming information, thus markedly reducing its volume.

Major functions of memory in brain information processing include its role as an archive (Spinnler, 1999), or a long-term database that stores and preserves compressed information for its future use; a short-term storage facility that compresses information and transfers it to long-term storage and also uses the information in the process of learning to recognize novel objects and actions and acquire new skills and habits; and a modular memory intimately involved in the

428

LOCALIZATION
OF CLINICAL
SYNDROMES IN
NEUROPSYCHOLOGY
AND NEUROSCIENCE

real-time processing of information via various recognition and action modules.

Since the original description of the amnestic syndrome in patients with chronic alcoholism (Korsakoff, 1887), researchers have presented clinical data related to memory disorders and have described these disorders as disturbances of immediate memory; short-term memory, also known as recent memory; and long-term memory, also known as remote memory. Disturbances in long-term memory are reflected in impairments of storage in and retrieval from the memory data base, while impairments in short-term memory are manifested as difficulties in saving information for 1–2 days, a considerably longer time than the several minute–long capacity of the short-term memory. The information is thus unavailable to the individual for help in day-to-day functioning or recognition and procedural learning and is unable to be consolidated for transfer to the database. Immediate memory is concerned with the preservation of information from 1 msec to 2–5 min or more, allowing for the amount of time needed for certain modules to recognize stimuli and to react in an appropriate manner. Disturbances of immediate or modular memory may often be seen in patients with agnosia, apraxia, or aphasia, manifesting as impairments in conventional and unconventional information processing. The term *immediate memory* is quite close to the term *working memory,* which is actively involved in the processing of information preserved for the time needed to complete certain operations in the process of recognition and action.

Declarative and Nondeclarative Memory.   Memory can be used as a long-term archive, or database, of events and knowledge and is organized in such a way that it may subsequently allow for retrieval for the processing of information in particular modules. This type of memory has also been described as *declarative memory,* which refers to the conscious recollection of facts and events and is termed declarative since its content can be declared (Cohen & Squire, 1980; Squire, 1994). Declarative memory may be further divided into *episodic memory* and *semantic memory.*

Episodic memory refers to the storage and retrieval of one's personal past, of the primarily social events connected with certain times and places in the subject's life, such as autobiographical data and public events. This type of memory is closely connected with the storage of self-image data, which is used for the formation and updating of an image of the self in its interaction with the social and physical environments. Disturbances of this type of memory are usually described by the clinical term *amnestic syndrome.*

Semantic memory contains the general, in some sense encyclopedic, knowledge of the world, for example, of a given society, a historical

429

*Memory Disorders:
Disturbances of the
Major Supportive
System of Brain
Information
Processing*

period, or a geographical site, including the names of foreign currencies, cities, famous subjects, the chemical formula for salt, and so on.

Nondeclarative memory includes the definitions of *procedural memory*, which includes skill learning (motor, perceptual, and cognitive skills), habit formation, and classical conditioning; and *priming*, which is the recognition of a stimulus following a previous first encounter with that item. Procedural memory and priming are difficult to express in verbal declaration, since recollection lacks conscious access to the memory of learning. Both types of nondeclarative memory, which are used by certain modules in the processes of learning, recognition, and action, may be considered as types of unconventional information processing.

The term *modular memory* for recognition and action covers a much wider set of memory functions, which includes procedural memory and priming. Modular memory is an important part of brain information processing that is used by various modules in the different stages of recognition and of action performance in both the physical and social environments. Modular memory is utilized in these environments in the process of describing objects, spaces, and features of actions, in interpreting combinations of these descriptions, in bidirectional comparison with the prototypes memorized in model storage, and for the ekphorization of the models of actions. Modular model storage for both recognition and action is similar to the databases of episodic and semantic memory but contains only a limited set of well-defined models, known as prototypes, which are used in the processes of recognition and of action production in real-time conventional information processing.

During the course of unconventional information processing, especially the processing of novel information, prototypes of objects, spaces, or actions must be adjusted to accommodate or to learn new information, as well as to add new models. (For more details, see chapter 2, section titled "Visual Agnosia.") The adjustment of the model stores may also be conducted more slowly using information stored in the database of both episodic and, especially, semantic memory.

While procedural memory and priming, as well as other parts of modular memory for recognition and action, tend to be preserved in patients suffering from amnesia of episodic and semantic memory, they are usually found to be disturbed in patients with apraxia and agnosia and are described as impairments in unconventional information processing. (For more details, see the corresponding sections in this book.)

Explicit and Implicit Memory.   The distinction between *explicit* and *implicit memory* is similar to that between declarative and nondeclarative memory (Schacter, 1994). Explicit memory refers to a subject's ability to recall and recognize material, while implicit memory corresponds to memory that cannot be consciously reached and is related to conditioning, the learning of skills, and so forth.

There are some similarities between the structures of episodic and semantic memory and model memory for recognition and action. Both types involve both long-term memory storage and short-term memory, which is used for the encoding of information. However, model storage in modular memory is used to compare the information from the outside world with the stored model either to allow for the recognition of actual stimuli or to use the stored information to form interactions with the outside world. This process is primarily implicit and does not have to be consciously recognized. At the same time, episodic memory and semantic memory are used to allow for communication between the self and the outside world, especially the social world, without comparison to any real stimuli in the outside world. This ekphorization of information related to past experience, or stored knowledge, must be explicit and in many instances must be verbally declared. While episodic memory is explicit in recollection and in bringing descriptions of past events and knowledge from corresponding database memory into consciousness, the retrieval is implicit, or automatic, when it is applied to the stored model in the course of real-time recognition and action in both conventional and unconventional information processing.

In clinical reality, the terms nondeclarative and implicit memory are not directly related to the term amnesia, and they extend into the areas of agnosia, apraxia, and aphasia, just like modular memory for recognition and action does. At the same time, the terms explicit and declarative memory, especially in terms of episodic and semantic memory, seem to cover the term amnesia in its clinical sense. The use of the information stored in the database for episodic memory, however, may be also implicit, especially during the course of updating and of interactions with modular memory.

Semantic Memory.   Semantic memory is defined as the memory structure devoted to assigning meanings to words, objects, and situations (Spinnler, 1999). It includes nodes that store the attributes, or important features, of things, such as their names and their functional and conceptual properties.

Warrington (1975) described a syndrome of semantic memory impairment not as a pure linguistic deficit but as a loss of semantic memory of the items related to object naming, word comprehension, and object recognition.

Semantic memory represents a knowledge of the meaning of perceived items, either verbal or visual. This knowledge includes the names

431

Memory Disorders:
Disturbances of the
Major Supportive
System of Brain
Information
Processing

of the items, their functional and conceptual properties, and so forth. Warrington (1981) stressed the division between the categories characterized by sensory properties compared to functional properties. The utilization of sensory properties (e.g., shape, pattern, color, or flavor) is required for distinguishing between a lion and a tiger, a carrot and a parsnip, or gold and silver. On the other hand, functional information, or information regarding how, where, or what the object is used for, is needed to distinguish between a screwdriver and a chisel, or an arm and a leg. Such a division is also reflected in terms of the ordinate, which corresponds with the use of sensory properties in recognizing the difference between a dog and a cat, and the superordinate, which corresponds with functional memory, or semantic memory, as when recognizing a vehicle or a tool. These categories are used in studies of object recognition.

Semantic memory represents a type of long-term memory organization that may be used in the course of unconventional information processing. Semantic memory may frequently be multimodal, especially when related to the descriptions of ideas and emotions such as love, hate, and happiness. It is possible that semantic memory is represented separately for objects, words, or actions, but that these parts are closely interconnected.

Storage for semantic information seems to be organized according to the functional or sensory properties of things, rather than their time gradation, for example, according to nodes containing various tools or furniture, living and nonliving objects, properties of the individual's particular culture, scientific knowledge, and so forth.

Long-Term Memory. Long-term memory may be considered to be a database that selects and preserves information about personal and public events in episodic memory and about knowledge in primarily semantic memory. This information is used in the process of forming and updating various modules of recognition and actions, including the self in its interaction with the physical and social environments. The memory database seems to be organized in time layers in accordance with the time in which the particular information was stored. This indexing of information may underline the limitation of retrograde amnesia to a particular number of years, for example, 1–2 years, 9–10 years, or 20 years, with a sparing of earlier years, so that the remote episodic memory remains undisturbed for the teenage and/or the early adult years. Time indexing also facilitates the retrieval of information related to corresponding time periods in the subject's life. It is possible that nodes of stored information, for example, of events related to school years, such as graduation, are coded in a way that allows for the separate storage and retrieval of information in different

432

LOCALIZATION
OF CLINICAL
SYNDROMES IN
NEUROPSYCHOLOGY
AND NEUROSCIENCE

modalities, verbal, visual, and other. This suggestion is supported by the presence of cases with an isolated loss of visual imagery. (For more details, see chapter 2, section titled "Loss of Visual Imagery.")

Another possible method of information retrieval may be achieved via a catalogue, or directory, that is built on the type of events stored in the database in a fashion that is similar to that of a catalogue in the library or a directory of information stored in a computer's memory. As with catalogues in a library, the organization of stored information may also include alphabetical addresses based on the first letter of the names of things or events. Such a possibility is supported by the well-known effect of clues in recalling names in patients with anomia. This catalogue may be based on semantic information, especially for semantic memory.

It is impossible to store and retrieve all of the information processed in everyday life and in the course of studies, even in a large memory storage database. The information must be compressed and coded in a way that is convenient for subsequent retrieval and use in brain information processing. Thus, the information stored in a memory database cannot be eidetic or echoic, since it would then be impossible to store and to retrieve the memory. It seems that the compression and coding of information begins in earlier stages of the process of information storage in the short-term memory, which may store and process information for ongoing brain information processing and discard it after the use of the stored information is completed. The individual's short-term memory may also prepare the information for further transfer to long-term memory by compressing and coding the information in a form that may be acceptable for long-term memory storage. Studies of short-term memory disturbances provide some understanding of the organization and function of the short-term memory.

Long-term memory cannot be represented by either eidetic or echoic types of information, since the preservation of such information would quickly exceed the capacity of any storage database and would be difficult, if not impossible, to retrieve. Thus, in order to prepare information for long-term storage in the database, the information must be compressed and coded in the short-term memory, which selects the most salient parts of the perceived information for storage in the database.

The compression of information before it is transferred to long-term memory storage may be achieved by the preliminary recognition of objects, spaces, and actions, and the possible translation of multimodal results in the coding of visual, auditory, or verbal modalities into a unitarian code that is adjusted for use in the storage database. Retrieval of information from the memory database, however, is usually achieved via verbal input, as in cases of autobiographical inquiry.

433

*Memory Disorders:
Disturbances of the
Major Supportive
System of Brain
Information
Processing*

Retrieval may be also performed in visual form, as in cases of visual imaging.

Certainly, some important information may be omitted or erased in the course of its storage or may be wrongly presented during retrieval, especially when affect is involved in the process. Clinical data points to better protection of old information compared to information that has been stored in the database relatively recently.

The process of selection of information for transfer to long-term memory storage seems to depend on the social and physical saliency of the event or knowledge, its frequency, and its informational value. It seems that affect may also influence what information is selected for storage in and retrieval from the database by enhancing the storage and preventing the retrieval of negative information, and by facilitating the retrieval of positive information. This possibility was discussed in detail via the psychoanalytic theory of suppression, which stresses the importance of the implicit use of database memory. This memory may also be used implicitly during the formation and functioning of modular memory. At the same time, long-term database memory is far more accessible for declarative, explicit retrieval than it is when the capabilities of modular memory are used.

AMNESTIC SYNDROMES

AMNESTIC KORSAKOFF'S SYNDROME

AMNESTIC KORSAKOFF'S SYNDROME was first described by Korsakoff (1887), who stressed that a common cause underlay the development of memory disorders and neuropathy in patients suffering from chronic alcoholism and suggested the term *psychosis polineuritica* to describe the condition. Researchers later found that an amnestic syndrome may develop in such cases without concomitant signs of neuropathy.

Clinical Aspects

The clinical symptoms of amnestic Korsakoff's syndrome include prominent disturbances in remote, long-term episodic and semantic memory, also known as *retrograde amnesia,* as well as marked impairments in the individual's short-term episodic and semantic memory, also known as *anterograde amnesia. Confabulations* are another frequent manifestation in patients with alcoholic Wernicke-Korsakoff's syndrome. Immediate memory that is used in the course of recognition and action is usually observed to be in the normal range, and other cognitive abilities, as well as consciousness, remain relatively preserved. Speech is found to be fluent, and no significant defects are noted in

434

LOCALIZATION
OF CLINICAL
SYNDROMES IN
NEUROPSYCHOLOGY
AND NEUROSCIENCE

the patient's comprehension. Insight, however, is usually limited, and patients seem to be apathetic and not interested in their surroundings. Those discrepancies between the almost or completely preserved level of intelligence, as well as the immediate memory, and the prominent disturbances of episodic memory and knowledge and recent and remote memory represent a hallmark of alcoholic Korsakoff's syndrome.

Disturbances of Long-Term Memory

Retrograde amnesia, or a disorder of remote memory, involves severe disturbances in the recall of past experiences, while more recently formed memories remain relatively preserved. In some cases, there is a clear cutoff point between preserved earlier memories of events that took place anywhere from 3–4 to 20–25 years ago, and severely disturbed memories of events that occurred later on in the course of the patient's life. In most cases, however, retrograde amnesia extends for a period varying from several years to the whole of the patient's life before the onset of the illness, making it difficult to sharply delineate a cutoff point. When presented with pictures of famous people, patients may demonstrate an inability to recognize the names of persons famous in a specific period before the onset of the amnestic disorder but remain able to recognize those famous persons that he or she was familiar with following the onset of the disorder. The patient also suffers from disturbances in the sequencing of past actions and experiences difficulties in attempting to recall whether a particular event preceded or followed another event.

Disturbances of Short-Term Memory

Anterograde amnesia is manifested as a severe disturbance of short-term recent memory, as well as difficulties in the ability to memorize and recall experiences, and in the ability to acquire and recall social and personal events that occurred after the onset of the disease. In cases of Korsakoff's syndrome, anterograde amnesia often involves an inability to recall recent events, for example, what food was served during breakfast or lunch in as little as 10–15 min following the meal, and especially several hours after the meal.

Confabulations refer to instances of false recall, or a feeling of memory gaps with a description of events that never happened in spite of their often vivid recall by patients and their insistence on the true nature of the false recall. In some cases, temporal sequences may be lost for the recall of true events in a patient's life.

Though anterograde and retrograde amnesia form the basic core of Korsakoff's syndrome, confabulations are not regularly noted in patients. Two distinctive types of confabulation have been described (Cummings, 1985a, 1985b; Stuss, Alexander, Lieberman, & Levine, 1985).

435

*Memory Disorders:
Disturbances of the
Major Supportive
System of Brain
Information
Processing*

The most common type is that which is based on a true memory, but the events have become distorted in context and/or displaced in time. Confabulations are not produced spontaneously; they must be provoked by asking the patient to recall the events of his or her life. Answers tend to be short and abrupt if the patient is not repeatedly encouraged to continue with his or her recollections. The second type of confabulation is rare and consists of spontaneously produced fantastic stories in which the patient describes, in terms of grandiosity, his or her own participation in events that clearly could not have taken place in the patient's life. Confabulations are often accompanied by a lack of insight. For a review, see Parkin (1984).

Disorders of orientation in time and place are often observed in patients with amnesia. Orientation in person, however, is disturbed only in more severe cases of amnesia. On the other hand, all three forms of orientation may be preserved in less pronounced cases of amnesia, giving the impression that disorders of orientation may result from some special lesion localizations. This is especially important when considering disorders of visuospatial orientation, including disorders of topographic memory.

*Amnestic Syndrome of Korsakoff's Type
in Various Disorders and Diseases*

Amnestic syndrome has also been described in patients who developed memory disturbances following a bilateral removal of the hippocampus. In addition to the development of retrograde and anterograde amnesia, the immediate memory of such patients is often disturbed, with impairments of predominantly verbal memory in patients with lesions of the left hemisphere, and of visual and auditory memory in patients with lesions of the right hemisphere. Confabulations are absent, and the amnestic syndrome is usually not accompanied by anosognosia.

Since its original description in patients with chronic alcoholism, various degrees of amnestic Korsakoff's syndrome have been frequently observed in various psychiatric and neurological diseases. The list of such diseases includes chronic alcoholism; cerebral tumors, including craniopharyngiomas and intracerebral tumors; confusional states produced by intracerebral hypertension in patients with cerebral tumors, or by toxic-metabolic or infectious causes; cerebrovascular accidents, especially hippocampal infarctions and either a rupture or the surgical repair of an anterior communicating artery in an aneurism; carbon monoxide poisoning; posttraumatic amnesia, including head injuries in boxers; cerebral infections, especially herpes simplex encephalitis and AIDS encephalitis; anoxia; hypoglycemia; electroconvulsive therapy; degenerative dementias, especially Alzheimer's disease;

436

LOCALIZATION
OF CLINICAL
SYNDROMES IN
NEUROPSYCHOLOGY
AND NEUROSCIENCE

posttemporal lobectomy status; and interictal status in epilepsy (Cummings, 1985b). Evidence of amnestic Korsakoff's syndrome, however, was rarely found in isolation in such cases and was frequently accompanied by other cognitive changes.

Amnesia may be less pronounced and may primarily consist of forgetfulness in patients with subcortical pathology, including Parkinson's disease, progressive supranuclear palsy, Huntington's disease, and prominent white matter hyperintensity. Amnesia may be also present in the more advanced stages of schizophrenia or be secondary to depression. The psychogenic origin of amnesia must be taken into account in patients with depression, severe stress, or histrionic personality disorders, or as a manifestation of malingering, especially in forensic cases.

Wernicke's Disease.   Wernicke's disease is characterized by an abrupt onset of ocular abnormalities and as ataxia and confusion in patients with chronic alcoholism or acute poisoning. Ocular abnormalities include nystagmus, paralysis of the extreme lateral and upward ocular movements, convergent strabismus, and diplopia. *Ataxia* has primarily been found to be limited to the gait, with a characteristic broad base and shuffling. Confusion is characterized by signs of hypokinetic delirium accompanied by apathy, indifference, and disorientation. The disease was first described by Wernicke (1881) in two male patients, each suffering from chronic alcoholism, and in one young woman who suffered from vomiting after ingesting sulfuric acid. All three patients eventually progressed to the stages of stupor, coma, and death. The pathological findings included punctuate hemorrhages in the gray matter around the Sylvian aqueduct, located at the third and fourth ventricles. The changes appeared to be inflammatory in nature, which was reflected in the term *poliencephalitis hemorrhagica superioris*. It was later shown that Wernicke's disease is usually associated with a thiamine deficiency in both alcoholism and other diseases. Treatment with thiamine has been found to be life saving, often resulting in a dramatic improvement, in many cases within 1–3 weeks, in ocular symptoms, confusion, and to some extent gait ataxia. Nystagmus and gait ataxia were frequently still present during the chronic stage. After recovering from mental confusion in the acute stage, the presence of amnestic Korsakoff's syndrome may become apparent in some cases.

Evidence of an amnestic syndrome may be observed in cases of Wernicke's disease, especially in its chronic stage, while ocular symptoms and ataxia are sometimes seen in cases of Korsakoff's psychosis. Thus, the term amnestic Wernicke-Korsakoff syndrome has been suggested to unite both clinical entities. Pathological findings have been found to be similar, if not identical, in both Wernicke's and Korsakoff's

437

*Memory Disorders:
Disturbances of the
Major Supportive
System of Brain
Information
Processing*

syndromes (Victor, Adams, & Collins, 1971). However, the insidious onset of amnestic syndrome remains the primary clinical feature of Korsakoff's syndrome. Wernicke's disease, on the other hand, is mainly characterized by the abrupt onset of the ocular and gait abnormalities, as well as the development of mental confusion, not by an amnestic syndrome in the acute stage of the disease. Researchers thus tend to prefer, at least for the time being, to continue to use the term amnestic Korsakoff's syndrome to describe the chronic stage of the amnestic illness, and Wernicke's disease to describe the acute stage.

Reduplicative Paramnesia. A disorder of orientation in place may also be presented as a reduplicative phenomenon, similar to disorders of body image with autoscopy, or the duplication of hands or heads. Patients with reduplicative paramnesia may claim that they are simultaneously present in two locations, for example, simultaneously in a hospital and at their apartment in their hometown (Benson, Marsden, & Madows, 1976; Fisher, 1982; Patterson & Zangwill, 1944; Ruff & Volpe, 1981).

Pick (1903) described a patient who insisted that he was in Pick's clinic in Prague and in a duplicate clinic in another city at the same time. Other cases include the one reported in Benson et al. (1976), involving a patient who believed he was being hospitalized at the Boston Veterans Administration hospital and that the hospital was located in a spare bedroom in his house in Great Falls, Montana; and the case reported by Patterson and Zangwill (1944), whose patient claimed to have recently made a journey from one location to another.

Reduplicative paramnesia may be considered as a type of delusion, since it is based on apparent disturbances in reality testing and is based on the false belief that a person may be present in two different places at the same time. The condition holds a more delusional disorientation in place than does a true amnestic disorder.

Fugues, Multiple Personality Disorders, and Psychogenic Amnesia. Patients suffering from these types of disorders demonstrate total amnesia for a certain period, during which they often experience a loss of identity, due to either psychogenic causes or brain pathology. Such experiences are frequently observed in patients with epilepsy. The learning of new information is usually preserved in such cases.

Transient Global Amnesia. Transient global amnesia (TGA) refers to profound memory loss for a limited period of time; in this way it is similar to psychogenic amnesia. TGA often persists for several hours at least, but usually for no more than 24 hours. Patients are unable to recall events in both anterograde and posteriograde periods of memory, but

438

LOCALIZATION
OF CLINICAL
SYNDROMES IN
NEUROPSYCHOLOGY
AND NEUROSCIENCE

they remain fully conscious and demonstrate preserved recognition of their one identity and of familiar people. The patients give the impression of experiencing a transient blockade of free recall, while recognition remains mainly preserved. The same question may be repeated many times, and patients often appear bewildered, though aware of their memory problems. A full recovery of memory is typical, and no further attack of TGA is reported in most patients. No neurological abnormalities are found during the experience of TGA.

TGA is reported following mental and physical strain in a vulnerable individual and may involve a variety of causes, including cerebrovascular disease, migraine, seizures and tumors. For a review, see Cummings (1985). The pathology underlying the development of TGA, however, remains unclear in most cases. Fujii et al. (1989) compared PET findings in four patients within 3 months of the initial onset of the attack of TGA, and seven patients with transient ischemic attacks (TIA). The TGA patients were found to have better preserved cerebral blood flow and metabolism than TIA patients. The authors concluded that TGA may be caused by a reversible circulatory and/or a metabolic disturbance of an unclear organic nature. In addition, indisputable epileptic activity observed via EEG in patients with TGA may be recorded only after the episode, and never during it, in cases with definite epileptic seizures (Jaffe & Bender, 1966). Amnesic episodes due to seizures are usually brief and repetitive and are followed by a longer period of postictal amnesia.

Anatomical Aspects

Anterograde and Retrograde Amnesia

Two major lesion sites in amnestic Korsakoff's syndrome include the mesodiencephalic region, primarily the mammillary bodies, the medial dorsal thalamic nuclei, and the hypothalamus. Lesions may also be located in the fornix, which connects the mammillary bodies and the hippocampus, and in the basal forebrain.

Mammillary Bodies and Thalamic Medial Dorsal Nuclei. Gamper (1928) studied the brains of 16 patients with Korsakoff's psychosis and found changes in various areas extending from the dorsal motor nuclei of the ninth nerve to the anterior commissure and involving the inferior colliculi, the central gray matter of the midbrain, the medial portion of the third nerve nuclei, and the walls of the third ventricle. The most persistent lesions presented were found in the mammillary bodies in every case, causing Gamper (1928) to conclude that those lesions were primarily responsible for the memory disorders in these cases.

Pathological changes in the mammillary bodies were later found in many cases of Korsakoff's psychosis. Grüntal (1939) reported a 40-

439

*Memory Disorders:
Disturbances of the
Major Supportive
System of Brain
Information
Processing*

year-old patient with progressive memory disorder, the result of a cra-niopharyngioma that had destroyed the mammillary bodies. Remy (1942) described a patient who had died from cancer of the larynx at the age of 60, 19 years after the onset of Korsakoff's syndrome. According to the autopsy, the patient's mammillary bodies were atrophic and gli-otic. Though the thalamus was small, it appeared to be intact upon a histological examination.

Pathological changes in the mammillary nuclei were described in a series of cases reported by Gruner (1956), Malamud and Skillicorn (1956), Kahn and Crosby (1972), and Brion and Mikol (1978). These changes also involved the brain stem nuclei, the periaqueductal region, and the tec-tum. For a review, see Brierley (1966).

Victor et al. (1971) reviewed the literature and carefully described postmortem data from 82 of their own cases of Wernicke's disease and Korsakoff's psychosis. The authors concluded that the pathological changes are essentially the same in both conditions and thus suggested that the two disorders be united under the name Wernicke-Korsakoff syndrome. In addition to lesions in the mammillary bodies, pathologi-cal changes were found in all cases in the medial dorsal nuclei of the thalamus, as well as the medial part of the pulvinar. Other affected regions included the anterior medial nuclei of the thalamus, the peri-aqueductal region, the floor of the fourth ventricle, and the anterior lobe of the cerebellum, though not in all cases. The authors found an absence of involvement of the medial dorsal nucleus of the thalamus in five cases without memory deficits, though the mammillary bodies were affected in all five cases. Based on these findings, Victor et al. (1971) concluded that memory deficits are related to lesions in the medial dorsal thalamic nuclei, and that lesions in the mammillary bodies are probably not critical with respect to the functioning of the memory.

Victor et al. (1971) found evidence of gross cortical atrophy in only 27% of 72 cases. Malamud and Skillicorn (1956) found no specific ab-normalities in the cerebral cortices of 70 patients with Korsakoff's syndrome, and some minor damage was found in only a few patients. Delay, Brion, and Ellissalde (1958) reported an absence of consistent cortical damage in 8 patients with Korsakoff's syndrome. However, cortical atrophy with frontal lobe involvement was found in a high pro-portion of the alcoholics' brains studied by Courville (1955), Neuberger (1957), and Lynch (1960).

The development of amnesia was also reported in cases with uni-lateral and bilateral thalamic infarctions in the territories of the tu-berothalamic, or paramedian, arteries in the vicinity of the dorsomedial nuclei, without direct lesions in the mammillary bodies (Goldenberg, Wimmer, & Maly, 1983; Graff-Radford, Damasio, Yamada, Eslinger, & Damasio, 1985; Guberman & Stuss, 1983; Mills & Swanson, 1978; Schott,

440

LOCALIZATION
OF CLINICAL
SYNDROMES IN
NEUROPSYCHOLOGY
AND NEUROSCIENCE

Mauguière, Laurent, Serclerat, & Fischer, 1980; Speedie & Heilman, 1982). Squire and Moore (1979) also observed memory dysfunction in a patient with a head injury that involved, according to CT data, the left mediodorsal thalamic nucleus as well as other structures.

Grüntal (1939) and Remy (1942), however, reported an absence of thalamic involvement in cases of amnesia. Brion and Micol (1978) reported lesions of the mammillary bodies in 11 cases of Korsakoff's syndrome. Mediodorsal thalamic nuclei were found to be damaged in only 7 of the 11 cases. At the same time, thalamic nuclei other than the mediodorsal nuclei were damaged in 3 out of the 4 remaining cases. Limited damage to the dorsomedial thalamic nuclei involving, according to MRI data, not more than 15% of the nuclei may also result in the absence of any discernable memory impairment (Kritchevsky, Graff-Redfford, & Damasio, 1987).

Studies in monkeys that exhibit delayed performance on the non-matching test support the connection between mediodorsal nucleus lesions and the development of amnesia. Aggleton and Mishkin (1983) reported the development of moderate memory impairment in monkeys after damage to the anterior part of the mediodorsal nucleus and the adjacent midline nuclei of the thalamus. No damage was done to the anterior nucleus, and no degeneration of mammillary nuclei was observed. Damage to the posterior portion of the mediodorsal nuclei with a preservation of the adjacent midline nuclei resulted in even more memory impairment in the patient than did a lesion of the anterior portion of the mediodorsal nuclei. In another study, Aggleton and Mishkin (1985) reported the development of almost negligible memory impairments following lesions of the mammillary nuclei in monkeys. These impairments were milder than those memory deficits caused by damage to the mediodorsal thalamic nuclei.

Hippocampal Formations. Bechterev (1900) described a 60-year-old man who was experiencing memory problems, as well as confabulation and apathy. An autopsy showed a softening of the uncinate gyrus, as well as a bilateral softening of the hippocampal gyrus. Glees and Griffith (1952) described memory disturbances in cases of dementia following a bilateral destruction of the hippocampus.

Scoville and Milner (1957) presented one of the most thoroughly studied cases of amnestic syndrome. The patient, H.M., was a 27-year-old man who developed profound and permanent amnesia following bilateral anterior temporal lobectomies that had been performed in an effort to control intractable posttraumatic seizures. The resected areas included both halves of the hippocampus and the amygdala, as well as the epileptogenic cortex of the anterior temporal lobes. H.M. subsequently suffered from complete anterograde amnesia and was un-

441

*Memory Disorders:
Disturbances of the
Major Supportive
System of Brain
Information
Processing*

able to recall any episodes of his daily life. His experience of retrograde amnesia, however, extended only to a period of several years preceding the surgery. The patient's IQ remained above the normal range. Corkin (1984) described H.M.'s amnesia 14 years postsurgery. At that point, H.M. remained disoriented in terms of his age, time, and place and was unable even to recall the food he had eaten earlier that same day. Retrograde amnesia was limited to the 2 years preceding the operation.

Penfield and Milner (1958) reported two other cases, patients P.B. and F.C., in whom pronounced amnesia developed after extensive resections of the left temporal lobe. A later autopsy of patient P.B. found evidence of preexisting pathology in the right temporal lobe (Penfield & Mathieson, 1974). Though the area appeared to be normal externally, the hippocampus was shrunken, and a microscopic look revealed evidence of neuronal loss in the pyramidal cell layer.

Memory loss has been reported to be due to bilateral lesions of the hippocampal formations (gyrus dentatus, hippocampus, and parahippocampal gyrus), as well as to the amygdala and the uncus, and has also been described in cases of viral encephalitis, primarily herpes simplex encephalitis (Brierley, Cosellis, Hierons, & Nelvin, 1960; Damasio, Graff-Radford, Eslinger, Damasio, & Kassel, 1985; Davies, Davies, Kleinman, Kirchner, & Taveras, 1978; Drachman & Adams, 1962; Rose & Symonds, 1960); systemic lupus erythematosus (Schnider, Bassetti, Gutbrod, & Ozboda, 1995); a posterior cerebral artery occlusion (Benson, Marsden, & Meadows, 1974); a bilateral infarction of the hippocampal region (DeJong, Itabashi, & Olson, 1969); a bilateral infarction of the hippocampal region with an involvement of the left amygdala (Kartsounis, Rudge, & Stevens, 1995); a bilateral infarction of the inferomedial portions of the temporal lobes, including the hippocampal formation and extending to the fornix and occipital lobes (Victor, Angevine, Mancall, & Fisher, 1961); and a unilateral large infarction involving the hippocampus, the hippocampal gyrus, and the matter beneath the fusiform gyrus on the left, and a small infarction limited to the middle and anterior portions of the right hippocampus (Woods, Schoene, & Keisley, 1982).

Severe memory impairment was also revealed by disturbances in matching to sample test in monkeys with bilateral resections limited to the hippocampus (Mahut, Zola-Morgan, & Moss, 1982; Mishkin, 1978; Squire, 1987; Squire & Zola-Morgan, 1985). Memory impairment was more severe when the damage involved the adjacent entorhinal and parahippocampal cortex. A further increase in the severity of memory impairment was observed when the lesion also involved the perirhinal cortex. No increase of severity for memory loss was observed when a lesion of the hippocampus was extended in an anterior direction to include the

442

LOCALIZATION
OF CLINICAL
SYNDROMES IN
NEUROPSYCHOLOGY
AND NEUROSCIENCE

amygdala. However, the amygdala may play an important role in affective memory, for example, in the conditioning of fear (Davis, 1986; Gallagher, Graham, & Holland, 1990).

Data obtained from four cases of amnesia in humans (L.M., R.B., G.D., and W.H.) demonstrated that damage limited primarily to the hippocampal region produces moderate and long-lasting anterograde amnesia. Additional damage involving the adjacent areas of the dentate gyrus, the entorhinal cortex, and the subiculum results in both the exacerbation of anterograde amnesia and the development of extensive retrograde amnesia (Rempel-Clower, Zola-Morgan, & Squire, 1994; Rempel-Clower, Zola-Morgan, & Squire, 1995; for a review see Zola, 2000).

Fornix. The fornix was originally deemed to be included in the memory circuit consisting of the hippocampus, fornix, and mammillary bodies, and a lesion of the fornix alone was considered by several authors to be a cause of memory impairment (Gaffan & Gaffan, 1991; Heilman & Sypert, 1977; Hodges & Carpenter, 1991; Sweet, Talland, & Ervin, 1959). However, a lesion of the fornix alone did not result in significant memory loss in several published cases of fornix sections or damage caused by tumors, head injury, or cerebral infarctions. Garcia-Bengochea et al. (1954) described cases with bilateral interruption of the fornix during surgery without the development of a permanent memory deficit. Sweet et al. (1959) reported the development of Korsakoff's syndrome after the removal of the fornices and of a third ventricular tumor. The memory loss in this case, however, was mild and may have resulted from the compression of, and damage to, the diencephalic structures, rather than a section of the fornices. Heilman and Sypert (1977) reported the development of Korsakoff's syndrome in a patient with a splenial tumor, believed to be a cause of isolated bilateral damage to the fornix. However, the supracallosal longitudinal striae and posterior cingulate bundles seem to have been involved as well. All three pathways were disrupted in a case of persistent amnesia described by von Cramon and Schuri (1992). At the same time, in a case reported by D'Esposito, Verfaellie, Alexander, and Katz (1995), a prominent case of anterograde and retrograde amnesia followed a traumatic bilateral fornix transection caused by a penetrating gunshot injury. According to the head CT data, the bullet track extended from the left posterior parietal lobe through the right lateral ventricles, both fornices, and the hippocampal commissure to the left posterior temporal lobe. A microscopic lesion of the adjacent hippocampal structures could not be excluded.

Fornix sections in monkeys resulted in no deficit in memory (Mahut et al., 1982) or any amount of minimal memory impairment

443

*Memory Disorders:
Disturbances of the
Major Supportive
System of Brain
Information
Processing*

(Bachevalier, Saunders, & Mishkin, 1985). This may be explained by the existence of additional projections from the hippocampus to the mammillary bodies through the enthorinal cortex to several subcortical and cortical structures (Rosene & van Hoesen, 1977). On the other hand, some of the fornix fibers originate not from the hippocampus but from other structures, including the cingulate gyrus, the septal area, and the hypothalamus (Nauta & Feirtag, 1986).

Basal Forebrain. The basal forebrain region includes the septum, the nucleus accumbens, the diagonal band of Broca's area, and the nucleus basalis of Meynert (substantia innominata). The region includes cholinergic neurons in the nucleus basalis and dopaminergic neurons in the nucleus accumbens that innervate the entire cortical surface. The medial septal nucleus and nuclei of the diagonal band of Broca's area provide cholinergic projections to the hippocampus.

The development of amnesia, mainly of the anterograde type, has been described in cases with damage to the basal forebrain region. Such damage has often been observed in cases with the development of amnesia after a rupture of anterior communicated artery aneurisms (AcoA; Damasio, Eslinger, Damasio, Van Hoesen, & Cornell, 1985; Gade, 1982; Lindqvist & Norlen, 1966; Talland, Sweet, & Ballantine, 1967; Volpe & Hirst, 1983). In addition to amnesia, the AcoA syndrome often includes confabulations and personality changes (Damasio, Graff-Radford, Eslinger, Damasio, & Kassel, 1985), which may be attributed to the extension of neural damage from the basal forebrain region to parts of the frontal lobe (Damasio, Graff-Radford, et al., 1985; DeLuca & Cicerone, 1991; Vilkki, 1985; for a review see Rajaram, 1997).

In the assessment of the anatomical sites producing amnesia in cases with AcoA syndrome, it must be taken into account that many structures adjacent to the basal forebrain region may be involved, including the anterior hypothalamus, anterior cingulate gyrus, gyrus rectus, head of the caudate nucleus, and columns of the fornices. However, according to a review of the literature by DeLuca and Diamond (1995), some of the cases with AcoA syndrome suffered damage to the core forebrain structures, with possible extensions limited to the gyrus rectus and to some portions of the anterior cingulate.

The primary role of damage to the basal forebrain region in the development of amnesia is also supported by cases of infarctions and tumors with more circumscribed lesions compared to cases with AcoA syndrome, but some extensions of lesions to areas adjacent to the basal forebrain region were reported in those cases. The postoperative MRI of several patients with amnesia caused by cerebral tumors showed focal lesions in the basal forebrain region with extensions to the anterior hypothalamus, the preoptic area, the paraterminal gyrus, the lamina

444

LOCALIZATION
OF CLINICAL
SYNDROMES IN
NEUROPSYCHOLOGY
AND NEUROSCIENCE

terminalis in a case of glioma (Morris, Bowers, Chaterjee, & Heilman, 1992), and the bilateral gyrus recti and the inferior portions of the cingulate gyri in a case of meningioma (Rajaram, 1997). The MRI scan of a patient suffering from profound amnesia following a cerebral infarction revealed an extension of the damaged area from the septal nuclei to the rostrum of the corpus callosum. At the same time, the traditional memory structures, mesodiencephalic structures, and medial temporal lobe structures were preserved in cases with tumors or cerebral infarctions as well as in many cases with AcoA syndrome. This stresses the role of damage to the basal forebrain region and adjacent areas in the development of amnesia.

Lesions in the septal region involve an area that projects cholinergic pathways to the hippocampus as well as to the neocortex through the nucleus basalis of Meynert. Severe neuronal loss in the basal forebrain cholinergic system, especially in the nucleus basalis of Meynert, was reported in amnesic patients with Alzheimer's disease (Coyle, Price, & DeLong, 1983; Whitehouse et al., 1982). These findings led to the suggestion that the development of amnesia from lesions in the septal area may be attributed to the impairment of the mediating role of cholinergic pathways on the memory structures in the hippocampus and other cortical areas related to memory function (see Damasio, Eslinger, et al., 1985; Rajaram, 1997). In addition to being related to the thiamine deficiency experienced by patients with Korsakoff's syndrome, damage to the diencephalic region may be related to the reduction in cholinergic supply because of significant damage to the nucleus basalis of Meynert (Arendt, Bigl, Arendt, & Tennstedt, 1983).

Studies of rodents and primates provide data that support the relationship between isolated damage to the basal forebrain cholinergic structures and memory disturbances. Researchers demonstrated that memory impairment may be produced by an isolated lesion in the septal area (for a review see Olton & Wenk, 1987; Wenk & Olton, 1987). However, some studies involving monkeys have shown that a large lesion of the basal forebrain did not produce prominent amnesia in the absence of additional damage (Aigner et al., 1984; Squire, 1987). This stresses the need for further studies of the role that the basal forebrain cholinergic system may play in the development of amnesia.

Frontal Lobe. Frontal lobe tumors may be manifested as memory deficits. Kolodny (1929) found evidence of memory disturbances in 43% of his patients with frontal lobe tumors. Strauss and Keshner (1935) reported memory disturbances in 57.5% of such cases. The authors stressed the role of attention disturbances in the development of amnesia in patients with frontal lobe tumors. Paillas, Bourdouresques, Bonnal, and Provansal (1950) noted memory disturbances in 28 of 72 patients with frontal lobe tumors. Paillas, insisted that a disorder of immediate memory was present in 26 of 28 patients. Hécaen and de Ajuriaguerra (1956) reported 9 cases of amnesia out of 80 cases with frontal lobe tumors.

Amnesia of fixation, or a disorder of immediate memory, was observed in seven of the nine cases reported by Hécaen and de Ajuriaguerra (1956). The typical Wernicke-Korsakoff's syndrome accompanied by retrograde and anterograde amnesia, as well as confabulation, was observed in only one of these cases. Strauss and Keshner (1935) reported no such cases with Wernicke-Korsakoff's syndrome in their patients with frontal lobe tumors. Hécaen and de Ajuriaguerra (1956) also found no evidence of Wernicke-Korsakoff's syndrome in any of 75 patients with temporal lobe tumors, probably because of the unilateral location of the tumors. At the same time, Wernicke-Korsakoff's syndrome may be noted in patients with mesodiencephalic tumors (Hécaen & de Ajuriaguerra, 1956).

Similar results were reported by Delay, Brion, & Derouesné (1964). These authors calculated the frequency of Wernicke-Korsakoff's syndrome in cases of brain tumors published in the literature from 1893 to 1958 and found 1,509 individuals who were suffering from mental problems. Evidence of memory disturbances was found in a total of 379 cases. More specifically, disturbances were observed in 31% of frontal patients, 56% of parietal patients, 20% of temporal patients, 26.5% of patients with occipital lobe tumors, 17% of patients with tumors in the hypophisis, 39% of individuals with tumors in the region of the third ventricle, and 23% of patients with tumors in the subtentorial structures. Wernicke-Korsakoff's syndrome was noted in only 12 cases, including 5 of 355 patients with frontal lobe tumors, 6 of 187 patients with tumors in the region of the third ventricle, and 1 of 101 patients with tumors of the hypophysis.

Stuss, Alexander, Lieberman, and Levine (1985) reported the development of moderate-to-dense retrograde amnesia together with confabulation in five patients with frontal lobe lesions, including two patients following head injuries, two patients following a surgical clipping of the anterior communicating artery aneurism, and one patient following a cerebral infarction. While the lesions were unilateral in four of the five patients, the extension of the damage was quite prominent in all cases.

Prominent retrograde amnesia usually develops after bilateral frontal lobe lesions in cases with less extensive damage. Della Sala, Laiacona, Spinnler, and Trivelli (1993) presented 16 cases with frontal damage, 6 of them with left frontal lesions, 6 with right frontal lesions, and

446

LOCALIZATION
OF CLINICAL
SYNDROMES IN
NEUROPSYCHOLOGY
AND NEUROSCIENCE

4 with bilateral lesions of the frontal lobes, all of which were confirmed by head CT data. As in cases with hippocampal amnesia, low scores in the autobiographical memory test were observed in all 4 patients who had suffered from bilateral frontal lesions. Unilateral frontal lesions resulted in low autobiographical scores in 1 patient with a right lesion and in 1 patient with a left frontal lesion. In the first case, a closed head injury was the cause of frontal damage, and an extension of the injury to the opposite hemisphere cannot be ruled out. The regions involved in all diseases included frontal poles and dorsolateral frontal areas, primarily in the subcortical white matter in all 16 cases, but with an encroachment to the cortex in 4 of the 16 cases. The localization of lesions within the frontal lobe did not differ in bilateral and unilateral cases. The orbital cortex was never involved. Frontal lobe lesions were caused by a stroke in 6 cases, closed head injury in 4 cases, open head injury in 1 case, posttraumatic hygroma in 1 case, glioma in 2 cases, and meningioma in the 2 remaining patients. It seems that amnesia, especially anterograde amnesia, did not reach the severity of the memory disturbances experienced in Wernicke-Korsakoff's syndrome in any of 6 patients with low scores on autobiographical tests. The authors did mention, however, that some type of anterograde amnesia manifested as everyday forgetfulness was present in 3 of 4 patients with bilateral frontal lesions and in 1 of 2 patients with amnesia and unilateral frontal damage. Thus, 5 out of 6 patients with retrograde amnesia showed some sign of anterograde amnesia. Everyday forgetfulness was observed in only 2 of 10 remaining patients who had not demonstrated any evidence of a disturbance on autobiographical memory tests.

Isolated Anterograde Amnesia

Anterograde amnesia is often profound in cases with hippocampal lesions, while retrograde amnesia is relatively moderate, extending 2 or 3 years before the development of anterograde amnesia (Parkin, 1984; Scoville & Milner, 1957). Duyckaerts et al. (1985) reported a case of a 36-year-old man who became amnesic after a transient state of confusion. The patient experienced primarily anterograde amnesia, as he suffered from an inability to remember events that had occurred since the onset of amnesia, while his retrograde memory remained relatively well preserved. The patient died 21 months after the transient state of confusion from Hodgkin's disease. An autopsy showed bilateral atrophy of the hippocampus with microscopic findings of almost complete neuronal loss restricted to the hippocampus and amygdala bilaterally.

Kazui et al. (1996) described two patients who developed both anterograde and retrograde amnesia during attacks of TGA. After the attacks, both patients recovered from retrograde amnesia, but anterograde amnesia persisted in both cases. Head CT and MRI scans were

447

*Memory Disorders:
Disturbances of the
Major Supportive
System of Brain
Information
Processing*

found to be normal in both cases. A SPECT scan performed in one of the cases during a TGA episode revealed reduced blood flow in the bilateral temporal lobes. This reduction was eliminated by the day after the TGA attack. The SPECT scan was normal during the TGA attack in another case. Kazui et al. proposed that the medial temporal lobes are important in retrieving the newer events in both autobiographic and public domains. These areas do not, however, play an important role in the retrieval of older events, that is, events that occurred more than just a few years ago.

Zola-Morgan, Squire, and Amaral (1986) described 52-year-old patient R.B., who developed anterograde amnesia after an ischemic episode following a cardiac bypass operation. Autobiographic recall was preserved, but some retrograde amnesia was observed for memories of events that had occurred a few years prior to the surgery. An autopsy revealed complete bilateral loss of cells through the full mediolateral and rostrocaudal extent of the CA1 field with a slight extension into the subiculum and the CA3 region in the caudal third of the hippocampus. No evidence of cell loss was found in any component of the mammillary complex. Subsequently, three more cases (L.M., G.D., and W.H.) with amnesia caused by damage to the temporal lobe were described by the same group of authors (for a review, see Zola, 2000). It was found that isolated anterograde amnesia may result from a lesion of the hippocampus limited to the CA1 field, while an extension of the lesion to the CA2 and CA3 fields and the enthorinal cortex may lead to the development of temporally graded retrograde amnesia in addition to the anterograde amnesia.

Evidence of relatively isolated anterograde amnesia was reported in most cases with damage to the basal forebrain. Retrograde amnesia was either mild or completely absent in those cases (see above on the basal forebrain).

Isolated Retrograde Amnesia

Researchers recently described several cases in which retrograde amnesia developed in either the complete absence of an anterograde memory deficit or the presence of only a mild degree of such a deficit (Andrews, Poser, & Kessler, 1982; De Renzi & Lucchelli, 1993; Goldberg, Mayer, & Toglis, 1981; Kapur, Young, Bateman, & Kennedy, 1989; O'Connor, Butter, Miliotis, & Eslinger, 1992).

Goldberg, Antin, Hughes, and Mattis (1981) described a patient who had suffered from an open skull fracture in the right occipito-parietal and temporal areas. During the course of recovery from dense anterograde and retrograde amnesia, the patient demonstrated marked improvement in the ability to remember recent events. The patient's retrograde amnesia remained unchanged. A CT scan revealed a region

448

LOCALIZATION
OF CLINICAL
SYNDROMES IN
NEUROPSYCHOLOGY
AND NEUROSCIENCE

of rarefaction in the right middle and posterior temporal areas, as well as a small region of rarefaction along the left middle-temporal convexity. A follow-up CT scan a year later showed additional hypodensity that extended from the ventral tegmental portion of the upper mesencephalon in a caudal direction to the ventral portion of the ponto-mesencephalic junction. Goldberg, Antin, et al. (1981) ignored the temporal lobe lesion and concluded that a lesion in the ventral tegmental region was the cause of the persistent retrograde amnesia. They also concluded that the mesencephalic reticular activation system of limbic structures is an important part of long-term memory retrieval.

De Renzi and Lucchelli (1993) described a patient who, following trauma, experienced brain hypoxia and developed isolated retrograde amnesia. While an MRI scan was found to be negative, a PET scan showed a bilateral reduction in the uptake of the tracer in the posterior-superior temporal areas.

Kapur et al. (1989) presented a patient who had suffered from focal retrograde amnesia after a severe closed head injury due to a fall from a horse. An MRI scan revealed bilateral damage to the temporal lobes, including the temporal poles, the anterior middle temporal gyri, and the parahippocampal gyrus of the right temporal lobe. MRI scans failed to show any hippocampal abnormalities. The authors proposed that the anterior temporal lobes are critical for recalling memories of past events.

Markowitsch et al. (1993) described a patient who suffered a traumatic brain injury and developed isolated retrograde amnesia after a horse-riding accident. MRI data showed bilateral damage to the temporal poles, as well as to the lateral part of the right temporal lobe. The medial temporal lobe structures, including the hippocampus, were spared. The lesion also involved the latero-ventral portion of the right prefrontal cortex and the cortico-subcortical area of the left temporo-parietal transition zone. The authors proposed that the anterior temporal regions are crucial for the retrieval of old episodic memories and may involve an interaction with the prefrontal cortex. They suggested that this damage may be dissociable from the medial temporal lobe damage that leads to anterograde amnesia.

Stracciari, Ghidoni, Guarino, Poletti, and Pazzaglia (1994) reported two cases of selective loss of episodic memory caused by a closed head injury. MRI and EEG data were found to be normal in the first case; EEG and CT data were normal in the second case. SPECT scans showed hypoperfusion in the left temporal lobe in the first case, and right parietal abnormalities in the second case.

Evans, Wilson, Wraight, and Hodges (1993) described a patient with focal retrograde amnesia following cerebral vasculitis. MRI scans revealed lesions of the bilateral frontal area, the left anterior temporal area, and the left parietal area. The authors suggested that the impairment of memory arose from multifocal neocortical damage.

Confabulations and Lack of Insight

Confabulations and lack of insight may be seen in patients with Wernicke-Korsakoff's syndrome caused by chronic alcoholism (Victor et al., 1971). These symptoms are usually observed in the acute stages of the disease and markedly diminish in frequency and severity in the chronic stages. Lesion localization in such cases includes the mammillary bodies (Kahn & Crosby, 1972) and the thalamus (Sprofkin & Sciarra, 1952; Watkins & Oppenheimer, 1962). However, the absence of confabulations and the preservation of insight were also reported in some cases with lesions in the dorsomedial thalamic nuclei without a prominent extension to the adjacent thalamic regions (Kaushall, Zetin, & Squire, 1981; Schott et al., 1980; Speedie & Heilman, 1982) and in a case with a unilateral lesion of the mammillary bodies (Assal, Probst, Zander, & Rabinowicz, 1976). Confabulations may also develop in patients with diencephalic tumors in and around the walls of the third ventricle (Delay et al., 1964; Sprofkin & Sciarra, 1952).

Hippocampal amnesia is usually not accompanied by either confabulations or a loss of insight. Zangwill (1966) suggested that a lack of insight and a tendency to confabulate are often present in Korsakoff's syndrome of diencephalic origin, while temporal lobe amnesia is characterized by an absence of these symptoms. Insight was preserved and confabulations were absent in cases of amnesia following a temporal lobectomy (Scoville & Milner, 1957) and following other types of lesions as well (Benson et al., 1974; DeJong et al., 1969; Victor et al., 1961; Woods et al., 1982).

Parkin (1984) reviewed a series of cases with diencephalic and temporal lobe amnesia. This author found that diencephalic amnesiacs show a lack of insight and concern about their memory disorder; they often confabulate as well. Temporal lobe amnesia leads to these symptoms in rare cases. Retrograde amnesia is typically more circumscribed in cases of temporal lobe amnesia, extending back for only a few years. It seems that temporal lobe amnesiacs forget new information more rapidly than those with diencephalic amnesia.

The frontal lobes may also be involved in patients who experience confabulations. Kapur and Coughlan (1980) described the development of marked confabulations in a 48-year-old right-handed man after a subarachnoid hemorrhage caused by a rupture of the anterior communicated artery aneurism. The aneurism was clipped through a right frontal craniotomy. One week later, head CT scans showed a low-density area involving the medial aspect of the left frontal lobe,

450

LOCALIZATION
OF CLINICAL
SYNDROMES IN
NEUROPSYCHOLOGY
AND NEUROSCIENCE

extending upward and backward along the distribution of the left anterior cerebral artery. Three months after the surgery, the patient exhibited poor memory and fantastic hallucinations. He claimed, for instance, to be engaged in imaginary business appointments, when in fact he was attending a day care center. The patient would take a cup of tea outside for his foreman, a man he had stopped working with several years earlier. Spontaneous confabulations subsided 7 months after the surgery, and his confabulations became momentary, reflecting actual events distorted in context, time, and spatial relationships. Based on this evolution from fantastic to momentary confabulations, Kapur and Coughlan suggested that these changes may be considered as a manifestation of a different degree of frontal lobe dysfunction rather than of differences in lesion localization.

Stuss et al. (1985) reported the development of spontaneous, fantastic confabulations in five patients, each with frontal lobe lesions confirmed by head CT scan data. Head CT data obtained 14 weeks after Patient 1 suffered from a closed head injury revealed multiple areas of decreased density in both frontal lobes, but more severely in the left frontal lobe. An enlargement of the third and lateral ventricles was also noted. Head CT data obtained from Patient 2 showed a deep left frontal infarct involving the caudate nucleus, the internal capsule, and the tip of the left temporal lobe. Patient 3 had a large medial frontal infarction. Patient 4 experienced a depressed left parietal skull fracture, and a CT scan performed 6 months after the injury showed mild bilateral frontal atrophy without a lesion of the temporal lobe. Patient 5 developed confabulations after a clipping of the right communicating artery aneurism. Five years later, head CT data revealed atrophy of the right frontal lobe, enlarged lateral ventricles, and persistent right porencephaly. In other cases, involvement of the frontal lobe in patients with confabulations was suggested on the basis that limited self-monitoring and self-criticism in such cases represent dysfunction of the frontal lobe (Shapiro et al., 1981).

Isolated Amnesia

Several cases of isolated amnesia have been described recently. Slowly progressive memory disorders remain isolated without manifesting any significant disorder of language, intelligence, praxis, or attention (Caffarra & Venneri, 1996). Isolated amnesia is often described as semantic amnesia since the disturbed memory is primarily related to difficulties in the recall of the meaning and conceptual and functional properties of words, objects, and events. Patients who experience isolated amnesia differ from those who suffer from Wernicke-Korsakoff's syndrome in that anterograde amnesia is less prominent, there is an absence of apathy, and there is a preservation of insight and of ori-

451

Memory Disorders:
Disturbances of the
Major Supportive
System of Brain
Information
Processing

entation in time, place, and person. Patients with isolated amnesia do have some similarities with hippocampal amnesic patients. While the etiology remains unclear, a degenerative process seems to be the most probable cause of memory disorders in such cases. Similar cases of isolated memory disorders were described as a focal onset of dementia of Alzheimer's type in several cases (Becker, Huff, Nebes, Holland, & Boller, 1988; Haxby, Raffaele, Gillette, Schapiro, & Rapoport, 1992; Weintraub & Mesulam, 1993).

Kritchevsky and Squire (1993) reported three patients, each with a 5–6 year history of isolated amnesia that extended back more than 20 years. Severe learning difficulties were observed in both verbal and nonverbal tests. MRI data revealed that the hippocampus was reduced in size in all three patients. Circular lucency on T1 weighted images was observed in the left inferior thalamus (a small subependimal cyst) in one of the cases.

Tanabe et al. (1994) described several patients with progressive isolated amnesia. SPECT data revealed hypoperfusion of medial aspects of the bilateral temporal lobes. CT and MRI scans showed different degrees of enlargement of the temporal horn, reflecting atrophy of the hippocampal region.

Lucchelli, De Renzi, Perani, and Fazio (1994) described a 69-year-old patient with amnesia characterized by insidious onset, slow progression and subsequent stabilization, impairment of knowledge of past events over the previous 2 or 3 years, and difficulties in the verbal recall of stories. CT and MRI scans did not reveal any brain atrophy. PET scan data revealed hypometabolism in the anterior and middle sections of the left thalamus as well as the temporal mesial region on the left.

For 8 years, Caffarra and Venneri (1996) followed the case of a 72-year-old patient with isolated memory disorders. The patient was tested via neuropsychological test batteries and obtained high standard scores on all tests assessing language, intelligence, short-term memory, and attention but failed all long-term memory tests. MRI scans revealed mild cortical and bilateral hippocampal atrophy, and a PET scan detected bilateral hypometabolism of the hippocampal regions and of the thalamus, the hypometabolism of which was more marked on the left.

Transient Global Amnesia

Stillhard, Landis, Schiess, Regard, and Sialer (1990) performed a SPECT scan on a patient both during and after a TGA attack and found evidence of transient hypoperfusion of both medial-temporal brain structures. Tanaba et al. (1991) also performed a SPECT scan on a patient both during and after a TGA attack and noted a reduction in cerebral

452

LOCALIZATION
OF CLINICAL
SYNDROMES IN
NEUROPSYCHOLOGY
AND NEUROSCIENCE

blood flow in the medial temporal lobes, including the hippocampus. Though cerebral blood flow returned to normal after the attack, an MRI scan detected a circumscribed lesion in the middle of the left hippocampus. Evans et al. (1993) reported the results of a SPECT scan of a patient with TGA. During the attack, the scan revealed a bilateral focal reduction in cerebral perfusion in the posterio-medial temporal lobe, though this reduction had been normalized 7 weeks after the attack. Lin, Liu, Yeh, Wang, and Liu (1993) reported the SPECT results of a patient 6 hours into a TGA attack. The scan indicated multiple perfusion defects in the medial temporal lobe, the left thalamus, and both occipital lobes. Perfusion defects returned to normal within 28 days post-TGA. Hodges (1994) reported a patient whose SPECT scan revealed focal left temporal lobe hypoperfusion during a TGA attack, though the problem had corrected itself in 3 months. Kazui et al. (1995) also found evidence via SPECT scans of hypoperfusion confined to the medial portion of the bilateral temporal lobes only, during TGA attacks in four patients.

Baron et al. (1994) performed a PET scan on a patient and noted a reduction in right frontal blood flow during the acute (early recovery) phase after a TGA attack. This was combined with some reduction of blood flow in the right thalamic and lentiform nuclei. Again, blood flow had returned to normal 3 months after the attack. The role of the hypoperfusion of the frontal lobe in TGA was not supported by the neuropsychological data reported by Hodges (1994). In Hodges's report, though the patient's anterograde memory was affected during the TGA attack, there was no accompanying disturbance in semantic memory nor any deficit in performance on tests known to be sensitive to frontal executive dysfunction (Hodges, 1994). Further, Regard and Landis (1984) and Evans et al. (1993) noted a discrepancy between profound loss of episodic memory and preserved semantic memory during TGA attacks.

Reduplicative Paramnesia

Malloy and Richardson (1994) presented anatomical data taken from reports of 18 focal cases that had been reported in the literature at that time. Neuroimaging data pointed to the involvement of the right hemisphere in 15 of the 18 cases. Lesions of the frontal lobe were reported in 9 cases, including 5 patients with bilateral damage and 4 patients with unilateral frontal lobe damage in the right hemisphere. In 7 of the 9 frontal lobe cases, the lesions extended to the posterior parts of the hemispheres, including the parietal, temporal, and occipital lobes. These extensions were noted in both hemispheres, but primarily in the right hemisphere. In 1 case only, the lesion was limited to the posterior parts of the right hemisphere without accompanying involvement

453

*Memory Disorders:
Disturbances of the
Major Supportive
System of Brain
Information
Processing*

of the frontal lobe, and an infarction was found in the right occipito-parietal area via neuroimaging (Fisher, 1982). Isolated damage to the frontal lobe was observed in 3 cases, including 2 cases with a unilateral right frontal lesion (Kapur, Turner, & King, 1988; Ruff & Volpe, 1981) and 1 case with a bilateral frontal lesion with more prominent involvement of the right hemisphere (Benson et al., 1976, Case 1). The lesions involved the right hemisphere in all 16 cases, including 5 cases with bilateral right and left hemisphere damage. No cases with unilateral damage to the left hemisphere were reported.

Thus, an analysis of the neuroimaging data on 16 cases of reduplicative paramnesia reported in the literature (Malloy & Richardson, 1994, see Table 1) revealed that lesions of the right hemisphere were involved in the development of amnesia in all cases. However, it remains unclear which damaged parts of the right hemisphere may be responsible for that development. Lesions in most of the cases extended from the frontal lobes to the temporo-parietal region, while isolated lesions of the frontal lobe were reported in 3 of the 16 cases and an isolated lesion of the occipito-parietal region was observed in one case. A possible role of general confusion in the development of reduplicative paramnesia must be considered, since most of the reported cases were observed in the acute stages of either cerebral hemorrhage or head injury. Further studies are needed.

CONCLUSIONS

1. Two major sites of neural damage have been described in patients with anterograde and retrograde amnesia. These sites include (a) the mesodiencephalic region, primarily the mammillary body and the thalamic medial dorsal nuclei; and (b) the medial temporal lobe, mainly the hippocampal nuclei. It seems that the amount of damage to the mediodorsal thalamic nuclei that produces amnesia has to exceed some baseline amount, and involvement of the anterior thalamic nuclei and the mammillothalamic tract may be required for the development of amnesia (Figure 8.1).

2. Damage to the fornix, which connects the anterior thalamic nuclei and the mammillothalamic tract, may also be found in cases of mild amnesia. However, memory disturbances may be completely absent in some patients with lesions of the fornix.

3. Bilateral frontal lobe lesions were also described in some cases of anterograde and retrograde amnesia. Nevertheless, amnesia in such cases may be secondary to a sense of apathy and a prominent loss of motivation, both of which are usually seen in patients with massive bilateral frontal lobe lesions. Lesions causing amnesia in patients with hippocampal or mesodiencephalic amnesia

454

LOCALIZATION
OF CLINICAL
SYNDROMES IN
NEUROPSYCHOLOGY
AND NEUROSCIENCE

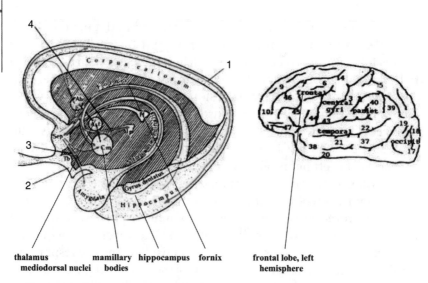

thalamus   mamillary hippocampus fornix   frontal lobe, left
  mediodorsal nuclei   bodies   hemisphere

FIGURE 8.1 Primary sites of lesion localizations in amnestic disorders. Frontal lobe lesions are often bilateral. H = habenula; Ip = interpeduncular nucleus; Tb = tuberculum olfactorium; Olf = bulbus olfactorius; Cm = corpora mamillaria; At = nucleus anterior thalami; Ah = nucleus anterior hypothalami; Sep = septum pallucidum; 1. = stria supracallosa; 2. = stria olfactoria lateralis; 3. = diagonal band of Broca; 4. = fasciculus medialis. Details are given in the text.

tend to be rather small in comparison with the large, extended lesions in patients with frontal lobe amnesia. In fact, memory disturbances and other signs of cognitive decline are often quite difficult to recognize in patients with less extended frontal lobe lesions. It is possible that the large amount of cerebral tissue in the frontal lobe allows for its use in long-term information storage, which may be destroyed via extended damage to the frontal lobes. At the same time, the mechanisms for the retrieval of information that requires a relatively small storage space may be located in the hippocampal and mesodiencephalic regions. Small lesions in these areas may result in disturbances of episodic and semantic memory due to an inability to retrieve particular items of information from storage in the frontal lobes.

4. The confabulations that tend to accompany amnestic syndromes result from lesions of the mesodiencephalic region. Confabulations have also been frequently described in cases of frontal lobe lesions.

5. Isolated anterograde amnesia frequently develops as a result of lesions in many sites of the memory circuit, often in response to relatively small lesions, such as lesions limited to the CA1 area of the hippocampus. The basal forebrain and its adjacent areas include

455

Memory Disorders:
Disturbances of the
Major Supportive
System of Brain
Information
Processing

another site in which lesions may result in anterograde amnesia. Cases of isolated retrograde amnesia have been observed most frequently in patients with bilateral temporal lesions, primarily of the anterior temporal lobe. These lesions usually involve either the hippocampal or the parahippocampal regions and are more extensive than those observed in patients with isolated anterograde amnesia (Zola, 2000).

6. According to CT, MRI, and SPECT scans, hypoperfusion and brain atrophy are usually detected in the hippocampi, in the temporal lobes, and in some cases in the thalamus in patients suffering from isolated amnesia, pointing to the location of lesions described in patients with more severe experiences of anterograde and retrograde amnesia.

7. A reduction in blood flow in the medial temporal lobes, the right frontal lobe, and the thalamus was observed on a SPECT scan during TGA attacks in the regions either adjacent to or inside the brain structures that are damaged in cases of persistent retrograde and anterograde amnesia. Yet blood flow had returned to normal at some point between 1 and 3 months after the attacks.

DISTURBANCES OF MODULAR MEMORY FOR RECOGNITION AND ACTION

THE FUNCTIONAL ROLE of modular memory significantly differs from the functional properties of episodic and semantic memory. Modular memory is involved in the recognition of real objects, words, and simple and complex features as well as their sequences. In other words, modular memory serves the operations underlying actions involving real stimuli in the outside world. The descriptions of the items stored in modular memory are compared with salient features of single items or their sequences in the course of recognition. This item recognition is an implicit process and occurs without conscious, explicit retrieval of those memory items in the process of recognition or in the course of action. The conscious part of this process includes only the actual recognition or action.

The functional roles of episodic memory and semantic memory are quite different. Episodic memory is used to store memories of events and semantic memory is used to store acquired knowledge. Both types of memories may be retrieved for conscious, explicit recall, usually verbal or visual, and used for the orientation of the self and one's interactions with the outside world.

Modular memory has its own long-term model storage capability that is used in the process of recognition and action. In order to

456

LOCALIZATION
OF CLINICAL
SYNDROMES IN
NEUROPSYCHOLOGY
AND NEUROSCIENCE

make recognition or action realistically possible, this storage must include a restricted number of models for the conventional information processing of high frequency items. Unconventional information processing—for example, the recognition of occluded objects, words, and sequences, and especially the recognition of novel information and the learning of new actions—requires an ability to adjust stored models in response to such operations as well as an ability to add new models to that storage. Modular memory is also involved in the process of describing features of items and comparing them with models stored at the different bidirectional stages of recognition and action.

Some of the operations involved in modular memory during the course of learning to recognize novel information and in reacting to the new information have been studied as part of research into procedural memory and priming.

DISTURBANCES OF PRIMING

Clinical Aspects

Priming may be considered to be an extension and clarification of two previously used terms: registration and immediate memory. Priming has been intensively studied and discussed in terms of patients with amnesia for episodic and semantic memories and has been at times described, especially in clinical studies, as long-term memory.

Priming is defined as the facilitation of object identification on a subsequent occasion due to prior exposure to the object (Schacter, 1995; Tulving, 1995). For instance, prior exposure to a target word significantly facilitates the task of judging whether a letter string constitutes real words or nonwords. In tasks of perceptual identification, the subject is asked to identify studied and nonstudied words that are presented quickly on the computer screen. Another example of priming is a fragment completion task, sometimes in the form of word stem completion. In such tasks, the subject studies a list of words and then is presented with both studied and nonstudied words in fragmented or word stem forms for completion by the subject (e.g., —NC—R, or ANC—, for ANCHOR). Normal subjects find this task much easier when the word fragments are incomplete versions of words that were previously studied rather than that were not previously studied.

Priming Disturbances

It may be suggested that priming in such tests facilitates recognition by limiting the choices of prototypes stored in modular memory. Rather than the word (or sometimes object) fragments being compared with a relatively large number of prototypes, the choices for comparison are limited to the few primed items. This may cause the subject to focus

457

*Memory Disorders:
Disturbances of the
Major Supportive
System of Brain
Information
Processing*

on the salient features of primed words or objects. In real-life situations, the facilitation of recognition via priming helps individuals detect and recognize occluded objects or words. This is reflected in such commonly used expressions as "giving a hint" or "knowing what you are looking for." The mental operations underlying priming may be especially helpful in patients with disturbances of object or word recognition related to impairments in the selection and description of features needed for the recognition of a particular item, especially an item with an incomplete set of available features. Disturbances in priming, however, have primarily been mentioned as somewhat unreliable experiences in amnesic patients, who usually exhibit disturbances in declarative memory accompanied by preserved priming capabilities, so to speak. Priming disturbances were consistently found in patients who had Alzheimer's disease, usually characterized by extensive cortical and limbic structural damage (Butters, 1978). However, no systematic studies of priming disturbances have yet been conducted in patients with relatively circumscribed cortical lesions.

Perceptual and word repetition priming has been used in a series of studies of working memory. A typical example of such a test is the auditory presentation of a string of digits, usually six in number. The subject is then asked to repeat the digits. When the digits are repeated correctly, the string is extended by 1 digit. Normal subjects are often able to repeat correctly up to 20 digits, usually in less than 15 trials (Squire, 1987). Those who have disturbances in working memory for words are often unable to repeat correctly a string of more than 6 or 7 digits. The patient with amnesia becomes unable to retain all of a previously learned string of 6 or 7 digits in working memory once a new set of digits is presented. In a study by Drachman and Arbit (1966), for example, researchers first read a list of 5 digits to five amnesic patients. The number of digits presented was then extended in subsequent trials. After 25 trials, none of the amnesic patients was able to recall correctly more than 12 digits. Similar priming tests have been used to study visual object memory.

Some preliminary data on priming disturbances have been collected in our studies of patients who have disturbances in the recognition of incomplete pictures of objects. We studied priming in such patients (Tonkonogy, 1997) using the subtest Recognition of Incomplete Pictures from our battery titled Brief Neuropsychological Cognitive Examination (BNCE). Each subject was asked first to identify four objects that were represented by incomplete pictures, then to identify complete pictures of the same objects. After this priming task, incomplete pictures of the same four objects were shown again (Figure 8.2). The number of correct and erroneous responses was calculated during each of the three stages of the task. Types of errors were also recorded.

458

LOCALIZATION
OF CLINICAL
SYNDROMES IN
NEUROPSYCHOLOGY
AND NEUROSCIENCE

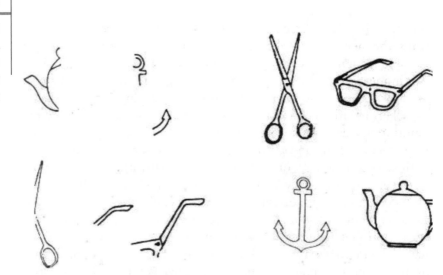

FIGURE 8.2 Left: Incomplete pictures of four objects. Right: Complete pictures of the same four objects, but arranged in a different manner. See text for further explanation.

The recognition of incomplete pictures has been found to be most prominently disturbed in patients with occipital and posterior-inferior temporal lesions caused by either a stroke or a tumor. We excluded from further analysis the findings obtained from some of the patients who suffered from visual object agnosia, and who thus found it impossible to recognize most of the complete pictures of the objects. Errors in the recognition of incomplete pictures often consisted of, for example, the erroneous recognition of a teapot as a shoe and an anchor as a traffic sign. Other errors included the erroneous recognition of a pair of glasses as a hockey stick and a pair of scissors as a screwdriver. During the next stage of testing, the patients recognized the complete pictures of the objects without difficulty. They were not required to memorize the images of these objects. The recognition of complete pictures usually improved during the third stage after priming during the second stage. The recognition of one or two and sometimes all four objects, however, was not facilitated by the priming characterized by the recognition of all four complete pictures of the objects. Recognition was instead probably related to the individual's inability to reconstruct the set of salient features needed to recognize an object in spite of a limited number of prototypes of the four objects. The recognition of these objects was possibly improved by priming. On the other hand, since the patients were able to recognize the complete pictures of all four objects using the full set of features needed for recognition, it may be suggested that priming was impaired as a way to facilitate the

459

*Memory Disorders:
Disturbances of the
Major Supportive
System of Brain
Information
Processing*

ability to reconstruct the missing features of the incomplete pictures of the objects. Such disturbances may certainly be modality specific and thus completely unrelated to the ability to recall all the objects presented during priming, as would be required for preserved declarative memory.

Another, rarer type of observed disturbances in priming is related to the inability to keep in one's memory the prototypes activated by priming. An example of such priming disturbances is provided by a patient, one of our own, who was unable to recognize any of the four incomplete pictures of objects but correctly recognized each of the full pictures. When confronted again with the same incomplete pictures, the patient was able to recognize the objects only via the comparison of the incomplete pictures of each object with the complete pictures of the four objects. This disturbance thus exemplifies impairment of priming in the activation of prototypes stored in modular memory.

Other studies have shown that priming, in addition to being used in the activation of stored memory, may be used during the course of implicit recognition of novel items that do not have preexisting representations, such as the nonword KHSF (Hamann & Squire, 1997; Keane, Gabrieli, Mapstone, Johnson, & Gorkin, 1995) or a newly associated pair of words. Instead of facilitating the recognition of studied words with prototypes already stored in memory models, priming leads to the formation of a new prototype in model memory, though probably only for the duration of the testing. This prototype may be constructed as a sequence of letters or words based on already existing models for the recognition of individual letters or words.

We also studied the formation of new prototypes during the course of priming via the use of the subtest Recurrent Figures from the BNCE (Tonkonogy, 1997). Each subject was asked to copy figures formed by sequences of triangular and rectangular shapes. After the subject finished copying the particular figure, the sample was removed and the subject was asked to draw the figure without seeing the sample again. The test is quite simple for the normal participant, as no difficulties were observed in normal controls. The copying of recurrent figures was frequently preserved in patients with Alzheimer's disease or Huntington's disease. The same patients, however, often incorrectly completed drawings of the figures after a 5-sec sample presentation. After a priming exercise of copying the figure, patient L.R., who had Alzheimer's disease, correctly drew the basic components of the figure—a triangular shape and a rectangular shape—but their sequence was incorrect (Figure 8.3).

Thus, patient L.R. was able to prime the basic components of the sequence using the prototypes of those components stored in memory. Priming was disturbed, however, when L.R. attempted to create

460

LOCALIZATION
OF CLINICAL
SYNDROMES IN
NEUROPSYCHOLOGY
AND NEUROSCIENCE

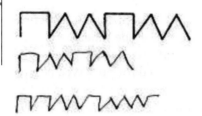

FIGURE 8.3 A drawing of sequences by a patient in the early stages of Alzheimer's disease. Top: Sample. Middle: A copy drawn while directly viewing the sample. Bottom: A copy drawn from memory after a 5-sec delay.

prototypes of the sequences of the components. L.R. was also unable to give a correct verbal description of the sequences. He described them as combinations of vertical and horizontal lines, despite his ability to draw correctly from memory a simple sequence of one rectangle and one triangle. This stresses the implicit nature of the test performance.

Another patient, J.M., had Huntington's disease and experienced difficulty attempting to directly copy recurrent figures. J.M. was also unable to prime the figures due to his inability to recognize the sequences used in the process of priming (Figure 8.4). It must be stressed that the task of drawing a copy of recurrent figures is based on operations that are different from those that are required for constructional praxis tasks, despite the relative complexity of the two tasks. J.M. was able to copy correctly the complex figure used in our constructional praxis subtest of the BNCE (Tonkonogy, 1986). These differences may be related to the fact that the repetition of sequences composed of two or three basic elements is different from a task of constructional praxis, in which the basic element is a line, rather than a sequence of two or three basic elements.

These difficulties in the priming of sequences were described by Luria (1966), who originally used the test of recurrent figures and demonstrated disturbances in the drawing of recurrent figures from memory after a delay of 5 sec or upon verbal instruction. Though Patient A, who had a tumor of the left frontal lobe, was able to copy single figures of circles and crosses, the patient could not draw correctly from memory the series of shapes (a circle-cross sequence was incorrectly drawn as cross-circle, and a triangle-circle sequence was incorrectly drawn as circle-circle).

In other cases, Luria observed disturbances in the drawing of single figures. A patient known as Step drew a minus sign as a small, elongated rectangle, while the patient known as Kur drew a dot as a small circle. We recorded these types of disturbances as demonstrated by patient J.G., who had Korsakoff's syndrome. The patient drew the sequences perfectly, but the comparative sizes of the figures were re-

Anatomical Aspects

Hamann and Squire (1997) studied patient E.P., who had bilateral damage to the medial temporal lobe as a result of herpes simplex encephalitis. E.P. was severely amnesic and exhibited prominent disturbances of declarative memory. The patient performed normally on the two priming tests—perceptual identification of words and word stem completion. Severe disturbances, however, were recorded for recognition tasks that examined declarative memory via two alternative forced-choice tasks and yes-no recognition tasks.

It must be stressed that priming is not the only way in which brain information processing facilitates recognition. This facilitation may be achieved even in the absence of priming, via semantic, functional connections between objects and words, for example, in the recognition of objects in a kitchen or of an expected word in sentences.

Some preliminary data point to the posterior neocortex as an anatomical locus of perceptual priming. Schacter and Bucjner (1998) found less activation in the posterior neocortex on both PET and fMRI (functional magnetic resonance imaging) scans for primed items than for unprimed items. Similar results were reported earlier based on the use of PET scans (Squire 1987). This decrease in activation is explained as a result of a diminished demand for resources needed to process material after priming has left a trace in the visual pathway (Squire & Knowlton, 1995).

However, since priming is involved in the operations of various modules, the localization of lesions may differ for priming disturbances in different tasks and modalities. Our data show that disturbances of priming in the recognition of incomplete pictures were usually observed in patients with posterior-inferior temporal and occipital lesions. (For more details, see chapter 2, section titled "Visual Agnosia.") It may be expected that priming for words will be disturbed in cases with superior-posterior temporal lesions. Frontal lobe lesions may also be responsible in some such cases, especially for the development of priming disturbances in tests with recurrent figures. Luria (1966) showed that patients with anterior frontal lesions developed disturbances in the ability to draw simple sequences from memory, while an extension of the lesion to deep subcortical structures, including the basal ganglia, led to a motor impairment in the drawing of single figures. We observed such a combination of disturbances in patient J.M. after priming the single figures and their sequences (Figure 8.4). MRI scans revealed atrophy of the caudate nuclei as well as mild cortical frontoparietal atrophy. In the drawings completed by patient J.G., another individual who had Korsakoff's amnesic syndrome with a probable lesion outside the cortical areas,

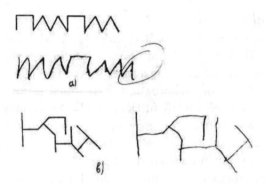

FIGURE 8.4 Drawings by patient J.M., who had Huntington's disease. (a) Th
of the sequence and the direct copy as drawn by the patient. Note that the nu
triangles increased from two to three in the patient's drawing. The first squar
omitted completely. (b) The sample figure used in the testing of constructiona
accompanied by the patient's correct drawing.

FIGURE 8.5 A direct copy of the simple
sequence of triangles and squares as drawn
by patient J.G., who had Korsakoff's amnesic
syndrome. Note the smaller size of the
triangles compared to the size of the squares
in the patient's drawing.

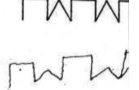

produced incorrectly—the triangles were smaller than the re
(Figure 8.5).

Changes in single figures may intensify difficulties in copyii
sequences. After priming, patient J.M., the patient with Hun
disease, was unable to draw a simple rectangle-triangle seque
drew instead an inverted rectangle.

The data described above show that priming is implicitly
in various operations of modules for recognition and actio
operations include the limitation of choices during the con
of features of objects or words with the prototypes stored i
lar memory, as well as the formation of prototypes during th
of unconventional information processing for either the rec
of novel items or the formation of new actions. These operai
implicit, or beyond the level of consciousness. It may thus be
that various types of priming may be preserved in patients w
disturbances in declarative memory.

463

Memory Disorders:
Disturbances of the
Major Supportive
System of Brain
Information
Processing

the comparative sizes of the single figures in the sequences were reflected incorrectly, while the actual sequences of figures were correctly reproduced.

Disturbances of Procedural Memory

The definition of procedural memory is closely related to that of the term *sensorimotor coordination*. This term was used in studies of conditioning and when considering disturbances of praxis, known as apraxia (for a review, see Luria, 1966; for more details, see chapter 6). Patients with amnesia of declarative, episodic, and semantic memory performed at a normal level on tasks for the evaluation of procedural memory. Procedural memory is thus considered to be independent from declarative memory (for a review, see Squire & Knowlton, 1995).

Procedural memory is based on the ability to learn a procedure after it is repeated a certain number of times. The procedure involves a particular motor program that is connected to a specific perceptual task. An example of procedural memory is a simple reaction task in which the subject must learn to rapidly press one of four keys as soon as a light above the particular key is illuminated (Nissen & Bullemer, 1987). In both normal subjects and amnesic patients, reaction time for key presses decreases and accuracy of performance increases after the sequence is repeated several times (for a review, see Squire, Knowlton, & Musen, 1993).

Another example of procedural memory tasks is the pursuit-motor tracking task, which requires the subject to keep a stylus within a circle measuring 2 centimeters in diameter. The circle is off-center on a rotating disc that is 25.5 centimeters in diameter and rotates and stops in 20-sec intervals. The subject completes six blocks of four trials, and the total time required for each of the four trials is recorded (Heindel, Salmon, Shults, Walicke, & Butters, 1989). The performance of amnesic patients on this task does not differ from that of normal subjects.

Disturbances in Sensorimotor Procedural Learning. The tasks described above are sensorimotor, skill-based tasks that require the preservation of the ability to form motor programs closely connected with sensory and visual information in the course of the learning and performance of actions. Disturbances in the learning of such actions have been described as being a result of striate lesions in patients with Huntington's disease (Heindel, Butters, & Salmon, 1988; Knopman & Nissen, 1991) and in patients with Parkinson's disease. Since these tests require the preservation of some primary motor skills, however, impairments in visual-motor coordination in simple reaction time tasks, and especially in pursuit motor-tracking tasks, may be mediated or perhaps even underlain by the dyskinesia experienced in Huntington's disease, or the bradykinesia experienced in Parkinson's disease. Pastpointing and tremors related to cerebellar involvement must be taken into account (for a review, see Thompson, 1990; see also chapter 3, on recognition of actions).

Lesions of the higher cortical visual and motor structures of modular memory, for example, in the parietal and frontal lobes, could also be responsible for disturbances in performance on the test described above. Based on studies of conventional information processing, for example, grasping in monkeys (Rizzolatti et al., 2000), it may be suggested that procedural memory tasks that use verbal descriptions consist of several operations directed to the formation of new prototypes in the storage of visual models and of motor programs or vocabularies of actions, as well as in the formation of connections between the prototypes in visual memory storage and the particular programs or "words" in the newly formed vocabulary of actions. (For more details, see chapter 6.) Disturbances in procedural memory tasks may thus result from impairments in the abilities (a) to form and use the new prototype in the visual memory storage, (b) to store new vocabularies of actions, and (c) to recognize their interconnections.

The role of disturbances in (a) is especially apparent in the mirror-tracing task, when the subject is asked to trace the outline of a star pattern reflected in a mirror. This task requires a preserved spatial orientation that may be disturbed by parietal and/or frontal lesions. The role of lesions of the frontal lobes and the deep subcortical structures in (b) has been demonstrated by Luria in his studies of the kinetic melody, which is based on such tests as the fist-edge-palm test and the fist-ring test (Luria, 1966). Disturbances in (c), sensorimotor connections, were explored in the massive amount of literature that focused on conditioning. However, the separation of those conduction disturbances from direct impairments of recognition and motor action processing remains difficult and is often illusive.

More abstract tasks used for the testing of procedural memory include, for example, probabilistic classification-learning tasks, in which the subject tries to predict one of two disease outcomes based on a set of one to four symptoms that are probabilistically associated with each outcome (Gluck & Bower, 1988). A learning task of artificial grammar rules requires the participant to view certain letter strings as he or she is told about the underlying rule system. Then the participant is asked to judge if the strings reflect or do not reflect the rules (Reber, 1989). These tasks are primarily targeted toward the perceptual component of procedural learning and are related to the learning of sequence recognition as a part of unconventional information

465

Memory Disorders:
Disturbances of the
Major Supportive
System of Brain
Information
Processing

processing, which is described in detail in chapter 3, section titled "Agnosia of Action."

Our own studies of procedural memory were conducted according to the schools of Pavlov and Bechterev and were derived from the concept of conditioning certain motor responses to simple stimuli and their sequences. These studies have been conducted in patients with circumscribed cortical lesions caused by strokes or, in some cases, by tumors.

The number of trials needed to form the correct response was scored, as was the stability of conditioning. Reaction times were not measured. These studies used the go–no go paradigm, in which the individual presses the button for an answer of yes and does not press the button for an answer of no in response to the auditory or visual signals. The examiner answers to the correct response by saying "correct," and to a wrong response by saying "error." At the end of each successful series of testing, the subject was asked to verbally describe the connection.

Auditory signals were based on a reference tone of 200 Hz, in response to which the subject had been instructed to push a button, and a different tone, such as 300 Hz, in response to which the subject had been instructed not to push the button. The number of trials needed for each subject to correctly perform the test without error was recorded. The task required the subject to memorize the reference tone using his or her auditory memory, and thus allowed researchers to examine disturbances in auditory procedural memory for tone pitch in patients with different localizations of brain lesions.

A disturbance in the number of learning trials required to successfully complete this task was first noticed in children with Wernicke's aphasia due to a lesion of the superior-posterior temporal lobe (Traugott, 1959). A similar increase in the number of trials was also reported in adult patients with Wernicke's aphasia that had developed after a cerebral infarction in the posterior T1 area (Dorofeeva & Kaidanova, 1969; Kabelyanskaya, 1957; Kaidanova & Meerson, 1961). Some of the patients tested by Kaidanova and Meerson (1961) were unable to learn the correct response or to differentiate between a tone of 200 Hz and a tone of up to 700 Hz. The number of trials required to achieve a response without error was generally two to three for patients with Broca's aphasia and seven to nine for patients with Wernicke's aphasia. This pointed to the role of disturbances in the procedural learning component of auditory memory due to a lesion in the left posterior T1 area, which is a lesion usually seen in patients with Wernicke's aphasia.

A similar increase in the number of trials needed to perform a task of differentiation between visual stimuli of varying orders of angles,

466

LOCALIZATION
OF CLINICAL
SYNDROMES IN
NEUROPSYCHOLOGY
AND NEUROSCIENCE

lines, and curves was recorded in patients with occipital lesions. Patients with Wernicke's aphasia due to a lesion of the posterior T1 area, however, performed at a normal level on these tasks. At the same time, the number of trials increased for the differentiation of a series of three tones in the last-mentioned group of patients (Dorofeeva & Kaidanova, 1969). The number of repetitions needed for the learning of visual sequences was high in patients with occipital lesions (11.5 ± 1.8 trials) but remained at a normal level for the same group in learning auditory sequences (3.6 ± 0.5). At the same time, the number of repetitions required to learn visual sequences was in the normal range for patients with Wernicke's aphasia (3.6 ± 3), while the learning of auditory sequences required a higher than normal number of repetitions (13.8 ± 1.8). Patients with premotor inferior-posterior frontal lesions of the left hemisphere learned to recognize both sequences, visual and auditory, after one or two repetitions for both visual sequences (1.7 ± 0.1) and auditory sequences (2.2 ± 0.33). Patients with parietal lesions required a higher than normal number of trials to learn both visual sequences (11.2 ± 1.3) and auditory sequences (12.2 ± 1.2).

WORKING MEMORY AND ITS DISTURBANCES

WORKING MEMORY WAS originally defined as the system for the temporary maintenance and manipulation of information, necessary for the performance of such cognitive activity as comprehension, learning, and reasoning (Baddeley, 1994; Baddeley & Hitch, 1974). The term was originally proposed by Baddeley and Hitch (1974) as an expansion of an earlier concept of a unitary short-term memory into a multicomponent working memory (Baddeley, 1998) that is capable of simultaneously storing and manipulating information while it is being processed. After processing is complete, the information is either wiped out or stored in long-term memory, thus helping to avoid overloading of the information capacities of the brain, which are daily exposed to enormous amounts of information.

While the terms priming and procedural memory reflect the final tasks of processing novel information by the modules for recognition and action, the term *working memory* refers to the operations conducted in the course of the processing of information by those modules, as well as those conducted during information coding for storage in long-term episodic and semantic memory. In this sense, working memory serves as an *operational* memory that operates with the information while it is stored for the duration of the operation. We used this term to describe disturbances of repetition in conduction aphasia as a result of a patient's inability to store and to process the information for the short time needed to translate acoustical to articulatory descriptions in order to allow the patient to repeat words and sentences.

CENTRAL EXECUTIVE AND SLAVE SYSTEMS OF WORKING MEMORY

ONE CRITICAL FUNCTION of working memory is that it helps to integrate sensory information that may arrive at different times via different channels, for example, taste and vision or sound and taste. Baddeley and Hitch (1974) proposed a model of working memory consisting of three parts, including a central executive or attention controller and two active slave systems: an articulatory system, also known as the phonological loop for speech-based information; and a visuospatial sketchpad, also known as the sketchpad for visuospatial information. The visuospatial sketchpad may be further divided into two subcomponents: pattern-based visual and spatial. Working memory is thus considered as a collection of temporary stores distributed over various cognitive subsystems but united under one central control system.

The Central Executive Part of Working Memory

The celebrated English neurologist Hughlings Jackson was probably one of the first to propose that the central nervous system functions as a vertical structure consisting of three major levels: information is represented first at a low level (spinal and brain stem), then re-represented at a middle level (motor and sensory areas of the cerebral cortex), and re-re-represented at the high level (frontal lobe region; Jackson, 1869, 1884). Goldstein (1934, 1948) later distinguished between the periphery of the cortex and the central cortex. While lesions of the cortical periphery result in disturbances of means or instruments of mental activity, damage to the central cortex leads to the impairments of abstract orientation and categorical behavior that represent the dynamic structures on the dynamic background, an idea that is in accordance with the gestalt viewpoint on the selection of figure from background. According to Goldstein, the central cortex includes primarily the frontal lobe, as well as the parietal lobe and the insula.

The concept of a central executive was advanced by Baddeley and may be considered an attempt to further develop ideas concerning the function of the "highest" or "central" level of brain information processing, in this case specifically related to the function of working memory. Following an influential article by Baddeley and Hitch (1974), the concept of working memory and the central executive as a part of working memory received special attention in subsequent publications. However, the article also provoked heated discussion, with

468

LOCALIZATION
OF CLINICAL
SYNDROMES IN
NEUROPSYCHOLOGY
AND NEUROSCIENCE

arguments against the acceptance of the central executive as a single entity (Parkin, 1998) and in support of the idea that working memory functions according to response selection rather than via a central executive (Kimberg et al., 1998).

Support for the central executive's role in working memory came from an early study by Baddeley and Hitch (1974). The memory performance of normal subjects was examined in this study in relation to digit preload. A drop in memory performance was observed when the digit preload rose above a certain level. The researchers concluded that the central executive was involved in such conditions and the results cannot be attributed to either of the slave systems. In another study, Baddeley (1988) examined disturbances in the coordination of information from separate subsystems by the central executive. Subjects were asked to memorize a span of digits while also performing pursuit tracking. Patients with Alzheimer's disease exhibited prominent difficulties in the coordination of the two tasks. Normal elderly subjects performed no differently than younger controls in the coordination of the two tasks.

Support for the existence of the an executive component of working memory was also based on Norman and Shallice's theory of the supervisory activating system (SAS), which hypothetically comes into operation when largely automatic, routine actions are insufficient. The SAS takes over in such cases and consciously redirects behavior, for example, in response to a situation of two competing routine behaviors (Norman & Shallice, 1986). Disturbances of the SAS may be used to explain signs of frontal lobe lesions such as perseveration, since dysfunction of the SAS may lead to an inability to interrupt an established response, as in the Wisconsin Card Sorting Test (WCST).

In addition to the WCST, it is claimed that disturbances of executive control have been revealed by other tests that measure the ability to overcome the routine, conventional type of response, such as the Trail Making test, Part B, from the Halstead-Reitan Neuropsychological Test Battery (Reitan & Wolfson, 1985). The test taker is required to alternate between the well-automatized sequences of numbers and letters of the alphabet. Overriding the routine is also required in the Stroop Test, when the color of the word competes with its use as a name for another color (e.g., the word *red* is printed in blue ink). Disturbances in performance on these and similar tests may be seen in patients with frontal lobe lesions. These disturbances have been considered as manifestations of *dysexecutive syndrome*.

Since dysexecutive syndrome has been frequently described as being a result of frontal lobe lesions, a critique of the concept of a central executive is primarily based on data showing that specific regions of the frontal lobe may be related to different types of tasks (Parkin,

469

*Memory Disorders:
Disturbances of the
Major Supportive
System of Brain
Information
Processing*

1998). The dorsolateral prefrontal cortex, for example, may be related to the delayed matching of visuospatial information (Goldman-Rakic, 1987), while the inferior convexity of the frontal lobe is involved in the processing of faces and specific objects (Wilson et al., 1993). The patient who has undergone a unilateral frontal lobectomy may demonstrate normal performance on dysexecutive tasks but may simultaneously suffer from disturbances in social functioning. Parkin (1998) has mentioned such examples based on functional imaging studies. Some authors have stressed the role of working memory in the various prefrontal functions, including executive control (Kimberg et al., 1998).

In answer to Parkin's conclusion (1998) that there is no localization evidence for a central executive and that different executive tasks are associated with different neural substrate[s], Baddeley (1998) departed from the traditional, more rigid understanding of the central executive as a system that is modulary and nonfractionable with a unitary anatomic location. He stressed that executive processes do not need to be unitary, referring to an article that differentiates at least eight executive subprocesses (Shallice & Burgess, 1996). Baddeley cited other current studies, such as the study of dual-task performance, that were directed to the breaking of the central executive system into components (Baddeley, Della Sala, Papagno, & Spinnler, 1997). Baddeley also extensively discussed the role of executive systems in various tasks that require the participation of attention, such as the role of the executive system in the separation of attention control from slave systems as well as in the focusing and switching of attention. Baddeley defended the use of the concept of an executive process in the question of their anatomical localization, while at the same time stressing that executive processes may be associated not only with the frontal region but also with other locations. He recognized that "patients with frontal lesions will not always show executive deficit" (Baddeley, 1998, p. 524).

Slave Systems of Working Memory

Baddeley and Hitch (1974) suggested that the central executive system integrates information from two major slave systems, which include the articulatory system, also known as the phonological loop, and the visuospatial sketchpad.

Special attention is given to the discrepancy between the ability of patients with associative agnosia and dementia to process objects, faces, and words at the presemantic levels and their inability to assign any meaning to the structural, semantic component of information. The subcomponents of the visuospatial sketchpad were considered as involved in the acquisition of pattern-based visual and spatial information.

470

LOCALIZATION
OF CLINICAL
SYNDROMES IN
NEUROPSYCHOLOGY
AND NEUROSCIENCE

The role of slave systems, however, seems to go far beyond the simple acquisition of modality-specific information. Two conclusions have been made from studies of agnosia; apraxia; aphasia; disturbances in the recognition of objects, scenes, and spaces; and impairments of actions in the physical and social world, especially for conventional information processing: These disturbances are often related to working memory disturbances at the level of well-learned operations of nonexecutive types; and they tend to result from limited lesions in the posterior hemispheres. These operations include intrinsic bottom-up processing, which leads to recognition and action and, finally, processing at the top-down level (see previous chapters). It is apparent that such a series of complicated operations could be defined as a function of slave systems. The role of the central executive seems to be directed toward the processing of unconventional information, which requires one to overcome the routine of well-learned operations. Such means are required, for example, in the process of recognition or action, which may be complicated by the occlusion of an object or scene, leading to an incomplete set of features for information processing. Special attention must thus be given to disturbances of information processing by operations in working memory, rather than to the simple acquisition or integration of information at the central and peripheral levels of working memory.

NEUROPSYCHOLOGICAL AND ANATOMICAL ASPECTS OF WORKING MEMORY DISTURBANCES

TO STUDY DISTURBANCES in information processing by operations of the working memory, we studied the processing of various types of simple and complex features of objects and sequences in patients with local brain pathology. Both unimodal and multimodal working memories were tested.

Working Memory for Simple Features
Unimodal Working Memory
   Auditory Working Memory.   To study disturbances of auditory working memory for simple features, we assessed the ability of participants to differentiate between thresholds of single tones when the pitch of a higher tone was decreased in varying intervals—from 300 Hz to 250 Hz, 220 Hz, 210 Hz, and 205 Hz—and while the reference tone remained at 200 Hz.

   An increase in the delay between tone presentation from 1 to 10 sec resulted in an increase in differential thresholds between the reference and comparison tones from 5 Hz to 18–20 Hz in patients with Wernicke's aphasia accompanied by a posterior-superior temporal le-

471

Memory Disorders:
Disturbances of the
Major Supportive
System of Brain
Information
Processing

sion. Thresholds remained at the level of 6–8 Hz in patients with Broca's aphasia resulting from a posterior F3 lesion (Kaidanova & Meerson, 1961; Tonkonogy, 1984, 1989; Tonkonogy, Dorofeeva, & Meerson, 1995). It is of interest that differential thresholds between the reference and comparison tones did not fall below 30 Hz in half of a group of 24 patients with Wernicke's aphasia studied by Dorofeeva and Kaidanova (1969). The same patients were able to recognize differences of 5 Hz between two single tones of 200 Hz and 205 Hz presented for direct comparison. (For more details, see chapter 3, section titled "Auditory Agnosia.")

An increase in differential thresholds for tone pitch in patients with Wernicke's aphasia in a condition requiring the participation of the auditory working memory may be explained by the existence of at least two parallel registers in the auditory memory for the purpose of parsing tones into corresponding small and large chunks. Auditory working memory parses pitches into small chunks of 5 Hz or less for unconventional information, and into larger chunks of 15–20 Hz for conventional information processing. Small chunks require a larger memory capacity that is less reliable and more vulnerable to destruction by a lesion in the superior-posterior part of the temporal lobe. Larger chunks of tone scale are easier to retain and much more difficult to destroy. The exact mechanisms and structures of these subdivisions of auditory memory, however, remain unclear.

Visual Working Memory. The differential thresholds method was also used in a study of visual working memory in 32 patients with visual agnosia, Gerstmann's syndrome, Wernicke's aphasia, or Broca's aphasia, each caused by infarctions in the left hemispheric occipital lobe, temporal lobe, parietal lobe, or premotor area of the frontal lobe (Meerson, 1986; Tonkonogy, 1973). Patients were asked to differentiate between angles presented with intervals of 0.5 sec, 2 sec, 5 sec, and 10 sec. Stimuli were presented on a tachistoscope screen for 0.5 sec each, and the patients were instructed to say whether two signals were identical or different. When a visual signal, such as an angle of a certain degree, was followed by a delay of 0.5 sec, 2 sec, 5 sec, or 10 sec before the presentation of another angle for comparison, the mean of the differentiation thresholds in a group of patients with occipital lesions increased to $9.6 \pm 1.4°$, 15.2, 18.0, and $22.6 \pm 7.2°$, correspondingly. In other groups of patients, the mean differential thresholds increased from 6–7° for a 0.5-sec interval to $7.6 \pm 0.08°$, $6.3 \pm 0.4°$, and $6.6 \pm 0.6°$ for a 10-sec interval in patients with parietal, posterior T1, and posterior F3 lesions, respectively. (For more details, see chapter 2, section titled "Visual Agnosia.")

The increases in visual thresholds in tests requiring the participation of the visual working memory may be explained, as in cases of

472

LOCALIZATION
OF CLINICAL
SYNDROMES IN
NEUROPSYCHOLOGY
AND NEUROSCIENCE

working memory and tone perception, by the existence of at least two subsystems of visual working memory, one of which may be disturbed by a lesion of the occipital lobe. One subsystem parses the signal into a large number of small chunks that are difficult to preserve in cases of damage. Another subsystem is more reliable, and parses signals into chunks containing 20°. In the event of damage, this subsystem is less vulnerable and better protected in the brain.

Multimodal Auditory and Visual Working Memory

Prisko (1963; an unpublished study later reported in details by Milner and Teuber, 1968) used Konorski's test to study working memory in patients who had undergone a frontal lobectomy. Subjects were asked to compare two same or different stimuli of the same modality separated by a defined delay, usually somewhere from 1 sec to 60 sec. Prisko used stimuli of visual and auditory modalities, including clicks, tones, flashes, colors, and irregular figures. Each stimulus had five values, to reduce the possibility of a verbal encoding. Patients with a unilateral right or left frontal lobectomy showed impairments in both visual (flashes and colors) and auditory (clicks and tones) modalities, while patients with a right temporal lobectomy demonstrated difficulties in the comparison of irregular figures. All tests were performed at normal levels by patients with a left temporal lobectomy. Prisko did not publish the data, however, and the results were never confirmed by the independent observers.

The results of Prisko's study may be explained by the role of a frontal lobe lesion in the development of polymodal difficulties of categorization for more complicated stimuli with increasing choices of basic values. A similar interpretation of the delayed test difficulties was suggested by Pribram and Tubbs (1967), who found that difficulties in delayed alternation tasks in animals with frontal lobe lesions may be overcome by introducing a 15-sec delay between the presentation of each pair of stimuli. The authors suggested that the delay allowed for the organization of information in the short-term memory into workable chunks, or categories. Further studies may well help to highlight the role of frontal lobe lesions in short-term memory disturbances related to the polymodal categorization of sensory information processing.

Stepien and Serpinski (1964) studied auditory and visual recent memory in five patients, each with a unilateral temporal lobectomy of 5–7 cm from the anterior tip and involving the hippocampal zone. The posterior third of the T1 area was preserved in most of the patients. Authors used a delayed pair comparison test adapted from a procedure widely used by Pavlov and his colleagues in a study of so-called delayed paired differentiation (Tonkonogy, 1973). Recent memory was studied by asking patients to differentiate between two compounded

473

*Memory Disorders:
Disturbances of the
Major Supportive
System of Brain
Information
Processing*

auditory or visual stimuli. Each stimulus was composed of two signals of the same sensory modality. When two signals in the stimulus were identical, the patient was to press the dynamometer connected to the recording instrument. The patient was instructed not to press the dynamometer when the two signals within the stimulus were different. Recent memory was tested both with and without intersignal intervals of 30 sec, 60 sec, and 120 sec. Participants were thus required to preserve the first signal in recent memory until the second signal was presented. Recent memory was also challenged by the insertion of a distraction signal in the interval between two signals.

Stepien and Serpinski (1964) found that the number of errors reached 45%–50% of trials for auditory and visual recent memory prior to surgery, an occurrence that was explained by prominent after-discharges in both temporal lobes as revealed via EEG. Recent memory deficits were completely eliminated following a unilateral temporal lobectomy, as were previously observed EEG abnormalities. The authors suggested that the bilateral hippocampal dysfunction reflected on the EEG may have been responsible for disrupting the neuronal circuit crucial for recent memory processing as well as for the recording of new information.

Some studies were limited to the testing of visual working memory and excluded auditory working memory, and vice versa, in patients who had undergone an anterior-posterior temporal lobectomy. Disturbances of working memory, however, were noted in both cases. Milner (1962, 1967) found some differences in auditory short-term memory for the perception of a series of tones in patients who had undergone a temporal lobectomy for the treatment of temporal lobe epilepsy. The lobectomy included the removal of a 4–8 cm area in the anterior-posterior parts of the temporal lobe along the base and Sylvian fissure, including the hippocampal formation. Superior-posterior parts of the temporal lobe remained preserved. Patients were presented with two series of three to five tones, presented one after another with minimal intervals between the tones, for comparison. After listening to the two series of tones, the patient was instructed to compare the varying pitches of tones. The pitches could be equal for all tones in both series or could differ in one or several tones. Patients were also asked to report the numbers of tones that differed in the two series. Though the mean number of errors did not change before or after the lobectomy, the number of errors was 23% higher in patients with a right temporal lobectomy than in those with a left temporal lobectomy. It should be stressed that this study was primarily directed toward the testing of working memory's role in tone pitch differentiation via masked noises rather than toward the comparison of sequences of tones with differences in the orders of higher and lower tone pitches.

474

LOCALIZATION
OF CLINICAL
SYNDROMES IN
NEUROPSYCHOLOGY
AND NEUROSCIENCE

Disturbances in auditory short-term memory in patients with anterior temporal lobectomies were less robust than those noted in patients with Wernicke's aphasia. Dorofeeva (1967) studied the differentiation between tones in a series that consisted of three tones. The second tone in both series ranged from 5 Hz to 150 Hz. Differential thresholds remained at 5–10 Hz in patients with Broca's aphasia but increased to 110–120 Hz in patients with Wernicke's aphasia. It is possible that the increases in the number of errors and differential thresholds in both studies are related to the masking of the tone pitch by the preceding and following tones in the sequences. Meerson (1986) studied visual working memory for angles of varying degrees in 22 patients with a right temporal lobectomy and 20 patients with a left temporal lobectomy. A resection was performed for the treatment of epilepsy and included a lobectomy from the pole of the temporal lobe to the vein of Labee. The differential thresholds for angles were 3.0 ± 0.2, 3.5 ± 0.3, and 3.5 ± 0.05 for interstimulus intervals of 0.1 sec, 5 sec, and 10 sec, respectively, in normal controls. The thresholds significantly increased for 5- and 10-sec intervals in patients with a temporal lobectomy. The differential thresholds were 3.6 ± 0.3, 8.2 ± 1.3, and 14.4 ± 2.3 for interstimulus intervals of 0.1 sec, 5 sec, and 10 sec, respectively. No significant differences were found between groups of patients with left versus right temporal lobectomies.

Working Memory for Complex Features, Geometric Figures, and Objects
Visual Working Memory. Disturbances in visual working memory for complex features composed of angles, lines, and curves of different degrees and orientations were found to be especially prominent in patients with lesions of the occipital lobe (Meerson, 1986; Tonkonogy, 1973). (These studies are described in more detail in chapter 2, section titled "Visual Agnosia.")

Visual working memory for more complex features, such as geometric figures and faces, was studied in two groups of patients: a group with right temporal lobectomies and another with frontal and parietal lobectomies. Patients were asked to find eight geometric figures, each of which had been presented earlier, from a set of 20 figures (Kimura, 1963). One condition involved comparing pairs of either identical or different geometric figures presented at increasing intervals (Prisko, 1963), while another required the patients to recognize the faces of 12 males and females, presented 1.5 to 2 min earlier, from a set of 24 photographs (Milner, 1967, 1968). Kimura (1963) found that the mean number of errors made in the recognition of geometric figures by patients with right temporal lobectomies was 1.5 more than that of patients with removed left temporal lobes, frontal lobes, or parietal lobes. The mean number of errors in patients with extirpations of the

475

*Memory Disorders:
Disturbances of the
Major Supportive
System of Brain
Information
Processing*

parietal lobe did not exceed that of a normal control group. In tasks of facial recognition (Milner, 1967, 1968), the mean number of correct responses in patients with right temporal lobectomies was 13%–18% higher than that of patients in other groups. Prisko (1963) observed that patients with right temporal lobectomies experienced difficulties in the recognition of geometric figures presented with increasing intervals of up to 60 seconds in the course of testing.

It was recently demonstrated that the prefrontal cortex contains several working memory domains, including spatial and object working memory (for a review, see Goldman-Rakic, O'Scalaidhe, & Chafee 2000). Using single-cell recording techniques, several authors found the localization for processing nonspatial information-form as well as color and spatial working memory to be in different areas of the prefrontal cortex in rhesus monkeys. Wilson et al. (1993) and O'Scalaidhe, Wilson, and Goldman-Rakic (1997) selected areas 12/45 below the principal sulcus on the inferior convexity of the prefrontal cortex for studies of nonspatial working memory in monkeys, since lesions in those areas produce disturbances in memory for the colors or patterns of stimuli (Mishkin & Manning, 1978; Passingham, 1975). Selective neuronal activity for geometric shapes and color, and more consistently for faces, was recorded in or around area 12 on the inferior convexity of the prefrontal cortex. This area was activated, for example, during a delay when the stimulus was a picture of a particular face. When monkeys had to recall the specific locations (one of eight) of small squares, the neurons that fired were located in another area above the principal sulcus, in the dorsolateral areas of 46 and 8A.

In human studies, fMRI and evoked potential recording studies showed selective activation of the inferior prefrontal cortex for the working memory of faces, as well as selective activation of the lateral and inferior prefrontal cortex for the working memory of features of objects (see e.g., Courtney, Ungerleider, Keil, & Haxby, 1997; Kelley et al., 1988). The recording studies also revealed hemispheric differences in the sites of inferior prefrontal activation. More specifically, the right hemisphere is activated when visual analysis is not aided by verbal encoding, and activation of the left inferior prefrontal area is observed with the engagement of verbal encoding (Grady et al., 1995; Kelley et al., 1988).

Goldman-Rakic et al. (2000) stressed that prefrontal areas in the inferior convexity of the prefrontal cortex involved in the visual working memory of faces and objects are connected to the TE in the inferotemporal cortex, which contains a number of cells that respond to the features of visual stimuli, including faces. The latter area is a major component of the ventral pathway for object recognition (Ungerleider & Mishkin, 1982). However, the role of these connections

476

LOCALIZATION
OF CLINICAL
SYNDROMES IN
NEUROPSYCHOLOGY
AND NEUROSCIENCE

and the differences in operations in the inferotemporal and prefrontal areas remain unclear. It is possible that the prefrontal area is used for intermittent storage in the course of more complicated operations in the other parts of the frontal lobe, including, for instance, the recognition of occluded objects or the recognition of faces in the processing of social gnostic tasks. In our studies of the recognition of occluded objects, we observed disturbances in patients with frontal lobe lesions; similar disturbances were observed by Luria (1966). (For more details, see chapter 2, section titled "Visual Object Agnosia.")

Working Memory for Speech and Language. Milner (1962, 1967) studied the memorization of two short stories and 10 pairs of words by patients with temporal, frontal, or parietal lobectomies carried out in the course of treatment for epilepsy. Patients were asked either to repeat the story or to recall the second word of the pair immediately following the presentation of the first word, 40–60 min before the surgery, and again after the lobectomy. The number of correct responses was lowest in the patients with left temporal lobectomies; the number was 50%–60% higher in patients with right temporal lobectomies. Similar results were reported in a study of dichotic listening in the same types of patients (Kimura, 1963). The patients with left temporal lobectomies were able to recall 149.9 out of 192 numbers presented, while the patients with right temporal lobectomies recalled 171.5 numbers.

Patients with aphasia (Tonkonogy, 1973) were asked to compare two vowels with interstimulus intervals of 2 sec and 15 sec. The number of errors made significantly increased in patients with Wernicke's aphasia, as well as in those with Broca's aphasia. This points to the role of efferent language systems in the working memory for speech stimuli. These systems are damaged in patients with Broca's aphasia.

Working memory appears to be specialized within the language system. The specialization of verbal working memory for assigning the syntactic structure of a sentence is discussed in detail by Caplan and Waters (1999).

Working Memory for Unimodal Sequences

Role of the Temporal and Occipital Lobes. Patients with local brain pathology exhibited differences in the differentiation of series consisting of three signals, tones with various pitches, for example, low (200 Hz), middle (1000 Hz), and high (2000 Hz) tones in a basic sequence and low (200 Hz), high (2000 Hz), and middle (1000 Hz) tones in differentiated sequences. A similar series of visual sequences included angles, lines, and curves (Meerson, 1986; Tonkonogy, 1973; Traugott & Kaidanova, 1975).

477

Memory Disorders:
Disturbances of the
Major Supportive
System of Brain
Information
Processing

Similarly, differences were noted in a subsequent series when working memory was tested after the patients learned to differentiate between sequences within either visual or auditory modalities. To test the working memory, the delay between basic and differentiated sequences was increased from 2 sec to 5 and 10 sec in subsequent series (Meerson, 1986; Tonkonogy, 1973). Both identical and differing pairs of sequences were presented in a random order. Each signal in the sequence was presented for a span of 1 sec. In patients with superior-posterior temporal lobe lesions in the left and right hemispheres, the number of errors in differentiating between three sequences of tones with a delay of 2 sec between sequences reached 15.8% and 12.5% respectively, while answers were at chance level for delays of 10 sec. No significant disturbances were recorded for visual sequences with any of the three delays. A relatively significant opposite pattern was observed in patients with left and right occipital lesions, with the number of errors for visual sequences reaching 14.8% and 10.6%, respectively, with delays of 2 sec. The numbers increased to chance level for delays of 10 sec.

Lesions of the superior-posterior temporal lobe thus resulted in unimodal disturbances of working memory for auditory sequences, while occipital lesions led to unimodal impairments of the working memory for visual sequences.

Working Memory for Multimodal Sequences
These disturbances were polimodal in patients with parietal lesions. Significant numbers of errors, 13.6% and 10.6%, were registered for visual sequences of angles, lines, and curves presented with delays of 2 sec in patients with lesions of the left and right hemispheres, respectively. A similar pattern, 14.3% and 10.6%, was noted for auditory sequences of tones, also with delays of 2 sec, in the same two groups of patients. However, an increase to delays of 5 and 10 sec did not result in a statistically significant increase in the number of errors. These multimodal, but less severe, disturbances of visual and auditory sequence differentiation were also observed in patients following a lobectomy of the right and left anterior-inferior parts of the temporal lobe (Meerson, 1986). The idea of multimodal disturbances in patients with lesions of the parietal lobe is also supported by data showing impairments in the differentiation of kinesthetic sequences in these patients.

Disturbances in the differentiation of auditory and visual sequences were more prominent in all test series in patients with lesions of the left hemisphere than in those with lesions of the right hemisphere. This may be to some extent related to the possibility of verbal encoding of the auditory and visual sequences. Such encoding may be partially impaired in patients with lesions of the left hemisphere.

478

LOCALIZATION
OF CLINICAL
SYNDROMES IN
NEUROPSYCHOLOGY
AND NEUROSCIENCE

At the same time, an increase in delay within the auditory or visual sequences did not result in a significant increase of errors made in a group of patients with parietal lobe lesions. The number of errors made did increase, however, for the differentiation of auditory sequences in patients with posterior-superior temporal lesions, and for the differentiation of visual sequences in patients with occipital lesions. This may point to the possible explanation of working memory disturbances in the differentiation of sequences of tones or colors. The differentiation of signals may be underlain by two mechanisms, the first being based on the working memory for the orders of single elements included in the sequence. This ability is impaired in cases of unimodal visual or auditory disturbances resulting from occipital or superior-posterior temporal lesions, respectively. The second mechanism includes operations that translate the description of sequences containing the orders of single auditory, visual, or kinesthetic elements into a single multimodal description of sequences that is easier to preserve in working memory and may thus be used in future operations, as in the differentiation between two sequences. Lesions in the parietal lobe or anterior-posterior temporal lobe may impair the operations or formation of such multimodal patterns of sequences, but once the pattern has been formed, it may be preserved during the delay between the presentation of two sequences, as has been shown in the study described above. At the same time, the formation of such patterns for translation into a multimodal description is impaired for auditory modalities as a result of superior-posterior temporal lesions, and for visual modalities as a result of occipital lesions. The differentiation of sequences is based on memorizing the orders of individual auditory or visual elements, which are difficult to preserve in the working memory during periods of delay. There is thus a marked increase in the number of errors during delays.

Working Memory for Space Position and Orientation
The role of damage to the frontal lobes in various disorders of working memory requires further exploration, especially in view of the suggestion that the frontal lobe plays a special role in the working memory of simultaneously presented multimodal stimuli (Baddeley, 1994). Some data point to the preservation of auditory and visual working memory in patients with Broca's aphasia, as well as in patients with lesions of the premotor region of the left frontal lobe. Patients with prefrontal lesions, however, have not yet been systematically studied in relation to possible disturbances of auditory or visual working memory.

Disturbances in the order of spatial working memory following lesions of the frontal lobe were first revealed via animal studies. Jacobsen

479

*Memory Disorders:
Disturbances of the
Major Supportive
System of Brain
Information
Processing*

(1935, 1936) showed that monkeys with frontal lobe lesions failed, after a delay, to select the box containing food from two covered boxes placed side by side in front of each monkey. Both of the uncovered boxes, with and without food, were situated in the same right-left position and shown to the monkeys prior to the delay. In a more complicated delayed alternation task, the food was placed in the alternate box during the delay if the previous response was correct. A series of studies echoed Jacobsen's original experiments, and the roles of attention, motivation, and lately kinesthetic disorders, rather than memory deficits, were suggested as an explanation of disturbances in the delayed alternation test (Konorski, 1967).

Jacobsen's studies concerning the role of the frontal lobe in spatial working memory were later continued using single-unit recording from neurons in Walker's areas 46 and 8A above the principal sulcus (for a review, see Goldman-Rakic et al., 2000). Rhesus monkeys were trained to store spatial information about the location of eight small squares for a brief period. At the end of the delay, each monkey was rewarded for shifting its gaze to the particular position that a square occupied. Neuronal activity in the various regions of the brain was recorded while the animal performed the task. It was found that the cells active only during the period of delay were located in prefrontal areas 46 and 8A above the principal sulcus (Funahashi, Bruce, & Goldman-Rakic, 1989).

Similarly, fMRI and evoked potential studies in humans showed that most active areas in spatial working memory seemed to be anterior to the frontal eye fields (Courtney, Petit, Maisog, Ungerleider, & Haxby, 1998; for a review, see Goldman-Rakic et al., 2000). These data support a multiple domain hypothesis of prefrontal functional architecture with superior localization of spatial processing and inferior localization of object processing, especially faces. The multiple domain hypothesis is also supported by human imaging studies showing that the lateralization of verbal processing tasks, including word generation, object naming, and word encoding, activate the inferior, insular, and anterior prefrontal regions in the left hemisphere (Kapur et al., 1994; Kelley et al., 1988).

However, some authors used PET to study orientation working memory for grating presented in the central visual field, showing that the maintenance of orientation involves not only the left and right superior frontal sulci but also the bilateral ventral prefrontal cortex (Cornette, Dupont, Salmon, & Orban, 2001). At the same time, the updating of orientation involved, according to this study, the dorsolateral prefrontal cortex and the medial superior frontal sulcus region. The most active areas also included the right superior parietal lobe and the bilateral precuneus.

Activation of the posterior parietal cortex was also recorded during spatial–working memory tasks in nonhuman primates (for a review, see Goldman-Rakic et al., 2000). Chaffee and Goldman-Rakic (1998) recorded the activation of neurons in both the prefrontal and parietal areas, using the same monkeys so as to eliminate individual differences between animals and the methods used in various studies. Similarities were found in delay period activity in both areas. The function of the superior prefrontal cortex was closely connected to that of the parietal cortex in the manipulation and maintenance of spatial information. No significant correlation was found between the ventro-lateral prefrontal cortex and the posterior parietal regions. It is not clear what specific roles are played by the parietal and prefrontal cortices in spatial working memory. Some authors suggest the role of the parietal cortex as providing storage buffers, while the frontal cortex may be involved in manipulative and executive functions, as well as rehearsal for the refreshing of the information stored in the parietal buffers (for a review, see Smith & Jonides, 1999). This singles out the frontal cortex areas as a main site for unconventional information processing.

However, in our studies of patients with local brain pathology, we found that parietal lobe lesions result in disturbances in the differentiation of angles with different orientations in space, an operation that may not require the use of spatial information stored in the buffer. Subjects were asked to assess whether the degrees of two differently oriented angles were the same or different. The differential thresholds in patients with parietal cortex lesions increased from the mean of $5.7°$ for the differentiation of angles with identical orientation to $13.5°$ for angles with different orientations. This increase remained insignificant for patients with occipital lesions (from $6.3°$ to $7.6°$), and for those with posterior-superior temporal lesions ($5.3°$ to $6.3°$). (For more details, see chapter 3, section entitled "Visuospatial Agnosia.")

It is possible that the superior prefrontal cortex plays a more prominent role in the processing of more complicated unconventional spatial information. The parietal cortex, on the other hand, processes relatively simple information. This may be accomplished by the constant rehearsal and updating of the information needed in the course of unconventional information processing by the prefrontal cortex. It must be taken into account that conventional, well-learned spatial information is processed primarily in the parietal cortex, and its various disturbances may manifest because of parietal lobe lesions. The processing of unconventional spatial information may also be observed in patients with parietal lesions. Certainly, the idea that impairments of spatial working memory are due to involvement of the frontal cortex requires further studies.

481

Memory Disorders:
Disturbances of the
Major Supportive
System of Brain
Information
Processing

CONCLUSIONS

1. Working memory disturbances may be observed as a result of lesions in various parts of the cortex. These lesions are not limited to impairments in the ability to use working memory as a slave system for the storage of information in the course of processing by the central executive. The disturbances actually involve not only the storage but also the processing of information by various operations at different levels of working or operational memory.

2. There is a clear tendency for impairments in unimodal working memory to develop as a result of lesions in the primary visual areas for disturbances of visual working memory, and near the primary auditory areas for disturbances of auditory working memory. For instance, occipital lobe lesions lead to disturbances in visual working memory for single and complex features of objects, as well as sequences of visual signals, while auditory working memory remains either preserved or only minimally disturbed. At the same time, lesions of the superior-posterior temporal lobe result in disturbances of auditory working memory for single tones and their sequences without impairing visual working memory.

3. Disturbances in multimodal auditory and visual working memory have been observed for sequences as a result of lesions in the parietal lobe, as well as in the anterior-inferior temporal lobe. Though some of the data point to multimodal types of working memory in the frontal lobes, such studies were limited to the visual modality, and no comparison with auditory working memory is available at present.

4. Differences in the localization of lesions in unimodal and multimodal disturbances of working memory may be explained by the role of a more anterior cortical structure in the processing of unconventional information that may be facilitated by the translating of visual or auditory descriptions into descriptions by a unitary code, for example, by an anterior-temporal lobe structure. Such a unitary code is probably used by the parietal and the frontal lobes in the description of spatial- and time-related information processed in the working memory. This unitary code is impaired because of damage to those structures manifesting as disturbances of working memory for spatial position and orientation and for the differentiation of auditory and visual sequences.

5. Disturbances of the central executive may be either unimodal or multimodal and are related to operations directed to overcome well-learned routine processing of conventional information and

482

LOCALIZATION
OF CLINICAL
SYNDROMES IN
NEUROPSYCHOLOGY
AND NEUROSCIENCE

to assist in the processing of unconventional information with incomplete features (see discussions in previous chapters).

6. Certainly, the differences in operations provided by working memory in the various cortical areas require further systematic studies, especially with regard to the role of the frontal lobe in comparison to the posterior cortical areas.

9

Disturbances of Regulatory Activity: Impairments of Visually Guided Attention

I T IS REASONABLE to suggest that brain information processing must include a system that activates and regulates the operations of various modules involved in recognition and action in the physical environment, and especially in the social environment. Such a system may provide substantial savings by excluding from activation the modules and operations that do not need to be activated for particular tasks of recognition and action. While general alertness is provided by another system along the sleep-wake axis, systems of regulation and activation are targeted toward more specific, particular operations participating in the interaction of brain information processing with both the outside and inside worlds. This includes regulation of recognition and action by attention, volition, and emotions. In pathological conditions, damage to the parts of such a system may manifest as disturbances in the activation of particular modules and operations. While the inner structures remain preserved in such cases, they cannot be used properly by brain information processing in the course of recognition, action, and communication.

DISTURBANCES OF VISUALLY GUIDED ATTENTION AND VISUAL AGNOSIA

B RAIN INFORMATION PROCESSING operates in a way that prevents an overloading of its capabilities by receiving information at low levels of sensory inputs, for example, retinal or cochlear cells. This system is based on the use of both simple and, especially, complex features in the process of object and scene recognition. Another way of preventing overload is based on the use of attention mechanisms to select particular information for subsequent processing. The major components of attention mechanisms are the shifting of the attention focus to the processing point, sustaining attention at the processing point for information processing, and the subsequent disengagement, unlocking the attention when information processing is complete (for a review, see Parasuraman, 1998; Ullman, 1996).

The operations performed by attention mechanisms may be summarized based on a review by Ullman (1996) in the following way: The shifting of the focus of attention may be primarily guided by parallel scanning directed toward the detection of the salient location at the scene. The properties that distinguish the salient location may include color, contrast, orientation, and some shape features. After the filtration of such properties from the surrounding noise, the focus of attention is shifted to the appropriate location and locked in there for selected information processing, for example, the recognition of letters or objects. When information processing is complete, the focus of attention is disengaged and unlocked, and may be shifted to another target in the scene. The shifting of the focus of attention is also facilitated by cueing the focus, which decreases the shifting time from the center of the fovea to the eccentric position of the target. It has been demonstrated that the focus of attention may be shifted either externally via eye movements or internally without such movements.

Disturbances of these described operations underlie the development of syndromes related to impairments in the sustaining and shifting of the visual processing focus of attention in, for example, Balint's syndrome, unilateral neglect, and disturbances in the filtration of a salient location from background noise.

Disturbances of attention have been discussed in a series of articles related to the role of executive control in brain functioning (for a review, see Posner & DiGirolamo, 2000). Norman and Shallice (1986) suggested two levels of executive control: *attention scheduling* for well-learned behavior and thoughts (compare to our "conventional information processing"); and the *supervisory attention system*, which intervenes and provides additional activation and inhibition when the situation is novel, is highly competitive, and/or cannot be solved by a routine operation of attention-scheduling mechanisms (compare to our "unconventional information processing"). According to Shallice (1994), involvement of the supervisory attention system is required for planning and decision making, error correction, novel responses, and dangerous or difficult situations, as well as for overcoming habitual responses. While researchers subsequently stressed that executive control is difficult to define since the term has been used in many ways, a discussion of attention mechanisms for stimulus and response elements may help to narrow the situation in which executive control is needed (Posner & DiGirolamo, 2000). The discussion in the following section is focused on disturbances of the attention system in overcoming well-learned, conventional responses.

DISORDER OF SHIFTING OF THE VISUAL PROCESSING FOCUS: BALINT'S SYNDROME

Clinical Aspects

Balint (1909) described a patient with what he called psychic paralysis of visual fixation. Hécaen and de Ajuriaguerra (1954) later noted three major elements of the syndrome. First, movements of the eyeballs were preserved. Problems were instead manifested as disturbances in voluntary gaze movements, since Balint's patient had to conjugate the deviation of his eyes to the right, and was only able to move them to the left when told in advance that his eyes were deviated to the right. The second element of the syndrome was optic ataxia. The patient had difficulties following the object with his gaze. He could follow the object with his right hand, but his hand was usually placed to the right of the object, and he was unable to touch or grasp the object. The third element was a peculiar disturbance of attention manifested as a difficulty in fixating on more than one object in his visual field; at the same time, the patient was able to recognize the object on which he was fixated.

Similar cases were subsequently described by Holmes (1918), Holmes and Horrax (1919), Kleist (1934), Hécaen and de Ajuriaguerra (1954), Luria (1959), Godwin-Austen (1965), Tyler (1968), Williams (1970), Kase, Troncoso, Court, Tapia, and Mohr (1977), and Girotti et al. (1982). The term *Balint's syndrome* was used by the majority of these authors.

Balint's Syndrome and Disturbances of Brain Information Processing

Disturbances in sustaining the focus of visual information processing and shifting it to a selected location underlie the development of Balint's syndrome. The three elements of Balint's syndrome originally described had been observed separately in "minor" manifestations of the disorder. Various researchers recognized that the syndrome might

486

LOCALIZATION
OF CLINICAL
SYNDROMES IN
NEUROPSYCHOLOGY
AND NEUROSCIENCE

also appear in incomplete minor forms (Hécaen & de Ajuriaguerra, 1954; Karpov et al., 1979; Luria, 1959; Tyler, 1968).

The first element of Balint's syndrome, which consists of disturbances in disengagement and locking out the visual processing focus using eye movements, was reported by Holmes (1918) in cases of spasmodic fixation of gaze. The second component, or optic ataxia, was described as difficulties in sustaining the fixation point of the gaze on the object, resulting in loss of the object from sight and an inability to grasp the object with the hand; at the same time, movement of the eyeballs was fully preserved in such cases. Luria (1959) reported two cases of a minor syndrome with optic ataxia revealed by the oculographic registration of ataxic eye movements by the Yarbus test. Using the Yarbus test for oculographic registration, we found difficulties in the fixation of gaze, as well as eye movements wandering around the point of gaze fixation, in five patients with occipital lobe lesions (Karpov et al., 1979); no other elements of Balint's syndrome were noted in these cases (Figure 9.1).

In some such cases, the object may be seen and recognized but then may disappear spontaneously (Karpov et al., 1979; Luria, 1959; Tyler, 1968). This may also be observed when the patient must follow the moving object (Girotti et al., 1982; Godwin-Austin, 1965; Karpov et al., 1979; see also Farah, 1990).

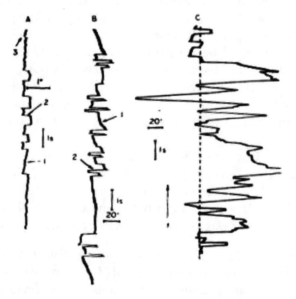

FIGURE 9.1 Recording of eye movements in patients with Balint's syndrome during fixation on a stationery target (a horizontal component). A. A normal fixation pattern. B. A fixation pattern in Case 2. Note the higher frequency and amplitude of the flicks. C. Inconsistent, ataxic fixation pattern in Case 1 (Karpov et al., 1979).

The third component manifests as an inability to see more than one object at a time. According to a review by Farah (1990), this inability to switch one's point of focus may be related to top-down disturbances in the visual system's ability to define an object. Luria (1959) described a patient who, when confronted with two objects on a tachistoscope screen, was able to see and correctly recognize one of two objects, ignoring the other. The impact of disturbances in the ability to identify an object was demonstrated in this case with the presentation of two overlapping triangles composing the Star of David. The patient saw the object and recognized that it was a star but was unable to comprehend the individual triangles. In the next task, the triangles were painted in different colors, and the patient was able to recognize the triangles only by fixing his attention on the color features, which outlined objects as rectangles in this particular case. The patient demonstrated an inability to overcome object identification based on color and to internally shift the focus of his attention to the star as a whole object. Similarly, the same patient was able to recognize a face only if it was drawn in one color. The ability to see and recognize the face as a whole became disturbed when various parts of the face were colored differently. The patient was also able to see and recognize an entire rectangle composed of dots, and to recognize these dots as stimuli, but was unable to count the dots, as he saw only one dot at a time.

Another explanation of these data may be related to disturbances in locking out and shifting the focus of attention internally without any eye movement. The patient sees one object at a time, unable to switch his or her attention to another object, in a fashion similar to spasmodic gaze fixation and optic ataxia of eye movements. Difficulties in the identification of objects may be secondary in such cases. The focus of attention may be chosen in the course of shifting from the conventional, more frequently used features, such as color, or the configuration of the sequences of dots. This focus is locked in tightly, making it difficult, if not impossible, to switch to a less conventional task, such as counting the dots that form a rectangle, or minimizing the role of color features in the recognition of a Star of David.

In cases of Balint's syndrome, the color features may actually augment gaze fixation, making it difficult for the patient to switch attention to another object, as, for example, in Luria's patient, for whom the focus of attention on the colored triangles composing the Star of David could not be shifted internally to the star as a whole object. Such a possibility is also supported by findings showing that additional objects may be seen and recognized when the stimuli are presented in spatially compact areas, such as central vision or small visual angles of 2 to 4 degrees. Under such conditions, patients who experience difficulties in perceiving more than one object at a time may be able to recognize more than one object at once (Girotti et al., 1982; Hécaen & de Ajuriguerra, 1954; Tyler, 1968; for a review, see Farah, 1990). The ability to identify a visual stimulus as an object appeared to have been preserved, and more than one object could be seen and recognized since the task did not require the internal shifting of one's focus in spatially compact areas. This explanation helps to describe Balint's syndrome as a syndrome of disturbances in the locking in, locking out, and internal shifting of the focus of visual attention, as well as in external shifting via eye movements.

Luria (1959) considered a disturbance in perceiving more than one object at a time to be an inability to see objects simultaneously; he subsequently proposed the term *simultanagnosia* for such cases. Wolpert (1924) had previously used the term simultanagnosia, describing impairments in the ability to appreciate the overall meaning of complex pictures, while the recognition of details was partially preserved. (For more details, see chapter 3, section titled "Agnosia of Action.") Farah (1990) supported this suggestion and made a distinction between ventral simultanagnosia and dorsal simultanagnosia. The terms reflect the ventral localization of lesions in the occipito-temporal region, and the dorsal localizations in the occipito-parietal region. According to Farah, both syndromes result in similar disturbances, which are characterized by a piecemeal recognition of complex visual stimuli. Patients with ventral simultanagnosia, as well as those with dorsal simultanagnosia, are generally able to recognize a single object but show disturbances in the recognition of more than one object or a complex picture.

Patients with ventral simultanagnosia can see multiple objects, while those with dorsal simultanagnosia are able to see only one object at a time. Farah (1990) reviewed in detail studies of patients with ventral simultanagnosia and those with dorsal simultanagnosia. Cases of dorsal simultanagnosia seemed to be secondary to the disturbances of disengagement and shifting of visual attention in those with Balint's syndrome, leading to an inability to see more than one object at a time in such cases. In cases of ventral simultanagnosia, as in Wolpert's description, the piecemeal perception of several objects and complex scenes is seemingly underlain by an inability to recognize the complex features of a scene. This shows similarity to cases of object agnosia, for which primary impairments are underlain by difficulties in the recognition of complex features of single objects. In this sense, the term simultanagnosia describes disturbances in the use of complex features, also known as gestalts, during the process of the recognition of scenes, objects, and written words, as well as in other tasks of recognition, while not directly reflecting clinically separate syndromes, such as visual object agnosia, prosopagnosia, agnosia of actions, or pure alexia.

Anatomical Aspects

Bilateral involvement of the occipito-parietal region was found in a case of Balint's syndrome. Bilateral lesions in this region were present in cases described by Hoff and Pötzl (1935), Hécaen et al. (1950), Hécaen and de Ajuriaguerra (1954), and Luria (1959). Gloning et al. (1968) found bilateral occipito-parietal lesions in two cases, a right occipito-parietal lesion and a left parietal lesion in one case, and a left occipito-parietal lesion and a right parietal lesion in another case.

At the same time, studies of primates did not show the possible participation of occipital areas in the shifting focus of eye movements, visual attention without eye movements, and optico-motor coordination, which is impaired in Balint's syndrome. Optical ataxia or disturbances of visually guided grasping has been produced by lesions of area 7 in monkeys. Area 7 covers the inferior parietal lobule. In primates, the area has been divided into five main structures—areas 7a, 7b, 7ip, 7op, and 7m (for a review, see Grüsser & Landis, 1991). Area 7ip is further divided into the lateral intraparietal area LIP and the ventral intraparietal area VIP. After suffering lesions of area 7, monkeys revealed prominent difficulties in visually guided reaching tasks performed by the contralateral fingers.

Single-cell studies show that neurons in area 7, primarily those in areas 7a and 7ip, contain fixation cells, which are activated when an animal gazes at a stationary target. Some of these cells may also be called attention neurons since they may be activated by a spatial shift in attention without a shift in gaze position. Tracking neurons, which are other types of neurons in the 7a and 7zip areas, are activated during pursuit eye movements, such as when a monkey follows the movements of an object. As in cases with involvement of the temporal lobe in visual object processing, these differences require further exploration. It must also be mentioned that area 7 in monkeys has no direct homologue in the human brain, which is characterized by the development of areas 39 and 40, where the supramarginal and angular gyri can be found. Lesions of these areas were found to produce a number of human-specific deficits, including acalculia, agraphia, constructional apraxia, alexia, and finger agnosia. It is possible that the occipital areas adjacent to the posterior inferior parietal lobe play some still-unspecified role in the regulation of eye fixation, the pursuit of movements, and the shifting of visual attention without eye movements.

In summary, according to clinico-anatomical data, lesions in cases with Balint's syndrome involve the lateral and superior surfaces of the occipital lobes and extend to the parietal lobes, while the mesial and the inferior occipital lobes may be not involved.

490

LOCALIZATION
OF CLINICAL
SYNDROMES IN
NEUROPSYCHOLOGY
AND NEUROSCIENCE

UNILATERAL VISUAL NEGLECT

UNILATERAL DISTURBANCES OF visual attention were first described for the left visual field by Anton (1898), Balint (1909), and Head and Holmes (1911). Poppelreuter (1917) reported visual inattention in one side of the visual field in patients who had suffered a head injury during World War I. Poetzl (1928) and Scheller and Seidemann (1931–1932) each presented cases with hemianopia of attention. Brain (1941) described in detail unilateral spatial agnosia, or neglect for one half of the body, as it is related to somatoagnosia. Unilateral neglect was also found to be related to agnosia (Hécaen & Angelergues, 1963) and followed Brain in its description as unilateral spatial agnosia (Hécaen & Albert, 1978). Gloning et al. (1968) stressed the frequent association of unilateral spatial agnosia with body image disturbances, as well as anosognosia of hemiplegia.

Clinical Aspects
Unilateral Neglect in Topographic Orientation
   Patients in these cases neglect one side of the space, usually the left side, when describing the layout of streets or the placement of buildings in well-known squares in their hometown. In other words, they completely omit the streets and landmarks that were on their left side. When the viewpoint of the individual's imagination is changed in such a way that the left and right sides are reversed (e.g., Now imagine you are standing facing the other direction), the patient reverses the neglected side accordingly, remembering and verbally expressing what is located on what is now the left side of the person.
   We observed evidence of unilateral neglect in a patient who lived in St. Petersburg, Russia. The patient was asked to name the streets that either merge or intersect with the main street, Nevsky Prospect, when he imagined walking down the street in one direction toward the railway station as opposed to when he imagined walking the other way down the street, toward the street's end at the Winter Palace Plaza. The streets and landmark buildings on the left side of the street were missing in each of the patient's accounts.
   Bisiach et al. (1979) asked their Milanese patients to imagine that they were viewing a central plaza in Milan dominated by a Gothic cathedral when looking first toward the cathedral, then when looking in the opposite direction, while standing on the steps of the cathedral. The patients usually omitted the landmarks situated on the left side of their viewing point. In some other cases, patients reportedly omitted left turns when describing a route, and were thus unable to accurately describe routes (Brain, 1941).
   Omission of the left side of their surroundings and visual field may also be observed when subjects are asked to draw a plan of their room

491

*Disturbances of
Regulatory Activity:
Impairments of
Visually Guided
Attention*

or hallway in a hospital, or in their house or apartment. The plan may be drawn without the wall on the left side of the room, or with most of the furniture on that side omitted. Similar unilateral neglect of the left side may be seen when patients are asked to draw the layout of the streets and the primary landmarks in their town of residency.

Interestingly, neglect of the left side of the space in topographic orientation in the imagination, rather than neglect of the right side of space, has been described in the literature. To the best of our knowledge, no cases have been reported of neglect of the right side of space in topographic orientation in real space.

Unilateral Neglect in Visual Orientation

Unilateral neglect may occasionally be experienced in the perception of a 3-D field. The condition may be observed when a patient without any sign of hemianopia is asked to verbally identify the object he or she sees while one object is held in the examiner's right hand and another in the examiner's left hand. A patient with unilateral neglect tends to miss or ignore the object in the experimenter's left hand, seeing only the object in the experimenter's right hand. This disturbance is known as visual extinction and may also be observed with tactile stimuli. Unilateral neglect in visual orientation may not be apparent when a patient is asked to describe the scene in his or her visual field of view.

An examination of the subject's orientation with special tests in the 2-D visual field may result in clearer and more convincing signs of unilateral neglect in visual orientation. Such special tests have been employed in numerous studies of unilateral neglect over the past few decades. Patients may demonstrate unilateral neglect, for example, in the test of line bisection, for which they may determine the central point of a line to be to one side, often to the right, thus ignoring the left side of the line (Bisiach, Capitani, Colombo, & Spinnler, 1976; Colombo, De Renzi, & Faglioni, 1976). In tests of cancellation of certain letters or of line crossing (Albert, 1973; Kartsounis & Warrington, 1989), the patient crosses out letters or lines on one side of the page but leaves the targets on the other side of the page. Similar unilateral neglect may be seen when patients are required to count the number of dots on a single line or page (Kimura, 1963; Warrington & James, 1967). Spontaneous writing, as well as writing in response to verbal dictation, may also demonstrate unilateral neglect when writing is confined to one side of the patient's space (McCarthy & Warrington, 1990).

Unilateral neglect in visual orientation in the 2-D visual field may be observed on either side of a space but is more frequent for the left side, especially for more complex tasks (Hécaen & Albert, 1978; McCarthy & Warrington, 1990).

492

LOCALIZATION
OF CLINICAL
SYNDROMES IN
NEUROPSYCHOLOGY
AND NEUROSCIENCE

Unilateral Neglect in Object Recognition and Drawing

Omission of the left side of the figure is striking in the drawing of a daisy by a patient with unilateral neglect. Similar disturbances may be seen in copies of other objects, such as houses or trees, when a patient may draw only the right side of the figure (Gainotti, Messerli, & Tissot, 1972; Hécaen & Albert, 1978; McCarthy & Warrington, 1990). Unilateral neglect may also be manifested when patients demonstrate failure to find a target on the left side of Poppelreuter's figures, in which drawings of objects overlap with one another (Gainotti, D'Erme, Montelone, & Silveri, 1986), or failure to read words located on the left side of a page (Kartsounis & Warrington, 1989).

Unilateral visual neglect may be accompanied by similar neglect in the auditory and tactile modalities (De Renzi, Faglioni, & Scotti, 1970) as well as by hemiasomatoagnosias and visuoconstructive deficits (Hécaen et al., 1956). In many cases, hemianopia in the neglected field does not accompany unilateral neglect. Gloning et al. (1968) found hemianopia congruent with the side of unilateral neglect in 61 of 101 cases.

Unilateral Neglect and Basic Operations
of Brain Information Processing

The basic deficit in cases of unilateral neglect has been viewed as a disturbance of attention (Heilman & Valenstein, 1979; Kartsounis & Warrington, 1989; Kinsbourne, 1977; Poppelreuter, 1923). Some attention theories have suggested disturbances in the spatial gradient of attention toward the intact, or undisturbed, side of space (Kinsbourne, 1977), while others have proposed an impairment of moving attention toward the neglected side of space, away from the normal side of space (Posner, Walker, Friedrich, & Rafal, 1984).

Some authors have suggested representational theories, which consider unilateral neglect to be a distortion of representation in the central map of space (De Renzi et al., 1970), or perhaps an inability to construct a mental image of the presented stimulus (Bisiach, Luzzatti, & Perani, 1979).

However, consideration of unilateral neglect as a disorder of basic operation in brain information processing may help to bring together both the attention and representational theories and to explain some basic clinical and experimental data of unilateral neglect studies, especially data concerning similar patterns of neglect for topographic orientation, visual orientation, object recognition, and constructive praxis. It is conceivable that the system of brain information processing uses a special operation of shifting the processing focus (Ullman, 1996), during which the patient scans from one hemispace to another as a simple way to avoid overloading the system with excessive information at the very first stages of information processing.

493

Disturbances of
Regulatory Activity:
Impairments of
Visually Guided
Attention

Such an operation of shifting the focus of processing may be task independent, since it can be used in a variety of different tasks, such as topographic orientation, visual orientation, object recognition, or the copying of objects. The individual is required to be able to shift the focus of processing externally in the visual field either with or without eye movements, as well as internally across representations of the topographic space and objects. It is possible that the operation of shifting the focus of processing extends to the different sensory modalities—auditory, tactile, and somatosensory—and is executed by a "shift controller," which may have a special preference for the right hemispace. Such shift controllers for the right hemispace may exist in both hemispheres, while the less-protected left hemispace is covered only by the shift controller in the right hemisphere. It is possible that the shift controller also performs operations related to the next stages of shifting the focus of processing to certain targets for further information processing. Such types of shifting from one object to another may be disturbed in cases of Balint's syndrome.

Anatomical Aspects

Right Versus Left Hemispheric Lesions

Unilateral visual neglect was originally considered to be the result of lesions of the right hemisphere (Brain, 1941). Hécaen and Angelergues (1963) found evidence of unilateral neglect for writing, copying, and drawing in 59 out of 413 patients with retrorolandic lesions. Lesions of the right hemisphere were found in 51 patients, lesions of the left hemisphere in 4 patients, and bilateral lesions in 4 cases. Left-handedess was noted in 3 of 4 cases with lesions of the left hemisphere. Spatial neglect of the left side was found in all of the 51 patients with lesions of the right hemisphere, and in 4 patients with bilateral lesions. The right side of space was neglected in all 4 cases with lesions of the left hemisphere. Gloning et al. (1968) reported the incidence of unilateral neglect in 31% of patients with lesions of the right hemisphere, compared to only 2% of patients with lesions of the left hemisphere. A prevalence of right hemispheric lesions in cases of unilateral neglect was also found by Weinstein and Cole (1963), Semenov (1965), and Zarit and Kahn (1974).

Some authors have studied the incidence of errors made in drawing, bisecting lines, and cancelling lines and found an almost equal percentage of cases with lesions of the right and left hemispheres. However, the severity of deficit was found to be significantly greater in the right hemisphere cases (Albert, 1973; Bisiach et al., 1976; Gainotti, 1968; Ogden, 1987). These results indicate that prominent unilateral visual neglect in the left hemispace develops in cases with right hemispheric lesions, while neglect in the right hemispace is usually mild in right-handed patients with left hemispheric lesions.

Parietal and Occipital Lesions

Riddoch (1935) observed unilateral neglect in cases with parietal lobe lesions. Hécaen et al. (1956) observed unilateral neglect in patients with restricted cortical ablations when the supramarginal gyrus, the angular gyrus, and the posterior portions of the first temporal gyrus were included in the resection. Hécaen (1962) also stressed the role of damage to the occipital lobe. Thus, posterior lesions of the right hemisphere with involvement of the parietal and occipital lobes seem to be the most frequent lesion sites in patients with unilateral visual neglect.

Frontal Lobe Lesions

Unilateral visual neglect has been described in some cases with frontal lobe lesions; Silberpfennig (1941) used the term *pseudo-hemianopia* to describe such cases. Deficits are noted in the initiation of eye movements contralateral to the site of the lesion in such cases. Albert et al. (1972) suggested that frontal neglect is most often the result of a right frontal lesion. Posner and Peterson (1990) recently suggested that a posterior attention network, which includes the posterior parietal lobe, is involved in orientation to sensory stimuli, while the location and detection of information is provided by the anterior attention network, which includes the anterior cingulate. In consideration of animal studies that have demonstrated the onset of unilateral neglect in monkeys following lesions limited to the oculomotor area, the role of the oculomotor area of the frontal lobe may also be suggested (Latto & Cowey, 1971).

Subcortical Lesions

Unilateral visual neglect has been observed in only a few cases with subcortical and thalamic lesions. Hassler (1979) demonstrated hemi-inattention in patients via pallidal stimulation during the course of stereotaxic surgery. Watson, Valenstein, and Heilman (1981) described neglect syndrome in a patient with a thalamic infarction as revealed by a CT scan. The legion sites involved portions of the posterior ventral nucleus, most of the medial group, and possibly the anterior pulvinar. Watson and Heilman (1979) reported three cases with thalamic hemorrhages and hemispatial neglect in a number of patients. However, the role of widespread edema cannot be eliminated in these cases. Similarly, unilateral neglect in some cases of putaminal hemorrhages may be related to compression of the internal capsule, causing hemisensory loss. Damasio et al. (1980), however, were able to confirm the possible role of subcortical structures by presenting two patients with hemispatial neglect caused by infarctions of the putamen and caudate.

495

*Disturbances of
Regulatory Activity:
Impairments of
Visually Guided
Attention*

ATTENTION DISTURBANCES IN THE DETECTION OF SIGNALS FROM NOISE

UNILATERAL NEGLECT AND Balint's syndrome are observed only occasionally in patients with cerebral lesions. One of the major manifestations of both of these conditions is a disturbance in the filtration of stimuli from other noise, a disturbance that may underlie the various types of attention disturbance that are usually noted during the course of cognitive evaluation. In healthy individuals, such filtration may be underlain by an ability to distinguish salient stimuli by using color, orientation, texture, and simple shape features.

Filtration of Figure Contour From Noise Composed of Different Textures

A typical example of such a disturbance is an impairment in the detection of object drawings against a background of textures. (For more details, see chapter 2, section titled "Visual Object Agnosia.") The detection of an object is relatively simple in such a task since the signals are drawings of objects, while the background noise is composed of textures that differ in their basic components—in the textons and dots defining the contours of objects, both of which make it easier to locate the targeted object as a focus of attention. The filtration of an object from background noise may be carried out by noting differences in the simple features of basic components such as textons and dots, as well as line orientation (Figure 9.2). Signal detection in such pictures is generally preserved in patients with visual object agnosia but has often been found to be significantly disturbed in patients who have visual hallucinations.

The role of single feature differentiation in the filtration of a signal from noise may explain the findings of some disturbances in patients with lesions of the occipital lobe in contrast to the insignificant

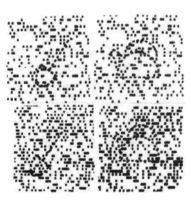

FIGURE 9.2 Contours of the objects against a background of noise formed by varying textures. Probability of black squares is $p = 0.25$ for the top pictures, and $p = 0.45$ for the bottom pictures. See text for further explanation.

496

LOCALIZATION
OF CLINICAL
SYNDROMES IN
NEUROPSYCHOLOGY
AND NEUROSCIENCE

number of errors made by patients with lesions of the parietal, temporal, and/or frontal lobes. At the same time, object recognition becomes difficult with the interference of background textures, which may occlude some of the salient features of object contours. Prominent disturbances in the filtration of a signal from background noise in this particular task were observed in patients with acute alcoholic delirium (Bajhin et al., 1975). The typical patient's gaze tended to wander across the picture with an apparent inability to visually fixate on the region of the object's location. This wandering of attentional focus may also underlie other cognitive disturbances typically noted in cases of delirium. (For more details, see chapter 12, section titled "Delirium.") In such cases, functional disturbances likely involve the occipito-parietal region, taking into account the localization of anatomical lesions in Balint's syndrome, which is characterized by disturbances in shifting of the focus of attention.

Detection When Signal and Noise Are Similar in Their Basic Components

Some tasks have examined the detection of a signal that belongs to the same category as the background noise and is thus theoretically more difficult to detect. In the cancellation test, popular in classic neuropsychology, the target is a letter that has to be repeatedly detected and crossed out within an array of other letters, which are the detractors comprising the background noise. Each subject is informed of the targeted letter in advance and is required to demonstrate an ability to read the letters of the alphabet without difficulty. The test provides an evaluation of the ability to shift the focus of attention from one letter to another, to filter target letters from the background noise of irrelevant letters, and to maintain concentration of attention on the task for its duration. Task performance is likely facilitated if the subject is able to use some simple features of the shape to distinguish the salient location for further recognition of the target letter. For example, the subject must be able to differentiate the letter X from other letters in the alphabet without needing to individually recognize each of the other letters. A more complicated type of task includes a target composed of sequences of target letters, such as the sequence AX. This allows not only for the scoring of the overall number of errors but also for an evaluation of the number of errors (missed target letters) on the right versus the left side of the paper, thus helping to demonstrate disturbances of visual neglect. We developed a cancellation test that uses numbers rather than letters as the basic components. This particular task is usually easier for subjects as it requires the recognition of only 1 of 10 numbers, instead of 1 of 26 letters in the alphabet. The task is thus suitable both for the

497

*Disturbances of
Regulatory Activity:
Impairments of
Visually Guided
Attention*

evaluation of patients with cognitive disturbances and for the testing of illiterate subjects (Figure 9.3).

DISTURBANCES OF ATTENTION SPAN

THE ABILITY TO sustain attention for an extended period of time is also known as concentration of attention, or attention span; its distractibility represents one of the most frequent findings of cognitive impairments in patients with various types of brain pathology. These impairments are often observed during the course of a regular mental status evaluation, manifesting as the inability of a patient to focus his or her attention on the content of discussion or testing for more than several minutes. The cancellation test is usually used to evaluate the ability of a patient to sustain his or her attention for the repeated detection of a specific letter, which is presented in dispersed fashion between other letters. In many cases, while the ability to detect and recognize one letter may be preserved, the repetition of the same task may be disturbed and overall performance may thus decline with time, revealing an impairment in the maintenance of attentional focus for an extended period of time.

These abilities are specially evaluated by the Continuous Performance Test (CPT; Rosvold, Mirsky, Sarason, Bransome, & Beck, 1956). A subject is presented with sequences of various letters appearing in succession on the screen of either a tachistoscope or a computer. The subject is instructed to press a key when the target letter appears on the screen. Various target stimuli have been used in this task, including sequences

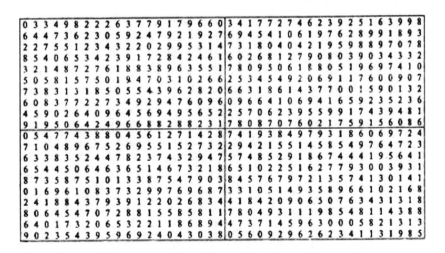

FIGURE 9.3 Number cancellation test. See explanation in the text.

498

LOCALIZATION
OF CLINICAL
SYNDROMES IN
NEUROPSYCHOLOGY
AND NEUROSCIENCE

of letters (e.g., *AX*), numbers, colors, and geometric figures. The entire task lasts for 14 min allowing for the examination of the subject's attention span. It has been shown that the CPT reveals impaired attention in patients with head injury, and especially in patients with either attention deficit disorder (ADD) or attention deficit hyperactivity disorder (ADHD) with a probable frontal lobe localization of lesion. (For a review, see Spreen and Strauss, 1998.) Several SPECT scan studies found that the CPT resulted in the bilateral activation of the mesial frontal lobes. A suggested research study would include the comparison of CPT findings in patients with different sites of circumscribed cortical and subcortical lesions.

DISTURBANCES OF FLEXIBILITY IN THE ATTENTION PROCESS

AUTOMATIC PERFORMANCE MUST often be reversed in tests that involve counting numbers, naming the months of the year, or reciting the alphabet, for example. These are all tasks that are usually automatic and may not require the use of attentional mechanisms. To count backward from 20 to 1, to name the months in reverse, or to recite the alphabet backward from Z to A, however, requires a person to overcome the well-learned automatic processing and focus attention on the reverse task. Such tasks are often used in clinical practice in the course of bedside mental status examination and are also included in some screening test batteries, such as the Brief Neuropsychological Cognitive Examination (BNCE; Tonkonogy, 1997). These tests are often used to evaluate the executive function as well. (For more details, see chapter 3, section titled "Agnosia of Action." Also, see Figure 9.4 for primary sites of lesion localization in patients with attentional disturbances.)

The Stroop Test (Stroop, 1935) is one of the most frequently used of such tests in neuropsychological clinical examination and research. The Stroop Test requires the subject first to read a list of color words (e.g., *red, blue, green*) printed in black ink. The next task is to read a list of words in which the printed words are congruent with the color of the ink in which they are printed (e.g., the word *blue* is printed in blue ink, the word *red* in red ink, and the word *green* in green ink). The subject is then asked to go through a list of words in which the printed words are incongruent with the color of ink in which they are printed (e.g., the word *blue* is printed in green ink, the word *red* in blue ink, the word *green* in red ink, etc.) and name the color of ink in which the word is printed, ignoring the word itself. Thus the task involves overcoming the more natural tendency to read the name of the word and instead naming the color of the ink. The subject's attention must thus be fixed on the target in such tests (e.g., the color of the ink of the printed word), while ignoring the background noise (e.g., the word itself). In

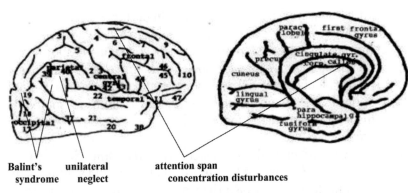

Balint's   unilateral   attention span
syndrome   neglect   concentration disturbances

FIGURE 9.4 Primary sites of lesion localization in patients with attentional disturbances.

other words, the tendency to read the word must be suppressed, inhibited by mechanisms of attention.

Impaired performance on the Stroop Test was noted in patients with various causes of brain damage, including head injury, various types of degenerative dementia, schizophrenia, and mood disorders. (For a review, see Spreen and Strauss, 1998.) Several neuroimaging studies found a midline activation of the cingula during the course of the testing of incongruent conditions. (For a review, see Posner and DiGirolamo, 1998.) Janer and Pardo (1991), however, administered the Stroop Test to a 34-year-old patient both 1 week before and 2 weeks after a bilateral anterior cingulotomy. The patient developed a significant deficit after surgery only in congruent conditions, pointing to the absence of a specific deficit in the incongruent conditions after damage to the cingula. Further studies in this area are certainly needed.

CONCLUSIONS

1. Anatomical data on disturbances in shifting and sustaining the focus of attention in cases of Balint's syndrome point to the role of occipito-parietal lesions, primarily in the right hemisphere, and to the role of lesions of the right parietal lobe in cases of unilateral neglect.
2. The localization of lesions in syndromes of visual attentional disturbances often overlaps with lesions of the occipito-parietal region in cases of visual spatial agnosia. It is possible that attentional operations are independent of, but located in close proximity to, the regions involved in spatial aspects of object and scene recognition, facilitating information processing in those regions.

500

LOCALIZATION
OF CLINICAL
SYNDROMES IN
NEUROPSYCHOLOGY
AND NEUROSCIENCE

3. Attentional mechanisms may play an important role in unconventional information processing by helping to overcome automatic, conventional types of information processing. In addition to the occipito-parietal region, the dorsolateral frontal lobe and the anterior cingula seem to be involved in these operations. Lesions of these areas may lead to disturbances in attention span or in the ability to sustain attentional focus for an extended period of time.

4. Involvement of both the subcortical areas and the occipito-parietal region may be key in disturbances in the shifting of attentional focus. These disturbances are secondary to the decrease in vigilance observed, for example, in the course of delirium. (For more details, see chapter 12, section titled "Delirium.")

5. As in working memory, attentional mechanisms likely represent the supportive operations that are primarily located in the dorsolateral regions, extending from the occipital lobe, through the parietal lobe, to the frontal regions.

10

Disturbances of Regulatory Activity: Impairments of Volition

AVOLITION, AKINESIA, AND NEGATIVE SYMPTOMS

WHILE THE ABILITY to recognize an object, scene, or action and to perform a particular movement or action may be preserved, the support and regulation for reaching the goals of brain information processing is disturbed by diminished or absent activation of particular actions caused, for instance, by apathy. The term apathy was used in the old psychiatric and neurological literature to define "the absence of feeling" as well as a "blunting or flattening of affective response" (Sims, 1988, p. 226). *Avolition*, also known as abulia, was defined as a loss of will, which is closely connected to the absence of emotions, or apathy, and motivation. This idea has been reflected in recent attempts to include the term avolition in the definition of apathy, which is defined as lack of motivation, or a decrease in the behavioral, emotional, and cognitive components of goal-directed behavior (Marin, 1996; Silva & Marin, 1999). Avolition is considered to be a more pronounced degree of apathy.

Historically, signs of apathy and avolition were often described as a major manifestation of frontal lobe syndrome in patients with massive lesions of the frontal lobe that had been caused by a brain tumor,

502

LOCALIZATION
OF CLINICAL
SYNDROMES IN
NEUROPSYCHOLOGY
AND NEUROSCIENCE

a head injury, or another neurologically defined disturbance. These terms were also used in the older psychiatric literature to describe the particular set of symptoms that now defines one of two principal groups of patients with schizophrenia. According to Kraepelin (1919), this group was characterized by "a weakening of those emotional activities which permanently form the mainstream of volition.... The result of this part of the morbid process is emotional dullness, a failure of mental activities, and a loss of mastery over volition, of endeavor, and of the ability to maintain independent actions" (pp. 74–75). Bleuler (1951) included the symptoms of flat affect, ambivalence, and autism, thus adding the so-called three-*As* syndrome to the list of the fundamental features of schizophrenia. This set of symptoms was originally defined in the psychiatric literature as apatho-abulic syndrome; the term *productive symptoms* was then used to describe the prevalence of delusions and hallucinations in a second principal group of patients with schizophrenia.

Throughout the years, the role of productive symptoms as the essential and defining feature of schizophrenia has been supported by the general acceptance of Schneider's description of first-rank schizophrenic symptoms, which include specific types of delusions and hallucinations that have been found to be typical, if not pathognomonic, for schizophrenia. Apatho-abulic syndrome, however, was considered to be an important feature of schizophrenic illness and almost completely disappeared from Western psychiatric and neuropsychiatric literature beginning in the 1950s and 1960s. Researchers found it difficult, however, to use the term *first-rank symptoms* to describe the chronic deterioration that leads to the development of the so-called deficit syndrome in patients with schizophrenia, and renewed interest in apatho-abulic syndrome steadily increased beginning in the 1970s.

Strauss, Carpenter, and Barko (1974) reintroduced the idea of apatho-abulic syndrome in 1974 under the label "negative symptoms" as one of the three major types of processes underlying schizophrenic symptoms. The other two categories included positive symptoms and disorder in relating. The terms *negative* and *positive symptoms* were first suggested by John Hughlings Jackson (1875), who described them using epilepsy as a model. The positive symptoms, manifested as delusions and hallucinations, were considered to be the result of a disinhibition of normal brain processing caused by a destruction of higher-level brain functioning, while the negative symptoms were underlain by a dissolution of higher-level brain functioning.

Jackson's (1875) terms were later used by Crow (1980a, 1980b). According to Crow (1980b), negative symptoms include flat affect, poverty of speech, and a loss of drive in patients with Type II schizophrenia, while positive symptoms encompass hallucinations, delusions, and thought disorder in cases of Type I schizophrenia. The positive symptoms observed in cases of Type I schizophrenia were considered by Crow to be the result of a biochemical imbalance, for example, an increase in dopamine-2 (D2) receptors. It was suggested that structural-anatomical abnormalities, which are revealed via brain imaging more frequently in patients with prominent negative symptoms than in those with positive symptoms, underlie the development of more chronic negative symptoms and thus often lead to prominent cognitive impairment. Individuals who proceed to this point are generally found to be unresponsive to various neuroleptic treatments.

APATHY, AVOLITION

Clinical Aspects

During the course of developing the Scale for the Assessment of Negative Symptoms (SANS) and the Scale for the Assessment of Positive Symptoms (SAPS), Andreasen (1982) classified negative symptoms into five groups: alogia (also known as aphasia), affective flattening, avolition (e.g., apathy), anhedonia, and attentional impairment. The positive symptoms included in SAPS were hallucinations, delusions, bizarre behavior, and positive formal speech disorder. Within the umbrella of negative symptoms, there is an apathy-avolition subscale, which consists primarily of symptoms of avolition, including poor grooming and hygiene, a lack of persistence at work or at school, and physical anergia. Affective flattening, not listed in the apathy-avolition subscale, includes signs of a lack of emotional reactivity. Flat affect was previously regarded as related to the major manifestations of apathy, such as paucity of facial expression and expressive gestures, a lack of vocal inflection, affective nonresponsivity, and poor eye contact. A subscale of anhedonia-asociality also incorporates signs that were previously included in the definition of apathy, including a loss of interest, a disturbance in the ability to feel a sense of intimacy and closeness, and disturbed relationships with friends and peers. While an advantage of this subscale approach is that it helps to assess more precisely the various manifestations of negative symptoms, we consider these manifestations together as apathy and avolition in order to facilitate the clinico-anatomical approach to these disturbances, which becomes almost impossible to conduct using the subdivisions suggested by Andreasen (1982).

In addition, an alogia subscale includes items such as poverty of speech and its content and blocking and increased latency of response,

504

LOCALIZATION
OF CLINICAL
SYNDROMES IN
NEUROPSYCHOLOGY
AND NEUROSCIENCE

which may be defined as speech akinesia for the purpose of clinico-anatomical analysis. The affective flattening subscale also incorporates some symptoms of speech akinesia, such as a decrease in spontaneous movements and a paucity of expressive gestures. It must be stressed that speech akinesia is often observed as a primary symptom with specific localization of lesion in patients with neurological diseases (Cummings, 1985).

In patients with negative symptoms, activity and functioning actually seem to level off, becoming stalled or inhibited. While the inner structure of a particular activity often remains preserved, patients are often unable to initiate activities and thus tend to have a habit of not following through with activities. A knowledge of grammatical structure may be demonstrated when patients are encouraged to speak, but the initiation of speech is markedly diminished. Patients tend to respond only to specific questions, often with phrases only one or two words in length; sometimes, however, patients may fail to respond in any manner. The patient's voice is often monotonous, reflecting the absence of the prosodic activity that usually accompanies the free flow of speech. The general inability to switch between particular functions is manifested as avolition, flat affect, social withdrawal, poverty of speech and speech content, and akinesia against the background of preserved alertness and an absence of drowsiness or lethargy.

Depression differs from apathy and avolition in that its sufferers tend to experience relatively highly intense negative emotions, such as depressed mood and sadness. Patients suffering from negative symptoms, however, generally experience a flatness of affect, avolition, and apathy. A comorbid experience of depression and avolition is possible, especially secondary to depression, but the core symptoms are certainly related to the high intensity of negative emotion in depression, and the low level of flatness of affect and bluntness of emotion in patients with negative symptoms.

Anatomical Aspects
Frontal Lobe Lesions

The role of a frontal lobe lesion in the development of aspontaneity, apathy, and affective flattening was first observed in patients with head injuries suffered during World War I. Feuchtwanger (1923) evaluated 400 patients with head injuries caused by bullets penetrating the skull. Apathy was frequently observed among 200 patients with frontal gunshot wounds. Kleist (1934) reported the results of a detailed study of patients with lesions of the frontal lobe, which had resulted from head injury in most cases. Kleist observed a wide spectrum of aspontaneity in various forms of activity, manifested as apathy, a loss of initiative, akinesia, a paucity of ideation and speech, and mutism. This set of symptoms usually resulted from bilateral lesions of the convex, including the first and second frontal gyri and their underlying white matter. Similar results were reported by Walsh (1956) and Faust (1955).

Shmaryan (1949) reported a case of head injury caused by a bullet penetrating the skull from left to right at the middle level of the frontal lobe. Surgery followed within several hours of the injury and consisted of the bilateral removal of the frontal poles. Apathy, a loss of activity, a tendency to social isolation, and aspontaneity of thinking all developed postinjury and were still present 7 years later. Blumer and Benson (1975) described a similar patient who became apathetic, often sitting alone and smoking most of the day, following an accident that necessitated the removal of the left frontal pole.

Apathy, inertia, and affective flattening were also reported in patients after prefrontal psychosurgery. Freeman and Watts (1943) found that prefrontal lobectomies or lobotomies were often followed by the development of apathy and aspontaneity, both of which lasted well beyond the first days after surgery in some cases. A loss of interest and drive, a decrease in social activity, and flat or shallow affect were observed by Greenblatt and Solomon (1966) following a patient's bilateral prefrontal lobotomy.

Further support for the role of frontal lobe lesions in the development of negative symptoms is provided by studies of patients with various localizations of brain tumors.

Shmaryan (1949) described psychiatric symptoms in 420 patients with brain tumors. Frontal lobe tumors were present in 180 of the cases. Apathy, aspontaneity, and paucity of thoughts were often noted in an unspecified number of patients with frontal lobe tumors. Shmaryan described some of these patients in detail, including a 2-year-old male who developed apathy, a loss of initiative, and slowness of motions and thinking. Surgery revealed and allowed the removal of a meningioma that was suppressing the pole of the right frontal lobe. After the surgery, the patient improved, becoming more active and less inhibited.

Hécaen and de Ajuriaguerra (1956) noted psychiatric manifestations in 229 cases out of 439 patients with brain tumors. Frontal lobe tumors were found in 54 of the 229 cases. A loss of initiative was the relatively isolated manifestation of psychiatric problems in 10 patients. Marked abulia was found to be present in some of those cases. All 10 patients were included by the authors in the larger group of patients in an "akinetic state," which was composed of 23 patients with frontal lobe tumors. An akinetic state was described as a profound loss of activity, and apathy was often combined with poverty of speech, also known as "akinetic mutism." The researchers did not specify any particular localization of tumors within the frontal lobes in cases of akinetic states.

506

LOCALIZATION
OF CLINICAL
SYNDROMES IN
NEUROPSYCHOLOGY
AND NEUROSCIENCE

Some researchers have stressed the relationship between a convexital localization of frontal lesions in cases of apathy and aspontaneity (Feuchtwanger, 1923; Kleist, 1934). Involvement of the frontal poles was reported in some cases with frontal pole lesions (Blumer & Benson, 1975; Shmaryan, 1949). In cases with a more posterior localization of frontal lobe lesions, akinetic mutism may become a leading manifestation of aspontaneity. Lesions in these cases usually involve the posterior parts of the first frontal gyri on the mesial surface of the frontal lobe, as well as the anterior parts of the cingular gyrus.

In general, negative symptoms of aspontaneity, loss of initiative, apathy, and flatness of affect combined with poverty of thought and speech have been observed in patients with frontal lobe lesions caused by head injury and brain tumors. An association between dorsolateral frontal lesions and aspontaneity and apathy was also shown, primarily in cases of head injury, but also in some patients with relatively circumscribed frontal lobe tumors, such as parasagittal meningiomas.

Subcortical Lesions

Recent advances in brain imaging have markedly enhanced the opportunity to study aspontaneity, loss of initiative, and apathy in cases of relatively circumscribed small subcortical lesions, primarily in patients with either medial thalamic infarctions or bilateral lesions of the globus pallidus.

Thalamic Lesions

Apathy, which includes a lack of motivation, a slowness of responses, and a general lack of concern about one's deficit(s), has been noted in cases of various types of injury, including a paramedian right thalamic infarction (Castaigne et al., 1981, Case 19) and a bilateral paramedian thalamic infarction (Castaigne et al., 1981, Case 2). Katz, Alexander, and Mandell (1987) observed apathy, a loss of motivation, and flat affect in six different patients: four cases of bilateral medial thalamic infarctions, and two cases of infarctions (in the left medial thalamus in one patient and in the left anterior central thalamus in the other). The researchers stressed various degrees of involvement of the subthalamic area and midbrain in all cases.

Bogousslavsky et al. (1988b) presented the case of a 72-year-old right-handed female who had developed manic delirium and who experienced periods of aspontaneity during which she would either remain in bed or sit in her chair without any drive to initiate goal-directed actions. A CT scan revealed a recent nonhemorrhagic infarction in the right paramedian thalamus with an involvement of the intralaminar nuclei, including the dorsomedial nucleus and the internal part of the ventral lateral nucleus. The left midbrain tegmentum was also noted to have been involved. A SPECT scan revealed a 50% hypoperfusion in the right thalamus in comparison to the left thalamus, and a 30% decrease of perfusion in the overlying left hemispheric cortex in comparison to the right hemispheric cortex, predominantly in the frontal region. Evidence of apathy and a striking lack of spontaneity and initiative were reported by Sandson, Daffner, Carvalho, and Mesulam (1991) in a 62-year-old right-handed female who had recently suffered from a left medial thalamic infarction, as demonstrated by CT and MRI scans. The lesion primarily involved the dorsomedial nucleus and extended to the adjacent internal medullary lamina, the mamillothalamic tract, and the ventral lateral nucleus. A SPECT scan showed a marked decrease in uptake in the left thalamus, as well as a 30% decrease in the left dorsolateral and anteromedial frontal lobe in comparison to that of the right. Aspontaneity with a loss of affective drive and psychic self-activation was also observed in a 29-year-old female (Lisovski et al., 1993). An MRI scan of the patient showed a left thalamic infarction that was limited to the territory of the left tuberothalamic artery.

Hypersomnia, fluctuating alertness, and cognitive deficits of various degrees were found to be common in patients with thalamic infarctions. These patients often have a tendency to fall asleep if left alone for a period of time, even in cases with a recovery of alertness and normal wakefulness (Katz et al., 1987). Cognitive deficits persisted for many months after the onset, primarily consisting of memory difficulties, especially in recalling the most recent events, as well as impaired attention. Hypophonia, dysarthria, and transient language difficulties were also noted in some cases (Castaigne et al., 1981; Katz et al., 1987; Sandson et al., 1991).

Lesions of the Globus Pallidus

Lesions of the basal ganglia may also lead to apathy, unconcern, aspontaneity, and a loss of drive. Laplane et al. (1989) presented evidence of psychic akinesia and obsessive–compulsive disorder in eight cases with bilateral lesions of the basal ganglia, primarily within the globus pallidus. Case 1 was reported by Laplane, Widlocher, Pillon, Baulac, and Binoux (1981); and Cases 2 and 3 were later published together with Case 1 (Laplane, Baulac, Widlocher, & Dubois, 1984). Laplane et al. (1989) later presented five new cases, as well as the three previously published cases. In addition to data obtained from MRI and CT scans, the results of PET studies were described in seven of the eight patients. The primary clinical manifestations in all eight cases were avolition, aspontaneity, inertia, a loss of drive, and a flattening of affect. Stereotyped activity with obsessive–compulsive components was demonstrated by some of the patients. Movement disorders, such as extrapyramidal symptoms, were mild or completely absent. Cognitive impairment was

508

LOCALIZATION
OF CLINICAL
SYNDROMES IN
NEUROPSYCHOLOGY
AND NEUROSCIENCE

largely restricted to the slowing of mental capabilities and the variability of attention. Remote and recent memory; orientation in time, space, and person; and verbal fluency all appeared to be preserved in most of the cases, though mental and motor shifting were found to be disturbed when patients were evaluated via the simplified version of the Wisconsin Card Sorting Test (WCST) and Luria's arithmetic, graphic, and motor series. Brain damage was caused by carbon monoxide poisoning in four of the eight cases; the causal factors for the other four cases included disulfiram poisoning, electroshock, a wasp sting, and cerebral anoxia during general anaesthesia. CT and MRI scans demonstrated lesions of the basal ganglia, primarily affecting the globus pallidus bilaterally in all eight cases. PET studies revealed a decrease in striatal glucose utilization and normal values of glucose utilization in the cerebral cortex. However, there was a significant reduction in glucose utilization in some parts of the frontal cortex as compared to the entire cortex, as well as relative hypermetabolism in the occipital cortex of several patients.

Patients with apatho-abulic syndrome caused by primarily pallidal lesions were also described by Ali-Cherif et al. (1984); Starkstein, Mayberg, Berthier et al. (1989); Lugaresi, Montagna, Morreale, and Gallassi (1990); Trillet, Croisile, Tourniaire, and Schott (1990); and De Poorter, Pasquier, and Petit (1991; see also the review by Starkstein and Manes, 2000). Apatho-abulia was often accompanied by varying degrees of parkinsonism, memory impairment, obsessive–compulsive disorder, or disorders of executive function. These varying comorbid experiences were probably dependent on the extent of the lesion outside the ventromedial and rostral portion of the globus pallidus and the adjacent white matter. Many patients experienced pallidal lesions following carbon monoxide intoxication (Figure 10.1).

Strub (1989) described social withdrawal, apathy, and a loss of motivation in a patient who had developed bilateral hemorrhages in the globus pallidus within minutes of reaching an altitude of more than 4,000 meters above sea level. The patient remained spatially oriented, and recall of remote and recent events was preserved. Performance on Parts A and B of the Trail Making Test was normal, and a full-length administration of the Wechsler Adult Intelligence Scale–Revised (WAIS-R) yielded a full-scale IQ score of 103. Cognitive impairments were limited primarily to verbal memory disturbances manifested as an inability to recall three of four words after a delay of 5 min, as well as difficulty in shifting sets in the WCST and the Stroop Test.

Habib and Poncet (1988) used the somewhat awkward term *athymhormia* to describe the syndrome observed in a similar patient. The original term, apathy-abulia, seems to be much easier to pronounce and to better reflect the clinical manifestations of the syndrome. The au-

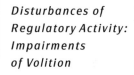

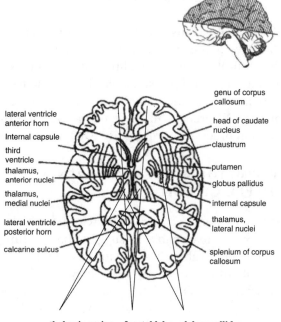

lateral ventricle
anterior horn

Internal capsule

third
ventricle

thalamus,
anterior nuclei

thalamus,
medial nuclei

lateral ventricle
posterior horn

calcarine sulcus

genu of corpus
callosum

head of caudate
nucleus

claustrum

putamen

globus pallidus

internal capsule

thalamus,
lateral nuclei

splenium of corpus
callosum

thalamic region   frontal lobe   globus pallidus

FIGURE 10.1   A horizontal section of the brain on the level of the anterior commissure. Localization of lesions in cases with apathy and avolition; lesions are often bilateral.

thors explained the SPECT findings of a mesial frontal hypoperfusion in their patient, which was the result of dysfunction caused by pallidal necrosis to the loop connecting the ventral pallidus with the anterior cingulate through the dorsomedial thalamus. Habib and Poncet (1988) stressed the absence of parkinsonism, amnesia, or cognitive impairment in their patient.

Conclusions

NEGATIVE SYMPTOMS CONSISTING of apathy, aspontaneity, avolition, loss of drive, and poverty of speech have been reported in relatively circumscribed lesions of the major cortical and subcortical areas, including the following.

1. The frontal lobe, especially in the dorsoconvexital region of Brodmann's areas 9 and 10, and involving the frontal poles, unilaterally and/or bilaterally.
2. The paramedian thalamic region, which is sometimes unilateral, but almost always bilateral.

510

LOCALIZATION
OF CLINICAL
SYNDROMES IN
NEUROPSYCHOLOGY
AND NEUROSCIENCE

3. The basal ganglia, primarily the bilateral globus pallidus.

The localization of lesions in cases with aspontaneity and avolition points to damage in the dorsolateral-prefrontal-subcortical circuit. However, the clinical pattern of avolition and aspontaneity seems to be similar if not identical for lesions within specific parts of the circuit. It is difficult to imagine that all those parts are performing the same operations. Differences in these operations and their roles in brain information processing will be discussed below.

Negative Symptoms in Schizophrenia and the DLPFC Circuit

Extrapolation from data in patients with identifiable neurological diseases makes it reasonable to suggest that dysfunction of the dorsolateral-prefrontal-subcortical circuit, also known as the dorsolateral-prefrontal cortex circuit (DLPFC), may be related to negative symptoms in schizophrenia. This suggestion may be supported by the findings of neuroanatomical and metabolic abnormalities in schizophrenia made possible by the advent of in vivo studies provided by constantly improving structural and functional brain imaging techniques. The most consistent findings of the neuroanatomical studies appear to be an increase in ventricular size, as observed via CT scans (Johnstone, Crow, Frith, Husband, & Krel, 1976; Weinberger & Wyatt, 1982; for a review, see Shelton & Weinberger, 1986) and MRI data (Kelsoe et al., 1988; Rossi et al., 1988). These findings point to the damage to subcortical structures that may be involved in the subcortical parts of the DLPFC circuit. Involvement of the cortical portion of this circuit may be implied by the *hypofrontality* revealed by PET scan studies of glucose metabolism and blood flow, especially during cognitive activation (Buchsbaum et al., 1984; Ingvar & Frazen, 1974; Weinberger, Berman, & Zec, 1986; Wolkin et al., 1985).

However, a comparison of the neuroanatomical findings with positive and negative symptoms has so far yielded inconclusive results. Some early reports have shown that signs of hypofrontality are related to negative symptoms. Ingvar and Frazen (1974) studied cortical blood flow using the intracarotid xenon technique and found that levels of blood flow were highest in the anterior cortical region of control subjects, while decreased levels of blood flow in that region, or hypofrontality, were observed in patients with schizophrenia. Interestingly, the degree of decrease in blood flow was found to be correlated with the severity of the patients' negative symptoms. Andreasen et al. (1982) studied schizophrenic patients using ventricular brain ratios (VBRs) measured via head CT scans carried out to study ventricular size, as well as using the positive and negative symptoms scales (SAPS and SANS) that were devised by Andreasen. The negative schizophrenia group was found to have larger VBRs than groups of patients with either positive or mixed symptoms. However, further studies based on CT scan data did not support these findings (Nasrallah et al., 1983; Pandurangi et al., 1988). Nasrallah et al. (1983) found no differences in VBRs or sulcal widening between the groups of patients with negative and positive symptoms. In another study, Owens, Johnstone, and Crow (1985) compared VBRs in a group of 192 subjects, including 110 patients with schizophrenia, who had been divided into pairs according to their age, gender, treatment, education, and the presence (or lack of presence) of positive symptoms in a defect state. No differences in VBRs were found within the pairs with or without the negative symptoms.

An MRI study by Olson, Nasrallah, Coffman, and Schwarzkopf (1991) of 75 subjects—41 male and 24 female—also failed to confirm statistically significant higher VBR in a group of female patients with a prevalence of negative symptoms, while a group of male schizophrenics had statistically significant higher VBR values for some of the negative symptoms. Contradictory results have also been reported in studies using measurements of relaxation times—T1 and T2. Williamson, Pelz, Merskey, Morrison, and Conlon (1991) examined 24 chronic schizophrenic patients, 10 of whom had a high rating for negative symptoms. No changes in T1 values for the left frontal white matter in these patients were confirmed. However, a statistically significant increase in T2 values was found for frontotemporal ratios in patients with negative symptoms.

Earlier reports by Ingvar and Frazen (1974) of a decrease in blood flow in the prefrontal area, or hypofrontality, were later confirmed by PET scan findings of lower glucose metabolic rates in the frontal cortex than in the posterior cortical region in patients with schizophrenia (Buchsbaum et al., 1982; Farkas et al., 1980; Widen et al., 1981). However, while some researchers found no correlation with clinical symptoms (DeLisi et al., 1985), others reported hypofrontality in patients with more prominent negative symptoms (Volkow et al., 1987). Studies of blood flow using the inhalation xenon technique in resting conditions and especially using activation tests (Berman, Weinberger, Shelton, & Zec, 1987; Weinberger et al., 1986) confirmed the results found by Ingvar and Frazen (1974) of decreased frontal blood flow in patients with schizophrenia. Ingvar and Frazen reported the results of studies that were specifically designed to test the dorsolateral prefrontal cortex to avoid the influence of other areas of the frontal lobes on the results. Activation tests included the WCST. A group of 25 normal controls showed an increase in DLPFC blood flow while taking the WCST; no activation was recorded in the groups of 20 medication-free schizophrenic patients and 24 neuroleptically treated patients. The authors did not study the correlations of decreases in blood flow with symptoms, negative or otherwise, but the study clearly points to the abnormal functioning of the DLPFC, which is known to be involved in the drive–emotion–speech (DES) activation system. This study stresses the role of the more precise targeting of an area of possible dysfunction, in this case the DLPFC, which is not commonly emphasized by other researchers. Further studies in this direction may be fruitful in establishing the relationship between DLPFC dysfunction and negative symptoms in schizophrenia. It should also be taken into account that a decrease in blood flow in the DLPFC was noted in patients suffering from depression (Baxter et al., 1989; Martinot et al., 1990), making the data from the blood flow tests even more difficult to use for localization studies in cases with negative symptoms. It is possible, however, that the involvement of the DLPFC may be related to the development of apathy, or a loss of interest, which is often seen in patients with depression.

Postmortem studies showed that parts of the DES system other than the DLPFC may also be implicated in the development of negative symptoms in schizophrenia. A reduction in the total number of neurons was reported in the mediodorsal thalamic nucleus of schizophrenic patients (Bäumer, 1954; Treff & Hempel, 1958). Bogerts, Meertz, and Schönfeldt-Bausch (1985) found a reduction in volume of the globus pallidus in a postmortem study of patients with schizophrenia. Thus, two subcortical parts of the DLPFC system may have anatomical abnormalities in patients with schizophrenia. The relationships between these abnormalities and negative symptoms, however, have not yet been studied in depth.

Changes in the cortical parts of the DES activation system have also been found in postmortem studies of cases of schizophrenia. In addition to the old reports of cortical atrophy, especially in the frontal lobe (Rawlings, 1920), a recent study revealed decreased cell numbers in Layer VI of the prefrontal cortex, Layer V of the cingular cortex, and Layer III of the motor cortex (Benes, Davidson, & Bird, 1984). However, a loss of neuronal cells, atrophy and dysmorphism have all been observed in other parts of the cortex, as well as in the limbic-diencephalic structures. (For a review, see Kirch & Weinberger, 1986.) The relationship of these changes to the clinical manifestation of schizophrenia, including negative symptoms, is quite difficult to study in a systematic manner, especially taking into account the fact that no pathognomonic lesion has been identified in cases of schizophrenia.

Dysfunction of the DES activation system may also be related to an imbalance in neurotransmitters, especially dopamine. The empirical grounds for this idea may include the following data: neuroleptic drugs are dopamine receptor blockers, and their use may induce parkinsonian and/or extrapyramidal symptoms, as well as apathy, a loss of drive, and a poverty of speech; and the mesocortical dopaminergic system, which is initiated in the ventral tegmentum, terminates predominantly in the frontal cortex, especially in the precentral motor area, and to a lesser extent in the prefrontal cortex, though this area still maintains a relatively heavy dopamine concentration. (For a review, see Fuster, 1989.) It can be inferred that the depletion of dopamine in the prefrontal cortex and the negative symptoms experienced are the result of an interruption of the mesocortical dopamine pathway. An enlargement of the ventricles in schizophrenic patients may reflect the presence of such an interruption. According to Berman et al. (1987), the hypofrontality assessed by blood flow measurements during the WCST correlates with the degree of ventricular enlargement in schizophrenic patients. These correlations reveal similarities with the results of a comparison between hypofrontality and levels of homovanillic acid (HVA), a dopamine metabolite, in the cerebrospinal fluid (CSF; Weinberger et al., 1988). These data allowed Berman and Weinberger (1991) to suggest that dopamine may be a common factor underlying neurobiological correlates of negative symptoms.

These results certainly require replication and confirmation in further studies, which should include an evaluation of the role of imbalances of various neurotransmitters in the development of negative symptoms. It is possible that a depletion of dopamine in the DLPFC plays a more significant role in the early stages of the development of negative symptoms in the progression of schizophrenia, while neuroanatomical destruction of the structures and their interconnections within the DLPFC-subcortical circuits may become the leading mechanism in the advanced stages, in which an irreversible deficit state is experienced.

In conclusion, recent studies using the brain imaging techniques provide subtle, but reliable, evidence in support of the neuroanatomical data on ventricular enlargement and metabolic abnormalities, pointing to hypofrontality, primarily in the DLPFC region, in cases of schizophrenia. The relationships between these abnormalities and negative symptoms have begun to be evaluated, and further clarification is expected concerning the correlations between the localization of lesion or injury, the type of brain pathology, and the clinical symptoms of schizophrenia, including the negative symptoms. Studies of these correlations may prove to be quite difficult to carry out, since the pathological process underlying the development of schizophrenia is probably heterogeneous in nature, varying from one case to another. The neuroanatomical or metabolic differences between groups are often subtle, frequently overlapping with normal controls and requiring the

514

LOCALIZATION
OF CLINICAL
SYNDROMES IN
NEUROPSYCHOLOGY
AND NEUROSCIENCE

use of complicated statistical analysis. Also, the results of one study are often not supported by the data from subsequent studies.

The difficulties of these studies are reflected in the prominent differences in neuroanatomical findings in schizophrenic patients with similar clinical manifestations. One of our own patients had a 26-year history of schizophrenia and prominent symptoms of a defect state with apathy, flat affect, avolition, marked poverty of speech, and prominent cognitive impairment. An MRI scan of the patient was read as perfectly normal by a neuroradiologist, and an EEG yielded negative results. Another patient with a similar defect state and a long history of schizophrenia was found to have marked enlargement of the lateral ventricles. It may be suggested that a malfunction of the DLPFC-subcortical circuits is heterogeneous and is probably related to the loss of brain tissue. More specifically, the loss of brain tissue involves neuronal cell loss in the second case discussed, while in the first case, the pathology may be caused by the dysmorphism of cells and the derangement of cellular connections not reflected directly or indirectly by the cerebral atrophy. Further research based on modern neuropathological techniques and thorough case studies would possibly be helpful in the elucidation of the differences in the DLPFC circuit pathology, which underlies the development of negative symptoms in schizophrenic patients.

AKINESIA

SEVERAL TYPES OF akinesia have been described in neurological and psychiatric illnesses. These include *bradykinesia* or a Parkinsonian type of akinesia, *pure akinesia, psychomotor retardation, akinetic mutism,* and *catatonia.*

Clinical Aspects

Bradykinesia and/or A Parkinsonian Type of Akinesia

The syndrome characterized by bradykinesia, muscular rigidity, tremor, and a loss of postular reflexes was first described by James Parkinson in 1817 as paralysis agitans. Later, the condition was termed *Parkinson's disease,* while the term *secondary parkinsonism* continues to be used to describe a similar syndrome in a variety of diseases and conditions of the nervous system, including encephalitis, head injury, brain tumors, degenerative disorders, and arteriosclerosis, as well as intoxication with neuroleptics and poisoning with carbon monoxide and/or heavy metals.

Primary Parkinsonism. The classical triad of parkinsonism is bradykinesia, rigidity, and tremor. Akinesia manifests as hypokinesia or bradykinesia, slowness and poverty of movement with difficulties in changing the position of the body, a lack of mobility of facial expression or face masking, infrequent blinking of the eyelids, and a loss of arm swing while walking. A slowness of oral motor movements may lead to dysphasia without choking and/or aspiration, especially in more advanced cases. Rigidity, or resistance to passive movements, is readily observable by passive movements of a limb, is implicated in stiffness of movements, and is often characterized by a fixed body posture. Patients often have an impairment or loss of postural reflexes. When the patient stands and walks, his or her center of gravity seems to be moved forward, as the trunk is bent forward, the head is bowed, and the arms and knees assume a flexed position. The arms protrude forward and do not move or swing while the patient walks. The gait is a small-stepped shuffle, reflecting a combination of postural abnormalities and rigidity. There is a tendency toward an acceleration of pace, known as a festinating gait, as well as errors of propulsion and retropulsion, which are difficulties in stopping, causing the patient to move forward or to take several steps backward. The patient's speech reveals bradykinesia and rigidity by becoming hypophonic (abnormally weak) or aprosodic (lacking, for example, normal variations in pitch or tone), with a tendency toward acceleration of speech (festination) and involuntary word repetition, also known as palilalia. Rigidity is also reflected in micrographia of the handwriting. Tremor, also known as "pill-rolling," is usually limited to the thumb and forefinger and is observed at rest with a frequency of 4 to 7 Hz. Autonomic disturbances include sialorrhea (increased salivary flow); hyperhidrosis caused by a hyperactivity of the sweat glands; and an oily, greasy appearance of the facial skin, resulting from an overactivity of subcutaneous glands.

Bradykinesia and rigidity may sometimes be overcome by the extreme stress caused by, for example, the sudden development of a fire in the house. The patient may begin to run with great speed, giving the appearance that his or her parkinsonism is functional, rather than related to structural brain damage. On the other hand, long-standing L-dopa treatment may result in an on–off phenomenon characterized by the sudden development of a frozen state, during which the patient loses his or her ability to move at all. The manifestations of Parkinson's disease may be markedly diminished with modern medications such as L-dopa and bromocriptine, but the general pattern of bradykinesia, rigidity, and fixed posture remains unchanged and is reduced only in the degree of impairment (Yhar, 1984).

Secondary Parkinsonism. Manifestations of parkinsonism may develop in a variety of nervous system diseases, intoxication, and poisoning. Drug-induced parkinsonism is a typical example of secondary

516

LOCALIZATION
OF CLINICAL
SYNDROMES IN
NEUROPSYCHOLOGY
AND NEUROSCIENCE

parkinsonism and is usually related to the use of neuroleptics. The primary features of this syndrome include rigidity of the limbs, face masking, and bradykinesia, as well as a slowness of movement, including oral-facial akinesia, leading to bradykinetic dysphasia and an increased risk of choking and aspiration (Bazemore, Tonkonogy, & Ananth, 1991). Fixed posture is limited to the poverty of the associated movements of the arms while the patient is walking. There is an absence of many of the symptoms typically observed in cases of Parkinson's disease, such as the bending forward of the trunk and the head, flexion at the elbows and knees, propulsion and retropulsion, and festinating gait. Speech often becomes dysarthric, though the characteristic hypophonia and festination are not present. Hypersalivation, as well as greasy facial skin, are also not noted in cases of neuroleptic-induced parkinsonism. This may partly reflect the milder degree of disturbances in secondary parkinsonism due to the timely use of benztropine as an antiparkinsonian agent, as well as a reduction in the dose of neuroleptics. The full pattern of primary parkinsonism, however, is not seen even in more severe cases of neuroleptic-induced secondary parkinsonism. It is of interest that clorazepam, a neuroleptic that does not induce parkinsonism or tardive dyskinesia, often elicits prominent sialorrhea in a manner that is usually more pronounced than the hypersalivation of patients with Parkinson's disease.

Parkinsonism has frequently been observed as a sequela of encephalitic lethargica, which spread around the world between 1919 and 1926. One of the manifestations of postencephalitic parkinsonism is the experience of oculogyric crises, which are spastic deviations of the eye(s) to the right, to the left, upward, or downward (Von Economo, 1931).

Steele, Richardson, and Olsewski (1964) described a disorder that included the clinical symptoms of supranuclear ocular palsy, extrapyramidal rigidity, bradykinesia, shuffling gait, ataxia, and resting hand tremor. The disorder is somewhat similar to parkinsonism but shows limited or no response to L-dopa (Steele, 1972).

Pure Akinesia

Pure akinesia is similar to parkinsonism but does not include tremor and rigidity. The syndrome was studied by Riley, Fogt, and Leigh (1994), who presented data suggesting that pure akinesia may represent a limited expression of progressive supranuclear palsy.

The gait of those with pure akinesia is characterized by a frequent freezing of motion, which the patient may overcome by stepping over an object. In a case presented by Riley et al. (1994), the patient walked with a wooden block attached by a short chain to a cane. He placed the block in front of the affected foot to overcome the frozen state. Hesitation, festination, and disequilibrium with frequent falls were also noted. Similarly, the patient's speech becomes marked with festination and freezing, as well as stuttering, stammering, hypophonia, and a loss of modulation. Handwriting also becomes festinated, and micrographia develops. Pure akinesia differs from parkinsonism in that there is an absence of rigidity while there is a cessation of movements of the eyelids accompanied by blepharospasms. The patient does not experience tremors or dementia during the progression of the illness. No response to L-dopa has yet been reported in any published cases.

Psychomotor Retardation

Psychomotor retardation was included in early descriptions of depression by Kraepelin (1913, 1919) and other authors at the turn of and in the early part of the twentieth century. The disorder is often present in patients suffering from depression, especially depression of the melancholic type. Akinesia seems to be the primary underlying feature of the syndrome of depression. Typical manifestations of psychomotor retardation include hypokinesia, a slowness of movements, face masking, and a decrease in associated arm movements while the patient walks. There is no rigidity, and no sign of fixed posture is present when the patient stands or walks. The patient's voice is hypophonic and bears no signs of festination or palilalia. However, evidence of depression in patients with Parkinson's disease may represent an early manifestation of a slowly progressing form of Parkinson's prior to the presence of more clear-cut symptoms, such as bradykinesia, rigidity, and fixed posturing. In such cases, it may be difficult to differentiate bradykinesia from psychomotor retardation of depression. Differentiation may be facilitated by findings of rigidity in the limbs, which may point to the possibility of primary parkinsonism.

Akinetic Mutism and Speech Akinesia

This syndrome was first described by Cairns, Oldfield, Pennybacker, and Whitteridge (1941), who reported a 14-year-old girl who had akinesia and mutism caused by an epidermoid cyst of the third ventricle. Fluid from the cyst was surgically removed, leading to remission. The syndrome closely resembles catatonia and may be due to brain tumors and cerebral vascular lesions.

Akinetic mutism is characterized by immobility and mutism, two features that are usually seen in catatonia. A patient may be lying in bed in a mute and immobile state but may be able to follow the examiner with his or her eyes and may appear to be in an alert state of wakefulness. This state has been called a "coma vigil" since the patient's consciousness seems to be preserved. Akinetic mutism is frequently observed when a patient is coming out of a coma and his or her sleep–wake cycles have begun again.

518

LOCALIZATION
OF CLINICAL
SYNDROMES IN
NEUROPSYCHOLOGY
AND NEUROSCIENCE

Speech akinesia is characterized by a preserved ability to speak. The typical patient is not as completely mute as one with akinetic mutism, but speech initiation is decreased and simplified, with frequent stops requiring encouragement of the patient to continue to talk.

Catatonia

Catatonia was first outlined as a specific syndrome by Kahlbaum (1874). The term was derived from a Greek word meaning "to stretch tightly." Kahlbaum's monograph was titled *The Tonic Mental Disorder or Tension Insanity,* to stress muscle spasms, particularly of the facial muscles, as the most prominent clinical feature of catatonia.

According to *DSM–IV* (American Psychiatric Association, 1994), "the clinical picture of catatonia is dominated by at least two of the following: (a) motoric immobility as evidenced by catalepsy (including waxy flexibility) or stupor; (b) excessive motor activity (that is apparently purposeless and not influenced by external stimuli); (c) extreme negativism (an apparently motiveless resistance to all instructions or maintenance of a rigid posture against attempts to be moved) or mutism; (d) peculiarities of voluntary movements as evidenced by posturing (voluntary assumption of inappropriate or bizarre postures), stereotyped movements, prominent mannerisms, or prominent grimacing; (e) echolalia or echopraxia" (pp. 288–289).

Abrams, Taylor, and Stoluarova (1979) postulated two catatonic subsyndromes in a factor analysis study of 55 catatonic patients. The first subsyndrome was characterized by mutism, negativism, and stupor, and the second by stereotypy, catalepsy, and automatic cooperation. The features noted for the first subsyndrome are similar to those of negativistic stupor and akinetic mutism and are frequently described in cases of neurological disorders and metabolic conditions and as side effects of toxic and pharmacological agents. Von Economo (1931) grouped the disturbances together as the amyostatic-akinetic syndrome and observed its presence during the acute stages of encephalitis lethargica. Though these features are somewhat similar to those of akinesia of parkinsonism, or pure akinesia, motor immobility is much more prominent in catatonia; and speech disorders do not reach the stage of mutism even in the more advanced cases of parkinsonian speech disorders.

The second subsyndrome of catatonia is often observed in patients with schizophrenia or affective disorder but is rarely mentioned in cases of patients with neurological diseases. This subsyndrome is characterized by a series of peculiar symptoms, including extreme negativism, or a resistance to movement; *gegenhalten,* or "going against" and resisting passive movements proportional to the strength applied; *mitgehen,* meaning "going with," in which an arm is raised in response to light pressure on the finger, despite instructions to act in a contrary manner; automatic obedience or exaggerated cooperation with an examiner's request; inappropriate and bizarre posturing, including catalepsy or the maintenance of an uncomfortable posture for prolonged periods of time; either waxy flexibility or extreme rigidity while an examiner tries to move the patient's extremities or trunk into different positions; stereotyped movements, including repeatedly touching, patting, or rubbing oneself; verbigeration, or the repetition of phrases and sentences; strange mannerisms such as walking on tiptoe or hopping; echopraxia; and echolalia (Taylor, 1990).

Catatonia is also characterized by a cycling from motor immobility to excessive and purposeless motor activity, also known as catatonic excitement. Kraepelin (1913) referred to this cycling as periodic catatonia.

The name fatal catatonia was introduced by Stauder (1934) to refer to cases with a sudden onset of extreme excitement, catatonia, and high fever. This is followed by a fast deterioration marked by autonomic instability, stuporous exhaustion, coma, cardiovascular collapse, and death. The treatment of choice for such cases is electroconvulsive therapy (ECT), which has been shown to help to prevent death in most cases (Taylor, 1990). Lethal catatonia resembles what is known as neuroleptic malignant syndrome. According to a review of 292 cases of lethal catatonia, 75% of such cases were characterized by hyperthermia in the early, pre–catatonic excitement phase, while the development of hyperthermia coincided with the onset of stupor in cases of neuroleptic malignant syndrome (Mann & Caroff, 1987; Mann, Caroff, & Bleiler, 1986). Other signs of catatonia, such as bizarre posturing or repetitions of the behavior of others, known as echophenomena, are generally absent in patients suffering from neuroleptic malignant syndrome (Taylor, 1990).

Catatonia was actually originally described as a form of bipolar disorder with the consecutive development of melancholy, stupor, and mania. Kahlbaum stressed the presence of seizure disorders in many of his cases, and he described severe pathological postmortem changes in some cases, particularly cases of tuberculosis. Several years later, Kraepelin absorbed the concept of catatonia into his general concept of dementia praecox. He and Bleuler, however, recognized the possible presence of catatonic symptoms in cases of depression and mania. Kirby (1913) described five women, each of whom suffered from a manic-depressive illness and exhibited typical catatonic symptoms, stressing that catatonia is more often seen in cases of manic-depressive illnesses than in cases of schizophrenia. Abrams and Taylor (1976) arrived at a similar conclusion based on an analysis of 55 consecutive admissions of cases with catatonia to a municipal hospital. Sixty-two percent of the patients were manic, while 11% had neurological illnesses, 9% were depressed, 5% had reactive psychosis, and only 7% had schizophrenia. Gelenberg (1976) extensively reviewed the literature and found

520

LOCALIZATION
OF CLINICAL
SYNDROMES IN
NEUROPSYCHOLOGY
AND NEUROSCIENCE

that, in addition to being connected with schizophrenia and affective disorders, catatonia as a syndrome may be connected with a variety of possible causes, including brain tumors, head injuries, vascular lesions, encephalitis, epilepsy, metabolic conditions, and toxic and psycho-pharmacological agents.

Anatomical Aspects

Primary and Secondary Parkinsonism

Lesions in cases of primary parkinsonism consist of idiopathic degeneration of the dopamine-producing nuclei of the substantia nigra. Other pigmented brain stem nuclei may be also involved. The formation of Lewy bodies is often observed in these affected areas. Clinical manifestations have been related to a lack of dopamine, which is needed to incite the dopamine receptors in the subcortical nuclei, especially the putamen and the globus pallidus. The localization of lesions in cases of secondary parkinsonism has been well studied in postencephalitic parkinsonism. As in cases of primary parkinsonism, there is cellular loss in melanin-containing neurons in secondary parkinsonism. There was no evidence of Lewy bodies, but neurofibrillary changes were observed in many of the nerve cells.

Progressive Supranuclear Palsy

The pathology of cases of progressive supranuclear palsy consists of neuronal degeneration, primarily in the midbrain structures—the substantia nigra, the pontine tegmentum, and the periaqueductal gray matter—as well as in the pallidum (Steele, 1972).

Pure Akinesia

PET scans in five cases of pure akinesia (PA) showed a reduced uptake of L-dopa in the striatum, as well as a decrease in the cerebral metabolism of glucose in the striatum and the frontal cortex (Taniwaki et al., 1992). Postmortem studies of eight PA patients revealed pathologic changes; neuronal depletion; gliosis; and neurofibrillary tangles in the globus pallidus, the subthalamic nuclei, and the substantia nigra (Homa, Takahashi, Takeda, & Ikuta, 1987; Matsuo et al., 1991; Mizusawa et al., 1993; Yuasa, Homa, Takahashi, Mori, & Nayashi, 1987). These findings were consistent with those for progressive supranuclear palsy (PSP), though three of the eight patients did not develop clinical evidence of PSP.

Akinetic Mutism

Tumors in the region of the third ventricle represent one of the most frequently described localizations of brain pathology in cases with akinetic mutism (Cairns et al., 1941; Daly & Love, 1958; Klee, 1961; Lavy, 1959;

Ross & Stewart, 1981). In cases of speech akinesia, the most frequently observed lesion is either bilateral or of the left hemisphere in the anterior cingulate gyrus and/or the supplementary motor area on the mesial surface of the frontal lobe. Lesions may be of vascular origin with an infarction in the vicinity of the anterior cerebral artery (Barris & Schuman, 1953; Damasio & Van Hoesen, 1983; Masdeu et al., 1978; Nielsen & Jacobs, 1951; Tonkonogy, 1986; Tonkonogy & Ageeva, 1961). Parasagittal tumors have also been implicated in cases of akinetic mutism (Arseni & Botez, 1961; Chusid, de Gutierrez-Mahoney, & Margules-Lavergne, 1954). Speech akinesia manifesting as akinetic mutism may be pronounced in some such cases, though usually without the complete immobilization typical of akinetic mutism.

Tonkonogy (1986, Case 7) reported a case of speech akinesia in which the cerebral infarction involved primarily the white matter of the anterior cingula and the posterior portion of the first frontal gyrus on the mesial surface of the hemisphere. The infarction was anterior to the paracentral lobule, corresponding to the supplementary motor area of Penfield. The infarction responsible for speech akinesia was located in the same area in another case (Tonkonogy, 1986, Case 8), but no visible changes were noted in the cingula or the corpus callosum.

Catatonia

The clinical manifestations of akinetic mutism strongly resemble major features of the first subsyndrome of catatonia, also known as Catatonia 1 (Abrams et al., 1979), including immobilization and mutism. Some researchers have pointed to the possibility of similar localizations of lesions in both conditions (Gelenberg, 1976; Johnson, 1993). As in akinetic mutism, lesions in cases of Catatonia 1 may be localized in the mesial frontal lobe and in the hypothalamic structures around the floor of the third ventricle. Freeman and Watts (1942) found cases of Catatonia 1 to be the result of a lesion localized in the frontal lobe in patients with traumatic head injury suffered during battle when a bullet passed through the frontal lobe. Similar results were found by Hillbom (1960) with regard to individuals who had suffered traumatic missile wounds, primarily in the frontal lobe, and by Joseph (1990), who experienced a frontal subdural hematoma after having suffered a beating to his head. A similar type of catatonia was described in patients with parasagittal prefrontal lobe tumors (Brain, 1965), frontal lobe infarctions (Belfer & D'Autremont, 1971), and atrophy of the frontal lobe (Ruff & Russakoff, 1980), and in those who had suffered an aneurism of the anterior cerebral artery.

Catatonia 1 was also reported in a 45-year-old male who had suffered bilateral infarctions of the parietal lobes (Tippin & Dunner, 1981).

522

LOCALIZATION
OF CLINICAL
SYNDROMES IN
NEUROPSYCHOLOGY
AND NEUROSCIENCE

During the acute period of stroke, the patient was alert but unresponsive, and was resistant to passive movements of his limbs. Tippen and Dunner examined the patient 6 months following his stroke. At that time, the patient was sitting rigidly in a chair, leaning toward the right. He exhibited no spontaneous motor activity and demonstrated negativism by resisting passive movements of his limbs. He was mute most of the time, except for occasional incomprehensible muttering. There was no sign of waxy flexibility, and a head CT scan showed low-density areas that were restricted to the parietal lobes in a bilateral fashion.

Other researchers, including Gelenberg (1976) and Johnson (1993), have used cases of akinetic mutism, which strongly resemble those of retarded catatonia, or Catatonia 1, to point to the role of diencephalic lesions in the development of catatonia. Involvement of the hypothalamic region may be especially significant in cases of lethal or fatal catatonia, which are characterized by autonomic symptoms as well as hyperpyrexia and cardiovascular collapse.

The role of the basal ganglia in disturbances has also been reported in some cases. Cravioto, Silverman, and Fergini (1960) described catatonic symptoms in a patient who had suffered a bilateral lesion of the globus pallidus, the result of poisoning with gas used for illumination. Similarly, Mettler (1955) found evidence of catatonia following bilateral lesions of the globus pallidus caused by surgical treatment for the relief of symptoms of Parkinson's disease. A catatonic stupor was described in cases of encephalitis lethargica by the terms *amyostatic-akinetic syndrome* and *epidemic stupor* and was noted as the third most common symptom experienced during the acute stages of the disease (Von Economo, 1931). Lesions in such cases involved primarily the basal ganglia, the diencephalic, and the upper brain stem regions.

The cerebellum and the brain stem form another region of possible involvement in cases of catatonia. Joseph, Anderson, and O'Leary (1985) presented the CT scan data on five catatonic patients and five matched control patients. Four of the five catatonic patients, as well as four of the five control patients, had been previously diagnosed with a neurological disorder, including Alzheimer's disease in two of the five patients in each group, and temporal lobe epilepsy in one patient in each group. Evidence of generalized cortical atrophy was present in both groups of patients. However, atrophy of the vermis and/or the brain stem was noted in all five catatonic patients; atrophy of the brain stem was not noted in any of the noncatatonic control patients, and atrophy of the vermis was found in only one of the control patients. Further support for these findings came from data presented by Wilcox (1991), who visually assessed the enlargement of CSF spaces in 17 patients with catatonia and an absence of neurological disorders, as well as in 30 non-catatonic schizophrenic patients, 20 patients with psychotic affective disorder, and 15 nonpsychiatric control subjects. Wilcox found evidence of mild cerebellar atrophy in 29% of the patients with catatonia and without other neurological disorders, in 8% of the noncatatonic schizophrenic patients, in 5% of those with psychotic affective disorder, and in none of the nonpsychiatric controls. However, cerebellar and brain stem atrophy was mild in all cases, and its role in the development of catatonia remains unclear.

The leading features of the second subsyndrome of catatonia, known as Catatonia 2 (Abrams et al., 1979), include extreme negativism, bizarre posturing of the body, and stereotypic movements and mannerisms. Catatonia 2 has usually been described in cases of schizophrenia and affective disorders, and data concerning the localization of lesions are based on PET scans and SPECT studies in single cases. Luchins, Metz, Marks, and Cooper (1989) described a 22-year-old female with schizoaffective disorder who developed psychosis and catatonia during a 3-week drug-free period, during which she exhibited mutism, odd posturing, waxy flexibility, and decreased psychomotor activity. After 17 days of treatment with lithium, the patient demonstrated no signs of catatonia. She underwent her first PET scan during the time of the onset of catatonia, which yielded a 1.18 ratio of left to right basal ganglia glucose metabolic activity. A second PET scan was performed when no evidence of catatonia was present, and the ratio of left to right basal ganglia glucose metabolic activity was down to 1.02. However, Early, Relman, Raichle, and Spitzmagel (1987) and Early (1990) performed PET scans on 10 noncatatonic schizophrenic patients and 20 normal control participants and found evidence of a relative increase in blood flow in the left globus pallidus in the noncatatonic schizophrenic patients as compared to the controls.

Satoh et al. (1993) presented the results of a SPECT study of regional cerebral blood flow (rCBF) in six patients with catatonic schizophrenia. All of the patients demonstrated manifestations of Catatonia 2, including bizarre posturing, odd mannerisms, negativism, catatonic stupor, and excitement. A control group consisted of four patients with disorganized schizophrenia, three patients with paranoid schizophrenia, six patients with undifferentiated schizophrenia, and seven normal individuals. SPECT imaging revealed a significant reduction of rCBF in the parietal lobes and, to a lesser extent, in the superior frontal lobes of both hemispheres in the patients with catatonic schizophrenia. No evidence of a reduction of rCBF was found in the noncatatonic schizophrenics or the normal controls. The data must be considered as preliminary, however, since low levels of rCBF have previously been recorded in the parietal lobe of some noncatatonic schizophrenic patients

524

LOCALIZATION
OF CLINICAL
SYNDROMES IN
NEUROPSYCHOLOGY
AND NEUROSCIENCE

(Kishimoto et al., 1987; Wiesel et al., 1987). These discrepancies in results are probably related to differences in medication status, which may significantly influence the SPECT and PET images, and also related to details of the anatomical localization technique.

Conclusions

1. Anatomic data in secondary akinetic disturbances point to the involvement of the following mesial frontal lobe areas: the area that corresponds with Penfield's supplementary motor area; the anterior cingula; the striatum; the pallidum, especially; and the hypothalamic region around the third ventricles. The role of the substantia nigra in reduced dopamine production is also stressed, especially in cases of parkinsonism, progressive supranuclear palsy, and pure akinesia.

2. The damaged regions in cases of akinetic disturbances overlap with those that are implicated in cases of apathy-avolition in one area—the pallidum. A difference between the two disturbances is that lesions of the frontal cortex are concentrated primarily in the dorsoconvexital areas in cases of apathy-avolition syndrome, and in the mesial frontal lobe and anterior cingula in akinesia syndromes. Thalamic lesions were only reported in disturbances of apathy-avolition, while hypothalamic areas seem to be involved only in akinetic syndromes. However, the involvement of these areas in apathy-avolition syndromes cannot be completely excluded.

APATHY, AVOLITION, AKINESIA, AND DISTURBANCES OF BRAIN INFORMATION PROCESSING

For many years, apathy, avolition, aspontaneity, and a general lack of concern have been described as manifestations of a "frontal lobe syndrome," thought to be related to lesions in the dorsolateral convexity of the frontal lobe. A similar syndrome appears to emerge following lesions of the dorsomedial nucleus of the thalamus and its surrounding structures, as well as of the globus pallidus. All three structures are included in the cortical-subcortical circuits that have been extensively studied in recent years.

At the turn of the twentieth century, Monakow (1904) demonstrated the great profusion of connections between the prefrontal cortex and the thalamus. These connections have been more recently studied in much greater detail (Fuster, 1989). It has been shown that reciprocal connections are especially prominent between the prefrontal cortex and the mediodorsal nucleus, and that the projections seem to reveal a topological order. The medial, magnocellular portion of the dorsomedial nucleus appears to be interconnected with the orbital and medial prefrontal cortex, while the lateral, parvocellular part projects to the dorsolateral prefrontal cortex.

According to studies involving monkeys (Goldman-Rakic & Porino, 1985; Kuypers, 1978), a topological organization may also be demonstrated in other thalamic nuclei projections to the frontal cortex. The more rostral part of the cortex receives afferent signals from the more medial thalamic nuclei. This may be compared with the development of negative symptoms in cases with prefrontal convexital lesions, as well as paramedian thalamic infarctions involving the mediodorsal nucleus.

The connections of the basal ganglia to the prefrontal cortex appear to differ from prefrontal-thalamic interconnections by the absence of afferent signals directly from the basal ganglia to the prefrontal cortex (Fuster, 1989). However, the prefrontal cortex emits profuse efferent signals to the caudate nuclei and the putamen. Efferent signals are also traced from the prefrontal cortex directly to the globus pallidus, and indirectly from the prefrontal cortex to the striatum, to the nucleus accumbens, and then to the globus pallidus. The precise topological organization of these projections within the caudate and the pallidum has not been firmly established, and various types of organization have been suggested (Alexander, DeLong, & Strick, 1986). Selemon and Goldman-Rakic (1985) observed that a central strip of the caudate, from the head to the tail in a monkey, receives efferent signals from the dorsolateral prefrontal cortex, while the ventromedial longitudinal strip receives projections from the orbital prefrontal cortex, the anterior cingulate cortex, and the superior temporal cortex. In turn, the central strip of the caudate projects to the parts of the globus pallidus, after which the signals reach the dorsomedial nucleus of the thalamus through the ventral pallidum, which is interconnected with the prefrontal cortex (Nauta & Feirtag, 1986). Thus, the development of apathy, aspontaneity, and unconcern as they are related to bilateral lesions of the globus pallidus may be considered as an interruption of the basal ganglia portion of the DLPFC, which also includes the dorsolateral prefrontal cortex, certain parts of the caudate nucleus, the globus pallidus, and the parvocellular area of the dorsomedial thalamic nucleus.

It may be suggested that a lesion of any part of the DLPFC-subcortical circuit will lead to identical negative symptoms manifesting as a deactivation of emotion, drive, motivation, speech, and concern (Cummings, 1993). In this case, the individual parts of the circuit must be involved in the identical co-processing of activation programs. However, the functional role of the circuit cannot be limited to a simple function of turning on motivation, drive, or emotion. The individual parts of the circuit may each play a specific role in the activation process, and a decision to turn the system on may be quite complicated, requiring a processing of information related either to the social and physical environment or to the inner conditions of the organism. Stuss and Benson (1986) demonstrated the role of dorsolateral frontal convexity in the assessment of social conditions and the planning of social behavior. The results of such assessments and actions may be gauged by a feedback mechanism located in the same region that is responsible for turning on the logistics, motivation, drive, emotions, and speech needed to proceed with actions. Injury to the dorsolateral frontal convexity may lead to the destruction of this feedback mechanism, followed by a termination of the sense of logistics, and thus may manifest as the negative symptoms of apathy, avolition, and unconcern. This is often combined with disturbances of planning, foresight, scheduling, and shifting, as well as disturbances of the ability to follow plans or schedules—disturbances that are frequently observed in patients with frontal lobe lesions. The negative symptoms thus seem to be part of a broad frontal lobe syndrome.

While a thalamic lesion may also turn off the activation system, the role played by the thalamic nuclei may be different. Negative symptoms in thalamic cases are often accompanied by various degrees of alertness disorders, from the more pronounced somnolentia (Castaigne et al., 1981) to excessive daytime napping (Katz et al., 1987), pointing to a connection between levels of consciousness and activation of drive and emotion. In general, an increase in alertness leads to the turning on of the activation system, providing the logistics needed for gnosis and actions. Though lesions of the paramedian thalamus damage this system of activation, their clinical manifestations differ from those of the frontal lobe syndrome, since negative symptoms in the thalamic syndrome are often accompanied by disorders of consciousness, decreased alertness, and somnolentia. The system of activation in the thalamus may also receive sensory somatic information, which helps to activate drive and emotions when no somatic problems are sensed by the thalamic sensory nuclei.

The basal ganglia area of the DES activation system seems to provide connections with the activity of movement. In spite of the fact that no significant deactivation of movements is observed in the cases described above as negative symptoms related to bilateral lesions of the globus pallidus (Laplane et al., 1989; Strub, 1989), it has been well established that movement deactivation, bradykinesia, and akinesia in combination with apathy and loss of drive are often observed in patients with subcortical diseases, Parkinson's disease, and progressive supranuclear palsy characterized by involvement of the basal ganglia.

It may be suggested that the dorsolateral part of the DES activation system gauges social actions, while the basal ganglia area is tuned to the action occurring in physical space, and the thalamic area provides feedback for one's state of consciousness and somatic conditions. Lesions disconnecting these three parts of the activation circuit may well produce various types of negative symptoms, depending on the localization of injury within the circuit.

The activation program of the circuit seems to combine a set of relatively independent components—drive, emotion, speech, and movement. The particular programs of each component are most likely located outside the circuit but may be activated as some form of package needed for the activation and feedback control of the actions in the social and physical environments. This helps to optimize the use of every component in the logistics of goal-directed behavior. The primary purpose of the circuit is probably to connect all three feedback mechanisms, gauging and exchanging the appropriate information to turn on the activation system. A malfunction in one of the feedback mechanisms or in one of their connections may lead to the inhibition of all systems, and thus to the development of negative symptoms.

11

Disturbances of Regulatory Activity: Impairments of Emotion

MOOD DISORDERS

ROLE OF EMOTIONS IN THE ACTIVATION AND INHIBITION OF ACTIONS

EMOTIONS ARE USED by the self as a specific language for a rough assessment of both the outward and inner conditions, helping to invoke typical responses to these conditions. The emotional language consists of six to seven basic words that help to limit the recognition of such conditions to several general positive or negative situations, and to facilitate information processing by the brain to choose the appropriate program of action. When the outcome of one's own actions is unsuccessful, for example, the outcome may be followed by the experience of depression, with its corresponding programs that may slow down or postpone future actions in order to avoid repeated failure, to gain the time needed for a reassessment of the cause of the failure and to develop an effective plan of future action. In conditions in which there is a more favorable outcome of one's own actions, the subsequent elation may encourage the continuation of these successful actions. Sometimes, however, such encouragement may cause a person to fail to anticipate obstacles, and his or her pattern of actions may become

530

LOCALIZATION
OF CLINICAL
SYNDROMES IN
NEUROPSYCHOLOGY
AND NEUROSCIENCE

erroneous: this has become known as dizziness from success. Threats that lead to either fear or anger may also direct a person's subsequent actions in response to the threat.

In normal conditions, one's emotional background is constantly fluctuating, and assessments of actions in which emotions have been involved are usually of short duration and may be replaced by other emotions and assessments depending on the dynamics of the actions. A minimally or fairly short-lasting depressed mood may, for instance, prevent the continuation of social actions in the wrong direction, providing an individual with some time to change the direction of a particular activity or attracting the individual's attention and thus evoking an appropriate response to, for example, evolving health problems.

Patients with mood disorders often experience emotions that may become rigid and long lasting, leading the patient to assess different situations using the same negative or positive emotion (e.g., depression, mania, anxiety, or fear) and to respond in a way that is dictated by a program of action related to the particular rigid emotion. Depression, for instance, may become long lasting and severe, and thus counterproductive. This precludes the negative assessment of any neutral or positive situations, invoking a program of action that includes a loss of interest, anhedonia, a loss of energy, and a loss of appetite, as well as feelings of guilt and thoughts of suicide in more severe cases. A depressed patient develops a slowness of mental and physical activity and a loss of interest and constantly blames himself for imagined failures. The onset of apathy, or loss of interest, may manifest as one of the symptoms of depression.

In contrast, a manic patient becomes hyperactive and excessively involved in social activities, initiates a series of new and risky actions compounded by a loss of awareness of social rules, suffers an inability to maintain an appropriate social distance or to properly assess the consequences of his or her own actions, and experiences a sense of grandiosity. Anxiety may become long lasting and rigid and may not subside with positive accomplishments, such as washing one's hands or closing the door.

In some cases, emotions may be short lasting but very intense and are often defined as certain subcategories of affect. A sudden explosion of anger, for example, may come to fit the definition of *rage* when a patient becomes aggressive and violent in response either to a minor provocation or to no provocation at all. Intermittent exacerbation of emotions may also be observed in cases of panic attacks in which one experiences an extreme fear of dying, and panic suddenly sets in accompanied by prominent signs of autonomic nervous system excitation, including tachycardia, tachipnea, and sweating, as well as a rise in blood pressure and temperature.

This chapter presents the types of mood disorders that may be described on the basis of available clinico-anatomical findings.

DEPRESSION

A DEPRESSED MOOD is an essential feature of various types of depression. According to *DSM–IV–TR* (American Psychiatric Association, 2000), the symptoms of major depression include the following: a loss of interest or pleasure; fatigue, or a loss of energy; difficulty concentrating; psychomotor agitation or retardation; feelings of guilt or worthlessness; thoughts of suicide; insomnia; a loss of appetite; and significant weight loss. In cases of dysthymic disorder or minor depression, most of the symptoms are less prominent, and some are not present at all, such as thoughts of suicide, feelings of guilt, and psychomotor retardation or agitation. In cases of depression with melancholic features, all of the manifestations of depression are more severe and persistent than in cases of regular depression, including feelings of guilt, psychomotor retardation, thoughts of suicide, and a loss of interest, energy, and appetite.

Primary depression is characterized the absence of any definite disease that may underlie the onset of depression, while *secondary depression* is diagnosed in cases with the presence of apparent brain disease or medical systemic conditions that may be related to the onset of depression.

Secondary Depression

Clinical Aspects

Secondary depression has frequently been reported in patients with epilepsy (Betts, 1981; Currie, Heathfield, Henson, & Scott, 1971; Robertson & Trimble, 1983). Mendez, Cummings, and Benson (1986) reported evidence of depression in 55% of 175 outpatient epileptics, and in 30% of matched control subjects. Depression in epileptic patients is often characterized as being of the endogenous or melancholic type, with evidence of paranoia and other psychotic traits (Betts, 1981; Mendez et al., 1986). Patients with epilepsy are 4–5 times more at risk for suicide compared to the general population (Barcliough, 1987; Hawton, Feagg, & Marsack, 1980; Matthew et al., 1980). Mendez et al. (1986) found that prior suicide attempts were reported by 30% of epileptic patients, compared to only 7% of control subjects.

Depression is frequently observed in patients with cerebral tumors (Baruk, 1926; Hécaen & de Ajuriaguerra, 1954; Keschner, Bender, & Strauss, 1936; Malamud, 1967). The reported frequency of depression in cases of posttraumatic stress disorder has varied from 25% to 50% (Kinsella, Moran, Ford, & Ponsford, 1988; McKinlay et al., 1981; Robinson & Jorge, 1994). Depression may develop during the acute stages following traumatic

532

LOCALIZATION
OF CLINICAL
SYNDROMES IN
NEUROPSYCHOLOGY
AND NEUROSCIENCE

brain injury, or later during the follow-up period (a year or more later). Poststroke depression has been described in a series of publications by Robinson, Kubos, Starr, Rao, and Price (1984) and Starkstein, Robinson, and Price (1987).

Depression in patients with multiple sclerosis (MS) is characterized by nonmelancholic features, including sadness, a lack of interest, excessive worrying about the future, disproportionate displays of anger, and difficulties in concentration (Minden, Orav, & Reich, 1989; Whitlock & Siskind, 1980). The prevalence of depression in MS patients is estimated by some to be in the range of 27% to 54% (Minden & Shiffer, 1990) and by others to be in the range of 10%–40% (Cummings, 1994). The rate of depression seems to be higher among patients with cerebral involvement than among those with spinal cord involvement.

Depression has also been frequently observed in patients with degenerative diseases of late onset, such as Alzheimer's disease, Huntington's disease, frontotemporal dementia, and Lewy body dementia.

Anatomical Aspects

Temporal Lobe. Hécaen and de Ajuriaguerra (1956) reported evidence of depression in 31 out of 229 cases of cerebral tumors with psychiatric manifestations. Depression was found to be more frequent in cases with temporal lobe tumors (10 out of 24, or 42%) and mesodiencephalic tumors (5 out of 61, or 8%). The percentage of cases with depression with other localizations was far lower, including 6 out of 80 (7%) cases with frontal lobe tumors, 5 out of 75 (7%) with parietal lobe tumors, 1 out of 24 (4%) cases of frontotemporal tumors, 1 out of 25 (4%) cases with occipital lobe tumors, and 3 out of 85 (4%) of those with subtentorial tumors.

Depression in patients with temporal lobe tumors was often characterized as melancholic with suicidal thoughts and attempted suicides, while depression in frontal lobe patients was usually transient, switching between states of euphoria and asthenia in three patients, and of the melancholic type in two patients.

The frequent development of depression in patients with temporal lobe tumors was also stressed by Baruk (1926), Bush (1940), and Pia (1953). Malamud (1967) reported 18 cases of individuals who were admitted to a state hospital with various psychiatric diagnoses and who, unbeknownst to the patients themselves, had intracranial tumors. Four out of 10 patients with temporal lobe tumors located in the hippocampal and amygdala regions were diagnosed with depression; suicidal thoughts were reported in two of those patients. On the other hand, none of the seven patients with tumors in the region of the third ventricle and none of those with tumors located primarily in the frontoparietal region of the cingula were diagnosed with depression.

Though interictal depression may be noted in patients with various forms of epilepsy, it is more frequently observed in epileptics with complex partial seizures and temporal lobe foci as recorded via EEGs (Altshuler et al., 1991; Bear & Fedio, 1977; Dongier, 1959/1960; Mendez et al., 1986; Roy, 1979; Victoroff, Benson, Grafton, Engel, & Mazziota, 1994), particularly in comparison with patients with either grand mal generalized epilepsy (Shukla et al., 1979) or juvenile myoclonic epilepsy (Perini et al., 1996). The role of temporal lobe lesions was also supported by a significant decline of up to 45% in the rate of depression following a temporal lobectomy for the treatment of temporal lobe epilepsy (TLE) in patients with a lifetime history of depression (Altshuler, Raush, Delrahim, Kay, & Crandall, 1999). Similar results were reported by Hermann and Wyler (1989) and Raush et al. (1998). At the same time, de novo development of depression was observed in approximately 10% of surgical patients (for a review, see Altshuler et al., 1999).

Frontal Lobe. Depression has been found to be less prevalent in patients with frontal lobe tumors than in those with temporal lobe tumors Keschner et al. (1935) reported evidence of depression in only 6 out of 85 (7%) cases with frontal lobe tumors, while Keschner et al. (1936) noted depression in 21 out of 110 (19%) patients with temporal lobe tumors. Paillas et al. (1950) stressed an absence of depression in 72 cases with frontal lobe tumors.

Studies of poststroke depression have pointed to the possibility that such depression may be connected to lesions in the premotor areas of the frontal lobes, the adjacent areas of the central sulci, and the temporal and the parietal cortices in the left and, in some cases, the right hemisphere (Robinson et al., 1984; Starkstein et al. 1987). The severity of depression was found to be correlated with a more anterior localization of a left hemispheric stroke, more specifically in the posterior parts of the frontal lobe. This severity of depression does not reach, however, the degree of melancholic depression that is primarily described in patients with temporal lobe tumors and temporal lobe epilepsy. Also, despite significant correlations of poststroke depression with an anterior location of the lesion, depression may also be observed in patients with other locations of stroke throughout the right hemisphere and the posterior left hemisphere. Several studies have also pointed to weaker, but significant, connections between the onset of poststroke depression and other factors, including subcortical atrophy, family and/or personal history of psychiatric illness (especially affective disorders; Starkstein, Robinson, & Price, 1988; Starkstein et al., 1989), functional impairment (Eastwood et al., 1989), and a nonfluent type of aphasia (Robinson & Benson, 1981; Signer, Cummings, & Benson, 1989). Mean

534

LOCALIZATION
OF CLINICAL
SYNDROMES IN
NEUROPSYCHOLOGY
AND NEUROSCIENCE

scores for major depression also show significant improvement during the second year after stroke (Robinson, Bolduc, & Price, 1987).

Carson et al. (2000) recently reported results of a meta-analysis of 35 studies of depression in stroke patients. The authors concluded that there were no statistically significant differences between the incidence of poststroke depression in the case of the anterior localization of a lesion and the incidence in patients with lesions localized elsewhere in the brain, including anterior versus posterior lesions and right anterior versus left anterior lesions. Bogousslavsky, Ferrazzini, Regli et al. (1988b) reached a similar conclusion based on a study of 64 stroke patients using both the standard depression scales and observations made by acute care nurses who monitored patients continuously throughout the day. The nurses were instructed to assess the patients' observable behaviors, such as overt sadness. Special attention was paid to the assessment of patients with aphasia, who often represent the majority of the left anterior lesion group and who have exhibited the most severe symptoms of depression in previous studies based on standard depression scales. However, Bogousslavsky did not provide data concerning the comparative severity of depression in relation to various localizations of lesions, while Robinson et al. (1984) stressed the increasing severity of poststroke depression with more anterior lesions of the left hemisphere.

No correlation was noted in multiple sclerosis patients between the severity of depression and the extent of cerebral demyelinization. Affectively disturbed MS patients, however, had significantly greater temporal lobe involvement than a control group (Honer et al., 1987). Ron and Logsdail (1989) reported a significant correlation between lesions in the temporo-parietal areas and a flattening of affect, as well as the presence of delusions and thought disorders.

Some authors have stressed the role of lesion localization in the development of depression following head injury. Lishman (1968) reported primarily frontal and parietal lesions in cases of depression that had developed following penetrating head injury, while Grafman et al. (1986) stressed the role of injury to the orbito-frontal area in depression. Jorge et al. (1993) presented CT scan findings from 66 closed head injury patients, 28 of whom developed significant symptoms of depression following damage to the dorsal-frontal and basal ganglia regions.

Psychosocial factors, premorbid personality, and history of psychiatric illnesses also play important roles in the development of depression after traumatic head injury (Lishman, 1968).

Some authors have found a significant correlation between depression scores and regional cerebral glucose metabolism as measured by PET scans in patients with Alzheimer's disease (Hirono et al., 1998), while others have either failed to show such a correlation (Craig et al., 1996) or have found a correlation between depression and Alzheimer's disease and glucose metabolic rates in the parietal lobe but not in the frontal lobe (Sultzer et al., 1995).

Irle, Peper, Wovra, and Kunze (1994) studied mood changes following removal of tumors in the cerebral cortex in 141 patients. The researchers evaluated the mood of patients via a questionnaire consisting of 123 adjectives, which described factor analysis results of vigor, fatigue, extraversion, irritability, anger, and anxiety/depression. They found that patients with temporo-parietal or ventral frontal lesions reported postoperative increases in levels of fatigue, irritability/anger, and anxiety/depression and decreased levels of vigor/extraversion. The postoperative mood states of these patients significantly differed from the mood states of the patients in the other lesion groups. A clinical control group of 29 patients after spinal surgery for herniated discs showed fewer negative mood changes compared to the previously mentioned ventral frontal and temporo-parietal groups. Another group with lesions of the motor and somatosensory cortices reported highly positive mood states. Contrary to previously reported data, Irle et al. (1994) found that dorsolateral frontal lesions led to the development of highly positive mood states, while negative mood states developed after ventromedial frontal lesions. These findings may be partly explained by the authors' expansion of the ventromedial region beyond the orbitofrontal area, including the frontal poles. No significant differences were found in any emotional measures in groups of patients with left hemispheric lesions (n = 43) versus groups of patients with right hemispheric lesions (n = 83). However, it should be noted that the group of patients with lesions of the left hemisphere was significantly smaller than that of patients with lesions of the right hemisphere (43:83), since some left hemispheric patients were excluded, either due to evidence of aphasia or other neurological disturbances or because of a refusal to complete the questionnaire. The authors combined anxiety and depression into one group and did not individually compare the manifestations of depression in groups with various localizations of lesion. Also, the extent and exact localization of the lesions within the groups require further clarification: for example, the ventral frontal group included eight patients with lesions limited to that region and 10 patients with an extension of the lesion to the lateral frontal cortex. Seven of those 18 patients had meningiomas, and 11 had lesions that lacked clearly outlined borders, including 8 patients with gliomas, 2 with metastasis, and 1 with gamartoma.

Beginning in the early 1980s, a series of systematic studies of poststroke depression were carried out by Robinson and colleagues (Robinson et al., 1984; Starkstein et al., 1987). Researchers have used various depression scales, including those of Hamilton and Zung as well as the Present State Examination (PSE), to measure the presence and

536

LOCALIZATION
OF CLINICAL
SYNDROMES IN
NEUROPSYCHOLOGY
AND NEUROSCIENCE

degree of depression and have compared the data with the results of head CT scan data. Robinson et al. (1984) performed a study that utilized rigorous exclusion criteria, including those who were left-handed, who had severe comprehension disorders, who had a history of alcohol and/or drug abuse, who had a family and/or personal history of psychiatric disorder, and who had clinical evidence via CT scans of previous brain injury and/or multiple lesion sites. Thirty-six patients were eventually chosen for the study, including 22 patients with stroke-inducing lesions of the left hemisphere, and 14 with stroke-inducing lesions of the right hemisphere. Out of these 36 patients, evidence of major depression was found in 6 patients with left anterior lesions versus 1 patient with a left posterior lesion. Starkstein et al. (1987) also found poststroke depression to be associated with left frontal and left caudate lesions. Robinson et al. (1984) reported that minor depression was more frequent in patients with left posterior lesions (3 patients) compared to those with left anterior lesions (1 patient). Depression was diagnosed in only 2 patients with lesions of the right hemisphere, both of which were posterior lesions. At the same time, hypomania was noted in 6 of 12 right hemisphere patients—5 patients with anterior lesions, and only 1 with a posterior lesion. These anterior lesions were no closer than 18%–20% of the anterior-posterior (A-P) distance to the frontal pole, and no further from the frontal pole than 40% of the A-P distance, and thus covered areas in front of the central sulci, often extending to the parietal lobe. Some overlap between anterior and posterior groups was therefore noted. The researchers stressed that they had evaluated lesions that covered approximately the middle two-thirds of the hemisphere, being either primarily anterior or primarily posterior. Such lesions are usually in the territory of the middle cerebral artery and located in the proximity of the upper end of the limbic system and subcortical structures.

Sinyor et al. (1986) attempted to replicate previous findings by studying depression following recent stroke in 35 patients—19 patients with left hemispheric lesions and 16 with lesions of the right hemisphere as determined by CT scans. The severity of depression was found to be more prominent with the increasing proximity of the lesion to the frontal pole in patients with lesions of the left hemisphere, findings that are similar to those reported by Robinson et al. (1984). However, a curvilinear relationship was noted in patients with right hemispheric lesions—depression was more prominent in cases of both more anterior and more posterior lesions. Eastwood et al. (1989), who examined patients who were admitted to a rehabilitation center after suffering a stroke, confirmed significant correlations between the depression score and the distance from the frontal pole to the left hemispheric lesion. Sinyor et al. did not find significant correlations between depression scores and locations of lesions in patients who had suffered strokes of the right hemisphere.

Morris et al. (1992) also found that the severity of depressive symptoms was significantly correlated with a stroke of the anterior left hemisphere, but only when patients with a prior history of depression were excluded. Depression scores of patients with right hemispheric strokes were not significantly correlated with the location of lesion within the damaged hemisphere. The results reported by Robinson et al. (1984) were therefore replicated in that Morris and colleagues found a correlation between the severity of depression and a more anterior location of lesion in patients who had suffered a stroke of the left hemisphere. No such correlation was confirmed for strokes of the right hemisphere.

Lesions of the Left Versus the Right Hemisphere

Left Hemisphere. The laterality of epileptogenic foci has been attributed to the development of depression in cases of temporal lobe epilepsy. Most studies have favored an association between left temporal lobe epileptogenic foci and depression (Altshuler, Devinsky, Post, & Theodore, 1990; Bear & Fedio, 1977; Dominian, Serafetinides, & Dewhurst, 1963; Mendez et al., 1986). Flor-Henry (1969), however, found that manic-depressive disorder is associated with the right temporal lobe epileptogenic region, while Mignone, Donnely, and Sadowsky (1970) and Rodin and Schmaltz (1984) found no differences between the laterality of epileptic activity and the frequency of depression in cases of temporal lobe epilepsy.

Poststroke depression was mentioned by Goldstein (1948), who observed the development of catastrophic reactions of sadness, anxiety, and agitation in aphasic patients with left hemispheric lesions. Goldstein (1948) and Fisher (1961) regarded the onset of depression as a psychological catastrophic reaction to a physical and cognitive deficit caused by stroke. Gainotti (1972) described a depressive-catastrophic type of reaction as significantly more frequent in patients with brain damage to the left side of the brain, while an indifferent reaction was more frequent among the patients with damage to the right side. Gainotti based his conclusion on a study of 160 patients—111 with vascular etiology and 49 with neoplastic and other etiology. No data were presented concerning the number of patients with tumors. An analysis of the results also yielded statistically significant differences between left- and right-sided lesions for catastrophic reactions, anxiety, tearfulness, refusal to be tested, anosognosia, jocularity, and general indifference. Though depressive moods were observed more frequently in patients who had suffered damage to the left hemisphere, these tendencies were statistically insignificant.

538

LOCALIZATION
OF CLINICAL
SYNDROMES IN
NEUROPSYCHOLOGY
AND NEUROSCIENCE

Robinson et al. (1984) found evidence of major or minor depression in 14 of 22 patients who had suffered strokes of the left hemisphere, and in 2 of 14 right hemispheric stroke patients. On the other hand, inappropriate cheerfulness was observed in 6 of 14 cases with lesions of the right hemisphere, but in none of the cases of stroke due to lesions of the left hemisphere.

In cases in which depression developed following closed head injury, some researchers found lesions more frequently in the left hemisphere, especially in the acute period after the injury. Jorge et al. (1993) studied 66 patients who had been admitted to a hospital for the treatment of acute closed-head injury. CT scans were performed within the first days after trauma, as well as 1–2 weeks later. The presence of diffuse versus local lesions was assessed via CT scans. Twenty-eight patients, primarily with closed head injury according to CT scan data of lesion location, were given quantitative depression ratings using the Hamilton Rating Scale. Acute-onset major depression was diagnosed in 17 patients, and delayed-onset major depression was reported in 11 patients. The authors concluded that acute-onset depression was associated with the presence of specific lesion locations, especially lesions of the left dorsolateral frontal and/or left basal ganglia areas. No such association was noted between lesion location and delayed-onset major depression. The latter group of patients also had significantly lower scores for social functioning than the acute-onset group. A limitation of the study, however, was in the use of CT scan data for the detection of posttraumatic nonhemorrhagic lesions; MRI scans have been shown to be more sensitive for the detection of such lesions.

Right Hemisphere. Folstein, Maiberger, and McHugh (1977) compared 20 stroke patients with 10 orthopedic patients and found 45% (9 out of 20) of the stroke patients to be depressed, compared to 10% (1 out of 10) of the orthopedic patients. Among those 9 patients with poststroke depression, Folstein et al. reported that depression developed much more frequently in patients with strokes of the right hemisphere compared to those with strokes of the left hemisphere. Sinyor et al. (1986) used CT scan data to determine the location of lesions in 16 patients with stroke due to lesions of the right hemisphere and 19 patients due to lesions of the left hemisphere and found no differences between the two groups in the frequency of depression.

Some researchers have stressed that lesions of the right hemisphere are primarily responsible for cases of depression after head injury. In cases with penetrating injuries, for instance, depression was found to be frequent in patients with lesions of the right hemisphere, especially with injury involving either the right frontal and parietal regions (Lishman, 1968) or the right orbitofrontal area (Grafman et al., 1986).

No Differences Between Left Versus Right Hemisphere Lesions. Victoroff et al. (1994) presented data in support of more complicated relationships between the frequency of depression and the laterality of epileptogenic foci. The researchers studied 53 patients with medically intractable complex partial seizures using video-electroencephalographic telemetry and fludeoxyglucose F 18 PET. Ictal onset was found to be lateralized in 41 of the cases—in the left hemisphere in 19 cases and in the right hemisphere in 22 cases. Depressive spectrum disorder was diagnosed in 15 of the 19 (79%) cases of left-sided ictal onset, and in 11 of the 22 (50%) cases of right-sided onset. These differences, however, were not found to be state dependent, since no significant association was observed between the Hamilton Depression Scale rating and the laterality of ictal onset. At the same time, patients with a previous history of one or more depressive episodes after the onset of seizures demonstrated left-sided predominance of ictal onset. PET scans showed unilateral temporal lobe hypometabolism in 36 of 53 patients with complex partial seizures, and a history of major depression was found to be more frequent in patients with left temporal lobe hypometabolism. The authors stressed that this asymmetry was relative, since a history of major depression was strongly associated with high degrees of both left and right temporal lobe hypometabolism. In general, other researchers have not reported differences between the frequency of depression in patients with tumors in the right versus the left hemispheres (Hécaen & de Ajuriaguerra, 1956; Malamud, 1967).

Subcortical Diseases

Parkinson's Disease. While some of the early studies, based on clinical diagnoses of patients with Parkinson's disease, reported relatively low rates of depression (4%–7%; Hoehn & Yahr, 1967), others reported rates as high as 67% (Strang, 1965). Studies that were based on broader definitions of depression and on the active use of rating scales yielded rates ranging from 25% to 70% (Cummings, 1992; Dooneief et al., 1992). Using scores from the Beck Depression Inventory (BDI), researchers reported higher rates of depression in patients with Parkinson's disease than in normal elderly patients, spouses of Parkinson's patients, and disabled individuals. Depression scores of Parkinson's patients were in the range of 8.1%–14.1%, while the mean scores of other subjects ranged from 3.8% to 7.1%. However, as in poststroke depression, the profile of depressive features in cases of Parkinson's disease differed from that of melancholic depression, being rather similar to the profile found in nonmelancholic depression and minor types of depression. Several researchers reported high levels of irritability, hopelessness, sadness, dysphoria, and suicidal statements (without actual suicidal intentions or attempts) in patients with Parkinson's disease (Brown, MacCarthy,

Gotham, Der, & Marsden, 1988; Huber, Paulson, & Shuttleworth, 1988; Levin, Llabre, & Weiner, 1988; Taylor, Saint-Cyr, Lang, & Kenny, 1986). While reports of melancholic depressive symptoms, including feelings of guilt, failure, self-blame, and punishment were low, anxiety symptoms were reported to be rather high (Gotham, Brown, & Marsden, 1986), in similar fashion to the leading features of the neurotic stage of hypertension and cerebral atherosclerosis as described in the older literature.

Though depression seems to be more common in patients with pronounced gait and postural changes than in Parkinson's patients with tremors (Huber et al. 1988), these correlations need further exploration, especially in relation to rates of depression and levels of dopamine. Torack and Morris (1988) found evidence of ventral tegmentum involvement in four depressed patients with Parkinson's disease, and of no such involvement in two nondepressed Parkinson's patients. Interestingly, the ventral tegmentum is known to be a source of dopaminergic projections to the mesocortical and medial temporal regions. The role of decreased dopamine levels in depression may also be supported by observations of greater depression during akinetic off stages in patients experiencing the on–off phenomenon (Freidenberg & Cummings, 1989; Nissenbaum et al., 1987). These observations may be compared with PET scan findings of lower glucose metabolic rates in both the orbitofrontal cortex and the caudate nuclei of depressed Parkinson's patients (Mayberg et al., 1990).

Kostic et al. (1987) and Mayeux, Stern, Cote, and Williams (1984) reported levels of CSF 5-hydroxyindolacetic acid (5-HIAA), a serotonin metabolite, to be lower in patients with both Parkinson's disease and major depression than in nondepressed Parkinson's patients, though the 5-HIAA levels were not found to correlate with the severity of depression (Kostic et al., 1987; Mayeux et al., 1984).

In summary, the development of depression in patients with Parkinson's disease is primarily related to a decrease in the levels of major neurotransmitters, including norepinephrine, dopamine, and serotonin (for a review, see Meyerson, Richard, & Kastenberg, 1997).

Huntington's Disease. A diagnosis of depression is given to approximately 30%–40% of patients with Huntington's disease (Caine & Shoulson, 1983; Cummings, 1994; Folstein, Folstein, & McHugh 1979), most mostly depression of the melancholic type accompanied by a high rate of suicide. Common symptoms of depression include psychomotor retardation, insomnia, and anorexia with weight loss; dysthymia is noted in approximately 5% of patients with Huntington's disease. Mood fluctuations are typical, resembling bipolar disorder in some cases. In some families, mood disorders and suicidal attempts may precede the development of other manifestations of illness (Folstein et al., 1990).

The location of cerebral atrophy in cases of Huntington's disease has been shown to extend beyond the caudate nuclei, involving the frontal and temporal lobes, especially in the more advanced stages of the disease. However, no anatomical data have been published concerning the relationship between these extended lesions and the development of depression. Yet Mayberg et al. (1992) presented PET scan data showing paralimbic frontal lobe hypometabolism, a decreased rate of glucose metabolism, in the orbitofrontal cortex of patients with Huntington's disease, which they compared to an absence of hypometabolism in that region in patients without mood changes (Mayberg et al., 1992). Though further studies are certainly needed to outline possible peculiarities in lesion location in depressed Huntington's disease patients, melancholic depression accompanied by high suicide rates apparently develops in patients with Huntington's disease because of anatomical changes in the caudate nuclei and their connections with frontal lobe structures.

Cerebrovascular Diseases

White Matter Hyperintensities, Arteriosclerotic Changes. The role of arteriosclerosis in the development of depression in the elderly was first stressed by Alzheimer (1902), who described the nervous form of mild arteriosclerosis as characterized by mental and physical fatigue, headaches, dizziness, and memory impairment. Severe progressive arteriosclerotic brain degeneration begins with symptoms similar to those of the nervous form as well. During the progression of arteriosclerotic brain atrophy, the emerging symptoms of affective disorders include a morose, tearful mood, sometimes tantrum of distemper, apathetic behavior, severe melancholic dysphoria, and violent anxiety states. Though Alzheimer did not consider affective disorders to be a type of pseudodementia, he did recognize the presence of a gradual development of profound and torpid mental impairment (for a review, see Förstl, Howard, & Levy, 1992). Postmortem studies revealed multiple small infarctions in the cortex, white matter, and basal ganglia, as well as ventricular enlargement and a loss of brain weight.

Alzheimer stressed that his findings were different from Binswanger's encephalitis subcorticalis chronica, which was characterized by exceptionally severe arteriosclerotic degeneration of the long penetrating vessels of the lenticulostriate, the thalamo-perforate, and the medullary arteries, which arise from cortical branches to supply deep portions of the hemispheric white matter. Dementia was mentioned as a major manifestation of Binswanger's disease. Recently, with advances in brain imaging, signal hyperintensities in T2-weighted MR images have been observed in the cerebral white matter of both elderly individuals and patients with various neurological disorders, including cerebral

542

LOCALIZATION
OF CLINICAL
SYNDROMES IN
NEUROPSYCHOLOGY
AND NEUROSCIENCE

arteriosclerosis, multiple sclerosis, and head trauma with a shearing injury. Similar observations of signal hyperintensities have also been made in the periventricular and deep white matter of patients with cerebral arteriosclerosis and are considered to be a reflection of the anatomical findings seen in Binswanger's disease.

In addition to the dementia described in patients with Binswanger's disease, however, there have been a significant number of reports of dementia in elderly patients with depression. Coffey et al. (1988) presented a study of leukoencephalopathy in 36 elderly patients who had severe melancholic depression. Each of the patients had been referred for electroconvulsive therapy (ECT), either because of a diagnosis of a drug refractory type of depression or because of an intolerance to antidepressants. MRI scans revealed periventricular and deep white matter hyperintensities in 31 of the 36 patients (86%). Figiel, Krishnan, Doraiswamy, et al. (1991) reported evidence of caudate and white matter hyperintensities in 60% of patients with late-onset depression, versus 11% of patients with early-onset depression. Similar changes have been reported in normal, age-matched elderly control subjects, though the changes are less frequent and smaller in size (Coffey et al., 1988; Figiel et al., 1990; Rabins, Starstein, & Robinson, 1991). These data were recently confirmed in a Rotterdam Scan Study, which included a sample of 1,077 nondemented elderly patients, among whom depression was found to be 3–5 times more frequent in a group of patients with severe white matter lesions compared to a group of patients with either mild or no white matter lesions (Groot et al., 2000). A significant correlation was also found between severe subcortical lesions and a history of late-onset depression.

The theory of an arteriosclerotic/ischemic origin of hyperintensities was supported by postmortem studies (Boyko, Alston, & Burger, 1989; Marshall et al., 1988) that revealed two different patterns in cases with hyperintensities of white matter. One type of pattern manifests as myelin pallor that is not associated with the myelin breakdown products in local reactive astrocytes, making it unlikely that the loss of myelin is secondary to demyelination; it is suggested that ischemia may be the cause of the myelin pallor in this pattern. The second type of pattern involves a central infarct cavity, local demyelinization, and astrogliosis. The swollen, reactive astrocytes characterized by increased water and protein content are presumably reflected in high signal intensity for proton density and T2-weighted images in MRI scans. This deep white matter ischemia may also involve the basal ganglia, leading to lacunar infarcts.

Stroke. Starkstein, Boston, and Robinson (1988) studied depression in 25 patients who had suffered either ischemic or hemorrhagic infarctions restricted to the basal ganglia or thalamus. Lesions of the basal ganglia included lesions in the head of the caudate nucleus and/ or the lenticular nucleus, either with or without an extension to the internal capsule. Thalamic lesions extended to the internal capsule in some cases. Depression was assessed by the researchers using the Hamilton Depression Rating Scale, the Zung Self-Rating Depression Scale, and the Present State Examination. The authors observed more frequent and severe depression in patients with lesions located in the left basal ganglia, mainly in the head of the caudate nucleus, compared to those with lesions in either the right basal ganglia or either side of the thalamus. For example, mean scores on the Hamilton Depression Rating Scale were 20.3 in 8 patients with lesions of the left basal ganglia, but only 8.2 in 17 patients with lesions either in the right basal ganglia or in the thalamus. Major depression was diagnosed in 7 of 9 patients with lesions of the left basal ganglia. None of the 10 patients with thalamic lesions were diagnosed with major depression, and only 2 were diagnosed with minor depression. At the same time, elevation of mood, also known as euphoria, has been reported in patients with thalamic lesions (Graff-Radford et al., 1985; Hays et al., 1966).

Lauterbach, Jackson, Wilson, Dever, and Kirsh (1997) reported evidence of major depression in 31 patients with either subcortical lacunar infarctions or lesions of white matter.

Mesodiencephalic Lesions and Endocrine Disorders

Mesodiencephalic Tumors. Hécaen and de Ajuriaguerra (1956) reported evidence of depression in 5 of 61 patients with mesodiencephalic tumors. Cleghorn, Garnett, & Nahmias (1989) similarly reported depression in 5 patients with mesodiencephalic tumors—2 suffered from melancholic depression with suicidal ideas and feelings of an upcoming catastrophe, and 3 from a mild, asthenic depression.

Spence, Taylor, and Hirsh (1995) described a case of primary major depressive disorder in a patient with craniopharyngioma. A depressive mood was accompanied by hypersomnolence (excessive sleepiness) and hyperphagia (excessive eating), pointing to the possibility of a diencephalic lesion. An MRI scan revealed a hypothalamic lesion with a cystic area filling the third ventricle. A histopathological examination following surgical removal of the lesion area confirmed the mass to be a craniopharyngioma.

Endocrine Disorders. The prevalence rate of depression may be as high as 60%–70% in patients with Cushing's syndrome (Popkin & Andrews, 1997; Kelly, 1996), a condition characterized by an increased secretion of adrenocorticotropic hormone (ACTH), a hormone that in turn stimulates the secretion of cortisol. Depression is also reported in cases of adrenal insufficiency, which is typical of Addison's disease

544

LOCALIZATION
OF CLINICAL
SYNDROMES IN
NEUROPSYCHOLOGY
AND NEUROSCIENCE

(Johnstone, Rundell, & Esposito, 1990), as well as in some patients with hypothyroidism or, more frequently, with hyperthyroidism (for a review, see Hutto, 1999). The comorbidity of depression and diabetes mellitus may reach a rate of 14%–32% but may be primarily related to the high risk of macrovascular and microvascular complications in patients with diabetes (Kovacs et al., 1995).

Systemic Medical Conditions, Drugs, and Pharmacological Agents

Coronary Artery Disease. Lespérance, Frasure-Smith, and Talajic (1996) reported a significant rate of depression in patients recovering from myocardial infarctions (MI). This rate approached 50% by one year post-MI. Other medical conditions with an increased risk of the development of depression include cancer, with reported depression rates ranging from 5% to 58% (for a review, see Popkin & Andrews, 1997), as well as end-stage renal disease, with rates of 5%–8% for major depression and 17.7% for minor depression (Popkin & Tucker, 1992).

Drugs and Pharmacological Agents. Antihypertensives, especially reserpine and beta-blockers (e.g., propranolol) are the medications most frequently cited as causes of secondary depression due to their role in the depletion of the central catecholamines (for a review, see Smith & Atkinson, 1997). However, several studies have reported no increased risk for persons treated with beta-blockers and diuretics compared to placebo controls. Depression also represents one of the major components of withdrawal syndrome in patients with addictions to alcohol opiates and such psychostimulants as cocaine and amphetamine.

CONCLUSIONS

1. The development of secondary depression in patients with cortical lesions is usually underlain by the involvement of the temporal lobe, especially in more severe cases. Temporal lobe tumors and temporal lobe epilepsy may lead to the development of severe depression of the melancholic type and may be accompanied by suicidal ideas and suicidal attempts. Depression is less prominent and relatively rare in patients with frontal lobe tumors, though apathy and asthenia may be confused with symptoms of depression in many such cases. However, lesions leading to major depression may be also observed in poststroke and head-injured patients with frontal lobe involvement. Depression has been reported in some cases of damage to the parietal lobe.

The severity of poststroke depression appears to be less prominent than depression in both patients with temporal lobe tumors and those with epilepsy. Signs of melancholic depression, suicidal ideas and attempts, psychomotor retardation, and feelings of guilt are frequently described in patients with temporal lobe tumors and those with epilepsy, though usually not at all in poststroke patients. Thus the localization of lesion in truly severe, melancholic types of depression is primarily related to lesions of the temporal lobe, probably in the vicinity of a limbic structure, such as the amygdala. Stroke data point to the role of left posterior frontal lobe lesions in the development of major depression, though usually not reaching the severity of melancholic depression. In cases with posterior location of stroke in the left hemisphere, minor depression has been usually described.

2. A series of studies of patients with epilepsy and stroke point to the prevalence of left hemispheric lesions in patients with depression. However, some authors have not found evidence of differences between the location of lesions in the left and right hemispheres in patients with brain tumors, stroke, or epilepsy as well as depression. There have also been several reports of a prevalence of right hemispheric lesions in patients who developed depression following a closed head injury. These differences in results may be explained by factors other than lesion location, including personal and family history of psychiatric illnesses, especially affective disorders.

3. The onset of depression has been frequently observed in patients with basal ganglia disorders such as Parkinson's disease, Huntington's disease, progressive supranuclear palsy, and in some cases in stroke patients. Depression has also been reported along with white matter disease in patients with probable cerebral atherosclerosis. More severe cases of major depression seem to be described especially frequently in patients with caudate lesions, including patients with Huntington's disease and stroke patients. Some researchers have reported severe cases of depression in stroke patients with left caudate lesions.

4. In some cases, for instance in response to the side effects of drugs or medications, or in patients with Parkinson's disease, the changes in the neurotransmitter levels seem to be responsible for the development of depression. In other cases, for example, in coronary artery disease or cancer, the role of intoxication caused by disease must be taken into account.

5. In summary, lesions of several cortical, subcortical, and mesodiencephalic areas have been observed in patients with secondary depression. These areas include the temporal lobe and prefrontal regions, the basal ganglia, and the hypothalamus. More severe melancholic depression has been reported in cases with temporal lobe involvement, primarily in the areas adjacent to the amygdala,

546

LOCALIZATION
OF CLINICAL
SYNDROMES IN
NEUROPSYCHOLOGY
AND NEUROSCIENCE

in the caudate nucleus, and in the hypothalamic region. Lesions in the prefrontal region seem to be related to the development of less severe depression, probably with the more prominent component of apathy, or loss of interest.

Further studies are certainly needed to clarify the role of cortical and subcortical lesions in the development of depression, with special attention to the more precise location of lesions and comparisons of injuries of the right versus the left hemispheres. The melancholic and nonmelancholic types of depression should be evaluated as separate groups in light of apparent differences between the clinical manifestations of the two types of depression. Special attention should also be paid to dysthymia, or minor depression, whose clinical manifestations often overlap with those of Alzheimer's arteriosclerotic neurosis. While the role of arteriosclerosis manifested as white matter hyperintensities and microinfarctions in the development of these types of depression is uncertain, it is known for its high comorbidity with anxiety disorders.

Primary Depressive Disorder and Bipolar Disorder
MRI Data

Subcortical Abnormalities: White Matter Hyperintensity in Bipolar Disorder. Dupont et al. (1987) found that younger patients with bipolar disorder had an increased volume of abnormal white matter manifested as white matter hyperintensity in comparison with both similarly aged patients with unipolar depression and normal control subjects. Dupont et al. (1987) used quantitative MRI analysis to study 36 patients with bipolar disorder, 30 patients with unipolar disorder, and 26 normal control subjects. The observed volume of abnormal white matter was as follows: 3279 ± 1187 voxels in bipolar patients, 2803 ± 1147 voxels in unipolar patients, and 2656 ± 1135 voxels in normal control subjects. Patients with bipolar disorder demonstrated abnormal white matter that was distributed in a more anterior fashion than in the other two groups.

Figiel et al. (1989) analyzed MRI data in 18 patients with bipolar disorder, 12 manic patients, and 6 depressed patients, as well as 18 age-matched control subjects; all the participants were less than 60 years of age. Deep white matter hyperintensity was found in 8 of 18 (44%) of bipolar patients, and in only 1 of 18 control subjects (6%). Four of 8 bipolar patients (ages 27, 26, 31, and 37) with white matter hyperintensity had large patchy confluences ranging in diameter from 5 to 16 mm. The number of hyperintensities ranged from one to five, and all were located in the deep white matter of the frontal and frontal/parietal regions. The only subject in the control group with deep white matter hyperintensity had four punctate lesions, each 2–5 mm in diameter. Lateral ventricle enlargement was noted in 8 of the bipolar patients. Assessments of such enlargements were recorded as follows: severely increased in 3 patients, mildly enlarged in 4 patients, and moderately increased in 1 patient. No correlations were found between the presence of white matter hyperintensity and ventricular enlargement. None of the control patients had enlarged ventricles. No significant differences were found between bipolar patients with or without white matter hyperintensities in regard to the patient's age, the age of onset, prior treatment with lithium, and atherosclerotic risk factors.

Altshuler et al. (1995) compared a number of T2 abnormalities in 29 patients with Type I bipolar disorder, 26 patients with Type II bipolar disorder, and 20 normal control subjects. Periventricular hyperintensities were found in 61% of the Bipolar I patients, 38% of the Bipolar II patients, and 30% of the normal control subjects. The mean age for each of the groups was 41.6, 40.0, and 35.2 respectively.

In spite of reported findings by some researchers, white matter hyperintensity remains a relatively infrequent MRI finding in younger patients with bipolar disorder. In our own experience, such findings were occasional and mild. Their presence and clinical significance, however, require further studies.

Cortical Atrophy and the Enlargement of Lateral Ventricles in Patients With Primary Depression. The enlargement of the lateral and third ventricles, as well as cortical atrophy, is often seen via CT and/or MRI scans of elderly depressed patients (Coffey et al., 1988; Coffey et al., 1993; Jacoby & Levy, 1980; Jacoby, Levy, & Bird, 1981; Pearlson et al., 1997; Shlegel & Kretzschmar, 1987). Using morphometric analysis, Bowen et al. (1989) showed a loss of cells in the pars opercularis and temporal poles of elderly depressed patients. Rabins et al. (1991) performed MRI scans on 21 elderly adults with major depression, as well as 14 age-matched normal with and colleagues found that elderly depressed patients had greater cortical atrophy in the vicinity of the limbic structures, including temporal sulcal atrophy, larger-than-usual temporal horns and Sylvian fissures, more atrophy of the lateral and third ventricles, and greater severity of subcortical white matter lesions, than did normal control subjects. This points to the involvement of paralimbic cortical areas and hypothalamic and subcortical lesions in the onset of depression in the elderly.

The presence of similar structural abnormalities in young depressive patients remains questionable (Shlegel et al., 1989). Hauser et al. (1989) compared MRI data with quantitative measurements of various cerebral areas in a group of depressed patients with a mean age

548

LOCALIZATION
OF CLINICAL
SYNDROMES IN
NEUROPSYCHOLOGY
AND NEUROSCIENCE

of 40.5 years compared to a normal control group with a mean age of 33.8 years and found a relative decrease in size of the temporal lobe. When 5 of the 17 depressed patients, all over the age of 50, were removed from analysis so that both groups had a mean age of 33.8 years, the difference remained statistically significant for cerebral areas in the left hemisphere only. However, the group of depressed patients had half as many males (5 out of 16) as the control group (10 out of 21), a significant difference, which allows for the possibility that this difference was responsible for the differences described.

Reductions of volume in particular brain regions were also found in a number of MRI studies of patients with mood disorders. These reductions were observed in the frontal lobe (Coffey et al., 1993), the temporal lobe (Altshuler et al., 1991), the left hippocampus (Bremner et al., 2000), the right hippocampus (Swayze, Andreasen, Alliger, Yuh, & Ehrhardt, 1992), the left amygdala (Pearlson et al., 1997), the brain stem and cerebellar vermis (Shah et al., 1992), and the caudate nuclei (Krishnan et al., 1992). A postmortem study of eight patients with mood disorders and eight control subjects found reduced volumes of the left amygdala, the right and left external pallidum, and the putamen in the depressed group compared to the control group (Baumann et al., 1999). And yet at the same time, a number of such studies have reported negative findings (Johnstone et al., 1989; Raine et al., 1992; Strakowski et al., 1993; Yates, Jacoby, & Andreasen, 1987).

Elkis, Freedman, Wise, and Meltzer (1995) reported the results of a meta-analysis of 29 studies of ventricular size and sulcal prominence in patients with mood disorders, primarily unipolar depression. Head CT scans were utilized in most of these studies, though some were based on MRI data. Eleven studies reported a greater degree of ventricular enlargement than controls ($p < 0.05$), 15 studies yielded statistically insignificant effect sizes, and 3 studies reported no indication of statistically significant differences. Sulcal prominence was found to be statistically significant in 3 of 10 studies ($p < 0.05$), a statistically insignificant prominent increase was found in 5 studies, and no statistical significance was indicated in 2 studies. A meta-analysis of 11 studies revealed that patients with schizophrenia tend to have larger ventricles than those with mood disorders.

As to the particular areas known to be related to the processing of emotion, MRI studies have yielded controversial and conflicting results. Some researchers have reported, for example, an enlarged amygdala in patients with bipolar disorder (Altshuler, Bartzokis, Grieder, Curran, & Mintz, 1998; Strakowski et al., 1993), while others have found the amygdala of such patients to be either smaller than that of normal control subjects (Pearlson et al., 1997) or the same size (Swayze et al., 1992). Similar inconsistent results have been reported for the hippocampus, the caudate nucleus, the thalamus, and the prefrontal cortex (for a review, see Strakowski et al., 1993).

In summary, some increase in cortical atrophy and a mild degree of ventricular enlargement have been reported in patients with primary depression. However, those abnormalities existed to a minimal degree, if at all, and were revealed primarily by quantitative studies with significant overlaps between groups of affected patients and groups of normal patients. Some authors have found a decrease in size of the particular areas of the brain that are involved in emotion processing in patients with bipolar disorder. A reduction of volume in the right and left hippocampus, the amygdala, the caudate, the thalamus, and the prefrontal cortex has been noted in some cases of depression. These reports roughly correspond to the sites of lesions found in patients with secondary depression.

Functional Brain Imaging

Blood Flow in Cortical Regions. PET has been used to study local cerebral glucose metabolism in depressed patients. In such studies, fluorodeoxyglucose (FDG) is injected intravenously, after which it enters the brain and is phosphorylated by brain hexokinase to the metabolic product F-2-deoxyglucose-6-phosphate (FDG-6-PO4). This product remains in the neuron for a short period of time, during which an image may be recorded by the scanner. Since glucose, along with oxygen, is the major energy supply for the brain, the metabolism of glucose reflects the functional demand for energy by both the brain as a whole and particular regions of the brain. Several studies have showed that demands for energy, especially in the prefrontal cortex, may be decreased in depressed patients.

Some authors have reported that global glucose metabolism is significantly lower in depressive states than in euthymic or manic states (Post et al., 1987). Baxter et al. (1985) studied 5 bipolar depressed patients, 3 bipolar mixed patients, 11 patients with unipolar depression, and 9 normal control subjects and found that bipolar and mixed patients had supratentorial whole brain metabolic rates that were significantly lower than those of both the normal controls and patients with mania. Using a xenon 133 inhalation technique, Sackeim et al. (1990) studied regional cerebral blood flow (rCBF) in 41 patients with major depressive disorder and 40 matched, normal control subjects and reported a marked reduction in global rCBF in the depressed group. This reduction was more prominent in the frontal, central, superior temporal, and anterior parietal regions. Baxter et al. (1989) also reported decreases in global blood flow in unipolar and bipolar depressed patients compared to individuals either without depression or with obsessive–compulsive disorders (OCD).

550

LOCALIZATION
OF CLINICAL
SYNDROMES IN
NEUROPSYCHOLOGY
AND NEUROSCIENCE

Buchsbaum et al. (1986) found no decrease in global glucose metabolism in a study of patients with affective illnesses, while clinical depression ratings correlated negatively with whole brain metabolic rates. Silfverskiold, and Risberg (1989), using the xenon 133 inhalation technique, reported normal blood flow levels in a group of 43 depressed patients and 30 manic patients in comparison with a group of normal control subjects. Eight of the depressed patients were examined during a euthymic state following the course of ECT. No significant blood flow changes were observed. A more detailed and systematic study by Nobler et al. (1994) showed that decreases in cerebral blood flow in cases of major depression were not reversed by successful ECT treatment, which showed, rather, additional reduction, especially in responders to the treatment. Cerebral blood flow was assessed via the xenon 133 technique in 50 depressed patients both before single ECT sessions and 50 min afterward, as well as during the week following the completion of the ECT sessions. The authors found that, relative to the treatment baseline, both depressed and manic ECT responders had reduced global cerebral blood flow (CBF) both in the acute periods following single treatments and during the week following the course of treatment. Decreases in CBF posttreatment were more prominent in the frontal and anterior temporal regions among depressed patients, especially during the acute periods following individual treatment sessions. The induction of hypofrontality was more marked in manic responders than in nonresponders.

Buchsbaum et al. (1984) used the PET-FDG technique to study glucose metabolism in 10 bipolar depressed patients and in 19 normal control subjects. In a subsequent publication, Buchsbaum et al. (1986) presented data from a PET-FDG study of 20 patients with affective disorders (16 with bipolar disorder and 4 with unipolar depression), compared to 24 normal control subjects. The authors found that patients with bipolar affective illness had significantly lower ratios of frontal to occipital metabolic rates, relative to hypofrontality, and decreased ratios of basal ganglia to whole brain metabolic rates compared to normal controls. Though unipolar depressed patients showed similar tendencies, researchers stressed the small number of cases examined. Buchsbaum et al. (1986) also suggested areas of metabolic increase in the superior temporal cortex and of metabolic decrease at the temporal pole in patients with bipolar disorder. Buchsbaum et al. (1997) then used MRI templates to increase the anatomic accuracy of previous findings. The authors observed a significant decrease in blood flow in the middle frontal gyrus and an increase in the major temporal gyri in patients with bipolar disorder compared to a group of patients with unipolar depression and a group of normal controls. Left prefrontal hypometabolism with left-right prefrontal asymmetry was also confirmed in a

PET-FDG study of 10 severely depressed patients (7 bipolar and 3 unipolar; Martinot et al., 1990).

Several researchers have found evidence of decreased global cerebral blood flow in depressed patients (Matthew et al., 1980; Sackeim et al., 1990; Warren et al., 1984). Others, however, have reported normal levels of global CBF in depressed patients compared to normal controls (Goldstein et al., 1985; Gur et al., 1984; Silfverski et al., 1989). Many researchers have found topographical variations in CBF in depressed patients. Matthew et al. (1980) used xenon 133 inhalation probes in 13 patients diagnosed with major depression and found significantly reduced blood flow in the left hemisphere, as well as a tendency for decreased flow in the right hemisphere, compared to normal controls. Uytdenhoef et al. (1983), on the other hand, found evidence of diminished right-posterior and increased left-anterior CBF flow in patients with major depression. Using SPECT to study cerebral blood flow, Devous et al. (1984) found that a group of 22 unipolar endogenous depressed patients had significantly lower levels of CBF in the right temporal and parietal lobes than 29 normal controls, while 13 bipolar depressed patients demonstrated significantly higher flow than normals in the same regions of the left hemisphere. Using PET scans, Drevets et al. (1992) studied CBF in patients diagnosed with familial pure depressive disease and compared currently symptomatic and asymptomatic patients. The authors found statistically significant increases in CBF in the left prefrontal cortex in both groups, and an increase of activity in the left amygdala only for the depressed group.

Lesser et al. (1994) performed SPECT measurements of CBF in cortical areas in 39 depressed patients with a mean age of 60.9 years and 20 healthy control subjects of the same mean age. The depressed patients were found to have significant bilateral decreases in CBF in the orbital frontal, inferior temporal, and parietal areas. Cerebral blood flow was also found to be lower in the high frontal, superior-temporal, and parietal areas in the right hemisphere of the group of depressed individuals, and, contrary to the data obtained in a study of poststroke mood disorders, the uptake of the tracer was more prominently reduced.

The involvement of the temporal region was reported by Post et al. (1987), who studied glucose metabolism in 13 affectively ill patients compared to 18 normal controls. The affectively ill group included 5 patients in the depressed stage of the illness, 6 in the euthymic stage, and 2 in the manic stage. Maximum glucose metabolism was divided by any other maximum in the same brain slice. These measures were significantly reduced in the right temporal lobe of depressed patients compared to normal controls. Baxter et al. (1989) found a similar decrease of glucose metabolism in the left anterolateral prefrontal cortex, but not in the temporal cortex, in both normal controls and in patients

552

LOCALIZATION
OF CLINICAL
SYNDROMES IN
NEUROPSYCHOLOGY
AND NEUROSCIENCE

with OCD compared to those diagnosed with primary depression. Three groups of patients with various types of depression—10 with unipolar depression, 10 with bipolar depression, and 10 with secondary depression compounded by OCD—were compared with a group of 14 OCD patients with no accompanying major depression, as well as 12 normal control subjects. The mean glucose metabolic rates for the left dorsal anterolateral prefrontal cortex were divided by the metabolic rates for the entire slice of the ipsilateral hemisphere. The metabolic rates of the left hemisphere (ALPFC/hem) were significantly lower for all three depressed groups than for either of the two comparison groups (normal controls and OCD patients without major depression). No significant differences were found for the right hemisphere. A significant correlation between Hamilton Depression Rating scores and the left ALPFC/hem was also found.

Hypoactivity of the frontal cortex was noted in patients with primary depression at rest, being more prominent in the left hemisphere than in the right (for a review, see George et al., 1994) and being proportional to the severity of depression (Baxter et al., 1989; Ketter et al., 1993). However, functional neuroimaging data of depressed individuals taken either during neuropsychological tasks or pharmacological challenges showed blunted activation of the right insula during attempted recognition of emotions from facial expressions (George et al., 1993), as well as markedly blunted anterior limbic activation following intravenously administered procaine (Ketter et al., 1993). Normal activation in the dorsoprefrontal cortex was noted in depressed patients during the Wisconsin Card Sorting Test (Ketter et al., 1993), and in the parietal cortex during spatial tasks. A PET study of a group of 11 patients diagnosed with depression and 11 normal control subjects matched for both age and gender who were examined while taking the Stroop Test revealed blunted left cingular activation and increased left dorsolateral prefrontal cortex and visual cortex activation in the depressed group compared to the normal group (George et al., 1997).

In summary, most cerebral blood flow studies in patients with primary depression have found a decrease of CBF in the prefrontal cortex, while some have reported an increase of CBF in the temporal lobe.

Changes of Blood Flow in Subcortical Regions

Thalamic Areas. Using MRI templates, Buchsbaum et al. (1997) studied PET scans in 9 patients with bipolar disorder, 36 patients with unipolar depression, and 23 normal control subjects matched for age and gender. The bipolar patients demonstrated the greatest decrease in blood flow in the medial areas of the thalamus, especially in the medial dorsal nucleus; the changes were more pronounced, however, in the lateral regions of the thalamus.

Limbic System. PET studies of healthy subjects have found that the limbic system is activated during transient sadness (George et al., 1995; Mayberg et al., 1992; Pardo, Pardo, & Raichie, 1993) and anxiety (Ketter et al., 1993; Parekh et al., 1995). Limbic system abnormalities, primarily cingulate hyperactivity, were found in resting studies of mood-disordered subjects (Drevets et al., 1992; Ebert et al., 1994; Wu et al., 1992). George et al. (1997) also used PET scans during a modified version of the Stroop Test, which included words with sad connotations, in 11 patients with depression and 11 normal control subjects matched for age and gender. They found that, in contrast to the healthy control subjects, patients with depression demonstrated slight activation of the left cingulate during the task, and increased activity in the left dorsolateral prefrontal and visual cortices. Buchsbaum et al. (1997) reported significantly lower metabolic rates for the cingulate gyrus and significantly higher metabolic rates for the entire striatum in patients with bipolar disorder than for both those with unipolar depression and normal control subjects.

CONCLUSIONS

1. A series of studies has shown that primary depression may often be observed against the background of persistent functional deficits manifested as global and regional CBF changes, primarily in the dorsolateral prefrontal region, to a lesser extent in the temporal lobes, and in some cases in the parietal lobe. Changes in blood flow in the limbic system, particularly in the cingula, were also reported. Though these changes were described as decreases in blood flow, other researchers observed increases of blood flow in the same region, especially in the temporal lobes, in patients with primary depression. Contradictory results have been reported from studies of global blood flow, which was assessed as normal by some of the authors and by others as having decreased.
2. There are some differences in the reported sites of blood flow change in primary depression compared to the typical site of lesion in cases of secondary depression. In patients with primary depression, the prefrontal cortex is the most frequently cited site of changes in blood flow, while lesions in the temporal lobe and caudate nuclei have been found to be prevalent in cases of secondary depression.

Notice that melancholic depression usually develops in cases of temporal lobe lesions, while the development of other types of depression, such as major and minor, is often related to lesions of the prefrontal, caudate, and hypothalamic areas (Figure 11.1).

554

LOCALIZATION
OF CLINICAL
SYNDROMES IN
NEUROPSYCHOLOGY
AND NEUROSCIENCE

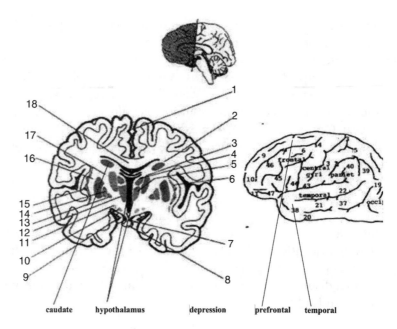

FIGURE 11.1   Primary sites of lesion localization in depression. Left figure: Subcortical structures on the coronal slice at the level of tuber cinereum. Localization of lesions in the caudate nuclei and hypothalamus. 1: Fissure longitudinalis. 2: Caudate nucleus. 3: Thalamus, lateral nucleus. 4: Anterior nucleus. 5 and 12: Medial nucleus. 6 and 15: Claustrum. 7: Infundibulum. 8: Hypophysis. 9: Nervus opticus. 10: Substantia nigra. 11: Corpus luisi. 13 and 14: Globus pallidus. 16: Capsula externa. 17: Capsula interna. 18: Corpus callosum. Right figure: Localization of cortical lesions in the left hemisphere.

Neurotransmitter Hypothesis.   Several hypotheses based on the therapeutic efficacy of antidepressants have been suggested to explain the mechanism of depression in the brain. One of the primary hypotheses was based on two observations: first, that antidepressants block the synaptic reuptake of either norepinephrine or serotonin, depending on the antidepressant, into the presynaptic neurons; and second, that there are decreased levels of the norepinephrine metabolite MHPG (3-methoxy-4-hydroxyphnylglycol) in the cerebrospinal fluid, urine, and plasma in patients with major depression. However, while the synaptic reuptake of antidepressants is immediate, the effects appear 10–15 days later. Some potent antidepressants, such as mianserin (not currently available in the United States), do not significantly block the reuptake of either norepinephrine or serotonin. In addition, the direct assay of norepinephrine itself recently became available, and studies employing this assay have revealed either normal or increased levels of norepinephrine in CBF and urine in patients with major depression.

Similar findings lead to the suggestion that the locus coeruleus–norepinephrine system is significantly activated in major depression (for a review, see Gold et al., 1981). The role of neuroendocrine abnormalities, especially hypercortisolism, in the development of depression has also been discussed in depth in the literature. Researchers have demonstrated that a significant percentage of patients with depression escape dexamethasone suppression, probably due to an increase in corticotropin-releasing hormone. Some have suggested that the corticotropin-releasing hormone and the locus ceruleus–norepinephrine system may reinforce one another's activities, and that these connections are disturbed in cases of major depression (Gold et al., 1981). The involvement of these changes in neurotransmitter activity and clinico-anatomical findings in the onset of depression requires further investigation.

MANIA

Mania IS DEFINED as a "persistently elevated, expansive, or irritable mood" (American Psychiatric Association, 2000, p. 362). The list of symptoms of mania include the following: inflated self-esteem and grandiosity; speech pressure; flight of ideas; racing thoughts; a decreased need for sleep; distractibility; excessive involvement in activities of questionable value, such as extreme shopping sprees; sexual indiscretion; and foolish business investments. *Hypomanic episodes* are identified as similar to manic episodes, but as not sufficiently severe to cause marked impairments in social and occupational functioning (American Psychiatric Association, 2000, p. 367).

Secondary Mania
Clinical Aspects
Secondary mania differs from *primary mania* in that the former includes the presence of an identifiable neurological disease. In most cases, secondary mania is characterized by features that are common in cases of primary mania, including hyperactivity, an excessive involvement in social activities accompanied by a loss of rules regulating social behavior, and disturbances in the planning and proper assessment of the individual's own position and achievements within the social environment. These disturbances are manifested as a lack of social distance; intrusiveness; an overfamiliar manner with others; tactlessness; hypersexuality; unusual sexual behavior; sexual disinhibition; sexual indiscretion; extreme promiscuity; marital discord; fatuous financial hyperactivity; foolish business investments; shopping sprees; elevated moods; extreme feelings of elation, euphoria, or irritability; hyperactivity of speech and thought; pressured speech; flight of ideas with a

556

LOCALIZATION
OF CLINICAL
SYNDROMES IN
NEUROPSYCHOLOGY
AND NEUROSCIENCE

preservation of logical sequence; racing thoughts; grandiosity; inflated self-esteem; inflated self-assessment of one's own social status; and unwarranted and perhaps extreme optimism. Hyperactivity is usually accompanied by insomnia, or a decreased need for sleep.

In some cases, secondary mania differs from primary mania in that the former exhibits the presence of empty euphoria, an idea that was originally described by Jastrowitz (1888) as *moria,* and by Oppenheim (1889) as *witzelsucht;* the term *fatuous euphoria* was later created to incorporate both terms. Specific features of fatuous euphoria include the following: empty euphoria, characterized by an absence of true elation; foolish euphoria; shallow affect; a lack of ability to experience pleasure; boastfulness; irritability; facetiousness; witzelsucht, or a tendency to exhibit pranks, jokes, and puns; childishness; and moria, or childish excitement. The concept of fatuous euphoria bears some resemblance to that of hebephrenic schizophrenia.

Bipolar disorder is characterized by the development of one or more manic episodes as well as one or more depressive episodes. Rapid-cycling bipolar disorder is defined as having four or more mood episodes within the previous 12 months. A mixed episode is diagnosed when a patient experiences rapidly alternating moods typical of depression and mania (American Psychiatric Association, 2000, pp. 362–365). When signs of depression prevail, a patient is in a gloomy mood, but psychomotor retardation is replaced by restlessness, motor excitation, and irritability, leading to an increased possibility of suicidal actions. In cases of mixed episode with a predominantly manic state, euphoria and elation may be combined with psychomotor retardation and an inhibition of mental processing, as defined by the term nonproductive mania.

Etiology

Secondary mania may develop in patients with brain tumors, stroke, epilepsy, or head injury, as well as in patients with degenerative brain diseases. It is most frequently observed, however, in patients with frontotemporal dementia and Huntington's disease. Secondary mania may also be observed in cases of viral encephalitis, as well as in general paresis, but is relatively rare in cases of Alzheimer's disease (for a review, see Cummings, 1985).

A list of systemic medical conditions that lead to mania includes some of the diseases that also result in the development of secondary depression, such as uremia, hemodialysis, cancer, hyperthyroidism, pellagra, and vitamin B12 deficiency, as well as postpartum conditions.

Mania may be induced by antiparkinsonian medications, antidepressants, psychostimulants, and several other drugs, including steroids. Psychostimulants represent one of the highest potentials for abuse among the drugs and pharmacological agents mentioned above (Cummings, 1985).

Anatomical Aspects

Frontal Lobe. The development of mania related to the frontal lobe was first noted in patients with general paresis caused by syphilis. Such patients were usually described as euphoric with a tendency toward jocularity and often demonstrated delusions of grandiosity, power, and fantastic wealth. Though grandiose symptoms were described most frequently in cases of general paresis during the first half of the 19th century (for details, see Hare, 1959; Lishman, 1978), they have since been reported less frequently, comprising a reported 7% (Fröshaug & Ytrehus, 1956), 10% (Dewhurst, 1969), and 18% (Hahn et al., 1959) of such cases. Pathology consists of inflammatory lesions throughout the cortex as well as cortical atrophy, especially in the frontal and parietal regions. Noguchi and Moore (1913) were the first to demonstrate treponema pallidum, a bacterium associated with sexually transmitted disease, in the brain tissue of patients with general paresis. The spirochets in such cases are found primarily in the frontal lobes.

Euphoria, mania, and a state of excitation have been frequently reported in patients with brain tumors in the frontal lobe and mesodiencephalic regions. Jastrowitz (1888) described euphoria, pressure of speech, and moria, or childish excitement, in several patients with frontal lobe tumors. Oppenheim (1890) defined these symptoms as witzelsucht, or prankish joking and punning.

Hécaen and de Ajuriaguerra (1956) reported the development of moria in only 2% of cases with frontal lobe tumors, while euphoria, also known as excitation, was observed in 17 of 80 (21%) patients with frontal lobe tumors, and 7 of 61 (11%) patients with mesodiencephalic tumors. Euphoria was noted in only 14 of the remaining 298 patients (5%) with tumors affecting other regions, including 3 of 75 (4%) patients with temporal lobe tumors, 2 of 24 (8%) patients with frontotemporal tumors, 5 of 75 (7%) patients with parietal tumors, 3 of 25 (12%) patients with occipital tumors, and 1 of 85 (1%) patients with subtentorial tumors. No cases of mania were observed in 11 patients with tumors of the central gyri, or in 11 patients with tumors of the corpus callosum.

Bush (1940) described a similar high proportion of euphoric excitation among patients with frontal lobe tumors through the presentation of 355 cases of individuals with brain tumors. Evidence of euphoria was noted in 21% of cases with frontal lobe tumors, and in only 10% of cases with tumors in other locations. Moria was observed in 6% of the 75 patients with euphoria. The reported percentage of cases with euphoria in patients with frontal lobe tumors has varied between 27% (Kolodny,

558

LOCALIZATION
OF CLINICAL
SYNDROMES IN
NEUROPSYCHOLOGY
AND NEUROSCIENCE

1927), 30% (Strauss & Keschner, 1935), and 21% (Paillas et al., 1950). The frequency of mania was not reported to be different between patients with tumors of the left and patients with tumors of the right hemisphere. Mania was also reported in four individual cases—with brain tumors in the frontal lobe in 3 cases (Starkstein et al., 1988) and in the frontoparietal region in 1 case (Oppler, 1950).

Euphoria and manic hyperactive behavior were also observed following the surgical removal of the frontal lobe in cases described by Brickner (1936) and Ackerley (1937). Rylander (1939) reported the onset of euphoria following frontal lobe surgery in 20 out of 32 patients. The orbitofrontal region had been removed in 18 of those 20 patients. Recently, Benjamin, Kirsh, Vissher, Ozbayrak, and Weaver (2000) described a 41-year-old right-handed patient who developed hypomania after undergoing a resection of the left frontal arteriovenous malformation (AVM).

Tisher et al. (1993) described a case of mania that developed in a 64-year-old nurse without any previous history of psychiatric illness. An EEG revealed periods of sharp and spike waves in the right frontal cortex. The patient initially demonstrated pressured speech, insomnia, hyperreligiosity, and a change of hand dominance from the right hand to the left hand. Staring episodes lasting from 30 to 90 sec were also noted. A head CT scan, a metabolic screen, a lumbar puncture, and a neurological examination were all negative. A SPECT showed an area of hyperperfusion in the frontal and posterior parietal regions of the right hemisphere, as well as the mesial temporal area of the left hemisphere. The patient showed marked improvements once on carbamazepine, and her family considered her symptoms to be under control. An EEG scan performed at that time read as normal, while a SPECT scan showed that the hyperperfusion had become limited to a small area of the right frontal region.

Temporal Lobe. Poststroke mania has been found to occur somewhat infrequently.Starkstein, Pearlson, Boston, and Robinson (1987) found only three cases of mania out of 700 patients who were being examined for symptoms of depression after having suffered a stroke. Lesions involving the temporal lobe have been recently reported in 4 patients, including a right temporal lobe hematoma (Cohen & Niska, 1980), a left temporo-parietal infarction, a right fronto-temporo-parietal infarction (Jampala & Abrams, 1983), and a right occipito-temporal infarction (Starkstein et al., 1988).

Mania has rarely been mentioned as an ictal, postictal, or interictal manifestation of epilepsy (Trimble, 1991), though focal abnormalities have been reported in some cases. Drake (1988) reported a bipolar patient whose EEG would change from normal in a euthymic state to a slower hypomanic state in the right temporal lobe and left temporal region during periods of depression.

Barczak, Edmunds, and Betts (1988) presented three cases in which hypomania developed following complex partial seizures in patients with right temporal lobe epilepsy. The authors stressed the significantly higher frequency of depression than mania in patients with epilepsy. Gillig, Sackellares, and Greenberg (1988) described a patient with complex partial seizures who exhibited emotional lability resembling mania during ictal periods. Manic behavior was also observed during ictal periods, during which EEG changes consisted of a nonrhythmic slowing of the right parietal and right posterior temporal areas.

Two cases of mania and hypergraphia in patients with temporal lobe epilepsy were reported by Sanders and Mathews (1994). In the first case, a 58-year-old right-handed man suffered a ruptured right middle cerebral artery aneurism, which required a craniotomy. The patient subsequently developed complex partial seizures characterized by unresponsiveness, staring, and automatisms. During interictal periods, the patient demonstrated hypergraphia, as well as several episodes of alternating manic and mildly depressive phases. An EEG revealed right midtemporal epileptiform activity, and a CT scan showed a low density area in the right temporal cortex. The second patient was a 38-year-old right-handed woman with a 25-year history of complex partial seizures with secondary generalization. During adulthood, the patient was hospitalized several times for manic behavior. She exhibited pressured speech euphoria, tangential thinking, and hypergraphia. An EEG study exhibited dysrhythmia in the right hemisphere, and a CT scan showed an area of decreased density in the right temporo-parietal region.

Frontotemporal Lesions. The development of secondary mania is relatively rare following head injury; the number of such cases is usually limited to 5%–10% of post–head injury patients. Tennent (1937) diagnosed mania in only 2 of 44 head injury patients, while Hillbom (1960) identified mania in only 7 cases out of a large number of head-injured Finnish war veterans. Recently, Jorge et al. (1993) diagnosed mania in 6 patients during the first year postinjury in 66 patients with closed head injury.

The exact lesion location is often difficult to determine in cases of head injury resulting from more diffuse types of brain pathology. Traumatic contusions are, however, often concentrated in the ventral aspects of the frontal and temporal lobes. Deshimaru, Miyakawa, & Suzuki (1977) described a patient who had developed a manic-depressive disorder following a head injury suffered at the age of 41. An autopsy following the patient's death revealed bilateral lesions of the orbitofrontal region. Shukla et al. (1987) reported 20 patients

560

LOCALIZATION
OF CLINICAL
SYNDROMES IN
NEUROPSYCHOLOGY
AND NEUROSCIENCE

who had mania after closed head injury. In many of these cases, the authors noted the presence of seizures with a prevalence of partial-complex or temporal lobe epilepsy. This may point to the involvement of the temporal lobe in cases of posttraumatic mania. Using a logistical regression method, Jorge et al. (1993) concluded that the presence of a temporal bipolar lesion was associated with a greater risk of mania development in patients with closed head injuries.

Subcortical and Diencephalic Lesions. Secondary mania has been reported in single cases with various subcortical and diencephalic localizations of brain tumors. The tumors were localized in dien-cephalic structures in 5 of 13 cases (Alpers, 1937; Guttman & Herrman, 1932; Malamud, 1967; Starkstein et al., 1988). Mania was also described in four patients with vascular thalamic lesions, two cases of infarctions in the right thalamus, one case of a right thalamocapsular infarction, and one case of right thalamocapsular bleeding (Starkstein et al., 1988). A frontal infarction in the right hemisphere was also reported in one case (Starkstein et al., 1988).

Lesions of the Right Versus the Left Hemisphere. Differences in mood change in relation to the involvement of the right versus the left hemisphere were probably first reported in patients recovering from the sodium amytal test (Wada test). The test was originally used to locate which hemisphere was dominant for language in order to avoid unexpected language disturbances following and because of brain surgery. It was observed that intracarotid injections to the nondominant right hemisphere were associated with euphoric-manic types of reactions, while inactivation of the dominant left hemisphere resulted in depressive-catastrophic types of reaction (Aléma & Donini, 1960; Aléma, Donini, & Rossi, 1961; Rossi & Rosadini, 1967; Terzian, 1964).

Neither Milner (1967) nor Tsunoda and Oka (1976) were able to confirm the differences in reaction type between dominant and nondominant hemisphere inactivation. However, Ley and Bryden (1981) did replicate previous findings, reporting the onset of euphoria following the inactivation of the nondominant right hemisphere.

Gainotti (1972) demonstrated similar tendencies in a comparison of 160 patients—80 patients with right hemispheric lesions, and 80 with left hemispheric lesions. Vascular etiology was diagnosed in 111 patients—53 of the left hemispheric patients, and 58 of the right hemispheric patients. Neoplastic and other nonspecified etiologies were noted in 49 patients—27 with lesions of the left hemisphere and 22 with lesions of the right hemisphere. Symptoms of indifference, extreme jocularity, and anosognosia as well as a minimization of deficits were three to four times more frequent in the right hemispheric patients compared to the left hemispheric patients, while some of the catastrophic reactions were noted approximately twice as frequently in the left hemispheric patients than in the right hemispheric patients. These catastrophic-depressive or indifferent reactions were observed in a minority of patients, specifically in 4 of 33 patients in total, and no such reactions were seen at all in the majority of the other 127 of 156 patients, supporting the suggestion that a unilateral lesion of the right or left hemisphere only increases the possibility for the development of particular manic or depressive reactions.

Sackeim et al. (1990) combined data from 119 published cases of pathological laughing and crying associated with destructive hemispheric lesions. The researchers found that pathological laughing was associated with predominantly right-sided brain damage in 25 cases, compared to 8 cases with lesions of the left hemisphere and 19 cases of bilateral damage. Pathological crying was found to be associated with left-sided lesions in 16 cases, right-sided lesions in 7 cases, and bilateral lesions in 3 cases. Pathological laughing or crying was associated with either bilateral or undetermined brain damage in the remaining cases.

Of the 19 hemispherectomy cases collected by the same authors, 12 of 14 right hemispherectomy cases were diagnosed as euphoric, while 1 was diagnosed as depressed, and 1 was determined to be normal (Sackeim et al., 1990). Out of 5 left hemispherectomy cases, 1 patient was determined to be depressed, 1 to be manic, and 3 to be normal. The authors also reviewed outbursts of laughing in 91 patients with gelastic epilepsy and in 6 cases of outbursts of crying, or dacristic epilepsy. They found the lateralization of the epileptic foci to be in the left hemisphere in 40 patients, and in the right hemisphere in 19 patients. The foci were bilateral in 18 patients and undetermined in 14 patients. In the cases of dacristic epilepsy, the localization of epileptic foci was found to be in the right hemisphere in 4 cases, in the left hemisphere in 1 case, and undetermined in 1 case. Sackeim et al. suggested that the association of pathological laughing with predominantly right-sided destructive lesions is related to the disinhibition of the contralateral left side of the brain, while direct excitation by the epileptic foci is responsible for gelastic epilepsy, an observation that is more frequently made in cases of left-sided epileptic foci. Gelastic epilepsy has also been described in cases of lesions involving the hypothalamus (Gumpert, Hansotia, & Upton, 1970; Louiseau, Cahadon, & Cahadon, 1971; Sher & Brown, 1976; for a review, see Cummings, 1985).

The high frequency of right hemispheric lesions in patients with secondary mania was also suggested by Cummings (1985), who reviewed 24 cases of secondary mania from the literature, as well as 2 of their own cases, in which the onset of mania followed right thalamocortical infarctions. Lesions of the right hemisphere were noted

562

LOCALIZATION
OF CLINICAL
SYNDROMES IN
NEUROPSYCHOLOGY
AND NEUROSCIENCE

in 12 of the 26 cases, and of the left hemisphere in 2 cases. The lesions were found to be bilateral in 7 cases and of the midline in mesodiencephalic structures in 5 cases. Starkstein, Robinson, and Price (1988) and Robinson et al. (1988) studied 17 patients with secondary mania after brain injury and found lesions to be frequently located in the right hemisphere. Seven of those 17 patients met the criteria for bipolar affective disorder. Starkstein , Robinson, Honig et al. (1989) replicated these findings in 8 patients with secondary mania. Seven of the patients had right-hemispheric lesions, and 1 had bilateral brain damage. Starkstein et al. (1992) stressed that secondary unipolar mania was associated in poststroke cases with the involvement of the orbitofrontal and basotemporal cortices, while bipolar affective disorder usually developed following right subcortical lesions, primarily in the thalamus and the caudate nucleus.

Berthier et al. (1991) described nine patients with bipolar affective disorder associated with cerebrovascular lesions. An episode of depression occurred first in eight of the nine cases, followed by mania-hypomania later in the course of the disease, usually around 8 or 9 months after the onset of the stroke. Two of the nine patients had a personal history of depression, and eight reported a negative family history of bipolar disorder. Mania was induced by fluoxetine in two cases. A rapid cycling type of bipolar disorder was observed in three patients. The mean age of the onset of poststroke affective symptoms was 51.2 years, with only one patient being younger than 40 years of age, and the oldest age of onset being 62 years of age. Neurological findings included left-sided hemiparesis in four patients, left-sided parkinsonism in one case, and left arm postural tremors in one case. MRI scans were performed on five patients and CT scans on four patients. Seven of the patients had lesions restricted to the right hemisphere, while the two remaining patients demonstrated bilateral hemispheric damage. Exclusive subcortical damage was seen in seven of the patients. The subcortical structures that were most frequently involved were the putamen (seven cases) and the periventricular white matter (six cases). Involvement of the internal capsule was reported in four cases, and the caudate nucleus was found to be damaged in three cases. The researchers presented one MRI film of Patient 7, showing multiple bilateral microinfarctions in the putamen and subcortical white matter, as well as prominent white matter hyperintensity. The date and type of stroke onset was not mentioned for any of the nine cases.

Conclusions

1. Secondary mania has been observed in patients with various localizations of brain tumors. The frontal lobes have been the most

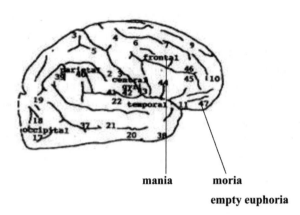

mania   moria

empty euphoria

FIGURE 11.2 Primary localizations of cortical lesions. Note that lesions are more often localized in the right hemisphere in patients with secondary mania. Lesions are less frequently found in the mesodiencephalic area. Note that cortical lesion sites often include the left hemisphere and frequently involve the temporal lobe in cases of melancholic depression, which is the most severe type of depression.

frequent site of brain tumor localization in such cases, reaching 20%–25% in different samples, while localization in the meszodiencephalic region was reported in 11%–38% of cases. Secondary mania was observed only in single-digit percentages of patients with temporal, parietal, and occipital lobe tumors, according to the literature. The development of euphoria after frontal surgery was also reported in many cases. **Moria** was observed only in 2%–6% of patients with secondary mania due to frontal lobe tumors. The role of an injury to the ventral aspects of the frontal and temporal lobes has been found in cases with the development of mania after head injury.

2. The development of mania in the interictal period in patients with epilepsy has been mainly reported in cases with EEG abnormalities, a slowing of electrical activity as well as paroxysmal activity, primarily in the right temporal lobe. In some cases, CT revealed a low-density area in the right temporal lobe.

3. A significant prevalence of right hemispheric lesions has been reported by many authors in cases of secondary mania following hemispherectomies and strokes and during the course of sodium amytal tests, as well as in cases of temporal lobe epilepsy. The development of secondary mania in patients with brain tumors has been observed by some to be relatively equally due to right and left hemispheric lesions, and by others to be due to lesions of the right hemisphere more often than lesions of the left hemisphere. A tendency to have suffered right hemispheric lesions due to stroke in patients with mania has been noted, as this was observed in seven

564

LOCALIZATION
OF CLINICAL
SYNDROMES IN
NEUROPSYCHOLOGY
AND NEUROSCIENCE

of nine cases in one particular report. Several cases of mania following a stroke in the thalamus, most frequently in the right thalamus, have also been noted.

4. Diencephalic tumors were reported in 5 of 13 (38%) individual cases, while the involvement of the frontal and temporal lobes was observed with a similar frequency, in 4 out of 13 (31%) cases. In one particular study, tumors were found to be right hemispheric in five patients, left hemispheric in one patient, and bilateral in three patients.

Primary Mania
Structural Brain Abnormalities

In contrast to the number of brain-imaging studies in depression research, few studies have been done in mania research. Using the quantitative analysis of CT scans, Pearlson et al. (1987) originally reported lateral ventricular enlargement in patients with mania. One of the first systematic studies of the subject was published by Nasrallah et al. (1982); in this study, structural brain abnormalities measured via CT scans were used to compare 24 manic patients, 25 schizophrenic patients, and 27 control subjects. All of the participants were males between the ages of 20 and 45. Both the manic and schizophrenic groups had significantly larger lateral ventricles than the normal control group. Sulcal widening was also found to be more prominent in patients with schizophrenia, while cerebellar atrophy was found to be more frequent in manic patients. Cerebellar atrophy in manic patients was also reported by Tanaka et al. (1982) and Standish-Barry et al. (1982). Tanaka at al. (1982) studied the CT scan data of 40 bipolar patients and 40 controls and found that in patients aged 49 or less, there was no significant difference in the measurements of the ventricular system, but there was a low length of the left septum-caudate distance in the bipolar group. Shlegel and Kretschmar (1987) examined CT scan data and found the third ventricle to be enlarged in affective patients.

Further data concerning the presence of some structural abnormalities in bipolar patients have been obtained via MRI studies. Hauser et al. (1989) compared the MRI data on 17 patients with affective disorder, 15 bipolar patients, 2 patients with unipolar depression, and 21 normal control subjects. The ratio of the temporal lobe to the cerebrum was significantly smaller in both hemispheres in the patients than in the control subjects. Altshuler et al. (1991) also found evidence via MRI data of reduced temporal lobe volume in bipolar patients.

Another interesting finding detected by MRI scans is the presence of subcortical signal hyperintensities in bipolar patients. Dupont et al. (1987) were the first to report this finding in 8 of 14 bipolar patients.

Swayze et al. (1990), also using MRI scans, confirmed the presence of signal hyperintensities in 9 of 48 bipolar patients, 5 of 54 patients with schizophrenia, and 2 of 47 normal control subjects. The mean age of the bipolar group was 41 years for men and 34.63 years for women. Signal hyperintensities in bipolar patients were localized on the lateral border of the ventricles in most cases and were bilateral in 4 cases. Signal hyperintensities were noted in 4 females and 5 males in the bipolar group. The researchers also measured the ventricular volume in all of the participants and found that ventricular volume was larger in the manic and schizophrenic patients than in the normal control subjects, with more apparent differences being noted in the male patients.

Functional Brain Abnormalities

Few functional imaging studies have been performed with patients with primary mania. Baxter et al. (1985), using 18-FDG PET scans, studied cerebral glucose metabolic rates in 11 patients with unipolar depression, 5 patients with bipolar depression, 3 patients with mixed depression, 5 patients with mania, and 9 control subjects. Global metabolic rates were found to be increased in the group of patients with mania in comparison with the group of patients with bipolar depression. No differences were found between the metabolic rates of those with mania and the normal control subjects.

Silfverski et al. (1989) studied rCBF with xenon-133 in 30 manic patients. The mean age of the mania group was 42 ± 12 years for the 20 males, and 43 ± 14 for the 10 females. There was no significant difference in either mean blood flow levels or regional distribution between matched normal control subjects and the entire group of manic patients, as well as with the male group of manic patients specifically. Significantly lower levels of blood flow, however, were found between the group of 10 female patients with mania and the normal control subjects.

Studies of blood flow in patients with mania in particular regions showed a decrease in prefrontal and basotemporal activity, and an increase in ventral singular activity. Each of these studies were conducted on a small number of patients with mania, usually with groups of no more than five or six subjects. Migliorelli et al. (1993), for instance, studied blood flow using SPECT in five female patients with mania and seven control subjects (six females and one male); the mean ages were 28 ± 5.8 years for the mania group and 25.2 ± 10.1 years for the control group. The manic patients demonstrated significantly lower cerebral blood flow in the right temporal basal cortex than the control subjects. The researchers explained the differences from previous findings as being due to the fact that three of the five subjects had not received psychotropic medications for at least a year prior to the study, while in

566

LOCALIZATION
OF CLINICAL
SYNDROMES IN
NEUROPSYCHOLOGY
AND NEUROSCIENCE

Baxter's group of patients (Baxter et al., 1985) a 7-day wash-out period was reported, and many of the patients studied by Silfverski et al. (1989) were on neuroleptics and other psychoactive drugs during the study. Blumberg et al. (1999) used high-sensitivity PET techniques to study regional blood flow in 11 patients with bipolar disorder, 5 patients with mania, 6 patients with euthymia in remission, and 5 normal control subjects. During a word generation test, decreased activation was registered in the right middle frontal gyrus (Brodmann's Area 10) and in the right orbitofrontal cortex (Brodmann's Area 11) in the manic group. In addition, decreased orbitofrontal activity at rest was noted in the manic group in comparison to the control group.

Nobler et al. (1994), however, measured cerebral blood flow with xenon-133 and demonstrated a decrease in blood flow levels 30 min prior to the first ECT session compared to 50 min after the fifth ECT session in 10 manic patients—6 females and 4 males. As in the group of depressed patients, larger global CBF decreases were found in responders to ECT treatment than in nonresponders to the treatment.

Conclusions

Brain-imaging studies of patients with primary mania showed some degree of increase in ventricular volume and the presence in some cases of white matter hyperintensity. Studies of cerebral blood flow revealed changes in global brain metabolic rates, an increase of which was recorded by some researchers and a decrease by others. In a manner somewhat similar to that of secondary mania, a decrease in cerebral blood flow was observed, primarily in the orbitofrontal cortex and the basal temporal cortex, and more frequently in the right hemisphere. The number of published studies is small, however, and further studies with larger samples are needed.

ANXIETY DISORDERS

In normal conditions, anxiety represents a normal, usually short-lasting response to various situations in the social and physical world that does not significantly interfere with the individual's functioning or cause marked distress (American Psychiatric Association, 2000). The anxiety and the related fear becomes excessive or unreasonable in cases of various types of phobia and anxiety disorders. Disturbances may manifest as general anxiety disorder, or sometimes as a specific phobia (simple phobia) if the experience of fear occurs in specific situations, as in a fear of close spaces, of open spaces at a high altitude, of staying at home or walking on the street alone, or of social situations (social phobia).

In this book, we discuss anxiety disorders in relation to relatively well-studied clinico-anatomical aspects. These include panic disorder, ictal fear in seizure disorder, and obsessive–compulsive disorder.

PANIC DISORDER

Clinical Aspects

According to *DSM–IV–TR* (American Psychiatric Association, 2000, p. 433), "panic disorder is the presence of recurrent, unexpected Panic Attacks followed by at least one month of persistent concern about having another Panic Attack, worry about possible implications or consequences of the Panic Attacks, or significant behavioral changes related to the attacks." The essential feature of a panic attack is "a discrete period of intense fear or discomfort that is accompanied by at least four or more of the following symptoms which develop abruptly and reach a peak within 10 min: palpitations; pounding heart, or accelerated heart rate; sweating; trembling or shaking; sensations of shortness of breath or smothering; a feeling of choking, chest pain or discomfort; nausea or abdominal distress; feeling dizzy, unsteady, lightheaded, or faint; derealization (feeling of unreality) or depersonalization (being detached from oneself); fear of losing control or going crazy; fear of dying; paresthesias (numbness or tingling sensations); and, chills or hot flashes" (p. 432).

Panic attacks may develop in patients with mesodiencephalic lesions in addition to those whose autonomic symptoms are usually found to be related to the temporal lobe. In such cases, the autonomic symptoms may also include goosebumps, polydipsia and polyuria, bulimia, increased blood pressure, increased or decreased body temperature, hiccups, excessive lacrimation, exophtalm with midriasis, excessive urination with colorless urine, and diarrhea at the end of paroxysm. The psychosensory symptoms of depersonalization and derealization have not been recorded in cases of panic attacks with mesodiencephalic origins (Davidenkova-Kulkova, 1959; Penfield, 1929; Scheffer, 1954).

Panic attacks resemble epileptic seizures in that they are abrupt, unexpected, and recurrent and are characterized by the development of paroxysm, which lasts approximately 10–15 min. The similarity of panic attacks to single partial seizures has also been stressed in the literature.

Signs of Panic Disorder in Patients With Seizures

Interictal panic attacks have been reported in a small percentage, specifically less than 1% (8 of 1,086), of patients with seizure disorders (Spitz, 1991). Weilburg, Bear, and Sachs (1987) described three cases

568

LOCALIZATION
OF CLINICAL
SYNDROMES IN
NEUROPSYCHOLOGY
AND NEUROSCIENCE

of concomitant seizure disorder and panic attacks manifested as either the aura of a complex partial seizure or interictal behavior. Wall, Tuchman, and Mielke (1985) recently reported episodes of panic attacks in a 33-year-old woman with a right temporal lobe arteriovenous malformation. Episodes of extreme fear and panic were associated with autonomic symptoms such as palpitations and a mild shortness of breath. An EEG revealed marked asymmetry between higher amplitudes and slower activity in the right hemisphere; sharp waves were present throughout the right hemisphere but were especially prominent in the central and parietal regions. Wall, Mielke, and Luther (1986) reported another case of panic attacks with autonomic manifestations in a 36-year-old woman with a history of encephalitis and mild left hemiparesis. This woman developed panic attacks 2 years following a right subtemporal decompression. The autonomic symptoms exhibited by the patient during such episodes included a rising sensation in the epigastrium, a burning feeling in the left upper extremities that spread to the left lower extremities, either excessive salivation or an extremely dry mouth, heart palpitations, hot flashes, and pleasant feelings that were described by the patient as resembling sexual gratification. A CT scan revealed a well-circumscribed decrease in density in the right parietal lobe, while an interictal EEG with nasopharyngeal electrodes showed epileptiform discharges of up to temporal leads.

According to Devinsky, Kelley, Porter, and Theodore (1988), the autonomic symptoms exhibited during simple partial seizures are identical to those experienced during panic attacks. Using video-EEG telemetry, the researchers studied the clinical and electroencephalographic features of simple partial seizures in 14 patients. Devinsky and colleagues observed 60 nonmotor seizures—26 autonomic seizures, 3 somatosensory seizures, 14 affective seizures, 1 cognitive seizure, and 16 mixed seizures. They usually found the EEGs to be normal in simple partial seizures. Ictal EEG changes were observed in only 9 (15%) of the nonmotor seizures, and in 18 (21%) out of all 87 simple partial seizures. The observed EEG changes consisted of localized spikes and paroxysmal theta activity over the temporal region.

In addition to developing during the course of panic attacks, autonomic symptoms may appear interictally in patients with panic disorder. We observed such symptoms in 11 patients, including bradycardia lasting about 46–48 min in 1 patient without cardiac pathology, irritable bowel syndrome in 2 patients, subfebrile temperatures in 1 patient, and dyspnea without signs of pulmonary pathology in 1 patient. A common manifestation of panic disorder in our patients was hypersensitivity to medium to high dosages of medications, which was observed in 8 out of the 11 patients. Fear accompanied by autonomic symptoms was reported in an additional three cases without panic attacks and local pathology of the heart, lungs, or gastrointestinal systems. Such cases have been identified as panic disorder without panic attacks, or diencephalic syndrome (Davidenkova-Kulkova, 1959; Scheffer, 1954).

Panic Attacks in Patients With General Medical Conditions, Especially Pheochromocytoma

Panic attacks may be observed without direct brain lesions as a result of intoxication via central nervous system stimulants, including cocaine and amphetamines, or in patients with various medical conditions such as hyperparthyroidism and cardiac arrhythmias (American Psychiatric Association, 2000, p. 437). Attacks are especially frequent in patients with pheochromocytoma, in most cases because of a tumor in the adrenal medulla. Pheochromocytoma produces, stores, and secretes the catecholamines with paroxysms, leading to episodes resembling panic attacks because of the sudden release of a large quantity of catecholamines. The autonomic symptoms in cases of pheochromocytoma are similar or identical to those noted in panic disorders and include tachycardia, diaphoresis, tac-hypnea, flushing, cold and clammy skin, severe headaches, angina, palpitation, nausea, vomiting, epigastric pain, visual disturbances, dyspnea, paresthesias, constipation, and a sense of doom. Hypertension is also a prominent feature in cases of pheochromocytoma; it is similar to that which occurs in cases of diencephalic seizures but occurs much more frequently than in diencephalic seizures. Hypertension in pheochromocytoma tends to be paroxysmal in 45% of cases and persistent in 50% of cases. Autonomic symptoms in such cases occur because of the secretion of catecholamines, including norepinephrine, epinephrine, and dopamine. This points to the possibility that panic attacks in patients without pheochromocytoma result from the hypersecretion of these hormones, which are stimulated by the seizure-like activity in specific brain regions such as the diencephalic and temporal lobe structures.

EEGs in Panic Disorders

Interictal Scalp EEGs. Beauclair and Fontaine (1986) recorded EEG changes in 27% of patients with panic disorder, 10% of patients with generalized anxiety disorder, and 3% of normal subjects. EEG abnormalities were defined as epileptic discharges. Stein and Uhde (1989) reported abnormal EEGs (defined as being laced with rhythmic midtemporal discharges and bilateral spikes) less frequently in patients with panic disorder (5 of 35, or 14%). Abnormal EEGs were reported primarily in patients with the psychosensory symptoms of derealization and depersonalization (4 of 15, or about 27%) as against those without these symptoms (1 of 20, or 5%). Similar frequencies were reported by Lepola, Nousiainen, Riekkinen, and Rimón (1990), who found abnormal EEGs in 13 of 54 patients (13%) with panic disorder. The EEG changes consisted of increased amounts of slow wave activity.

The Role of Subdural Recording.   Subdural recording is especially useful in studies of EEG abnormalities in patients with panic attacks. The role of subdural recording in the study of such disorders may be highlighted by the case of a 13-year-old girl who experienced episodes of fear while experiencing seizures (Devinsky et al., 1989). Video-telemetry did not reveal any changes in the scalp EEG. While subdural electrode recordings from the inferomedial temporal region showed epileptiform discharges, no changes were observed in the data obtained via electrodes placed over the lateral convexity of the temporal lobes.

Ictal EEG Changes During Panic Attacks.   Weilburg et al. (1993) described two cases with ictal EEG abnormalities. EEGs in Case 1 showed rhythmic 4.5 Hz sharp, but low amplitude theta, primarily in the temporal regions. Changes in Case 2 consisted of bursts of 3–4 delta activity over the right temporal region.

Ictal EEG changes seem to be similar during simple partial seizures and panic attacks. Ajmone-Marsan and Ralston (1957) found ictal changes during less than 50% of seizures, while Gastaut et al. (1956) reported such changes in 70% of seizures, and Thomas, Reagan, and Klass (1977) reported EEG abnormalities in 17 of his 19 patients with simple partial seizures. Using video-telemetry, Devinsky et al. (1988) found ictal EEG changes to be significantly less frequent, more specifically in 21% of simple partial seizures, including 33% of motor simple partial and 15% of nonmotor simple partial seizures. The data presented by Devinsky et al. (1988) show an almost identical frequency of EEG changes in panic disorders and simple partial seizures.

Anatomical Aspects
Amygdala and Temporal Lobe

The role of the amygdala in the conditioning of fear has been demonstrated in a series of animal studies. Kapp, Frisinger, Gallagher, and Haselton (1979), for example, showed that lesions to the central nucleus of the amygdala in rabbits disturbed the conditioning of the fear reaction as measured by heart rate. They also demonstrated that the amygdala is involved in responses to aversive events, leading to the experience of fear and to a conditioning to the stimuli that predict those threatening events (Blanchard & Blanchard, 1972). The role of neurons in the amygdala was later studied via single-cell recording in the macaca fuscata (Ono & Nishijo, 2000).

Subsequent studies described the projections from the central amygdala to the regions involved in the expression of fear. The lateral hypothalamus, for example, is involved in conditioned blood pressure increases, either through the tonic vasomotor center in the rostral ventral medulla (LeDoux, Ciccetti, Xagoraris, & Romanski, 1990) or through the supraoptic and periventricular nuclei of the hypothalamus, which contain the endocrine control structures (see LeDoux, 1995). Further studies have pointed to the role of the lateral nucleus of the amygdala as a key interface, which receives sensory inputs and transmits them to the central amygdala via intra-amygdala connections. LeDoux et al. (1990) also demonstrated that auditory input to amygdala may be destroyed by lesions in the medial geniculate bodies as well as the auditory thalamus.

Human studies using PET and fMRI (functional magnetic resonance imaging) scans have recorded activation in the amygdala while subjects were viewing aversive pictures or films (Cahill et al., 1996; Irwin et al., 1996) or fearful facial expressions (Breiter et al., 1996; Morris et al., 1996), as well as in response to stimuli that predict a conditioned fear to aversive stimuli, such as visual cues (e.g., squares) as predictors of a shock (LaBar, Gatenby, Gore, LeDoux, & Phelps, 1998) or neutral faces as predictors of an aversive noise (Büchel, Morris, Dolan, & Friston, 1998). Adolphs, Russel, and Tranel (1994) and Calder et al. (1996) also observed that patients with bilateral lesions of the amygdala exhibited difficulties in the recognition of facial expressions of fear but were able to accurately recognize other emotions from examining facial expressions. Several subsequent studies, however, were unable to replicate these findings. It has been stressed that while difficulties in the recognition of fearful facial expressions points to the role of the amygdala in affective information processing, these fearful faces may not induce emotions in the subject who is actually perceiving the pictures (Whalen, 1998).

Studies of complex partial seizures have also provided information on the role of temporal lobe structures in the generation of fear. Though no one has yet been able to pinpoint the exact primary localization of paroxysmal activity in such cases, some have demonstrated the role of activation in adjacent to amygdala structures of the inferomedial temporal lobe.

Fear has been described as an ictal symptom in TLE. The experience of fear in such cases is usually brief, lasting only a few seconds, in anywhere from 10%–15% (King & Ajmone-Marsan, 1977; Silberman, Post, Nurnberger, Theodore, & Boulenger, 1985; Strobos, 1961) to 35% (Bingley, 1958) of patients.

Hermann, Wyler, Blumer, and Richey (1992) identified the location of the epileptogenic foci of 15 patients during presurgical evaluations. Twelve patients were examined via invasive EEG monitoring with

572

LOCALIZATION
OF CLINICAL
SYNDROMES IN
NEUROPSYCHOLOGY
AND NEUROSCIENCE

subdural strip electrodes, and 3 via noninvasive EEG scalp monitoring. Of the 15 patients, 13 exhibited a right temporal lobe origination of ictal fear. This pointed not only to the role of temporal lobe epileptogenic foci in the generation of fear, but also to the specific right hemisphere localization of such foci. The idea that a right hemispheric epileptogenic focus is responsible for the generation of ictal fear in humans certainly requires further studies before it can be confirmed.

Mesodiencephalic Region: Diencephalic Autonomic Seizures

Penfield (1929) described autonomic epilepsy in a patient with an encapsulated cholesteatoma of the third ventricle that was pressing on the dorsal anterior nuclei of the thalamus. At the beginning of the seizure, the patient would become restless, and an abrupt onset of flushing in the distribution of the cervical sympathetic chain was noted, as well as a sudden rise in blood pressure, lacrimation, diaphoresis, sweating, and tachycardia, as well as a marked retardation of the patient's respiratory rate and salivation, and transient exophtalm. A dilation or contraction of the pupils was followed by the disappearance of hot flashes and a decrease in blood pressure, hiccupping, transient chills, and goosebumps, and the transient increase of body temperature to 37.7 degrees was followed by a decrease below normal range but rarely by urinary incontinence. Neither convulsions nor a loss of consciousness were typically observed during the course of the seizure. Penfield assumed that an epileptic discharge would have originated in the vicinity of the dorsal nucleus of the thalamus, either unilaterally or bilaterally, and would spread through the collections of gray matter in the wall of the third ventricle, for example, the nucleus paraventricularis of Malona, the supraopticus, the tuberis, the mamilloinfundibularis, the corpus mamillare, and the corpus subthalamicum.

Penfield and Jasper (1954) later presented cases of mixed seizures, autonomic and somatic, that were caused by infiltrating tumors of the temporal lobe and basal ganglia. Engel and Aring (1945) described autonomic seizures in a case with a cyst in the region of the right dorsomedial nucleus of the thalamus. The hypothalamic attacks would begin with anxiety and would consist of symptoms including chills, fever, nausea, vomiting, abdominal cramps, oliguria, fluctuating hypertension, and tachycardia.

Scheffer (1954) and Davidenkova-Kulkova (1959) observed diencephalic epilepsy in a series of cases of patients with brain tumors. As in the cases described by Penfield, Scheffer and Davidenkova-Kulkova reported disturbances of respiration and thermoregulation, vasomotor disorders, and changes in heart rate and blood pressure during the course of the seizures. In addition, 40% of their patients were suffering from gastrointestinal disorders, including increased peristalsis, an imperative urge to defecate, often with diarrhea at the end of the paroxysm, and an unpleasant sensation of pain in the epigastric area. Polyuria was often observed at the end of the paroxysm. Transient increases of serum glucose and lactic acid levels were reported in several cases. The researchers stressed that diencephalic paroxysms differ from cortical autonomic seizures (seizures with temporal lobe origins) in the richness and diversity of the autonomic disturbances, as well as in the symmetrical distribution of those manifestations.

Wilcox (1991) presented a female patient who suffered from pituitary adenoma and panic attacks. The patient reported episodes of intense anxiety accompanied by tachycardia, shortness of breath, palpitations, and a feeling of dread. No loss of consciousness was observed during these episodes. A CT scan of the sella turcica revealed microadenoma of the left anterior lobe of the pituitary gland. A transphenoidal resection of the pituitary gland resulted in the cessation of the panic attacks.

Brain-Imaging Findings

Head CT Scans. Kellner and Uhde (1988) reported the CT findings on 8 patients with panic disorders. They observed mild to moderate cerebral atrophy in 5 out of the 8 patients (62.5%). Less drastic results were reported by Lepola et al. (1990), who found incidental CT changes in 6 of 30 patients (20%); the changes included mild cerebral atrophy in 4 cases and small lacunar infarcts in subcortical structures in 2 cases.

Brain MRI Scans. Fontaine et al. (1990) reported brain atrophy in 40% of a group of patients with panic disorder.

PET Scans. Reiman, Raichle, Butler, Herscovitch, and Robins (1984) and Reiman et al. (1986) found focal asymmetries in the parahippocampal gyrus in patients with panic disorder (Figure 11.3).

Treatment

Though anticonvulsants may be helpful in the treatment of simple partial seizures with autonomic signs, no positive effect has been noted in patients with panic disorder. At the same time, the combination of imipramine and benzodiazepines has been shown to be highly effective in the treatment of panic disorder. This points to a probable intermittent neurochemical imbalance as a major cause of panic attack, in a fashion similar to cases with pheochromacytoma. It seems that an increase in norepinephrine levels via the intake of the antidepressant imipramine may actually suppress the excess of other catecholamines in cases of panic attacks.

574

LOCALIZATION
OF CLINICAL
SYNDROMES IN
NEUROPSYCHOLOGY
AND NEUROSCIENCE

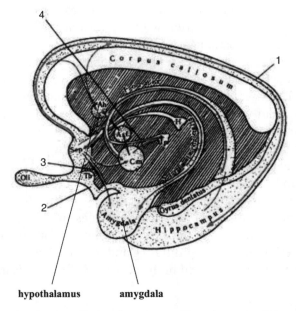

hypothalamus   amygdala

FIGURE 11.3 Localization of lesions in patients with panic attacks. Abbreviations are as follows: H—habenula; Ip—interpeduncular nucleus; Tb—tuberculum olfactorium; Olf—bulbus olfactorius; Cm—corpora mamillaria; At—nucleus anterior thalami; Ah—nucleus anterior hypothalami; Sep—septum pallucidum; 1. stria supracallosa; 2. stria olfactoria lateralis; 3. diagonal band of Broca; 4. fasciculus medialis.

Obsessive–Compulsive Disorder (OCD)

Clinical Aspects

Obsessions are defined by *DSM–IV–TR* (American Psychiatric Association, 2000, p. 462) as "recurrent and persistent thoughts, impulses, and images that are experienced, at some time during the disturbance, as intrusive and inappropriate and that cause marked anxiety and distress; the person attempts to ignore or suppress such thoughts, impulses, and images, or to neutralize them with some other thought or action." Examples of common obsessions include "repeated thoughts about contaminations (becoming contaminated by shaking hands), repeated doubts (. . . having left a door unlocked), . . . aggressive and horrific impulses (e.g., to hurt one's child or to shout an obscenity in church)" (p. 457).

Compulsions are defined as "repetitive behaviors (e.g., hand washing, ordering, checking) or mental acts (e.g., praying, counting, repeating words silently)" (American Psychiatric Association, 2000, p. 457). The *DSM–V–TR and Statistical Manual* (American Psychiatric Association, 2000, pp. 461–462) stresses that the goal of compulsions is to prevent or reduce anxiety or distress, not to provide pleasure and gratification as in eating disorders, sexual behavior (for example, paraphilias), and pathological gambling and substance use.

The difference between obsessions and compulsions seems to be to some extent artificial, since the repetitive behavior typical of compulsions usually accompanies obsessions. The existence of OCD symptom factors has been demonstrated (Baer, 1994), and each of these factors includes both obsessions and compulsions. Leckman et al. (1997), for example, reported that factor analysis revealed four main factors: aggressive sexual and religious obsessions with checking compulsions; symmetry obsessions with ordering, arranging, and repeating compulsions; contamination obsessions with washing and cleaning compulsions; and hoarding, saving, and collecting compulsions.

Compulsions differ from stereotyped movements, which are repetitive, seemingly nonfunctional motor behaviors (e.g., head banging, body rocking, self-beating). In order to differentiate between obsessions and specific phobias, *DSM–IV–TR* (American Psychiatric Association, 2000, p. 457) recommends, for instance, that a diagnosis of hypochondriasis should be used if the distressing thoughts are related to a fear of having a serious disease based on a misinterpretation of bodily symptoms. If the fear of illness, however, is accompanied by excessive washing or checking and attempts to be evaluated by an endless set of various tests, an additional diagnosis of OCD may be indicated. Thus the term *obsessive–compulsive disorder* is often preferable to the term obsessions, which may facilitate the differentiation between some types of specific phobias and obsessions. Obsessive–compulsive behavior is usually accompanied by a repetitive behavior or similar action of mind.

OCD has been described both as a primary psychiatric disturbance and a manifestation of other primary psychiatric disturbances, such as schizophrenia or depression. OCD has also been reported in a number of neurological disorders, including postencephalitic parkinsonism, Tourette's syndrome, cerebrovascular disease, brain tumors, brain injury, Pick's disease, and Huntington's disease, as well as being the result of amphetamine toxicity and levodopa therapy in patients with Parkinson's disease.

It should be stressed that the term compulsions was used in the old neuropsychiatric literature to describe egosyntonic, repetitive behavior with an absence of insight into the abnormal nature of the repetitive movements. The term was used, for example, to describe the repetitive movements in neurological disturbances, as in patients demonstrating sequelae of von Economo encephalitis. According to this previous definition, the term obsessions included not only obsessions per se but also compulsions and included only the egodystonic types of repetitive thoughts and actions. The poor insight that is typical for

576

LOCALIZATION
OF CLINICAL
SYNDROMES IN
NEUROPSYCHOLOGY
AND NEUROSCIENCE

egosyntonic repetitive behavior is actually mentioned in *DSM–IV–TR* (American Psychiatric Association, 2000, p. 458) as a specifier that "can be applied when, for most of the time during the current episode, the individual does not recognize that the obsessions or compulsions are excessive or unreasonable." In our view, the use of that specifier may be especially important for outlining some peculiarities of obsessive–compulsive disorder in cases with secondary OCD due to frontal lobe lesions, as well as in patients with Tourette's syndrome, Pick's disease, or Huntington's disease. It seems that the preservation of insight is one of the basic features of primary OCD.

Anatomical Aspects

Secondary Obsessive–Compulsive Disorder

Basal Ganglia.   Structural changes in the striatum, especially in the caudate nuclei, have been described in several cases of OCD. Laplane et al. (1981) reported a case of a previously healthy 53-year-old man who developed encephalopathy after being stung by a wasp at the age of 41. The most prominent psychiatric consequences included apathy, a lack of motivation, and inactivity. Two years after the wasp sting, the patient began to develop tendencies of compulsive mental counting, often accompanied by finger movements. He would count, for example, from 1 to 12, then begin again from zero, or perhaps count in multiples of three. He also liked to repeatedly switch the light on and off. Head CT scans revealed bilateral low-density areas in the anterior-medial part of the putamen and likely in the adjacent area of the pallidum as well. Other small low-density areas were observed in the head of the right and left caudate nuclei. Weilberg et al. (1989) reported a case of compulsive hand washing in a young college student. Brain MRI scans found changes in the striatum, probably of perinatal anoxic origin. The lesion appeared to be unilateral and left-sided and occupied the head of the caudate nucleus and the putamen. Ward (1988) described three cases of patients with transient compulsions, one of whom was a 62-year-old woman with lacunar infarcts in the left basal ganglia and the right superior cerebellar peduncle (Case 3). An EEG revealed abnormalities in the left temporal lobe.

We described the case of a 34-year-old gym teacher who developed compulsive hand washing spurred by compulsive thoughts concerning cleanliness and a fear of contamination (Tonkonogy 1989, 1994). The patient would also ride escalators without touching the handrails, go through revolving doors without putting her hands on the door, and take her coat off without using her hands. She washed credit cards before and after use and washed 10 loads of laundry per week. She washed her hands for 8–15 min at a time, 12–18 times a day. She used tissues whenever situations required her to touch or pick up anything. Insight into her repetitive actions was poor. She did not seem to be troubled by these actions, or to see them as excessive or unreasonable. Brain MRI scans revealed bilateral caudate atrophy (see Figure 11.4). Though the patient's fear of contamination and compulsive hand washing did diminish and eventually disappear about a year later, the disturbances then manifested as prominent pica compulsions, in which she had a desire to eat traditionally inedible items. At that time, head CT scans showed the progression of caudate atrophy, as well as the development of atrophy of the frontal poles and the bilateral medial surfaces of the frontal lobes. (For more details, see Figures 11.4 and 12.1.)

The figures 11.4 and 12.1 point to the role of caudate lesions in the development of egodystonic obsessive–compulsive hand washing, which disappeared following increasingly progressive frontal lobe atrophy. It also stresses the role of frontal lobe lesions in the development of compulsions similar to hypermetamorphosis, which is one of the primary manifestations of Kluver-Bucy syndrome and is characterized by a compulsive exploration of objects in the environment. Hypermetamorphosis was first observed by Klüver and Bucy (1937, 1939), together with hyperorality, or the oral exploration of objects, in adult rhesus monkeys with bilateral ablations of the temporal lobe anterior to the vein of Labbe. In our case, however, the lesion involved

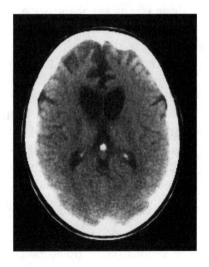

FIGURE 11.4 Head CT scan of a patient who had a fear of contamination and thus had obsessive–compulsive hand washing in the early stages of Pick's disease. The scan was performed 8 months after the onset of the obsessive–compulsive symptoms. Notice the butterfly-like appearance of the enlarged anterior horns of the lateral ventricles, reflecting bilateral caudate atrophy. Minimal frontal lobe atrophy is also seen. Marked progression of the atrophy involving the frontal lobes and the anterior temporal lobes was noted on a CT scan performed 3 years after the onset (see Figure 12.1). At that stage, the patient's fear of contamination and obsessive hand washing disappeared, after which the patient developed a prominent compulsion to eat inedible items, a disorder known as pica. Though the symptoms of OCD remained present during the course of frontal lobe and caudate atrophy progression, their structure had changed from egodystonic with a fear of contamination manifested by hand washing to egosyntonic with pica compulsions, probably related to the frontal lobe lesion.

578

LOCALIZATION
OF CLINICAL
SYNDROMES IN
NEUROPSYCHOLOGY
AND NEUROSCIENCE

the caudate nuclei and the frontal cortex, while the temporal lobes appeared to be spared when viewed via an MRI scan. An explanation of this substantial discrepancy may be related to the clinical peculiarities of hypermetamorphosis with hyperorality, which is characterized by a tendency toward oral exploration without eating the explored items, while a compulsive eating of inedible items, known as pica, was noted in our patient. The pica disappeared in our case with an accompanying development of prominent apathy, lack of spontaneity, and extension of cortical atrophy within the frontal lobe and adjacent areas of the temporal lobe. The diagnosis of Pick's disease, which had been suggested earlier in the course of the disease, seemed to be supported by the development of cortical atrophy limited to the frontal and anterior temporal lobes.

The patient continued to deteriorate. She developed recurrent pneumonia with frequent exacerbations, which eventually led to her death. The patient died 5 years after the initial onset of the disease. An autopsy revealed severe lobar atrophy involving the anterior frontal and inferomedial temporal lobes. Coronal sections showed a striking atrophy of the anterior putamen and the head, body, and tail of the caudate nucleus. The cingulate gyrus and the amygdala were atrophic. A microscopic examination revealed Pick's bodies in the striatum, substantia nigra, nucleus basalis of Meinert, and locus ceruleus.

Weiss and Jenike (2000) reported two cases of late-onset OCD. Case 1 was a 70-year-old woman who had developed obsessive–compulsive symptoms at the age of 53. Her symptoms included a fear that something terrible would happen while she was sleeping, which led to checking rituals, especially before bedtime. She would repeatedly check the stove, the sink, and the drain, for example, and would turn the light switch on and off several times until she was sure that she had "put it out right." Head CT scans revealed mild cortical atrophy with the focal area of attenuation in the head of the left caudate, consistent with a lacunar infarct of unknown age. Case 2 was a 70-year-old man who had developed a fear of contamination and infection at the age of 62, leading him to wash his hands approximately 20 times per day. A head CT scan revealed bilateral hypodense areas in the caudate nuclei, consistent with lacunar infarcts of an unknown age.

Frontal Lobe. OCD has been reported in several cases of frontal lobe lesions. Ward (1988) noted transient feelings of compulsion in two patients, with glioblastoma in the right frontoparietal region in one patient (Case 1) and left frontal glioblastoma in another (Case 2). Swoboda and Jenike (1995) described a 70-year-old man with hypertension and diabetes mellitus. At the age of 62, the patient was suddenly unable to recall a name of an actor, whom he had previously recognized with ease, while watching a television program. The patient began to experience extreme anxiety, calling several acquaintances, and eventually the television network, to get the answer. The patient then began to fear forgetfulness. To overcome the threat of forgetfulness, the patient began to memorize the names of songs and their composers, newspaper headlines, and the names of famous athletes and would collect lists of such items for future reference when needed. Insight into all of these activities was either limited or totally absent. A head CT scan revealed a wedge-shaped infarct in the posterior frontal lobe with extensions into the deep subcortical white matter. A SPECT scan revealed hypoperfusion in and around the damaged area but did not demonstrate any definite involvement of the right caudate nucleus. In another case, described by Volle, Beato, Levy, and Dubois (2002), a 40-year-old man developed a forced collectionism of electrical appliances following surgical removal of the olfactory meningioma, which resulted in a large porencephalic defect with bilateral involvement of the medial gyri in the orbitofrontal region with a bilateral extension into the middle and superior frontal gyri, as well as involvement of the frontal poles.

A case described by Donovan and Barry (1994) involved a 22-year-old man who had been involved in a motor vehicle accident and suffered an infarction of the right frontal lobe, a left subfrontal contusion, and fractures of the anterior and basilar areas of the skull. Against the background of apathetic syndrome with loss of initiative and social awareness, he developed a compulsion to count by odd numbers on the left and right sides of any object, ending on either the number seven or a multiple of seven. While driving in his car, the patient would travel only at speeds ending in the number seven and would read every license plate in view and every word on the passing billboards.

Checking rituals revolving around the number three were reported by Kim and Lee (2002) in a 66-year-old male patient who suddenly developed a fear that something wrong was going to happen. He began to lock and unlock every door in his house three times to confirm that the doors were locked, and to turn every faucet in the house on and off to confirm that the taps were not leaking. He also tied his shoes in the doorway several times a day. A brain MRI of the patient revealed a single infarct located in the medial portion of the left orbitofrontal cortex and involving the left gyrus rectus and the left medial orbital gyrus.

Forced thinking is manifested as a repetitive mental act that a patient feels forced to perform during an aura prior to a seizure. Jackson (1876) described an intellectual aura as a type of psychic seizure that begins with an alteration in thinking. Hill and Mitchell (1953) defined forced thinking as a psychic aura that is characterized by intrusive thoughts produced by epileptiform activity. Forced thinking was later separated

580

LOCALIZATION
OF CLINICAL
SYNDROMES IN
NEUROPSYCHOLOGY
AND NEUROSCIENCE

from psychic auras by Penfield and Jasper (1954), who related the origination of psychic auras to temporal limbic lesions and attributed forced thinking to the frontal lobe lesions. Other authors have related forced thinking to the temporal limbic structures (Brickner & Stein, 1942; Gloor et al., 1982). *Déjà pensé,* a separate temporal limbic psychic phenomenon, was described as a feeling that a thought had been previously experienced (Brickner & Stein, 1942).

Mendez et al. (1996) described three patients who were experiencing forced thinking as a result of left frontal lesions. In Case 1, a 36-year-old patient felt forced to think of the phrase "tell me yes" at the onset of partial complex seizures. An MRI scan revealed a neoplasm in the left frontal lobe, while an EEG revealed polymorphic delta changes in the left frontal area. An oligodendroglioma was partially resected during surgery, after which the patient's problems of forced thinking and seizure were resolved. Case 2 was a 29-year-old male who, during the onset of partial complex seizures, felt that his mind was talking to [him]. The phrases "why don't you tell them how you feel" and "why don't you have a seizure" also repeatedly came to the patient's mind, in a way he described as similar to a broken record. An MRI revealed a large neoplasm in the left anterior frontal area with extensions to the corpus callosum and the basal ganglia, and an EEG showed intermittent rhythmic delta activity, maximally in the left frontal area. The patient underwent a subtotal resection of a large low-grade glioma in the left anterior frontal pole. The patient in Case 3 was a 56-year-old woman who, at the beginning of her seizures, would experience the thought that she needed to "grab something." An MRI revealed nonenhancing areas of decreased signal intensity in the left frontal lobe, which had not changed in comparison to neuroimages obtained 6 years earlier. A possible old infarction was considered. An EEG showed slowing and electrographic seizures arising from the left frontal region.

In all three cases, attempts at vocalization with orobuccal movements, along with postictal (postsurgical) language difficulties, were observed during forced thinking, pointing to the possibility that motor language difficulties underlie the forced thinking from the left frontal lobe. Similar speech disturbances or speech arrests accompanied by left frontal lobe lesions were described in other cases of forced thinking (Penfield & Jasper, 1954; Ward, 1988). Temporal limbic cases differ from forced thinking in that they are characterized by experiential immediacy and the presence of vivid, out of context features, for example, a need to think about the onset of a specific story, "number 2," or a chain of words beginning with "esoteric" (Brickner, Rosner, & Munro, 1940; Gloor et al., 1982; Hill & Mitchell, 1953; for a review, see Mendez et al., 1996). Since obsessions and compulsions have been described in some patients with seizure disorders, an obsessive–compulsive component cannot be excluded from the overall picture of forced thinking (Kettl & Marks, 1986; Kroll & Drummond, 1993; Mulder, 1953).

Anterior Cingula. The role of the anterior cingula in the mechanisms of OCD has been demonstrated via cingulotomy, a surgical treatment in which the cingulate gyrus is disabled with the goal of alleviating the OCD symptoms. Whitty et al. (1952) were probably the first to report positive results from this procedure and did so in 4 out of 5 patients with OCD. The positive results of the cingulotomy were subsequently reported in approximately one-third of the patients. Kullberg (1977) noted a significant improvement in 4 out of 13 patients with OCD following the procedure. Similar results were reported by Baer et al. (1995), who performed cingulotomies to treat intractable OCD in 18 patients. The lesions were placed bilaterally in the anterior cingular cortex under the control and direction of MRI stereotactic guidelines. The lesion was 0.7 cm lateral to the midline in both hemispheres, 2 cm posterior to the most anterior portions of the frontal horn, and 1.0 mm above the roof of the ventricles. Positive results with the significant alleviation of OCD symptoms were noted in 5 of 18 patients (28%) during a postsurgical follow-up 26.8 months after the procedure. In addition, 3 patients met the criteria of "partial responders." Though Baer et al. did not statistically analyze the predictors of positive outcomes, they mentioned that the only predictors of such outcomes were preoperative obsessions with symmetry and compulsions of ordering and hoarding.

The reaction of amygdala neurons to various visual inputs was first studied via single-cell recording by Nishijo, Ono, Nakamura, Kawabata, and Yamatani (1986) and Nishijo, Ono, and Nishino (1988). Researchers have found that more than half of the vision-responsive neurons responded consistently to both familiar food and aversive nonfood objects associated with either an electric shock or a syringe. Similar responses were recorded from anterior cingulate (AC) neurons, though some significant differences were found between AC and amygdala (AM) neurons in the bar-press phase of the recordings (Ono & Nishijo, 2000). Some AC neurons responded when bars were pressed to obtain food, while other neurons were activated when bars were pressed to avoid an aversive stimulus such as an electric shock. No such bar phase–related neuronal activation was observed in the AM neurons. These results point to the role of the AC in motivation for movements, for which neurons are projected from the movement-related areas of the AC, through the anatomical connections to the motor and premotor cortices as well as the basal ganglia (Royce, 1982; Yeterain & Van Hoesen, 1978). Ono and Nishijo (2000) suggest that the AM may be involved in the evaluation of incoming external sensory inputs, while the AC receives and integrates inputs from the AM, the prefrontal cortex, and other emotion-related areas, then transforms the results of integration into appropriate motor behavior by sending the results of integration to the executive motor centers.

Clinical data support the role of the anterior cingula in the activation of motor behavior. Lesions in this area result in the inhibition of motor activity (see chapter 10 on disturbances of volition, motivation, and negative symptoms). It is also possible that the anterior cingula mediates conscious feelings of emotions, since its lesion leads to emotional flatness and apathy.

Subcortical Connections. At the same time, the interruption of the caudate and other subcortical connections had been used to treat OCD. A subcaudate tractotomy was introduced by Knight in 1963 to be used for the treatment of OCD and mood disorders. The lesion was placed in the region of the substantia innominata to interrupt the white matter tracts connecting the subcortical structures and the orbitofrontal cortex. Early reports showed an improvement in 50% of patients with OCD and 68% of patients with depression (Knight, 1965). Subsequent results, however, were less promising. Hodgkiss, Malizia, Bartlett, and Bridges (1995) reviewed the effectiveness of stereotaxic subcaudate tractotomy in the treatment of refractory OCD and mood disorders in 254 patients at the Geoffrey Knight National Unit of Affective Disorders in London between 1979 and 1991. One-year follow-up visits demonstrated either full recovery or significant improvement in 33% of the patients who had had OCD and 34% of those who had had depression. The results paralleled those that had been reported in the treatment of OCD via cingulotomy. A limbic leucotomy, which is a combination of a subcaudate tractotomy and a cingulotomy, is claimed to result in a much higher percentage of improvement, reaching 89% for patients with OCD and 78% for those with depression, according to some authors (Mitchell-Heggs, Kelly, & Richardson, 1976). More recent reports, however, have suggested more modest results of the procedure (Poyton, Kartsounis, & Bridges, 1995).

More promising results seem to come from an anterior capsulotomy, which interrupts the frontothalamic connections in the anterior limb of the internal capsule between the head of the caudate and the putamen. A more careful analysis of the preoperative states of patients treated with an anterior capsulotomy may certainly lead to less exciting, though still encouraging, positive results. Indeed, a recent report of a gamma knife–induced bilateral anterior capsulotomy in 23 OCD patients showed a 40% rate of much and very much improvement (Rasmussen, Greenberg, Mindus, Friehs, & Noren, 2000).

Primary Obsessive–Compulsive Disorder

Brain-Imaging Studies

PET Scan Data. Most of the early functional imaging studies showed increased glucose metabolic rates in the orbitofrontal regions, the cingulate cortex, and the caudate. Using PET scans, Baxter et al. (1987) found increased metabolic rates in both the caudate nuclei and the left orbitofrontal cortex in 14 OCD patients, including 9 patients with concurrent depression. Normal rates in those areas were observed in 14 patients with depression alone, as well as in 14 normal control subjects. Subsequent studies demonstrated increased metabolic activity in the orbitofrontal cortex but reported less consistent changes in the caudate, anterior cingulate, and thalamus (Perani et al., 1995; Sawle et al., 1991; Swedo et al., 1989).

PET studies have also shown that metabolic activity in both the caudate and orbitofrontal areas decreases following the effective treatment of OCD (for a review, see Saxena, Bota, & Brody, 2001). Benkelfat et al. (1990) observed a significant decrease in glucose metabolic rates in the left caudate and the orbitofrontal cortex (OFC) following OCD treatment via clomipramine. Swedo et al. (1992) found similar bilateral decreases in the OFC. Baxter, Schwartz, and Bergman (1992) observed a decrease in metabolic activity in the right caudate following OCD treatment with either fluoxetine or cognitive–behavioral therapy. Saxena et al. (2001) reported a decrease in metabolism in both the right caudate and the right OFC after OCD treatment with paroxetine. Some researchers, such as Perani et al. (1995), found a decrease in metabolic rates in the cingulate gyri following treatment with selective serotonin reuptake inhibitors (SSRIs). Successful treatment has been shown to lead to the disruption of the pretreatment correlation of metabolic rates in the left OFC and the left thalamus, the right caudate and the right thalamus (Benkelfat et al., 1990), the orbitofrontal cortex and the caudate, and the orbitofrontal cortex and the thalamus (Schwartz, Stoessel, Baxter, Martin, & Phelps, 1996).

Head CT and MRI Scans. Head CT scans have revealed increased ventricular volume in patients suffering from OCD with childhood onset (Behar et al., 1984). No such enlargement of the ventricles was observed in patients with adult onset OCD. Brain MRI studies have yielded controversial results thus far. While one group of researchers revealed a significant increase in the volume of the caudate nuclei in OCD patients (Scarone et al., 1992), others have reported decreases in volume (Jenike et al., 1996; Robinson et al., 1995). These discrepancies may be partly explained by differences in basic symptoms and underlying pathology in various groups of OCD patients (Figure 11.5).

584

LOCALIZATION
OF CLINICAL
SYNDROMES IN
NEUROPSYCHOLOGY
AND NEUROSCIENCE

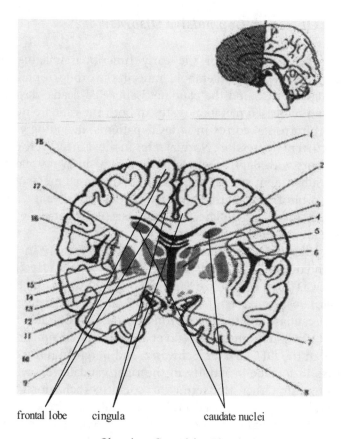

frontal lobe   cingula   caudate nuclei

Obsessive–Compulsive Disorder

FIGURE 11.5 Primary sites of lesion in cases of OCD. Subcortical structures on the coronal slice at the level of the tuber cinereum. Lesions in the caudate nuclei and the hypothalamus. 1: Longitudinal fissure. 2: Caudate nucleus. 3: Lateral nucleus of the thalamus. 4: Anterior nucleus of the thalamus. 5 and 12: Medial nucleus. 6 and 15: Claustrum. 7: Infundibulum. 8: Hypophysis. 9: Nervus opticus. 10: Substantia nigra. 11: Corpus luisi. 13 and 14: Globus pallidus. 16: Capsula externa. 17: Capsula interna. 18: Corpus callosum.

CONCLUSIONS

1. Obsessive–compulsive symptoms developed in six reviewed cases against the background of caudate lesions, three of which were bilateral and three of which were unilateral and of the left side only.
2. Various types of OCD were related to involvement of the frontal lobe in five reviewed cases. Orbitofrontal lesions were reported in two cases, with an extension of the lesion to the large areas of the convexital frontal cortex in one of the two cases.
3. The positive results of cingulotomies, subcaudate tractotomies, and anterior capsulotomies point to the role of the anterior cingula

and the connections between the orbitofrontal region, the anterior cingula, and the subcortical structures in the mechanisms of OCD. Some clarification of the roles of these areas may be discussed based on the results of brain imaging in patients with OCD.

4. Studies utilizing PET scans demonstrated the role of abnormalities in the caudate nuclei and orbitofrontal cortex in the development and treatment of primary OCD. The involvement of the anterior cingula and thalamus have also been observed and reported by some researchers.

5. Primary OCD is characterized by preserved insight with prominent anxiety underlying the development of OCD. Poor insight without signs of anxiety is often described in secondary OCD. These differences may be partly explained by the sites of lesions either in the frontal or the caudate regions. To the best of our knowledge, no cases of frontal lobe lesions have been described with such common symptoms of OCD as hand washing and obsessive mental counting. In our own case of an OCD patient with Pick's disease, compulsive hand washing eventually disappeared with the progression of atrophy from the caudate nuclei to the frontal lobes. Hand washing in this case eventually disappeared, being replaced by compulsive eating of both food and nonfood items, a symptom that is not usually seen in patients with OCD. It seems that OCD is characterized by more stereotypic, ritualistic, egosyntonic types of symptoms with either limited or absent insight in patients with frontal lobe lesions, while fear and anxiety, especially egodystonic fears of contamination and/or poisoning, underlie the formation of obsessive–compulsive symptoms in patients with caudate lesions.

Another explanation, however, may be derived from PET scan data. There are significant differences in the types of metabolic abnormalities described between cases of primary and secondary OCD. In one particular group of patients with primary OCD, an increase in metabolic activity was observed in structures involved in the development of OCD prior to treatment, accompanied by a decrease in metabolic activity in these structures following effective treatment of primary OCD. The metabolic activity in such cases was probably either absent or diminished in and around the structures involved in cases of secondary OCD.

PATHOLOGICAL ANGER, AGGRESSION, AND RAGE ATTACKS

ANGER IS A basic emotion that may be seen as a normal manifestation of a reaction to situations in the social and/or physical worlds.

586

LOCALIZATION
OF CLINICAL
SYNDROMES IN
NEUROPSYCHOLOGY
AND NEUROSCIENCE

Anger in pathological cases may reach extreme degrees, manifesting as episodes of aggressive, violent behavior that may be defined as either actual, attempted, or threatened attempts to inflict damage on a person or piece of property.

Aggressive, violent behavior may develop as a manifestation of extreme anger during the course of *rage attacks*. Other types of pathological anger leading to aggressive, violent behavior may also be observed. These behaviors may be secondary to the general agitation in the course of psychotic episodes or may reflect a persistent state of hostility or anger in a psychiatric patient. Like rage attacks, such types of aggression usually develop in response to either minor provocation or no provocation at all. Aggressive, violent behavior may also be of a prearranged, predatory type. Such behavior may still be based on anger, but with a delayed aggressive reaction in some cases. In other instances, the behavior is completely unrelated to anger and is motivated by other considerations, such as monetary reward or theft, or delusions in pathological cases.

It must be stressed that aggressive, violent behavior may be related to sociopsychological problems. These problems have been studied extensively by many researchers, who have shown that these types of aggression represent the major factor underlying violence in human society. However, there is a growing body of evidence that aggressive, violent behavior may develop as a peculiar manifestation of brain pathology. We concentrate on one of the types of pathological aggression manifested as a rage attack, since it has been studied extensively via both clinical and anatomo-physiological methods.

Clinical Aspects

Rage attacks have been described in detail by researchers who have studied such attacks in patients without any signs of primary mental illness. This type of aggressive behavior was reported by Mark and Ervin (1970) and Elliot (1976, 1982, 1992) as *episodic dyscontrol* in nonpsychiatric patients with minimal brain dysfunction. Dysfunction was found to be caused by either developmental or acquired brain defects characterized by soft neurological signs, seizure disorders, and learning disabilities. Elliot (1982) found evidence of either developmental or acquired brain defects in 94% of 286 patients with a history of recurrent rage attacks.

Episodes of dyscontrol were found to be characterized by the development of preictal anger and anxiety followed by an abrupt onset of rage characterized by severe violent, aggressive behavior with a senseless infliction of damage to people or property. Consciousness is usually partially preserved during such spells, and patients may react to some questions. Episodes generally lasted for 10–20 min, ending abruptly with feelings of remorse and regret, as well as fatigue, depression, or mania, and sometimes hyperphagia. The recollection of ictus was usually partial. These characterizations of episodic dyscontrol are similar to descriptions of *intermittent explosive disorder* in *DSM–IV–TR* (American Psychiatric Association, 2000). Differences between the two disorders include observations of a preictal sense of tension or arousal and the exclusion of partial amnesia from *DSM–IV–TR* descriptions.

The *DSM–IV–TR* (American Psychiatric Association, 2000, p. 664) stresses that a "diagnosis of Intermittent Explosive Disorder is made only after other mental disorders that might account for episodes of aggressive behavior have been ruled out (e.g., Antisocial Personality Disorder, Borderline Personality Disorder, a psychotic Disorder, a manic Episode, Conduct Disorder, or Attention-Deficit/Hyperactivity Disorder. . . . The aggressive episodes are not due to the direct physiological effects of a substance (e.g., a drug of abuse, a medication) or a general medical condition (e.g., head trauma, Alzheimer's disease)." However, the point of interest in this chapter is the description of the clinical signs and anatomo-physiological correlations of rage attack as a specific type of psychopathological phenomenon of pathological aggression that may be observed across the spectrum of different brain disturbances, much like the observation of delusions or hallucinations in various brain diseases.

In addition to minimal brain dysfunction, Elliot (1977) included in a list of illnesses with manifestations of episodic dyscontrol almost all known neurologically defined brain diseases and stressed the role of local and generalized brain pathology rather than specific diseases in the development of pathological anger and "episodic dyscontrol." Elliot's list included various types of encephalitis; sequelae of head trauma, stroke, and metabolic encephalopathy; such degenerative diseases as Alzheimer's disease and Huntington's disease; mental retardation; and brain tumors.

Cummings (1985) added the primary psychiatric disorders to the list of illnesses with episodic dyscontrol, stressing that personality disorders account for the largest number of outbreaks of violent behavior in psychiatric patients. The absence of a strong association between aggressive behavior in patients with primary psychiatric disorders and such clinical manifestations of those disorders as commanding hallucinations and delusions has also been demonstrated (Hellerstein, Frosh, & Koenisberg, 1987; Kay, Wolkenfeld, & Murrill, 1988; Shore et al., 1989). Statistical models for predictions of violent behavior based on these psychiatric symptoms have not exceeded a 42%–52% chance level (Cocozza & Stedman, 1976; Kay et al., 1988). Interestingly, the accuracy of violence prediction improved when a history of violent crime was included in the list of symptoms (Convit, Jaeger, Lin, Meisuer, & Volavka, 1988; Shore et al., 1989).

588

LOCALIZATION
OF CLINICAL
SYNDROMES IN
NEUROPSYCHOLOGY
AND NEUROSCIENCE

Anatomical Aspects

Major sites of lesions in cases of pathological aggression include the temporal lobe, especially the amygdala region; the frontal lobe, primarily the orbitofrontal area; and the hypothalamus (for a review, see Benjamin, 1999; Tranel, 2000; Volavka, 1995).

Temporal Lobe

Temporal Lobe Epilepsy and Rage Attacks. Seizure disorders, especially TLE, have been frequently observed in patients with aggressive, violent behavior. Lombroso (1911) was probably one of the first to suggest that most criminals suffer from epilepsy. While this view did not get much support in the following years, the relationship between seizure disorders and crime and violent behavior has been increasingly studied in recent decades.

Mark and Ervin (1970) surveyed 400 prisoners with a history of violent assaults and found the prevalence of epilepsy (38 cases, or 9.5%) to be 10 times more common among criminals than in the general population. The researchers noted that half of the prisoners experienced a phenomenon, resembling rage attacks, including an altered state of consciousness and warning stages that preceded the abrupt onset of violent acts, as well as sleep and lassitude, or drowsiness, following the acts of violence. A less frequent prevalence of epilepsy in the incarcerated population was reported by Whitman et al. (1984), who found the prevalence to be 2.4% in men entering the Illinois state prison system, a rate lower than that which was reported by Mark and Ervin (1970) but is still four times higher than in men aged 20–39 in the general population. Tardiff (1983) reported that assaultive patients from a state hospital system were two and a half times more likely to be suffering from a seizure disorder than were their nonassaultive counterparts.

According to some researchers, TLE may be observed more frequently among patients with seizure disorder. Serafetinides (1965) reported prominent physical aggressiveness in 36 of 100 patients with psychomotor epilepsy who had been referred for a temporal lobectomy (Serafetinides, 1965). Lewis, Pincus, Shanok, and Glaser (1982) noted psychomotor epilepsy in 18 of 97 incarcerated delinquent boys with a history of violence. Devinsky and Bear (1984) described five cases with TLE and various types of aggressive behavior, while Bear (1979) stressed that generalized tonic-clonic seizures may indirectly stimulate the development of secondary focus in the amyloid structures and hippocampus.

It must be stressed that direct aggression during a seizure is very rare, and murder and manslaughter are nearly impossible to commit during epileptic automatism. It seems that a loss of consciousness and an associated disorientation during a psychomotor seizure rather protects the patients from the ability to recognize the situation or to organize and focus their aggressive motor actions toward a purposeful target with destruction of property or physical damage to a person in mind. This was demonstrated in a special report of an international panel of epileptologists (Delgado-Escueta et al., 1981), who reviewed the telemetry data of 19 patients during partial seizures. Aggression was observed in 7 patients and included kicking, boxing, and grabbing the target. The aggressive actions, however, were "short-lived, fragmentary, stereotyped and unsustained, and were never supported by a consecutive series of purposeful movements" (p. 715).

While the preservation or partial loss of consciousness during rage attacks caused by temporal lobe paroxysmal activity may be used by a patient to direct aggressive, violent actions, such direction is practically impossible when consciousness is lost during a psychomotor seizure. The primary manifestations of rage attacks are actually identical to those of complex partial seizures, including abrupt onset and termination, similar warning and postictal signs, and a length of episode of several minutes to 1–2 hours. At the same time, rage attacks resemble simple partial seizures in the absence of a complete loss of consciousness during the spell, and in a lack of complete amnesia of the attack. It is thus possible to compare rage attacks with Jacksonian seizures, which are manifested with psychomotor phenomena such as aggression and violence instead of the convulsions or sensory phenomena typical for simple partial seizures.

The possible role of paroxysmal activity in rage attacks is supported by the data presented by Heath (1971, 1980), who recorded such activity via amygdala-hippocampal depth electrodes during episodes of aggressive outbursts in his patients. The electrical stimulation of the amygdala through the depth electrodes may also produce the outbursts of rage, as well as other types of aggressive behavior (Egger & Flynn, 1981; Mark & Ervin, 1970). Egger and Flynn (1981) showed that the modulation of aggressive behavior caused by stimulation of the ventromedial hypothalamus may be decreased by stimulation of the dorsomedial amygdala and increased via stimulation of the ventrolateral amygdala.

Mark and Ervin (1970) described a female patient, "Julia," who would experience rage attacks with a partial loss of consciousness and yet would later have relatively good recollection of the episode. During the attack, she looked in a restroom mirror and saw a distorted image of the right side of her face, developed intense fear mixed with anger, withdrew a knife from her pocket, and stabbed another girl who was looking in the same mirror; Julia believed that she had acted in self-defense. Julia's behavior was subsequently studied using deep electrodes inserted into her amygdala. When Julia played the guitar, the electrical stimulation of the amygdala electrodes led to an aggressive act, hitting the wall with the guitar; Julia did not lose consciousness during this time. The electrodes

590

LOCALIZATION
OF CLINICAL
SYNDROMES IN
NEUROPSYCHOLOGY
AND NEUROSCIENCE

showed paroxysmal activity in the amygdala-hippocampal leads during this episode. The role of such activity in the development of aggressive behavior was also mentioned by Benjamin (1999), who stated that "the behavior may be caused by subictal epileptic activity. Deep limbic discharges may be measured by depth electrodes in the absence of an abnormal pattern on scalp EEG in some cases" (p. 155).

EEG Data. The role of seizure activity in the development of rage attacks and other types of aggressive behavior has also been supported by EEG data. Abnormal EEGs laced with slow waves and spikes have often been reported in aggressive psychiatric patients and criminal offenders. Sayed, Lewis, and Brittain (1969) found changes in EEG in 21 (65%) of 32 "insane" murderers. Bach-Y-Rita, Lion, Climent, and Ervin (1971) reported EEG changes in 46% of 79 violent patients. Lewis, Pincus, Feldman, Jackson, and Brad (1986) described EEG abnormalities in all 10 of a group of juveniles on death row. It has also been stressed that motiveless homicide is strongly associated with abnormal EEG (Hill & Pond, 1952; Okasha, Sadek, & Moneim, 1975).

Though a predominant site of electrical abnormalities was not stressed in these studies, some researchers have stressed the temporal lobe foci, usually in relation to the presence of TLE in patients with aggressive behavior. Devinsky and Bear (1984) described five cases of aggressive behavior, TLE, and abnormal EEGs. Paroxysmal activity over the right temporal lobe was observed in all five cases, with additional involvement of the left temporal lobe in two of these cases. Serafetinides (1965) and Taylor (1969) reported paroxysmal activity at the temporal leads in patients with TLE and aggressive behavior. This activity was observed predominantly in the left temporal lobe.

Epileptic activity may be recorded via scalp EEGs in many cases with rage attacks and other types of aggressive behavior, but with no history of seizures at all. The number of such cases far exceeds the prevalence of TLE or generalized seizures in patients or prisoners with aggressive behavior. Mark and Ervin (1970) found EEG changes in 140 of 400 (35%) prisoners with a history of violent assaults; the prevalence of epilepsy, however, was only 9%. Bach-Y-Rita et al. (1971) studied EEGs in 79 violent patients from a larger group of 130 patients who were exhibitors of violent behavior. EEG abnormalities were noted in 37 of 79 (46.8%) of the patients, while TLE was reported in 22 of 130 (16.9%) patients.

Forced Normalization and Treatment With Anticonvulsants. The tight control of seizure activity may cause a psychotic exacerbation that was referred to as forced normalization by Landolt (1958). A series of cases of forced normalization has been reported since these early observations by Landolt (Roger, Grangeon, Guey, & Lob, 1968; for a review, see Trimble, 1991). Though the patients in such cases suffered primarily from complex partial seizures (Glaser, 1964; Landolt, 1958), generalized seizures were observed in some instances (Landolt, 1963).

The anticonvulsants taken by patients with manifestations of forced normalization have usually consisted of medications used in the treatment of complex partial seizures, such as succinimides (Trimble, 1991) and a new class of antiepileptic drugs that includes topiramate, lamotrigine, and vigabatrin. We also observed a sharp increase in psychotic behavior and aggression in several psychiatric patients who were taking Neurontin. The development of forced normalization may be observed with low dosages of succinimide. Valproic acid and carbamazepine, on the other hand, have been shown to help diminish aggressiveness and affective instability without the exacerbation of psychosis (Tonkonogy, 1991; Tonkonogy & Gaulin, 1992).

It has been suggested that forced normalization may be the result of an increase in dopamine and gamma-aminobutiric acid, which is caused by both succinimides and some of the newest anticonvulsants (Pollock, 1987), while such anticonvulsants as valproic acid and carbamazepine have not been shown to significantly alter the level of monoamines. Valproic acid is often preferable to carbamazepine due to the lower frequency of side effects, such as hyponatremia, which is a typical side effect of carbamazepine.

According to our own research, however, both valproic acid and carbamazepine may fail to control the rage attacks in some patients. We have followed a series of such treatment-resistant psychiatric patients residing at a state hospital. Severe rage attacks accompanied by abbreviated seizure episodes without complete loss of consciousness were developing daily in one of these patients. The patient, a 42-year-old woman, was treated with high dosages of valproic acid, which reached 3500–4000 mg daily, but experienced no sign of relief. The patient was then put on phenobarbital, an old psychiatric remedy that had been a commonly used treatment in the preneuroleptic era. When the dosage of phenobarbital reached a daily level of 200 mg, both the rage attacks and the seizures stopped, and it became possible to prepare the patient for transfer into the community program after 12 years of inpatient treatment in the state hospital. The same highly positive outcome was reached in several patients with similar medical backgrounds. Contrary to widely held beliefs, the phenobarbital did not produce behavioral disinhibition in these patients; it rather caused some drowsiness in the first days after the initial intake of the medication, followed by subsequent adjustment without accompanying side effects such as hyponatremia or drops in white blood cell counts, which are common side effects of carbamazepine and valproic acid treatments. It is of interest that in these cases, as well as in other cases of a similar nature,

592

LOCALIZATION
OF CLINICAL
SYNDROMES IN
NEUROPSYCHOLOGY
AND NEUROSCIENCE

the patients had first been given various neuroleptics without any sign of a decrease in the rage attacks. This supports the notion that episodes of aggressive behavior in such cases are related to paroxysmal activity, rather than to the customarily suspected neurochemical imbalance, which would theoretically require the use of neuroleptics.

Lesion Studies. While seizure activity mediating the development of rage attacks may be caused by relatively small lesions within the amygdala, more extensive lesions that damage the amygdaloid complex, especially bilaterally, may lead to a significant decrease in aggressive behavior. This was in fact observed by Klüver and Bucy (1937, 1939), who performed bilateral ablations of the temporal lobe anterior to the vein of Labbe on adult rhesus monkeys. The ablation areas included both the hippocampal and amygdaloid complexes. Following the procedure, the monkeys developed "tameness," or a significant decrease in reaction to objects that were usually fear inducing. In addition to tameness, the monkey's condition, known as the Kluver-Bucy syndrome, included hypermetamorphosis, or the extensive exploration of one's cage, as well as hyperorality, or the oral exploration of small objects within reach. Hypersexuality was also noted in the monkeys with Kluver-Bucy syndrome. The tameness seemed to reflect a loss of adjustment to the social environment, since monkeys with similar ablations demonstrated an inability to assume their role in the social hierarchy when present in the group once again.

The bilateral ablation of amygdala-hippocampal complexes in humans has been shown to produce some elements of the Kluver-Bucy syndrome, including hypersexuality, bulimia, and memory loss (Bailey, Green, Amador, & Gibbs, 1953). Terzian and Dalle Ore (1955) described a 19-year-old patient who had psychomotor and generalized tonic-clonic (grand mal) seizures and paroxysms of aggressive and violent behavior. The bilateral removal of the anterior portion of the left temporal lobe anterior to the vein of Labbe and including the hippocampus and the amygdaloid complexes resulted in the complete disappearance of psychomotor seizures; grand mal seizures, however, reappeared 2 months later. After the surgery, the patient no longer manifested the slightest rage reactions but developed several symptoms typical of Kluver-Bucy syndrome, including hypermetamorphosis and stopping everyone he met to ask them four or five elementary questions. He picked up objects around him, inspecting them with his hands, but without any attempts at oral exploration. Prominent amnesia, paraphasia, and obsessiveness were also noted. The patient also developed signs of hypersexuality and bulimia.

The symptoms reported in this case have been frequently described in cases of human Kluver-Bucy syndrome in patients with Pick's disease, Alzheimer's disease, herpes, toxoplasmic encephalitis, head trauma, and bilateral temporal infarctions (for a review, see Lilly et al., 1983). The tameness and loss of fear in monkeys was described in the human version of Kluver-Bucy syndrome as blunted affect and apathy (Lilly et al., 1983). A diminution of aggressive behavior had also been reported earlier following the surgical unilateral or bilateral destruction of amygdaloid nuclei in violent psychiatric patients (Heimburger, Whillock, & Kalsbeck, 1966; Kiloh et al., 1974; Narabayashi et al., 1963). The surgery, however, was unsuccessful in many cases, and sometimes actually led to the exacerbation of aggressive, violent behavior, especially in patients with mental retardation.

It is possible that, in normal conditions, the amygdaloid nuclei in one hemisphere inhibit the release of programs of violent behavior in the amygdala of either the opposite hemisphere or other parts of the limbic structures. This release may be disinhibited by the unilateral destruction of the amygdala and amplified by seizure activity in the remaining, still intact area of the amygdala on the opposite side. Our own data support the possibility that unilateral, relatively extensive lesions of the amygdala and surrounding structures may underlie the onset of rage attacks in psychiatric patients, which are probably due to seizure activity in the contralateral amygdala-hippocampal complexes (Tonkonogy, 1991). Using head CT and brain MRI scans, we found a loss of tissue in the anterior-inferior temporal lobe in a group of five psychiatric patients, each with a history of frequent episodes of aggressive, violent behavior. Lesions were localized either in the amygdala-hippocampal region or in the areas adjacent to the region. The role of seizures in the onset of rage attacks in these cases was supported by the presence of seizure disorders in four of the five cases, and paroxysmal activity shown by EEGs in three of the patients.

A typical case is that of a 48-year-old right-handed female who was referred for an evaluation of episodes of rage and of setting fire to various objects (Tonkonogy, 1991, Case 1). The episodes were characterized by a rapid onset of unprovoked rage with assaultiveness toward relatives and staff and destruction of property, as well as setting fire to objects during some of the episodes. Consciousness was partially preserved during the attacks, and the patient was able to recall some of the events that had happened during the episodes. The rage attacks each lasted from about 10 to 20 min and occurred approximately 2–3 times a month.

The patient's problems developed as a complication of meningitis, which had followed surgery for a brain abscess at the age of 16. She demonstrated mild spasticity and weakness in the muscles of the left upper and lower extremities, as well as slurred speech. A cognitive evaluation yielded an IQ of 57. The patient had experienced tonic-clonic

594

LOCALIZATION
OF CLINICAL
SYNDROMES IN
NEUROPSYCHOLOGY
AND NEUROSCIENCE

seizures, which were controlled by anticonvulsants. An EEG revealed intermittent sharp waves, which were especially prominent in the left temporal lobe. A head CT scan showed a large area of low density in the cortical and subcortical white matter of the anterior two thirds of the second and third temporal gyri, spreading to the amygdala-hippocampal area in the right hemisphere (Figure 11.6).

Thus, in this case of frequent rage attacks, the destruction of the amygdala in the right hemisphere was accompanied by prominent paroxysmal activity involving the same area in the left hemisphere and underlying the development of prominent and frequent rage attacks.

The mechanism described may explain the failure of unilateral amygdalotomies in the treatment of aggressiveness in some cases in which seizure activity is eliminated in the destroyed amygdala on one side but continues to be contralaterally active in the intact half of the amygdala. At the same time, while the bilateral destruction of the amygdala may be more successful in decreasing aggressiveness, it may lead to the development of serious disturbances of behavior and memory, as in cases of Kluver-Bucy syndrome. The use of amygdalotomies for the treatment of aggressive behavior was thus eventually abandoned due to medical and ethical considerations. The surgical treatment of TLE, however, continues to be performed with positive results, especially in cases of predominantly unilateral seizure activity in the temporal lobe. Decreased aggressiveness following a unilateral amygdalotomy has been observed in some such cases.

Hypothalamus

Posterior Hypothalamus. The role of the posterior hypothalamus in aggressive behavior was first demonstrated in animal studies. Bard

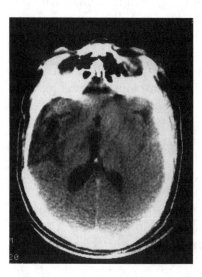

FIGURE 11.6 Head CT scan of a 48-year-old patient, called L.R. The patient was experiencing episodes of rage and fire setting. L.R.'s medical history included a craniotomy for treatment of a brain abscess at the age of 16. The loss of tissue in the right anterior-inferior temporal lobe region involves the amygdala-hippocampal region. It is suggested that paroxysmal activity involving the same region in the left hemisphere was responsible for the fire-setting episodes, while a lesion in the right hemispheric amygdala-hippocampal region facilitated the activation of the same region in the left hemisphere.

(1928) was able to produce sham rage in cats via a surgical transection of the upper brain stem anterior to the caudal hypothalamus. The cats displayed periodic fits of savage behavior characterized by hissing, autonomic excitement, arching of the back, and extensions of the claws. The sham rage phenomenon was not abolished by the subsequent removal of all neocortex and telencephalic structures located rostrally, dorsally, and laterally to the posterior hypothalamus. An additional transection caudal to the posterior hypothalamus effectively eliminated these rage attacks, pointing to the specific role of the posterior hypothalamus in the activation of aggressive behavior in cats.

Researchers subsequently demonstrated that the electrical stimulation of the posterior hypothalamus in cats using implanted electrodes resulted in the development of sham rage similar to the episodes of attacking behavior observed in Bard's experiments. It has been shown in both animals and humans that electrical stimulation of the ergotonic triangle in the posterior hypothalamus produces the autonomic responses necessary for the execution of aggressive behavior. These responses include a rise in blood pressure, tachycardia, and pupillary dilation. At one point, the ergotonic triangle was surgically destroyed in the treatment of patients with violent outbursts of various etiologies (Sano, Mayanagi, Sekino, Ogashiva, & Ishigma, 1970; Schwarcz, Theilgaard, Owen, & White, 1972). According to the researchers, the results were nonsatisfactory, especially in patients with mental retardation. The procedure was eventually abandoned because of ethical controversies.

Ventromedial Hypothalamus.   Animal studies point to the role of the ventromedial hypothalamus (VMH), which is adjacent to the floor of the third ventricle, in the inhibition of aggressive behavior. The destruction of the VMH decreases the threshold for aggressive behavior in rats and monkeys. At the same time, the stimulation of the juxtaposed lateral hypothalamus leads to the development of ferocious behavior and hyperphagia in animals (for a review, see Reeves & Plum, 1969).

Reeves and Plum (1969) described a young woman who developed outbursts of rage consisting of hissing, biting, scratching, and throwing objects at attendants, as well as visual and auditory hallucinations. The patient also suffered from diabetes insipidus, bulimia, and obesity. The patient died 2 months after an exploratory craniotomy that revealed a tumor at the base of the third ventricle. An autopsy revealed a hematoma occupying both ventromedial hypothalamic nuclei and partially spreading to both the lateral hypothalamic region and the caudal portion of the anterior hypothalamus. Flynn, Cummings, and Tomiyasu (1989) presented a case in which intermittent rage attacks were found to be associated with damage to the ventromedial thalamus.

596

LOCALIZATION
OF CLINICAL
SYNDROMES IN
NEUROPSYCHOLOGY
AND NEUROSCIENCE

In one series of cases, the development of rage attacks was mediated by hypothalamic tumors involving the floor of the third ventricle, with probable involvement of the ventromedial hypothalamus and an extension of the tumor to both the lateral and posterior hypothalami. Alpers (1937) presented a case of rage attacks accompanied by diabetes insipidus, urinary incontinence, and memory loss. An autopsy of the patient revealed a teratoma filling the cavity of the third ventricle and extending from the anterior commissure to the middle portion of the mesencephalon. Episodes of outbursts of rage were also described in a case of craniopharyngioma with hypothalamic-hypophyseal involvement (Killefer & Stern 1970; Malamud, 1967). We reported two cases of episodic rage outbursts that markedly diminished in one patient and completely disappeared in another patient following the removal of a craniopharyngioma that was extending out of the sella and extended in a supracellar direction to the chiasm in both cases (Tonkonogy & Geller, 1992). See Figure 11.7.

While the destruction of the VMH increases aggressive behavior, the inhibitory impulses from the VMH can also be diminished by paroxysmal activity. Such activity was prevented in two cases of patients with craniopharyngiomas. Seizure activity, however, has been infrequently noticed or reported in other cases of hypothalamic rage reported in the literature. It is possible that such a rage is often produced by the disinhibition of lateral and posterior hypothalamic nuclei that occurs, for instance, when the ventromedial nuclei are destroyed. In an opposite situation, the destruction of the posterior hypothalamus may amplify the impulses from the ventromedial nuclei, thus eliminating the aggressive behavior.

Somatosensory Information and Hypothalamic Rage. The experience of hyperphagia in both animals and humans with hypothalamic rage points to the role of satiety-hunger feelings controlled by the hypothalamus in

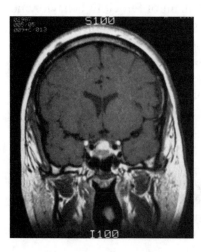

FIGURE 11.7 Brain MRI of a 21-year-old male known as Patient G. The image shows a craniopharyngioma extending beyond the sella toward the floor of the third ventricle.

the mechanisms of aggression. Hunger usually leads to the search for food and to the aggression that is necessary in order to find and obtain the food. In such cases, the hypothalamus mediates the response through somatic signals such as the need to get food. A similar mechanism would certainly be more sophisticated in humans and would be controlled by various guidance programs in the upper parts of the limbic and frontal lobe structures. However, the most primitive mechanism as noted in animals may surface in humans in pathological conditions, in which the presence of hyperphagia may facilitate the development of rage outbursts. A similar explanation may be applied to the development of aggressive behavior in patients with low glucose value on the glucose tolerance test (Benson, 1988; Yaryura-Tobias & Neziroglu, 1975). For reasons other than the hunger-satiety continuum, abnormal somatic information may also mediate the development of aggression in patients with high testosterone and low progesterone levels.

Frontal Lobe

Pathological aggression has been described primarily in patients with orbitofrontal syndrome. Clinical manifestations of this disorder include a lack of inhibition, hyperactivity with so-called empty euphoria, a loss of adherence to social norms, and sexual promiscuity. Aggressive behavior in such cases may be seen as a secondary manifestation of the syndrome rather than as a truly high-intensity rage attack in patients with amygdala and hypothalamic involvement. Benjamin (1999) stresses that the patient with frontal dysfunction is usually emotionally shallow, and his or her anger during aggressive episodes is typically short lived and poorly planned and may occur in response to trivial situations. An occasional aggressive outburst may also be observed in patients with dorsolateral frontal lesions. Most of the time, however, patients who experience such episodes are characterized by apathy, abulia (a loss of ability to make decisions), loss of motivation, and decreased overall activity.

A typical example of pathological aggressiveness is that of our 19-year-old patient with a history of a closed head injury suffered during a car accident when the patient was 14 years old. The patient lost consciousness for several hours following the accident. The patient quickly regained full consciousness but subsequently developed behavioral problems characterized by hyperactivity, a loss of awareness of social norms, recklessness, and sexual promiscuity, with episodes of aggressive behavior that eventually brought him to a psychiatric hospital. While in the ambulance, he became aggressive and tried to rape the female nurse who was attending him on the way to the hospital. Following admission into the hospital, the patient became calm and unconcerned, exhibiting signs of empty euphoria. A head CT scan revealed a prominent scar 15 mm in length and 2 mm in width in the left orbitofrontal region (see Figure 11.8).

598

LOCALIZATION
OF CLINICAL
SYNDROMES IN
NEUROPSYCHOLOGY
AND NEUROSCIENCE

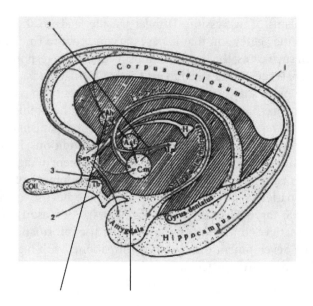

posterior hypothalamus amygdala

FIGURE 11.8   Primary sites of lesion and origination of paroxysmal activity in rage attacks. Another site implicated in some cases, but not shown in this figure, is the orbitofrontal region. Abbreviations for different areas of the brain are as follows. H: habenula; Ip: interpeduncular nucleus; Tb: tuberculum olfactorium; Olf: bulbus olfactorius; Cm: corpora mammillaria; At: nucleus anterior thalami; Ah: nucleus anterior hypothalami; Sep: septum pallucidum. 1. stria supracallosa; 2. stria olfactoria lateralis; 3. diagonal band of Broca; 4. fasciculus medialis. See text for more details. Note that the localization of lesions is almost identical to those in patients suffering from panic attacks. It is possible that the development of panic in one case and of a rage attack in another case is the result of differences in lesion localization within the hypothalamus and amygdala.

CONCLUSIONS

1. Attacks of rage are characterized by an acute onset of extreme anger compounded by aggressive, violent behavior. These episodes differ from psychomotor seizures in the partial or full preservation of consciousness and are thus similar to partial simple Jacksonian seizures. The difference lies in the manifestations of the two conditions: attacks of rage are characterized by extreme rage and aggression, while partial simple Jacksonian seizures are characterized by convulsions, sensory phenomena, or discharges of the autonomic nervous system. (For more details, see above, section titled "Panic Disorder.")

2. Paroxysmal activity in the temporal lobe, especially in the amygdala areas, is frequently recorded during rage attacks and during

interictal periods in patients with a history of such attacks. The removal of these areas may decrease the frequency and severity of such rage attacks and episodes of aggressive behavior, as has been demonstrated by neurosurgical data.

3. The posterior hypothalamus, located in the so-called ergotonic triangle, and in some cases the VMH are other localizations of lesion related to rage attacks. The stimulation of the ergotonic triangle in both animals and humans may lead to the development of sham rage characterized by increased blood pressure, tachycardia, and pupillary dilation. While the surgical removal of the ergotonic triangle has resulted in a decrease in aggressive episodes in some patients, no improvement has been noted in other cases.

4. While some patients with rage attacks are found to have lesions of the frontal lobe, especially in the orbitofrontal region, their attacks are usually less severe and easier to control.

5. Abnormal somatosensory information may mediate the development of rage attacks in some patients.

6. Anticonvulsants, especially medications that are effective in the treatment of complex partial seizures, may lead to forced normalization and an increase in psychotic behavior. At the same time, some anticonvulsants, such as carbamazepine and valproic acid, may markedly diminish the severity and frequency of rage attacks, thus pointing to the role of subclinical paroxysmal activity in the development of such attacks. Phenobarbital may be especially successful in controlling rage attacks, as it remains one of the most powerful anticonvulsants.

MOOD DISORDERS AND DISTURBANCES OF BRAIN INFORMATION PROCESSING

THE FUNCTIONAL ROLE OF EMOTIONS AND COGNITIVE IMPAIRMENT

THE PRIMARY FUNCTIONAL role of emotions is regulatory in its nature. Emotions are not included in the internal structure of information processing in recognition and action modules. The functional role of emotions consists of an external regulation of the functioning of these modules by initiating, accelerating or inhibiting, and decelerating information processing in them. When a subject becomes depressed, the situation, whether internal or external, is assessed as not being favorable for successful action. The subject's self-assessment also reaches a low point as he or she underestimates his or her ability to

600

LOCALIZATION
OF CLINICAL
SYNDROMES IN
NEUROPSYCHOLOGY
AND NEUROSCIENCE

overcome the difficulties of action in an existing situation. As a result, the speed of a subject's processing of relevant information markedly decreases, often approaching a complete stop in decision making. This helps to minimize interactions with unfriendly environments in order to avoid errors and losses, whether the threats are imagined or real.

The opposite happens in cases of mania, which are characterized by hyperactivity and an overestimation of the ability to successfully navigate the situation. The subject may have difficulty due to his or her inability to properly assess the situation and the resulting actions that are outside the limits of socially accepted norms of behavior.

The onset of anxiety is accompanied by an activation of systems within the subject's body that prepare the individual to respond to the threat, whether it be from the social or the physical environment. An individual may benefit from trying to focus his or her attention on regulating such vital signs as pulse, blood pressure, and breathing. In pathological cases, for example, during panic attacks, this regulation becomes impossible, and the patient develops tachycardia and a sharp increase in blood pressure to above normal levels and experiences concentration and attentional difficulties. In cases of pathological anger, the socially accepted response to threats is exaggerated and becomes out of control, resulting in rage attacks.

In all the cases described, the inner structure and function of the recognition and action modules remain preserved for the most part. A formal cognitive evaluation may show relatively high scores if the patient is evaluated during the interictal period between spells of panic or rage and is given enough time to overcome the inhibition or excitation signals that are the result of information processing caused by emotional disturbances in cases of depression or mania, respectively. This suggestion is supported by the clinical experiences of practicing physicians and psychologists, which point to primarily functional disturbances of cognition in patients with mood disorders manifesting as impairments in the initiation and speed of mental processing and as attentional disturbances. It has been consistently observed that psychomotor retardation represents one of the more frequent findings in patients with depression (for a review, see Newman & Sweet, 1992). This retardation may manifest as a depressive deficit on tasks requiring psychomotor speed, sustained effort, and concentration. Memory problems in depressive patients may also be secondary to depression since memory function has been found to return to normal levels in the stages of symptom remission (Frith et al., 1983; Johansen, Gustafson, & Risberg, 1985; Sweet, 1983). An absence of significant cognitive impairments was also found in patients with various types of anxiety disorders (for a review, see Orsillo & McCaffrey, 1992), as well as in patients with mania.

Cognitive impairments, however, may be more prominent in some patients with mood disorder. This may be related to the common pathological process that underlies the development of mood disturbances and cognitive problems. Disturbances may be observed in patients with various neurological illnesses such as degenerative dementia, vascular dementia, Parkinson's disease, brain tumors, sequelae of head injury, and multiple sclerosis.

EMOTION AS A LANGUAGE

EMOTIONS MAY BE considered as a supportive tool used in brain information processing for the cognitive assessment of both the external and internal worlds and for the selection of actions in response to the results of that assessment. An emotional language, which includes approximately 6–7 words that define basic emotions, is usually used in conventional information processing. Responses to unconventional, novel, social situations, however, may require terms that lie beyond the limited vocabulary that categorizes in a simple manner the responses of the self to typical situations in both the external and internal worlds. Such unconventional information processing may be based on more complicated information processing that necessitates the use of special types of higher-level emotions, as well as more complicated forms of social gnosis and praxis.

Given the fact that emotions are reflected and communicated via facial expressions, voice prosody, and gestures and body posture, the language of emotion is involved in social communication. In many cases, this language helps to communicate messages to others in various social interactions. In some sense, emotions represent a simple international, global language that may be used in communication without requiring a special knowledge of foreign languages, as well as in communication between infants and their parents or caretakers prior to the infants' acquiring the ability to talk and to understand verbal language. In some situations, attempts are made to conceal the external manifestations of emotions in order to hide one's true emotions from competing participants in various social situations. The seemingly effortless ability to express and to recognize particular emotions may be disturbed by brain lesions, especially when these lesions are located in the right temporal lobe. Such disturbances are discussed in chapter 5, section titled "Emotional Agnosia."

Emotions are usually reflected in the consciousness of the individual, who is usually able to appreciate and to report both specific emotions experienced in the past and those currently being experienced. Emotions may be present, however, only on a subconscious level, in response to which an individual may behave accordingly. This

602

LOCALIZATION
OF CLINICAL
SYNDROMES IN
NEUROPSYCHOLOGY
AND NEUROSCIENCE

subconscious level of emotion is probably responsible for so-called gut feelings.

EMOTIONS AND UNDERLYING BRAIN CIRCUITRY

THERE MUST, THEORETICALLY, be a functional and anatomical structure that contains and operates programs of actions for various types of emotions, a structure that is similar to the models used in the storage, recognition, and performance of actions. Such a structure may be either activated or suppressed via the influence of neurochemicals as well as damaged by brain lesions. The program of operations executed by the structure may be transmitted to other structures, for example, suppressing interest, energy, and appetite in cases of depression. This transmission may be conducted either through anatomophysiological connections or via neurochemical means. In order for depression, mania, anxiety, fear, or anger to develop, the neurochemical abnormalities of the various conditions must influence some of the basic brain structures that are related to the use of emotions.

Though it is unclear exactly how this system or circuit is organized, clinico-anatomical data does point to some possibilities. It is apparent that particular mood disorders may be caused by lesions in different parts of the brain. For example, lesions in the temporal lobe, primarily in the prefrontal cortex, caudate nuclei, and hypothalamic region of the left hemisphere, may lead to the development of depression. In cases of mania, the sites of lesions may include the frontal lobe, primarily the orbitofrontal cortex, the temporal lobe (primarily of the right hemisphere), the thalamus, and the mesodiencephalic structures. The experiences of fear and anxiety, as well as panic attacks, have been described as being related to electrical and blood flow abnormalities in the amygdala, the anterior cingula, and the mesodiencephalic region. Episodes of intermittent anger and rage have been seen in cases in which the amygdala and hypothalamic region are involved. Lesion localizations in cases of OCD include the caudate nuclei, the anterior cingula, and the prefrontal cortex.

Lesions that lead to various forms of emotional disturbances have been considered as being the major components of the limbic system (for a review, see Mega, Cummings, Salloway, & Malloy, 1997). The term *cerebri limbus* was introduced by Willis (1964) to describe the cortical border around the brain stem. Broca (1878) suggested that a ring of olfactory processing includes the anterior olfactory region, the hippocampus, and the anterior cingula. Broca considered this border zone to be le grand lobe limbique. Subsequently, the cingula and other medial structures were related to the mechanisms of emotions and their disturbances (Papez, 1937); the term limbic system was introduced to describe those structures and their role as a system in the processing of emotions (MacLean, 1952). The number of structures listed in Broca's *le grand lobe limbique* were joined by several additional structures considered to be components of the limbic system, including the amygdala, the anterior temporal lobe, the cingula, the septal nuclei, the anterior thalamus, and the hypothalamus. The number of structures included in the limbic system continues to grow, and some (Brodal, 1969) have suggested abandoning the term, as the limbic system concept has begun to encompass the majority of brain regions. Despite the survival of the term limbic system, researchers have begun to move their focus to the roles of various components in this system that are involved in the mechanisms of emotions and their disturbances, especially the roles of the amygdala and hypothalamus.

It may be suggested that all sites of lesions or electrical and blood flow abnormalities in patients with mood disorders perform different functions within the circuits. It seems redundant to construct the systems underlying the use of emotions from several identical parts. Logically, these parts should thus provide at least some variance in operations that contribute in specific ways to particular systems. For instance, since melancholic depression, the most severe form of depression, has been primarily reported in patients with temporal lobe lesions, it may be speculated that the stored model of the program of depression is localized in the temporal lobe, probably at the upper end of the limbic system in the areas of the amygdala and hippocampus. The program may be transmitted to the appropriate areas of the brain, such as the dorsolateral prefrontal cortex, thus evoking the suppression of motivation and underlying the development of the major symptoms of melancholic depression.

The program is also transmitted to the caudate nuclei, which may be responsible for the motor components of depression, such as psychomotor retardation. The hypothalamic region may be responsible for reporting the negative assessment of somatic signals, leading to the activation of the depression program in the amygdala region. At the same time, a nonamygdala lesion, for example, in the frontal lobe, may result in a loss of interest, known as apathy, which could be transmitted to the temporal lobe and lead to feelings of depression in some cases. The feelings of depression, however, would be less prominent in such cases than in those with direct lesions of the temporal lobe structures.

THE ROLE OF RECIPROCAL PROGRAMS

LESIONS IN CASES of mania have been observed primarily in the frontal lobe, especially in the orbitofrontal area, pointing to the probable

604

LOCALIZATION
OF CLINICAL
SYNDROMES IN
NEUROPSYCHOLOGY
AND NEUROSCIENCE

role of lesions in that area in the development of manic behavior. The temporal lobe contains another localization of lesions that is observed in patients with mania. Such lesions are more frequently localized in the right hemisphere in cases of mania, and in the left hemisphere in patients with depression. It is possible that the release, or activation, of certain emotional programs is inhibited by opposite programs, as in depression versus mania. In cases of brain lesions, the inhibiting program may be damaged. A lesion in the left hemisphere, for example, causes the program of depression stored in the right hemisphere to become disinhibited, while a lesion in the right hemisphere results in the disinhibition of mania programs in the left hemisphere. This may explain why unilateral ECT applied to the temporal lobe of the right hemisphere may help to treat depression in cases of bipolar disorder and schizophrenia (Balonov & Deglin, 1976). Reciprocal relationships between orbitofrontal areas and both the anterior cingula and the temporal lobe in the left hemisphere may also help to explain why damage to the orbitofrontal area may lead to the disinhibition of mania programs. Such programs are probably located in the cingula, as well as in the temporal lobe of the left hemisphere.

In a fashion similar to those of depression, mania programs may be transmitted to the corresponding areas of the cerebral cortex that are responsible for the development of hyperactivity, racing thoughts, flight of ideas, and grandiosity, all of which are typical of mania. On the other hand, thalamic lesions may influence alertness by facilitating the development of mania by increasing alertness itself, or by suppressing alertness via apathy and abulia.

Reciprocal programming could explain why aggressive behavior is disinhibited by the destruction of the ventromedial hypothalamus and suppressed by lesions in the dorsolateral and posterior hypothalamus. Mesodiencephalic lesions may also transfer false somatic signals to the central emotional structure, initiating the invocation of depressive or manic programs as well as a hypochondriacal fear of having certain diseases.

Disturbances in the Transmission of Emotional Programs

NEUROTRANSMITTERS MAY PARTICIPATE in evoking and transmitting described information, thus bringing another dimension to the functioning of the structure and its disturbances in various diseases that are not directly responsible for damage to the corresponding brain structures. Psychosocial stressors may also change the neurophysiological and neurochemical conditions required for the normal functioning of emotional information processing.

The proposed model of emotional processing may explain the development of depression or mania in some neurological disorders, which can occur not only because of direct damage to certain areas of the temporal lobe, basal ganglia, thalamus, or mesodiencephalic region but also because of damage to the pathways that transmit important signals of the emotional programs. Some cases of depression, for example, may be related to the development of white matter hyperintensity, cerebral microinfarctions, or demyelinization plaques in multiple sclerosis.

Reciprocal relationships between the areas responsible for the operations related to the programs of mania and depression may explain fluctuations around the unimodal scale, with mania at the upper end of the scale and depression at the lower end of the same scale. It is possible that there is a special mechanism that regulates these reciprocal relationships in a manner somewhat similar to the regulation of temperature, pulse, or blood pressure. The exact type and anatomical site of such a mechanism, however, remains unclear.

THE ROLE OF DIFFERENT SITES OF LESIONS IN THE DEVELOPMENT OF MOOD DISORDER

ABNORMALITIES IN ELECTRICAL activity and blood flow point to the role of the amygdala region in the development of fear, anxiety, and panic attacks, as well as pathological aggression, especially rage attacks. It is possible that the amygdala and temporal lobe structures are primarily responsible for the recognition of and response to the information from the outside world, primarily signs of danger that may initiate the fight-or-flight reaction in cases of aggression, and cases of fear, panic, or anger. These reactions may be abnormal in cases of the destruction or electrical stimulation of certain areas in the amygdala. At the same time, hypothalamic areas may be connected with the feedback of somatic needs, the autonomic nervous system involvement in the fight-or-flight response, and hunger-satiety responses. Interestingly, however, the anterior cingula seems to mediate motor responses in emotional reactions involving fear and anxiety. While the role of the frontal lobe in the programs related to fear and aggressiveness remains unclear, it likely provides the motor component of aggressive behavior, as well as decision making in cases of unconventional information processing of incomplete and novel information.

According to data obtained via single-cell recording, the absence of anxiety termination at the completion of certain actions may be related to lesions of the caudate nuclei, while the repeated excitation of

606

LOCALIZATION
OF CLINICAL
SYNDROMES IN
NEUROPSYCHOLOGY
AND NEUROSCIENCE

the same movements seems to be mediated by lesions of the anterior cingula. Lesions of the frontal lobe probably mediate the onset of a special type of egosyntonic OCD that is not directly related to anxiety disturbances.

In general, it seems that temporal lobe structures, especially the amygdala, and the hypothalamus represent the primary site for programs involved in the recognition of situations in the external and internal worlds. The use of emotions for the regulation of behavior mediates the use of these programs in motor and somatic activities in the actions defined by particular emotions. The special role of the temporal lobe in the recognition of emotions is also supported by the development of emotional agnosia in cases with right temporal lobe lesions. Further studies and theoretical considerations are certainly needed.

Mood Disorder and Social Agnosia

It has to be stressed that mood disorders may exert significant influence on the cognitive ability of the self to correctly recognize situations in the social world and to choose the appropriate action in response to these situations. This assessment may reach a delusional quality when severe depression manifests as delusions of guilt, or when prominent mania is accompanied by delusions of grandiosity. The cognitive processing of information in the physical world may remain either preserved or only mildly disturbed in such cases. On the other hand, prominent cognitive impairments in cases of dementia may lead to an inability to appropriately assess social situations, thus facilitating the development of responses guided by abnormal emotions and leading, for example, to episodes of anger and aggression.

12

Generalized Cognitive Disturbances

DELIRIUM

THE TERM *DELIRIUM* is Latin and literally means "getting out" (*de*) "of a track or furrow" (*lira*). It implies an acute or subacute deviation from the ordinary rut. Though various definitions of delirium have been suggested and numerous attempts have been made to replace delirium with other terms, such as *acute confusional state*, *clouded state*, and *acute brain syndrome*, delirium has remained the most frequently used term in psychiatric literature. The term acute confusional state, or simply confusion, is still widely used in clinical practice (for a review, see Lipowski, 1983).

Delirium is usually identified as a combination of disturbances of awareness and attention and is accompanied by multiple cognitive disturbances and either hypo- or hyperactivity, as well as a disruption of normal sleep-wake cycles (Lipowski, 1983). The development of delirium is usually either acute or subacute and represents a common feature of many medical illnesses and intoxications. Its duration is short, in many cases not exceeding several days or 1–2 weeks. Delirium is underlined in most cases by a reversible cerebral tissue dysfunction that does not have lasting anatomical changes. Such cases are often seen in patients with various types of dementia.

608

LOCALIZATION
OF CLINICAL
SYNDROMES IN
NEUROPSYCHOLOGY
AND NEUROSCIENCE

CLINICAL ASPECTS

ACCORDING TO *DSM–IV–TR* (American Psychiatric Association, 2000), the diagnostic criteria for delirium include a "disturbance of consciousness (i.e., reduced clarity of awareness of the environment) with [a] reduced ability to focus, sustain, and shift attention" that is accompanied by "a change in cognition (such as memory deficit, disorientation, language disturbance) or the development of perceptual disturbance that is not better accounted for by a preexisting, established or evolving dementia. . . . The disturbance develops over a short period of time (usually hours to days) and tends to fluctuate during the course of the day" (p. 143). The onset of delirium is marked by an acute or subacute onset of abnormalities in the patient's florid mental status, disturbances of consciousness, a misperception of the environment, disorders of attention and memory, visual hallucinations (usually), delusions, and extreme irritability and agitation. It is stressed that delirium may be caused by the direct physiological consequences of a general medical condition, substance intoxication, or medication side effect experienced either separately or in combination.

Hyperactive and Hypoactive Delirium

Two major types of delirium include disorientation accompanied by hyperactive behavior, known as delirious behavior, and a hypoactive type known as acute confusion, or torpor. Lipowski (1983) described these two types under one term—delirium. Meager and Trepacz (2000) stressed the role of motoric presentation in the clinical manifestations of delirium and divided delirium into two categories—the hyperactive motoric subtype and the hypoactive motoric subtype. Lipowski (1980) also described a third, mixed type of delirium. In general clinical practice, the most frequently used terms are acute confusion for hypoactive delirium, and delirium for hyperactive delirium. In this book, the term *hypoactive delirium* is used interchangeably with acute confusional state, and the term delirium is used interchangeably with the term *hyperactive delirium*.

Hyperactive delirium has many manifestations in common with those of hypoactive delirium, including disturbances in sustaining and properly shifting the focus of attention, as well as related impairments of recognition and orientation in time and space. Illusions, hallucinations, and delusions are often present in hyperactive delirium, and usually absent in hypoactive delirium.

Hypoactive delirium is characterized by the acute or subacute onset of confusion characterized by disorientation, with partial alienation from the surrounding world, incoherence, and an inability to follow simple commands or repeat gestures. The individual also demonstrates decreased alertness, a tendency to withdraw, a general unawareness, and an apathetic outlook. His or her speech activity is decreased, and speech is slow and simplified, with sentences consisting of two or three words. Frequent episodes of arrested speech, during which the individual makes no attempt to continue to talk, are typical. Comprehension is frequently disturbed, and the patient is often somnolent and gives the impression of a loss of awareness of both the internal and external worlds.

*Common Clinical Manifestations of Hyperactive
and Hypoactive Delirium*

A diminished or complete loss of awareness, manifested as a detachment from both the inside and outside worlds, represents one of the major manifestations of both types of delirium. The individual becomes unable to sustain his or her attention on a particular object, scene, or set of actions. Instead his or her attention wanders around, and the individual is often easily distracted and cannot be directed at will. This leads to disturbances in awareness of the external word and in the ability to follow the static and dynamic features of the environment. These difficulties are especially prominent in unconventional information processing, for example, when a patient must detect a signal against a "noisy" background. In our study of 15 patients, each in the initial stages of recovery from delirium tremens (Bazhin, Meerson, & Tonkonogy, 1973), the patients demonstrated prominent disturbances in locating the drawing of an object shrouded by background noise. At the same time, patients with visual agnosia resulting from occipital infarctions were able to correctly locate the object but experienced difficulties in the recognition of the object itself.

A patient with delirium is detached from the external world, performing actions without really being aware of his or her actual state. Attentional disturbances also lead to difficulties in establishing and sustaining connections between the various modules and the self of the internal world. These disturbances of awareness are similar to the experience of drowsiness that is experienced by many normal individuals, but they differ in that an individual with delirium suffers a disturbed connection with the self, leading to inability to appreciate his or her problems of diminished awareness and to overcome them with voluntary actions, even if only temporarily. Such a state of disturbed awareness is often called a clouding of consciousness and is considered to be underlain by disturbances of attention, which represent a major denominator of all cognitive disturbances in delirium (Lipowski, 1967, 1983; Morse & Litin, 1971).

These disturbances are accompanied by multiple cognitive impairments whose clinical manifestations are quite peculiar. A delirious

610

LOCALIZATION
OF CLINICAL
SYNDROMES IN
NEUROPSYCHOLOGY
AND NEUROSCIENCE

patient, for instance, may demonstrate a preservation of unconventional information processing, while conventional information processing may be disturbed. In cases of delirium, cognitive disturbances also develop with equal severity in both social and nonsocial information processing, while in cases of dementia, the disturbances primarily involve social information processing alone.

Speech and thought processing are disorganized in many cases. The individual's speech is incoherent and consists of mumbled sentences and exclamations that are short and difficult to understand. Disturbances in naming manifest either as an inability to recall the correct name of an object, or as nonaphasia misnaming, a condition resembling verbal paraphasia and one in which all items are named according to a specific theme, such as the individual's illness (Cummings, Hebben, Obler, & Leonard, 1980; Curran & Schilder, 1935; Geschwind, 1964; Weinstein & Kahn, 1952). Comprehension of gestures and spoken language is limited and is subject to false interpretations.

In cases of delirium, difficulties in object recognition are often manifested as illusions. Such disturbances are only distantly related to the shape or sound of the visual or auditory signal. For example, a curved crack in a wall or a fold in the sheets of a bed may be perceived as a snake, while a short-lasting sound in the room is recognized as a gunshot. The presence of visual and, less frequently, auditory hallucinations may be another manifestation of gnostic disturbances in cases of delirium. These include various images ranging from simple flashing spots or loud noises to frightening images of wandering dead bodies, monsters, animals and bugs, violent scenarios, fights, and funerals. Though patients sometimes watch such scenes with curiosity, as if they are watching a movie, more often they try to run away, either in fear or in an effort to defend themselves. Tactile hallucinations, such as those of bugs crawling over the patient's body, and olfactory hallucinations, such as the foul smell of a deceased body, are less common in cases of delirium. Illusions and hallucinations, especially those involving frightening images, may be accompanied by fluid, nonsystematized persecutory delusions that usually develop around immediate false images.

It is difficult to bring a patient's attention to the evaluation of his or her memory. The patient seems unable to concentrate on his or her surroundings, to appreciate the ongoing events of day-to-day life or social events, or to actively recall his or her own biographical data. The patient's orientation in time is either partially or completely lost, and he or she is unable to recall the month, year, day of the week, or exact date. Space agnosia is also apparent in such cases. A patient may, for instance, insist that he or she is at home or in another city altogether, when in reality he or she is in a hospital ward demonstrating a repeated inability to find the bathroom, the dining room, or his or her own room and bed, thus requiring constant observation and help in activities of daily living.

Mood swings are prominent in patients with delirium, ranging from fear and panic to irritability and then euphoria. A patient's facial expressions tend to reflect tension, and his or her gaze is often wandering or staring. The patient is restless, often trying to get out of bed and run, and resists restraining attempts.

Peculiar disturbances of conventional motor actions may also be observed in cases of delirium. For example, a patient who follows commands to point his or her right hand to his or her left ear may choose a strange, somewhat bizarre direction of movements, trying to follow the command by moving the right hand to the back of the neck, then reaching the left ear from that position, which is, as you may imagine, quite awkward. One of our patients who was suffering from relatively mild hypoactive delirium was unable to follow verbal commands or to copy a model of tandem walking, often demonstrating in such cases a slow, pacing walk forward without putting her lower extremities in the crosswalk position (no ability of tandem walking). At the same time, however, the patient's motor praxis of the hands was preserved. A prominent tremor is typical in cases of delirium due to alcohol withdrawal; the term delirium tremens is used to describe such cases. Other motor system abnormalities in patients with delirium include asterixis and myoclonus.

Autonomic disturbances may develop during the course of delirium. These include tachycardia, diaphoresis, shortness of breath, and pupillary dilation, heralding a possible failure of vital functions and thus death, especially in cases of delirium due to alcohol and/or drug withdrawal. Death may also result from a variety of the underlying conditions that led to the development of delirium.

One typical sign of delirium is a fluctuation of mental status throughout the day, during which the patient may become lucid and attentive, sometimes being able to regain, at least partially, his or her orientation and contact with the surrounding world, sometimes for a period of minutes or even hours. Delirium lasts for hours, days, and in some cases weeks. The patient's memory of a delirious state is usually either partial or totally absent.

Delirium and Dementia

In some sense, a patient in delirium often resembles a person who has just woken up from a very deep sleep and is unable to grasp what is going on around him or her or to act appropriately. This type of confusion helps to differentiate delirium from both dementia and depression. A demented patient is alert and usually tries to be involved with the surrounding world but is unable to recognize the sequences of

612

LOCALIZATION
OF CLINICAL
SYNDROMES IN
NEUROPSYCHOLOGY
AND NEUROSCIENCE

ongoing activities and their relationships to time and space, especially in conditions in which unconventional information processing is necessary. In a hospital ward, for instance, a patient with dementia may be able to find his or her room or bed by looking for and reading the signs on which his or her name is printed, signs that may be attached to the entrance door of the room or to the wall above the headboard of the bed. A delirious patient, on the other hand, would not pay any attention to such signs and clues, and would instead wander aimlessly from one room to another or perhaps lie down on someone else's bed. In general, cognitive disturbances in demented patients are characterized by the development of disturbances of unconventional information processing in milder cases, with subsequent disturbances of conventional information processing as the dementia continues to progress.

While many disturbances of brain information processing have been described in patients of alert and vigilant states, the leading clinical manifestations of delirium may be characterized as disturbances of the individual's sleep-wake cycle. In normal conditions, the 24-hour sleep-wake cycle consists of three major stages: wakefulness; alertness, usually for 15 to 17 hours, followed by a short period of drowsiness; then 7–9 hours of sleep. Drowsiness accompanied by a short period of sleep may interrupt one's levels of alertness during the period of wakefulness. Awareness of and attention to the outside world and, to some extent, the inside world is almost completely absent in sleep. Such awareness is also diminished in drowsiness, underlying the slowness and difficulties of cognition in this stage.

The stages of drowsiness and sleep may become more prominent and prolonged with the development of fatigue, as well as in cases of various medical illnesses or drug intoxication. In other cases, sleep may become more difficult to achieve and to sustain in cases of insomnia, which is a manifestation of many psychiatric and medical disorders, as well as of intoxication due to drugs.

The normal sleep-wake cycle is often reversed in cases of delirium. It is known as sundown syndrome in such cases and is characterized by the presence of stages of drowsiness and sleep during the day, and the awake and alert stage during the night. The patient is often agitated during these wakeful nighttime periods.

Delirium and the Dreamy or Oneiroid State

Abnormalities of the sleep-wake cycle may manifest as a so-called dreamy or *oneiroid* state. Such a state lasts for a short period of time, usually only 1–2 hours. A patient in an oneiroid state sits quietly in a chair, often with closed eyes, and "watches" the dream-like events that he or she is experiencing. Following a return to an alert state, one of our patients reported that she had been watching and participating in a soap opera with movie star Robert Redford. While in the alert state, the patient had no awareness that her experience was all part of a dream. The patient insisted that she had been able to invite the actor to visit her and was expecting to see him in the hospital. This patient had mild mental retardation with infrequent seizures of the temporal lobe epilepsy (TLE) type. An EEG revealed frequent bouts of slow theta activity in the bilateral inferior-posterior temporal leads. Despite some resemblance to hallucinations in cases of delirium, the patient's dreaming state was more systematized compared to hallucinations and was less fuzzy and more coherent. She was fully alert for most of the day, and she experienced dreamy states only rarely, usually once over the course of several days. Treatment with Depakote eventually eliminated the dreamy states in this patient. Dreamy states have also been described in patients with primary psychiatric illnesses, such as schizophrenia.

Delirium in Various Diseases

Delirium may be observed in a wide variety of conditions involving the nervous system, including infections, intoxication, barbiturate use, withdrawal from alcohol or other substances, cerebrovascular diseases, head injury, epilepsy, postoperative confusion, migraines, cerebral edema, anoxia, and vitamin deficiencies. Delirium is often the result of an extracerebral cause, such as one of a number of infections, a cardiac infarction, cardiac insufficiency, cardiopulmonary failure, uremia, dehydration, or hepatic encephalopathy (for a review, see Lishman, 1978; Cummings, 1985). Pneumonia, rarely accompanied by fever (afebrile), and urinary tract infections frequently underlie the development of delirium in geriatric patients. Delirium is rarely seen in primary psychiatric disorders such as schizophrenia, bipolar disorder, and depression. Intoxication caused by medications, especially the anticholinergic side effects of such medications, is often responsible for the development of delirium in psychiatric patients with primary mental disorders or degenerative dementia.

ANATOMICAL AND PHYSIOLOGICAL ASPECTS

IT IS DIFFICULT to imagine that delirium accompanied by disturbances of consciousness and prominent impairments of cognition, mood, and behavior can be caused by a single localized lesion. Brain anoxia, intoxication, encephalopathy, and infections underlying the development of delirium each involve a series of brain structures and, though they do not cause irreversible anatomical damage, lead to the malfunctioning of a number of information processing systems.

614

LOCALIZATION
OF CLINICAL
SYNDROMES IN
NEUROPSYCHOLOGY
AND NEUROSCIENCE

Anatomical lesions underlying the development of delirium in brain disease may be studied in patients with brain disease characterized by the development of local brain pathology, as in stroke cases.

Occipito-Temporal and Parietal Lesions

Several cases have been described in which delirium develops after a stroke with infarctions primarily being found in the inferior occipito-temporal region, including the hippocampus, the fusiform gyri, the lingual gyri, and the calcarine cortex. Profound dementia was usually noted in such cases after the signs of delirium had subsided.

Glees and Griffith (1952) described the case of a 58-year-old woman with delirium. She was agitated and disoriented, cried often, and repeatedly tried to strip the other patients' beds. After the agitation subsided, she remained severely demented. An autopsy showed bilateral symmetrical infarctions in the hippocampus with partial extensions to the fusiform and lingual gyri.

Horenstein, Chamberlain, and Conomy (1967) reported the sudden development of agitated delirium accompanied by partial or complete vision loss in nine patients with unilateral and bilateral infarctions of the fusiform gyri, lingual gyri, and calcarine cortex. In some cases, the infarctions extended to the hippocampal formation and the inferior temporal gyrus.

Medina, Rubino, and Ross (1974) described a 78-year-old male who had suddenly developed left hemiparesis, left homonymous hemianopia, and hemihypesthesia. Though the patient improved, the hemianopia remained. No changes in personality, behavior, or cognition were noted. Three months later, the patient suddenly became confused and was found standing in his bedroom, extremely disoriented and using foul language. He became agitated and combative, striking his niece and biting both the ambulance driver and his physician while en route to the hospital. Once admitted, the patient was agitated and repeatedly screamed, swore, spat, and bit. Doctors found him to be blind, as he would not blink in response to menacing movements, but he demonstrated preserved pupillary reactions. An EEG showed a bilateral diffuse slowing. One month later, the patient was still blind and was showing signs of profound dementia with agitation. The patient would shout without reason and though he could and would answer simple questions, he could not remember his own first name or those of his father or mother. He shouted all his answers, sometimes with an angry facial expression but usually with an unexpressive face. No delusions or hallucinations had been noted. The patient died 5 months after suffering from a second stroke. An autopsy revealed encephalomalacia of the cortex and underlying white matter of the posterior three fourths of the parahippocampal gyrus, the posterior one fourth of the fusiform gyrus, the entire lingual gyrus, and the calacarine sulcus in the left hemisphere. The encephalomalacia in the cortex and white matter of the right hemisphere included the superior temporal gyrus, as well as the supramarginal and angular gyri.

Medina, Chokroverty, and Rubino (1977) described three patients who suffered sudden visual impairment accompanied by preserved pupillary reactions and followed by agitated delirium one to three days later. The delirious state lasted for anywhere from 4 days to 2 months. During the acute state, the patients were found to be markedly excited, confused, and aggressive, with behavior marked by frequent shouting and swearing. Two of the three patients experienced visual hallucinations. In Case 2, the patient saw pipes sticking out of both his own head and that of his wife and subsequently tried to remove the pipes from his wife's head. An EEG showed focal slow waves in the left temporal region, with an extension to the occipito-parietal region in this case and to the temporal lobe of the opposite hemisphere in Case 3. Following recovery from acute agitation, some visual and cognitive deficits remained in all three patients. In Case 1, a head CT scan revealed areas of mixed density in the right occipito-temporo-parietal and left medial occipital regions. Head CT scans showed an infarction in the left medial occipito-temporal region in Case 2, and large areas of low density in the right Sylvian area and in the bilateral medial and occipito-temporal regions in Case 3.

Mesulam, Waxman, Geschwind, and Sabin (1976) described the sudden onset of an acute state of confusion in three patients. Though agitation was noted in all three cases, it did not persist for more than a few hours. No shouting or other forms of extreme reactions to external stimuli were noted. Disorientation, incoherence of stream of thought, and inattentiveness were observed in all three cases. A technetium brain scan revealed an area of increased uptake in the right occipito-parietal region in Case 1, and in the right parieto-temporal region in Case 2. A head CT scan showed an infarction in the right inferior frontal gyrus in Case 3. The absence of persistent extreme agitation in all three cases may be explained by the relatively small size of the infarction in each of the three cases, and the frontal lobe localization of Case 3.

The inferior parietal region has been found to be the primary area involved in some cases. Boiten and Lodder (1989) described six patients who developed delirium following a stroke that primarily involved the right inferior parietal lobule. Mesulam et al. (1976) presented several cases of delirium that developed following infarctions in the right parietal and right prefrontal regions, as well as in the ventro-medial and occipito-temporal areas.

Delirium has been also observed in cases of seizure disorders, especially in patients with temporal lobe seizures (Helmchen, 1976).

616

LOCALIZATION
OF CLINICAL
SYNDROMES IN
NEUROPSYCHOLOGY
AND NEUROSCIENCE

Subcortical Lesions

The development of delirium has also been observed in patients with relatively circumscribed subcortical lesions. Delirium developed in one case of a strangulation victim who suffered anoxic bilateral injury to the putamen and the caudate nuclei. Electroconvulsive therapy (ECT) may induce delirium in patients with basal ganglia and white matter changes, as well as in patients with parkinsonism (Figiel, Hasen, Zimbovski et al., 1991; Figiel, Krishnan, Breitner et al., 1989).

Special attention must be given to thalamic involvement in the development of delirium. Bogousslavsky, Ferrazzini, et al. (1988) described the development of hyperactive delirium following a paramedian infarction of the right thalamus. Delirium was also observed in 8 of 16 patients with bilateral thalamic infarctions (Acta Neurologica Scandinavica, 200), and in multiple patients with anteromedial thalamic infarctions (Friedman, 1985; Santamaria, Blesa, & Tolosa, 1984).

Possible Role of Thalamocortical Relay Neurons

EEG data also point to the possible role of thalamic abnormalities in the development of delirium. EEG data from the pioneering work of Romano and Engel have shown a slowing down of electrical activity in the brain, which has been recognized as an important finding in delirium research (Engel & Romano, 1959; Romano & Engel, 1944). These data were confirmed later via quantitative EEG in a comparative study of delirious and nondelirious elderly patients. The study showed an increased theta and delta power, a reduction in alpha percentage, and a reduced ratio of fast-to-slow band power (Koponen et al., 1989; for a review, see Jackobson, Fant, & Jerrier, 2000). EEG findings may consist of prominent fast beta activity against a background of low amplitude of electrical activity in delirious patients experiencing alcohol and benzodiazepine withdrawal (Kennard, Bueding, & Wortis, 1945; Pro & Wells, 1977).

The decrease in electrical activity may be related to the disinhibition of thalamocortical relay neurons, leading to the development of a thalamocortical oscillatory rhythm, such as delta activity, which is usually observed in non-REM (NREM) sleep (Hofle et al., 1997; Maquet et al., 1997; for a review, see Hobson, Pace-Schott, & Stickgold, 2000). A similar disfacilitation of the thalamocortical relay center may be responsible for the slowing of electrical activity as observed via EEG data, as well as the suppression of gnosis and awareness, in delirious patients.

DELIRIUM AND DISTURBANCES OF BRAIN INFORMATION PROCESSING

Delirium and Disturbances of the Sleep-Wake Cycle

It remains unclear exactly what mechanism underlies delirium, which develops in response to many different factors originating both inside and outside the brain, including various forms of intoxication, infections, brain hypoxia, and side effects of medications. One of the possible mechanisms that may be suggested in cases of delirium is a disturbance in the regulation and control of brain information processing via the sleep-wake cycle.

In normal alert conditions, the brain processes ongoing changes in both the outer and inner worlds. This is reflected by the roles of awareness and consciousness, which are used as screens to help the individual observe, recognize, and react to environmental changes via movements and actions. The stage of sleep permits one to turn off the connections with the external world, and with the internal world to some degree, and either to slow down or to temporarily deactivate the many modules that are involved in the processing of incoming information. This provides time for the biochemical and neurophysiological processes that are necessary to keep each of the brain's modules in full working capacity until the brain returns to full alertness. During sleep, some of the brain information processing continues and is reflected in dreaming, which is based on information already stored in the brain. While an individual is dreaming during REM sleep, the features of processed information are fused, incongruent, unusual or impossible, disconnected, and often confabulatory. Consciousness and awareness are reduced, leaving the individual without a clear spatio-temporal frame or the ability to self-reflect (Hobson, Pace-Schott, & Stickgold, 1998). Emotional overtones such as fear and anxiety may often accompany dreams during sleep.

In cases of brain or somatic disease, the sleep-wake cycle responds in an adaptive manner to the negative influence the diseases have on brain functioning by increasing the drowsiness-sleep stages of the cycle, thus inhibiting brain information processing and protecting it from disturbances inflicted by regular activity in the unfavorable conditions caused by disease. In clinical terms, this is described as an increase in drowsiness and somnolence in patients with various forms of infection, intoxication, brain hypoxia, and so on.

During the course of disease, however, the normal adaptive response may become pathological, manifesting as a decrease in brain metabolic activity beyond the level of normal sleep and leading to the development of sopor with a loss of consciousness but a preserved ability to be aroused by strong stimuli. This is followed by a coma, characterized by a complete loss of consciousness, during which a patient cannot be aroused at all. A less prominent decrease in brain metabolic activity may lead to the development of hypoactive delirium.

Hypoactive Delirium, Acute or Subacute Confusional State

It may be hypothesized that a decrease in cerebral metabolism in cases of hypoactive delirium reflects the deactivation of the reticular

618

LOCALIZATION
OF CLINICAL
SYNDROMES IN
NEUROPSYCHOLOGY
AND NEUROSCIENCE

activation system (RAT), resulting in the disinhibition of thalamocortical relay neurons, as observed in NREM sleep (Hofle et al., 1997; Maquet et al., 1997; for a review, see Hobson et al., 2000). Global cerebral metabolism decreases as the depth of NREM sleep increases. As in cases of delirium, this decline is correlated with increased delta activity (Hofle et al., 1997).

Decreases in brain wave activity, however, may also be observed in a nondelirious patient who has a deep midline tumor and has experienced a frontal lobe stroke. In addition, the clinical manifestations of hypoactive delirium resemble drowsiness rather than sleepiness. A patient in a state of hypoactive delirium is usually somnolent, with decreased attention and awareness. At the same time, somnolence in cases of hypoactive delirium differs from normal drowsiness in the inability to voluntarily make oneself more alert, to concentrate on a task, and to return to a normal state of mind after a period of sleep. Typical fluctuations of mental state in cases of delirium are not voluntary and generally do not fully restore one's mental alertness. Thus, there exists an abnormal type of drowsiness in cases of hypoactive delirium, which may be underlain by disturbances that alter the normal sleep-wake cycle via a pathological influence on the normal activity of both the RAT and the thalamocortical relay centers, which are both involved in the normal mechanisms of NREM sleep and, most likely, the stage of drowsiness.

Hyperactive Delirium

In cases of hyperactive delirium, the deactivation of certain regions of the brain is often accompanied by the activation of other brain regions in a way similar to Stage V of sleep, which is characterized by REM. There is no complete loss of activation, as is observed in cases of sopor and of coma. Delirium is similar to dreaming during sleep in the detachment of brain information processing for the outside and inner worlds. The development of dream-like hallucinations is similar to dreaming during REM sleep in its fusion, incongruence, and presence of threatening images. Detachment, however, is partial and incomplete, and a delusional person walks with eyes open, avoiding obstacles and often answering questions, giving the impression of being awake. The individual even tries to process information from the outside world, though these attempts are often unsuccessful, revealing multiple cognitive disturbances that are likely produced by modules that are already either inhibited or shut off, as in sleep. Consciousness and awareness of the outer and inner worlds are also attenuated and disturbed in such conditions. Since the delirious patient is able to move and walk, the emotional overtones of his or her hallucinations, such as anxiety or anger, may result in aggressive behavior and assaultiveness.

Many researchers once considered hallucinations and the general state of loss of awareness in cases of hyperactive delirium to be a type of disordered sleep—the dreams of walking persons (Lipowski, 1980). Similarities between generalized EEG slowing in delirium and sleep have been stressed in support of a relation between hyperactive delirium and dreaming (Kennedy, 1959).

The global cerebral energy metabolism in REM sleep is usually either equal to or greater than that of walking (Braun et al., 1997; Buchsbaum et al., 1989). According to PET and SPECT imaging studies, cerebral blood flow (CBF) is higher during delirium tremens in cases of delirium (Hemmingsen et al., 1988), while cortical CBF is found to be higher and subcortical regional CBF is either higher or lower in cases of delirium in traumatic brain injury (Deutsch & Eisenberg, 1997).

PET imaging studies performed during REM sleep (Braun et al., 1997; Maquet et al., 1997) have demonstrated a preferential activation of the limbic and paralimbic regions of the forebrain accompanied by a simultaneous significant deactivation of the dorsolateral prefrontal cortex (Hobson et al., 2000, p. 1346). Such studies have also served to emphasize the role of the pontine brain stem in REM sleep generation. The list of the areas that are activated during REM sleep compared to NREM sleep and waking states includes the pontine tegmentum, the anterior hypothalamus, the caudate nucleus, the amygdala, the parahippocampal cortex, and the anterior cingulate; the dorsolateral prefrontal cortex and the posterior cingulate are among the areas that are deactivated during REM sleep (Braun et al., 1997; Nofzinger, Mintun, Wiseman, Kupfer, & Moore, 1997). Other areas that are deactivated during REM sleep include the primary visual areas in the occipital cortex, while the visual association areas in Broadmann's areas 37 and 19 are usually among those activated during REM sleep. Based on these findings, Braun et al. (1997, 1998) suggested that, during REM sleep, internal information is processed between the deactivation of input via the primary visual cortex and the deactivation of output via the frontal cortex.

Similar patterns of activation and deactivation of various brain regions may be suggested in cases of hyperactive delirium. There are, however, significant clinical differences between hyperactive delirium and sleep. A patient with delirium is not only a person who dreams while walking but also one who is able to retain some contact with reality, for example, to continue to be able to recognize some objects or to develop illusions that are based on an incorrect perception of reality. Motor hyperactivity is another sign that may distinguish

620

LOCALIZATION
OF CLINICAL
SYNDROMES IN
NEUROPSYCHOLOGY
AND NEUROSCIENCE

delirium from normal sleep. These differences may be related to the differences in the patterns of activation and deactivation in delirium and REM sleep.

It may be hypothesized that input via the primary visual and auditory cortices and output via the frontal cortex are only partially deactivated in cases of hyperactive delirium, and that this underlies the patient's ability to walk around and to avoid obstacles. These areas are further deactivated during REM sleep. At the same time, regions of activation may overlap during both hyperactive delirium and REM sleep, resulting in the development of hallucinations and dreams, respectively. Further studies are certainly needed, especially concerning patterns of activation and deactivation in cases of delirium.

The similarities and differences between hyperactive delirium and REM sleep may be related to the pathological influences of various causative agents on the structures that are responsible for the regulation of the normal sleep-wake cycle. However, it remains unclear why those causative agents lead to normal variations of sleep in some cases and delirium in others. The effects of lesions in the temporal lobe, thalamus, and subcortical nuclei point to the role of such damage in the onset of abnormal adaptive responses involving the sleep-wake cycle. It is also possible that the structures responsible for the regulation of the sleep-wake cycle are especially sensitive in some cases to changes in the metabolic processes caused by various causative agents that respond with an abnormal adaptive sleep-wake pattern similar to that which underlies the development of delirium. The origins of this sensitivity may be related to prior subtle anatomical damage, as in patients with a history of alcohol abuse or one of various other dementing illnesses.

Special attention must be paid to the fluctuation of a patient's condition, as well as to the transient nature of delirium, which usually lasts for several days. This points to the primarily pathophysiological mechanisms that underlie the development of delirium, while anatomical changes in certain areas may only mediate the pattern of emerging metabolic and clinical manifestations in patients with delirium. When pathophysiological and metabolic changes either subside or disappear completely during the course of recovery from an infectious disease, intoxication, and so forth, the delirious condition terminates, despite the persistence of the anatomical damage that had mediated the development of delirium in the first place. In some cases, brain metabolic activity has been found to continue to decrease during the course of disease, leading to pronounced pathophysiological changes manifesting as either sopor or a coma. Such changes may still be reversed, as in cases of brain injury, or progress to the cessation of brain activity and death.

DEMENTIA

S INCE ITS ORIGINAL introduction by Pinel (1809) and Esquirol (1814), the term *dementia* has frequently been used in clinical literature to describe a primarily progressive decline in the level of occupational and social functioning. The definition of dementia, however, continues to be debated, as scholars differ over the extent of emphasis to be given to the primary components of the cognitive and behavioral changes that are typical of dementia. Since dementia includes impairments in multiple cognitive abilities, many researchers have stressed the primary role of memory disturbances in the overall clinical picture of global decline in intellectual functions. Others, however, have described dementia as an inability to solve problems of day-to-day living accompanied by a loss of social skills. A loss of perceptual–motor skills has been described as agnosia and apraxia in patients with dementia.

It has been generally accepted that patients with dementia are vigilant and alert, while patients with delirium are characterized by a clouding of consciousness. Dementia and delirium differ in that consciousness and self-recognition remain relatively preserved in cases of dementia, while contact with the environment may be almost completely lost in some cases of delirium. Delirium characteristically develops following a sudden onset of acute or subacute conditions with a prominent loss of cerebral function, and with either relatively small cerebral lesions or no structural brain lesions at all. Periods of delirium typically last for a limited amount of time, usually anywhere from a few days to 1–2 weeks.

The term dementia reflects a chronic disease course with extended structural lesions in the cerebral cortical and subcortical regions. The onset and progression of dementia are often irreversible in cases of underlying progressive degenerative diseases, they but may be at least to some extent reversible with the treatment of nonprogressive underlying disorders, for example, the sequelae of head injury, encephalitis, stroke, and brain anoxia.

The course of dementia may be insidious, characterized by a slow deterioration over an extended period of time, such as is observed in cases of Alzheimer's disease, Pick's disease, or schizophrenia. Dementia may also develop following a sudden onset of acute conditions, as in cases of cerebral anoxia, brain trauma, or encephalitis. In such cases, an acute period of obtundation, stupor, coma, or delirium may be followed by the subsequent emergence of chronic dementia, with the condition remaining relatively stable and unchanging for a long period of time.

The *Diagnostic and Statistical Manual* (American Psychiatric Association, 2000) lists several major types of dementia: dementia of

622

LOCALIZATION
OF CLINICAL
SYNDROMES IN
NEUROPSYCHOLOGY
AND NEUROSCIENCE

Alzheimer's type, vascular dementia, dementia due to other medical conditions, substance-induced dementia, dementia due to multiple etiologies, and dementia not otherwise specified. The "other medical conditions" mentioned include HIV disease, head trauma, Parkinson's disease, Huntington's disease, Pick's disease, dementia with Lewy bodies, Creutzfeldt-Jakob disease, normal pressure hydrocephalus, hypothyroidism, brain tumor, vitamin B12 deficiency, and intracranial radiation. The substances responsible for substance-induced persistent dementia may include alcohol, inhalants, sedatives, hypnotics, anxiolytics, and unknown substances. Examples of multiple etiologies are head trauma accompanied by chronic alcohol use, or dementia of Alzheimer's type with the subsequent development of vascular dementia. It is stressed that in cases of dementia of the not-otherwise-specified type, there is insufficient evidence to allow the establishment of a specific etiology.

CLINICAL SYNDROMES OF COGNITIVE IMPAIRMENTS IN DEMENTIA

ACCORDING TO *DSM–IV–TR* (American Psychiatric Association, 2000), dementia is defined as "the development of multiple cognitive deficits that include memory impairment and at least one of the following cognitive disturbances: aphasia, agnosia, apraxia, or a disturbance in executive functioning. These cognitive deficits must be sufficiently severe to cause impairment in occupational or social functioning and must represent a decline from a previously higher level of functioning" (p. 148). Disturbances in dementia usually develop as a prominent poverty of social information processing that interferes with social and occupational functioning and activities of daily living and is manifested as social agnosia and social apraxia.

Dementia may be considered to be an impairment in occupational and social functioning underlain by any one of a number of specific cognitive clinical syndromes, primarily social agnosia and social apraxia. These impairments are accompanied by disturbances in other modules of recognition and action, as well as in the supportive systems of memory and attention. The role of episodic memory disturbances in dementia remains unclear, considering, for instance, that patients with Korsakoff's amnestic syndrome experience severe episodic memory disturbances but experience preserved social gnosis and social praxis. This points to the possibility that cognitive disturbances in dementia may not be directly related to impairments in episodic memory, especially long-term memory. However, the registration and working memory that serve the invididual's social gnosis and praxis both during day-to-day social activities and in short-term episodic memory may be disturbed in dementia, manifested as difficulties in appreciating both the conventional and unconventional changes in social situations and in adjusting to these changes.

The term *cognitive impairment* may be used to describe various types and degrees of cognitive decline. Dementia may be considered to be mild, moderate, or severe depending on the degree of cognitive impairment. Impairments are usually centered around conventional information processing for moderate and severe degrees of dementia, and unconventional information processing for mild dementia.

Cognitive disturbances in dementia include a series of clinical impairments in modules of recognition and action, as well as in the supportive systems of memory, attention, and emotions.

Social Agnosia and Social Apraxia

Impairments in social and occupational functioning may be characterized as social agnosia and social apraxia. A patient with dementia loses the ability to plan and execute social actions and becomes unable to recognize or appropriately respond to evolving social problems, thus displaying the primary manifestation of dementia. Though it is quite difficult to see a full picture of dementia in the early stages of dementia, some early signs may point to the upcoming onset of prominent social agnosia and social apraxia, which are more typical in the more advanced stages of dementia. A patient may continue to be involved in his or her regular occupational and social functions, but a decline from previous levels of functioning begin to be noted by the patient's colleagues and relatives, and sometimes by the patient him or herself. The patient often demonstrates difficulties in following job-related conversations, in planning daily activities while at work, especially with regard to more complex jobs, and in properly understanding and following instructions.

In the case of a patient who holds a complex job, for example, as a manager or a lawyer, social agnosia and social apraxia may be appreciated earlier in the course of progressive dementia, as such jobs require a preserved ability to process unconventional information in order to recognize and to adjust to changing situations and to plan and to execute appropriate actions. Some patients may try adapting by moving to a less challenging job, still unaware of a slowly progressive dementia. One patient of ours, V.B., continued to drive a school bus in a timely manner, on the correct routes, and without any major mistakes while in the early stages of Alzheimer's disease. This individual was referred to us by his wife, who complained that her husband was slowly developing a progressive loss in the ability to participate in discussions concerning family problems and to react appropriately to these discussions. A head CT scan performed at that time showed

624

LOCALIZATION
OF CLINICAL
SYNDROMES IN
NEUROPSYCHOLOGY
AND NEUROSCIENCE

moderate cerebral atrophy. The patient was immediately suspended from his job as a school bus driver. The patient's reaction was surprise, as he was unable to recognize his cognitive problems. He continued to demonstrate a progressive cognitive decline with the development of prominent dementia of Alzheimer's type accompanied by social agnosia, social apraxia, agnosia of time and space, and anterograde amnesia followed by retrograde amnesia.

Social agnosia and social apraxia become more prominent with the progression of dementia and are manifested as disturbances in the ability to continue simple activities, with the patient eventually requiring help in performing activities of daily living. This is amplified and compounded by other types of agnosia, apraxia, aphasia, and memory disturbances. Prosopagnosia, or agnosia of faces, is one symptom that may be manifested in cases of social agnosia in dementia. Recognition of the faces of familiar relatives, friends, and medical staff, however, is usually preserved in cases of mild and moderate dementia. Yet the progression of dementia may eventually lead to symptoms of prosopagnosia, and the patient loses the ability to recognize even the faces of his or her close relatives.

A neuropsychological evaluation usually does not directly target the symptoms of social agnosia and social apraxia. Operations involving the orientation of time and space, memory, and executive functions also underly the functioning of social gnosis and social praxis. Special neuropsychological tests for the direct evaluation of social agnosia and social apraxia have been used relatively infrequently in dementia studies. Such tests involve the recognition of emotions, the theory of mind, and the recognition of social actions. The Picture Arrangement subtest of the Wechsler Adult Intelligence Scale–Revised (WAIS-R) for example, may be used to test the recognition of social actions. An examination of the recognition of emotion using a prosodic pattern of spoken language and facial expressions has been performed in several studies of patients with Alzheimer's disease (Albert, Cohen, & Koff, 1991; Allender & Kazniak, 1989; Cadieux & Greve, 1997). Testa, Beatty, Gleason, Oebelo, and Ross (2001) found that patients with mild Alzheimer's disease have significant impairments in the ability to comprehend the emotional components of speech. Such impairments increase with the progression of dementia. A comparable aphasic deficit of language comprehension has been observed only in patients with severe dementia. Results point to the role of disturbances in recognition of the emotional component of social gnosis in the formation of the dementia syndrome. Some researchers have observed associations between prosodic-emotional impairments and mood and behavioral disturbances in Alzheimer's disease (Roberts, Ingram, Lamar, & Green, 1996). Future studies may concentrate on direct neuropsychological examination of the recognition and formation of sequences of social actions in dementia cases using, for instance, theory of mind tests and thematic action picture tasks. This may help to improve the understanding and clinical evaluation of dementia, for example, in disturbances of social functioning.

Researchers also consider that social gnosis and social praxis, especially for unconventional information processing, may be assisted by some of the operations that underlie the recognition and action functions in the physical world that are defined as executive functions. Some tests directed toward the study of executive functions may reveal disturbances of such operations in dementia, including agnosia and apraxia of sequencing. Such tests require the individual to filter the basic components of sequences from background noise, to recognize the patterns of succession in the formation of sequences, and to recognize the shifting of basic components during the course of the testing. Examples of these tests include the Wisconsin Card Sorting Test (WCST), other card sorting tests, Part B of the Trailmaking Test, the Stroop Test, and the Object Alternation Test. Disturbances in performance on these tests have been observed in patients with relatively mild forms of cognitive impairment, primarily caused by frontal and temporal lobe lesions, as well as in cases of subcortical dementia. These disturbances may well also be noted in patients with moderate and severe cases of dementia.

We systematized some similar subtests as a study of unconventional information processing in Part II of the Brief Neuropsychological Cognitive Examination (BNCE; Tonkonogy, 1997). Though these subtests do not directly evaluate social gnosis and social praxis, they may reflect some changes that underlie the development of social agnosia and social apraxia. The subtests in Part II include the Shifting Set, which requires the recognition of simple sequences and the ability to preserve them in working memory. The recognition of sequences may underlie the basic operations involved in the recognition of actions, including social actions.

The Attention involves alternating connections of upward and backward rows of numbers and is designed to test the ability to alternate attention between the two rows while preserving a certain operation in working memory. One such operational task includes counting up from the number 1 and down from the number 12 in an alternating manner (e.g., 1, 12, 2, 11, 3, 10, etc.). The subtest targets the ability to overcome the well-learned, automatized tendency to count in an upward direction only, as well as the ability to plan and construct the sequence of backward counting alternating with upward counting. The subtest is similar to the widely used Part B of the Trailmaking Test from the Healsted-Reitan Battery (Reitan and Davison, 1974) but differs in that it uses only numbers, thus preventing subject exclusion due to illiteracy, and in that it is somewhat more difficult due to the inclusion of the

626

LOCALIZATION
OF CLINICAL
SYNDROMES IN
NEUROPSYCHOLOGY
AND NEUROSCIENCE

alternating forward and backward number count. Disturbances in the performance of such an executive function test may underlie impairments in the recognition of complicated sequences of social activity and the corresponding appropriate responses, which are important markers of mild cognitive disturbances (for more details, see chapter 13).

Personality and Mood Changes in Dementia, Disturbances in the Relationship of the Self to the Social Environment

Dementia, especially at the moderate and severe stages, is often accompanied by personality changes, depression, and, though less frequently, mania. A patient becomes apathetic, disinterested, disinhibited, and promiscuous with a loss of self-control. A patient may leave home or disappear from a shopping mall, for example, without warning his or her spouse or other accompanying individual. One of our patients with Alzheimer's disease, known as L.R., was an 83-year-old former college professor who unexpectedly left the doctor's waiting room while waiting for an appointment. He was later found sitting next to a nearby pond. When asked what happened, the patient answered that he had decided he wanted to get some fresh air. He stated that he did not remember leaving the doctor's office and going to the pond and did not know his way back to the office or to his home. On another occasion, the same patient left home and was found an hour later wandering around on a neighboring street. When he was found, L.R. created a confabulation that he was a lecturer and was walking to the place of his lecture. He could not explain the topic of this lecture nor where it was scheduled to take place. The confabulation in this particular case seemed to be related to his work many years earlier as a university professor of mathematical statistics.

It is apparent that prominent memory disturbances and absence of insight in such cases contribute to the tendency to wander. However, some patients with frontotemporal dementia may begin to wander during relatively early stages of dementia without demonstrating other obvious signs of spatial agnosia, temporal agnosia, or memory disturbances. Other frequent and quite troubling manifestations of personality and affective changes in cases of dementia include aggressiveness, anger, and assaultiveness in response to either no provocation or provocation of only a minor nature.

Changes in personality and mood in cases of dementia may be related to disturbances in the relationship between the self and the social environment. Such disturbances may manifest as an overinflated self-awareness, an overestimation of the ability to properly assess the results of one's plans and actions, a state of empty euphoria, and a loss of awareness of social rules and limitations and have been observed in patients with orbito-frontal lesions. This may also be related to either limited or completely absent insight in patients with dementia, especially at the moderate and severe stages. A patient refuses to acknowledge his or her apparent disturbances of memory and orientation and changes in personality, insisting that such disturbances are absent or perhaps only minimal and probably age related.

In other cases of dementia, symptoms such as apathy, loss of interest, and depression may develop secondary to either mesial frontal lobe involvement or temporal lobe involvement. The intermittent agitation and aggressiveness that often develop in patients with dementia may be related to lesions of the limbic system, especially in the amygdala and related regions.

These changes in personality and mood may appear in the initial stages of dementia without significant cognitive impairments, for instance, in cases of frontotemporal dementia. The subsequent onset of cognitive decline usually exacerbates the changes in personality and mood, making self-control of behavior more difficult.

Memory Disturbances

Social agnosia and social apraxia may be accompanied in the early stages of dementia by the development of anterograde amnesia manifested as recent memory problems, forgetfulness, and difficulties in the recall of previously well-known names. Retrograde amnesia then becomes apparent with further advances in cognitive decline. Anterograde amnesia is manifested as, for example, difficulties in the ability to recall recent visits by relatives or friends or difficulties in remembering to turn off the stove. Such a patient becomes unable to follow precisely the daily schedule of washing and food intake. These changes may be mild and are often difficult, in the early stages of dementia, to differentiate from age-related declines in memory and cognitive functioning. Retrograde amnesia involves difficulties in recalling the major events in the patient's life, especially the chronological succession of these events in time. An 83-year-old patient of ours, suffering from advanced Alzheimer's disease, knew that he was a professor who had taught at a university, but could not recall the subject he had taught. Despite having been retired for more than 15 years, the patient insisted that he was still a professor, but he was unable to recall the correct name and geographic location of the university. Retrograde amnesia is also manifested as an inability to recall the names of famous people in a specific order, for example, the names of the last four U.S. presidents. The patient's memory may be only slightly disturbed for more difficult-to-recall items, such as the U.S. president who came between Nixon and Carter, or the U.S. president who was assassinated in Ford's Theatre. It often remains unclear whether these difficulties are age related or are secondary to one's lower level of education, for

628

LOCALIZATION
OF CLINICAL
SYNDROMES IN
NEUROPSYCHOLOGY
AND NEUROSCIENCE

example. The Presidential Memory test is often used in screening batteries to uncover signs of retrograde amnesia. (For more details, see chapter 13.)

Memory disturbances in cases of dementia usually involve immediate memory and registration, which is preserved in cases of Korsakoff's amnestic syndrome. Social gnosis and praxis are also generally preserved in Korsakoff's syndrome, pointing to the possibility of the primary role of impairments in registration and working memory in mediating the onset of social agnosia and apraxia in dementia. It is especially important to take this into account in the early stages of dementia, when social agnosia and apraxia dominate the clinical manifestations of cognitive decline, while memory disturbances become an important component of dementia in more advanced stages.

In many cases, as in patients with Alzheimer's disease, the onset of social agnosia and social apraxia in dementia may be accompanied by agnosia of time, spatial agnosia, and memory disturbances. In other cases, as in patients with frontotemporal dementia, prominent social agnosia and social apraxia may manifest as primary disturbances in the planning and execution of actions as well as a loss of cognitive flexibility and executive functions. Memory and the recognition of physical space and time remain only mildly disturbed in such cases, especially in the early stages of the disease. Memory disturbances and temporal and spatial agnosia, however, become prominent later in the progression of dementia.

It must be taken into account that while some disturbances are often considered to represent memory problems, they are actually manifestations of prosopagnosia, which occurs when a patient is in the advanced stages of dementia and is unable to recognize his or her relatives, and topographic agnosia, which occurs when a patient experiences impairments in the orientation of familiar spaces.

Agnosia of Space

A patient may get lost in a familiar space, being unable to find the way home or to find the appropriate hospital room and bed. Disturbances in verbally mediated orientation in space may be revealed when a patient is asked to name the town of his or her residency, or the name of the institution in which he or she is presently resides, for example, hospital, outpatient clinic, or school. Prominent disturbances of topographic positioning systems are also manifested by the inability to point to the location of major cities on the map of a particular country.

Agnosia of Time

Agnosia of time is revealed by difficulties in the ability to correctly answer questions about the current date, month, or day of the week. The correct answer may sometimes be facilitated by any one of a number of clues, such as a limitation of choices (e.g., "Are we in the month of October, November, or December?" or "Are we in the year 1999, 2000, 2001, or 2002?"). This limitation of choices does not aid the patient who is in the more advanced stages of dementia.

Visual Object Agnosia

Conventional visual agnosia for objects is usually absent in patients with mild or moderate dementia. However, difficulties in object recognition may be observed when a patient is asked to recognize a partially occluded object characterized by an incomplete set of features. Tasks involving such skills include Gaulin's pictures, the Perceptual Closure Task (Snodgrass & Corwin, 1988), and the Incomplete Picture subtest of the BNCE. While these difficulties have also been observed in patients with visual object agnosia due to circumscribed cortical lesions, according to our observations the priming effect of object drawing with a complete set of pictures is usually not observed in patients with dementia but has been shown to facilitate recognition in patients with visual object agnosia resulting from local brain pathology, primarily in the occipito-parietal region. It is possible that priming is preserved in patients with visual object agnosia due to the local and limited nature of the cortical lesion, while multicognitive impairments in cases of dementia involve disturbances of priming in which the technique cannot be used to restrict one's choice in order to facilitate the recognition of objects and the subjects of social actions. Difficulties in the recognition of occluded objects mirror the impairments of social gnosis in social situations with incomplete sets of features needed for recognition. Disturbances of priming may prevent the facilitation of recognition in patients with social agnosia.

Motor Apraxia

Motor apraxia for conventional motor actions is usually absent in moderate dementia, and patients may show either no signs or only mild signs of ideational and ideomotor apraxia, a disorder of unconventional information processing in which a patient is asked to repeat sequences of movement. Such a task is required, for example, in Luria's fist-edge-palm test (for more details, see chapter 6). A patient with moderate dementia may still be able to dress himself or herself in the morning, undress at bedtime, wash his or her hands, or take a shower without assistance. L.R., a patient of ours with moderate dementia of Alzheimer's type, demonstrated prominent anterograde and retrograde amnesia, agnosia of time and space, agnosia of the recognition of incomplete drawings of objects, and prominent anomia. He was, however, able to pretend how to stir the sugar into a cup of tea, to hammer

630

LOCALIZATION
OF CLINICAL
SYNDROMES IN
NEUROPSYCHOLOGY
AND NEUROSCIENCE

a nail into the wall, and to comb his hair. Patient L.R. was able to undress himself, but required a degree of verbal help from his wife when getting dressed and could not repeat the sequences of movements in the fist-edge-palm test. These difficulties may reflect similar difficulties in the planning and execution of social actions or social apraxia.

Motor apraxia becomes more prominent with the progression of dementia. A patient with severe dementia may still be able to walk around a hospital ward but loses the ability to maintain personal hygiene: this includes the loss of such abilities as taking a shower, combing the hair, and dressing and undressing. The last to go is the ability to eat using utensils without assistance.

Motor apraxia is compounded by the development of urinary and, eventually, stool incontinence. In general, a patient with severe dementia completely loses his or her independent functioning and requires assistance in the performance of almost all activities of daily living. With further progression of the disease, prominent gait apraxia and ataxia lead to the patient's confinement to bed.

Aphasia

According to the appropriate subtests of the BNCE and the Mini-Mental State Examination (MMSE), language disturbances may manifest as moderate or prominent anomia with fluent speech and either completely preserved or only mildly disturbed comprehension. Naming difficulties may be observed only for words of relatively low frequency, such as *earlobe* and *eyelashes*. Anomia in cases of dementia also differs from aphasic anomia in the absence of naming facilitation when phonological clues in the form of the first two or three phonemes of a word are provided to a patient with dementia. This points to disturbances of the connections between various parts of the nodes connecting the linguistic, semantic, and visual information on particular objects in the physical world or subjects in the social world.

The preservation of fluent speech in cases of dementia differs from the laborious, effortful speech of patients with Broca's aphasia. Certainly, in moderate and, especially, more advanced dementia, a careful evaluation reveals the poverty or emptiness of expressive speech. Speech, however, has no specific prevalence of nouns or functional words as in cases of Broca's or Wernicke's aphasia, respectively.

The preservation or mild impairment of comprehension makes these language disturbances different from transcortical sensory aphasia. Comprehension disturbances in cases of dementia may also differ from those in cases of classical aphasia. While the comprehension of commands is usually disturbed in patients with various types of aphasia (Tonkonogy, 1986), a demented patient with preserved comprehension of commands may demonstrate an inability to understand the meaning of spoken language. Patient L.R., for instance, was able to follow both simple and complex commands without error and was able to understand the main point of a discussion with his wife that was related to the installation of an alarm system. However, the patient was completely unable to realize that the underlying idea of the planned actions was that this installation was needed to prevent his repeated wandering out of the apartment. It seems that disturbances in the comprehension of spoken language in such cases are secondary to general semantic impairments or an inability to understand the underlying point of a planned action. Such a disturbance may be considered as a manifestation of social agnosia of actions. At the same time, disturbances in cases of aphasia are often related to impairments in comprehension of the linguistic, nonsemantic meanings of words and sentences, while such mechanisms may be preserved in some cases of dementia.

In many cases, such as patients with Alzheimer's disease, the onset of social agnosia and social apraxia in dementia may be accompanied by agnosia of time, spatial agnosia, and memory disturbances. In other cases, for example, in cases of frontotemporal dementia, prominent social agnosia and social apraxia may manifest mainly as primary disturbances of planning as well as an inability to execute planned actions, a loss of cognitive flexibility, and a decline in executive functions. Memory and the recognition of physical space and time remain relatively mildly disturbed, especially in the early stages of the disease. Nevertheless, memory disturbances and temporal and spatial agnosia become prominent in the course of dementia progression.

All this is compounded by the development of urinary and, eventually, stool incontinence. In general, a patient with severe dementia may completely lose his or her independent functioning, requiring help and assistance in almost all activities of daily living. With further progression of the disease, prominent gait apraxia and ataxia lead to the patient's confinement to bed.

Delusions and Hallucinations

Delusions and hallucinations frequently develop during the course of dementia. Typical delusions include those of theft and of jealousy. A patient believes that somebody, often a spouse or daughter, has somehow managed to open a drawer, despite the fact that a locksmith has recently changed the lock, and has stolen items from the drawer. Delusions in cases of dementia are often nonsystematized, differing from delusions in schizophrenia in their concreteness and concentration on topics related to everyday life.

Hallucinations in patients with dementia are frequently visual, though auditory components are present in some cases. Hallucinatory

632

LOCALIZATION
OF CLINICAL
SYNDROMES IN
NEUROPSYCHOLOGY
AND NEUROSCIENCE

images generally include those of either people or animals. An elderly individual with dementia, for example, claimed that an unknown, vaguely described man "visited" with her, and that several men frequently sat on the porch of her house, often discussing "something" and then suddenly disappearing. Another patient described a rat that frequently appeared in his apartment near his bed. The rat would "disappear," however, when the patient called his neighbors to come and see it. In fact, the patient came to believe that an elderly woman living next door would bring the rat to his apartment just for the purpose of harassing him. The patient complained to his landlord, and became agitated and hostile when he was given an "evasive" and "unsatisfactory" answer.

CLINICAL AND ANATOMICAL ASPECTS OF DIFFERENT TYPES OF DEMENTIA

DEMENTIA MAY BE divided into cortical, cortico-subcortical, and subcortical types according to the prevalent localization of lesions. A comparison of the signs of mental decline and the localization of lesions in different types of dementia may help to elucidate some of the clinico-anatomical correlations.

The major manifestations of cortical and cortico-subcortical dementia include various impairments of memory, agnosia of time and space, social agnosia and social apraxia, and poor judgment and planning, leading to serious disturbances in social and occupational functioning. Cortical dementia has been extensively studied, especially in patients with Alzheimer's disease and Pick's disease, which was recently included in the larger category of frontotemporal dementia.

Cortical Dementia

Alzheimer's Disease

Dementia in cases of Alzheimer's disease, as well as in other diseases with extended cortical and subcortical pathology, differs from the classical syndromes of local brain pathology, such as aphasia, agnosia, and apraxia, because it involves disturbances in the recognition of actions and their subjects in the social world. Such disturbances thus underlie the development of dementia with disturbances in occupational and social functioning. These disturbances of social gnosis and praxis may be either primary, as in cases with prominent frontal lobe lesions, or secondary to agnosia of time, space, and registration, as well as impairments in working memory, which are caused by pathology in the temporo-parietal region including the hippocampal areas. Typical signs of parietal lobe pathology such as constructional apraxia, motor apraxia, agraphia, and acalculia may be absent in some cases at the moderate stages of dementia. The prominent pathology in certain areas of the parietal lobe appears primarily in the early stages of Alzheimer's disease with presenile onset, and related pathology appears in cases of posterior cortical atrophy, which is described in the following paragraph.

It is important to stress that memory disturbances may mediate the onset of social agnosia and social apraxia in cases of dementia, but that this mediation is limited since social gnosis and praxis can be preserved for the most part, while memory disturbances can be quite severe in patients with Kosakoff's amnestic syndrome.

Delusions and hallucinations are often observed over the course of the progression of Alzheimer's disease. The delusions are uncomplicated, simple, and often persecutory and involving theft or jealousy. The hallucinations are primarily visual, with auditory components in some cases.

Mood changes are primarily manifested as depression compounded by anger, irritability, episodes of agitation, and aggressiveness. Wandering may be observed during early stages of dementia in patients with Alzheimer's disease, while memory disturbances may be accompanied by confabulations, all of which may lead to dangerous wanderings out of the house into nearby areas—woods, city streets, a highway, and so on.

In the two original cases described by Alzheimer in 1906 and 1911, the age of onset was 51 in the first case and 54 in the second case. Aphasia, agnosia, and apraxia were noted in the early stages of the rapidly progressive state of dementia. Postmortem macroscopic and histopathological examinations revealed diffuse pathology of the entire cortex that is especially prominent in the parietal and temporal lobe of both hemispheres, which are damaged more severely than the frontal lobes. In typical cases of senile dementia the frontal lobes are, by all means, considerably more pathologic compared to our cases (for a review, see Tonkonogy & Moak, 1988). Thus, Alzheimer stressed that the more prominent posterior cortical pathology was manifested by the development of aphasia, agnosia, and apraxia in the early stages of progressive dementia. He considered that such cases are unique and are different from senile dementia, a condition that was later included in the broader spectrum of Alzheimer's disease.

Subsequent studies have shown that in cases of Alzheimer's disease with either senile or presenile onset, neuropathological changes are manifested as cortical atrophy, reflecting neuronal degeneration and loss in the temporo-parietal cortex, and to a lesser extent in the frontal cortex, sparing the primary motor and somato-sensory areas and, in most cases, the occipital cortex (Corsellis, 1976; Jervis, 1937; Tomlinson, 1977). The topographic pattern of histological changes usually repeats the pattern of atrophy that is observed during a macroscopic

634

LOCALIZATION
OF CLINICAL
SYNDROMES IN
NEUROPSYCHOLOGY
AND NEUROSCIENCE

examination. These changes include senile plaques, neurofibrillary tangles, and to a lesser extent granulovacuolar degeneration (Brun & Gustafson, 1978). In accordance with Alzheimer's original descriptions, these changes may be especially prominent in the temporo-parietal region in patients with a presenile onset of Alzheimer's disease manifesting as temporo-parietal symptoms.

Memory impairments have been described as one of the early signs of Alzheimer's disease. Corresponding hippocampal abnormalities, especially neurofibrillary tangles and granulovacuolar degeneration, are usually seen in the early stages of Alzheimer's disease (Corsellis, 1976).

The primary localization of lesions of the grey matter regions of the cerebral hemispheres has been described as a hallmark of Alzheimer's disease. However, white matter lesions, primarily of vascular origin, have recently been described in patients with Alzheimer's disease (George et al., 1986; Kosaka, Ikeda, Matsushita, & Iizuka, 1986). According to Blennow, Wallin, and Gottris (1994), white matter changes are noted mainly in patients with Alzheimer's disease of senile onset, specifically in 10 of 11 such patients compared to 5 of 15 patients with presenile onset.

A head CT scan of an Alzheimer's patient shows diffuse cerebral atrophy with ventricular and cortical sulci enlargement (Cummings, 1985; Donaldson, 1979). However, no direct correlation may be found between the severity of dementia and the degree of atrophy as revealed by a CT scan (Fox, Topel, & Huckman, 1975; Wu, Schenkenberg, Wing, & Osborn, 1981). Studies utilizing PET and SPECT scans have demonstrated that an abnormal perfusion pattern in cases of Alzheimer's disease is noted as a bilateral temporo-parietal defect in most cases (Foster et al., 1983; Friedland et al., 1983; Homan, Johnson, Gerada Carvalho, & Satlin, 1992; Jagust, Budinger, & Reed, 1987). A frontal lobe defect is also present in 40%–45% of patients with Alzheimer's disease, but a temporo-parietal defect is observed at a much more frequent rate of 82% in patients with Alzheimer's disease (Homan et al., 1992), reflecting the previously reported neuropathological findings. Brain MRI scans show that, in addition to gray matter encephalopathy, a prominent white matter hyperintensity is often observed in patients with Alzheimer's disease, pointing to the probable frequent association of Alzheimer's cortical pathology with white matter lesions of probable vascular origin.

Frontotemporal Dementia, Pick's Disease

Frontotemporal dementia is relatively rare compared to Alzheimer's disease. Frontotemporal dementia is characterized by the presence of prominent frontal and/or temporal lobe atrophy. Microscopic changes include neuronal loss and gliosis in the affected cortical regions (Brun, 1987). Atrophy and histopathological changes are usually concentrated in the orbito-frontal, anterior, and medial temporal cortex, sparing the central gyri and the posterior one-third of the superior temporal gyrus (Corsellis, 1976; Tissot, Constantinidis, & Richard, 1975). The hippocampus may be spared, especially in the early stages of Pick's disease (Steiberger et al., 1983; Tissot et al., 1975). Involvement of the parietal lobe involvement has been described in rare cases of Pick's disease. Atrophy of subcortical structures, especially the caudate nucleus and substantia nigra, has also been frequently noted via pathologic examinations (Akelaitis, 1944; Tissot, 1975; Tonkonogy et al., 1994).

Approximately 60% of cases with frontotemporal dementia are classified as cases of Pick's disease (Jervis, 1971; Tissot et al., 1975) based on the presence of inflated neurons with argentophilic cytoplasmatic inclusions, or Pick's body (Corsellis, 1976), which was first described by Alzheimer in 1911. Senile plaques and neurofibrillary tangles, the hallmarks of Alzheimer's disease, are usually absent in cases of frontotemporal dementia. An absence of Pick's body in cases with subcortical gliosis and a neuropathological picture similar to Pick's disease was described by Neumann (1949) and Neumann and Cohn (1967) as Type II Pick's disease. Recently, a series of cases with lobar frontotemporal atrophy with the absence of Pick's body were included in the broader entity defined as frontotemporal dementia (Brun, 1993; Gustafson, 1993; Kumar & Gottlieb, 1993; Neary, Snowden, Norsen, & Goulding, 1988). This entity includes three major types of pathology—Pick's disease, nonspecific frontal degeneration, and frontal degeneration with anterior spinal loss (Huiette & Crain, 1992; Mendez et al., 1996; Neary, Snowden, & Mann, 1993).

A peculiar form of frontotemporal dementia with parkinsonism has been reported lately under such names as pallidopontonigral degeneration (Wszolek et al., 1992) and familial multiple system tauopathy with presenile dementia (Murrell et al., 1997). A linkage to chromosome 17, specifically a mutation in the gene for the microtubule-associated tau protein, has been found in several cases of families with frontotemporal dementia and parkinsonism (Foster et al., 1997). Postmortem brain examinations in such cases are characterized by a widespread accumulation of cytoplasmic tau. The abnormal tau protein is also selectively deposited in other neurodegenerative disorders, including corticobasal degeneration, progressive supranuclear palsy, and Pick's disease (Komori, 1999; Litvan et al., 1999; Maturanath et al., 2000).

Head CT scans (see Figure 12.1) reveal disproportionate frontal and/ or temporal atrophy in patients with Pick's disease, as well as in patients with other forms of frontotemporal dementia (Cummings & Duchen, 1981; McGeachie, Fleming, Sharer, & Hyman, 1979; Tonkonogy et al., 1994; Wechsler, Verity, Rosenschein, Fried, & Scheibel, 1982).

636

LOCALIZATION
OF CLINICAL
SYNDROMES IN
NEUROPSYCHOLOGY
AND NEUROSCIENCE

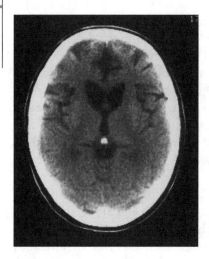

FIGURE 12.1 Head CT scan of patient M.S. with Pick's disease. Cortical atrophy extends from the frontal poles and mesial surface of the frontal lobes to the anterior two thirds of the temporal lobe, sparing both the posterior part of the temporal lobe and the occipital lobe. Subcortical atrophy is also found in this particular case. The early onset of caudate atrophy sometimes develops at the onset of Pick's disease. See a more detailed description of patient M.S. in chapter 11, section titled "Obsessive–Compulsive Disorder (OCD)."

An abnormal perfusion pattern is found to be different in patients with Pick's disease compared to Alzheimer's disease. Hypoperfusion is often observed in the frontal, and sometimes temporal, regions (Jagust, Reed, Scab, Kramer, & Budinger, 1989; Kamo et al., 1987; Miller et al., 1991; Risberg et al., 1993).

The manifestations of dementia may be quite similar in cases of Alzheimer's disease and frontotemporal dementia, especially in their advanced stages. This includes severe disturbances of occupational and social functioning underlain by such major disturbances of basic cognitive functions as social agnosia and social apraxia, poor judgment and planning, and various memory disturbances. These cognitive disturbances are usually present in any type of dementia, underlying the disturbances in executive functions. Their absence makes a diagnosis of dementia questionable, since relatively isolated disorders of language, praxis, gnosis, moderate amnesia, and personality change may be noted in nondemented patients.

At the same time, the predominant involvement of the frontal lobe and the anterior parts of the temporal lobes in cases of frontotemporal dementia may result in some significant differences in clinical manifestations compared to those in Alzheimer's disease. These differences are underlined by a more extended cortical lesion in Alzheimer's disease that involves, in addition to the frontal and anterior temporal regions, the posterior areas of the cortex, including posterior parts of the temporal lobe and hippocampus, and the parietal lobe in some cases. At the same time, the involvement of the frontal lobes may be more severe in cases of frontotemporal dementia (see Figure 12.2).

Prominent frontal lobe atrophy results in more prominent signs of frontal lobe involvement in frontotemporal dementia characterized by the development of personality changes, apathy, loss of motivation,

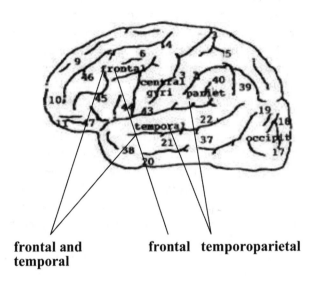

**frontal and
temporal**   **frontal   temporoparietal**

FIGURE 12.2   Left hemisphere. Primary localization of cortical atrophy in Alzheimer's disease and frontotemporal dementia; the atrophy is usually bilateral and symmetrical. Frontal lobe atrophy is usually more severe in cases of frontotemporal dementia.

primary disturbances of social gnosis and praxis, disinhibition with restlessness, wandering, and euphoria with inappropriate jocularities (Gustafson, 1993; Lishman, 1978; Mayer-Gross, Critchley, Greenfield, & Meyer, 1937–1938; Miller et al., 1991; Neary et al., 1988; Wechsler et al., 1982). Involvement of the anterior temporal lobe may produce some features resembling Kluver-Bucy syndrome, including bulimia, hyperorality with a tendency to eat inedible objects, and hypersexuality (Cummings & Duchen, 1981; Schneider, 1929; Tissot et al., 1975; Tonkonogy et al., 1994). Obsessive–compulsive disorders as a result of caudate atrophy are also described in the early stages of Pick's disease (Tonkonogy & Barreira, 1989; Tonkonogy et al., 1994).

Memory may be relatively preserved due to the preservation of the hippocampus, especially in the early stages of frontotemporal dementia. It was recently demonstrated that 16 patients with Alzheimer's disease showed a significantly greater impairment of memory in comparison with neuropsychological tests of executive functions, while 15 patients with frontotemporal dementia were characterized by an opposite pattern (Pachana, Boone, Miller, Cummings, & Berman, 1996).

In cases of frontotemporal dementia, language disorders are similar to those observed in Alzheimer's disease; they are characterized

638

LOCALIZATION
OF CLINICAL
SYNDROMES IN
NEUROPSYCHOLOGY
AND NEUROSCIENCE

by anomia, empty speech, circumlocution, and progressive deterioration of comprehension and may be related to temporal lobe pathology (Binns & Robertson, 1962; Klages, 1954; Kosaka, 1976; Wechsler et al., 1982). Some of the clinical manifestations of language disorders, however, point to the role of frontal lobe pathology in the formation of language disorders in frontotemporal dementia. Word-finding difficulties, for example, may appear early in the course of frontotemporal dementia; a patient often stereotypically uses the same general term as a substitute for a word that is difficult to find (Robertson, Le Roux, & Brown, 1958). Speech often includes stereotyped verbal output, with a tendency to repeat the same sentence or short story against a background of reduced speech initiation (Mayer-Gross et al., 1937–1938). This may eventually progress to mutism in the end stages of the disease (Cummings & Duchen, 1981; Gustafson, Hagberg, & Ingvar, 1978; Lowenberg, 1936; Tonkonogy et al., 1994).

Relatively preserved visuospatial orientation related to parietal spearing in cases of Pick's disease contrast with prominent space and time disorientations in Alzheimer's disease. A patient with Alzheimer's disease becomes disoriented in space and is often unable to find his or her way back home in the early stages of the disease. The patient eventually loses his or her sense of orientation in his or her own home or on a hospital ward (Brouwers et al., 1984; Gainotti et al., 1980). A relative preservation of orientation is usually observed in patients with frontotemporal dementia. Such patients may wander around without losing their way back home, and orientation in space is preserved when patients are in their homes or in a hospital ward, even in moderately advanced stages of the disease (Brun & Gustafson, 1978; Cummings & Duchen, 1981; Robertson et al., 1958; Sjögren, Sjögren, & Lindgren, 1952).

Conventional ideational and ideomotor apraxia are frequent observations in the advanced stages of Alzheimer's disease (Della Sala, Lucchelli, & Spinner, 1987; Hughes, 1970; Sjögren et al., 1952) but may be either mild or completely absent in cases of moderate dementia. Apraxia related to the activities of daily living, such as dressing, shaving, and bathing, develop later during the course of Alzheimer's disease. While patients with frontotemporal dementia do not suffer from conventional ideational or ideomotor apraxia, unconventional apraxia, or difficulties in repeating sequences of movements, may be observed in relatively early stages of frontotemporal dementia, as well as in cases of Alzheimer's disease. Apraxia related to the activities of daily living may appear only in the end stages of both types of dementia (Tonkonogy et al., 1994).

Preservation of the parietal lobe in cases of frontotemporal dementia is usually manifested by significantly better performance on construction and calculation tasks by patients with frontotemporal dementia than patients with Alzheimer's disease characterized by relatively frequent involvement of the parietal lobe (Johansen & Hagberg, 1989; Mendez et al., 1996; Wechsler et al., 1982).

Posterior Occipito-Parietal Cortical Atrophy

Involvement of the posterior cortex may extend to occipito-temporal and occipito-parietal lobe junctions, manifesting as visual agnosia in cases of Alzheimer's disease (Sjögren et al., 1952). In some cases, relatively isolated occipito-parietal cortical atrophy develops in the initial stages of progressive dementia. Benson et al. (1988) described five patients with progressive dementia and early onset of visual and spatial agnosia, alexia with subsequent development of Ballint's syndrome, Gerstmann's syndrome, and transcortical sensory aphasia. Head CT and/or MRI scans found evidence of prominent occipito-parietal atrophy in such cases.

In most of the more recently reported cases of posterior cortical atrophy, the clinical manifestations are similar to those reported by Benson et al. (1988). These manifestations include the development of visual object and topographic agnosia, alexia, agraphia, and occasional prosopagnosia in the initial stages of the dementing illnesses with subsequent development of apraxia, components of Balint's and Gerstmann's syndromes, and transcortical sensory aphasia (Ardila, Rosseli, Arvizu, & Kuljis, 1997; Berthier et al., 1991; Jagust, Davies, Tiller-Borcich, & Reed, 1990; Kyosawa et al., 1989; Levine, Lee, & Fisher, 1993; Mendez et al., 1996; Rogelet, Delafosse, & Destee, 1996). Either no significant memory loss (Benson et al., 1988) or a limited degree of memory impairment has been reported in most cases of posterior cortical atrophy (Croisile et al., 1991).

Neuropathological studies have shown that the etiology of posterior cortical atrophy may include not only Alzheimer's disease but also other pathological entities, including Creutzfeldt-Jakob disease and subcortical gliosis. Three of five of Benson et al.'s (1988) cases were examined via autopsy (Victoroff et al., 1994). Subcortical gliosis was noted in one case, Creutzfeldt-Jakob disease in another case, and Alzheimer's-type changes in the third case. One case of Creutzfeldt-Jakob disease and one case of Alzheimer's disease were also noted via an autopsy of two cases with posterior cortical atrophy (Renner, Morris, Storandt, & La Barge, 1992). In most cases of posterior cortical atrophy, however, Alzheimer's-type changes were noted on neuropathological postmortem examinations (Levine et al., 1993; Victoroff et al., 1994) and biopsies (Berthier et al., 1991; Rogelet et al., 1996). Though head CT scans may be normal in the initial stages of posterior cortical atrophy (Rogelet et al., 1996), predominantly occipito-parietal atrophy emerges with the progression of the disease (Ardila et al., 1997; Benson et al., 1988; Rogelet et al., 1996).

640

LOCALIZATION
OF CLINICAL
SYNDROMES IN
NEUROPSYCHOLOGY
AND NEUROSCIENCE

It is important to stress the similarities between the clinical manifestations of agnosia, apraxia, aphasia, presenile onset, and the neuropathological findings in presenile dementia as described by Alzheimer and presenile dementia with posterior cortical atrophy. The most recent descriptions of posterior cortical atrophy in cases with Alzheimer's-type changes in histopathological examinations also point to the need for further studies of possible histopathological differences between Alzheimer's disease of presenile onset and of senile onset.

Slowly Progressive Isolated Aphasia

Mesulam (1982) described eight cases of slowly progressive aphasia of various types. Other cognitive functions were preserved, and no evidence of dementia was observed in these cases at that time. However, dementia eventually developed in some of these cases. No specific neuropathological process was reported following a postmortem examination of one case. Similar cases of relatively isolated aphasia were described in two cases of Pick's disease with diagnoses proven via autopsies (Holland et al., 1985; Wechsler et al., 1982). Kirshner et al. (1984) found status spongiousus in the left perisylvian region in two of three postmortem cases with similar isolated aphasia. Mandell, Alexander, and Carpenter (1989) presented a case of Creutzfeldt-Jakob disease with isolated aphasia. Slowly progressive aphasia was also described in several cases of Alzheimer's disease (Poeck & Luzzati, 1988; Pogacar & Williams, 1984).

Vascular Dementia and Cortical Lesions

Alzheimer (1898, 1902, 1904) described ischemic cortical atrophy and perivascular gliosis as the result of ischemia caused by small-vessel arteriosclerosis. He distinguished between a neurotic phase produced by a mild degree of arteriosclerosis of small cortical vessels and vascular dementia resulting from prominent ischemic cortical atrophy and perivascular gliosis. Binswanger's disease (see section titled "Subcortical Dementia," below), or arteriosclerotic subcortical enecephalopathy, was considered an example of such pathology in the subcortical region produced by arteriosclerosis of the small penetrating intracerebral arterioles, leading to the development of ischemia and/or small infarctions.

Alzheimer also recognized the role of cortical and cortico-subcortical infarctions due to either thromboembolism or atherosclerosis of the medium-sized and large feeding vessels, such as the carotid or cerebral arteries. He actually was the first to describe the syndrome in relation to thrombosis of the carotid arteries. In subsequent years, however, primary emphasis was placed on cerebral arteriosclerosis as a main causal factor in the development of vascular dementing illnesses

(Mayer-Gross, Slater, & Roth, 1960; for a review, see Emey, Gillie, & Ramdev, 1994).

In the late 1960s and early 1970s, the role of cerebral vascular disease in the onset of vascular dementia was considered to be mainly limited to the presence of cerebral infarctions, both small and large, produced by pathology of the medium and large extra- or intracerebral arteries (Hachinski, Lassen, & Marshall, 1974). Such infarctions due to cortical thromboembolism may also be produced by a variety of cardiac diseases, including atrial fibrillation, myocardial infarction, endocarditis, and valvular pathology. As a result of this approach, the concept of multi-infarct dementia emerged as an alternative to that of cerebral arteriosclerosis (Hachinski et al., 1974). A simple score was suggested for the assessment of the clinical correlates of multi-infarct dementia. The items that make up the score include symptoms that are related to the development of cerebral infarctions, such as step-wise deterioration and focal neurological findings.

Cortical vascular dementia may reflect extended cortical lesions that are caused by a number of cortical infarctions (multi-infarct dementia) associated with medium and large vessel atherosclerosis, rather than progressive chronic ischemia. The multi-infarctions may be prevalent in the different focal areas of the cerebral cortex, resulting in symptoms of aphasia, agnosia, and apraxia (for a review, see Chui, 1989). Dementia is often absent when cerebral infarctions are limited to the specific anatomical distribution resulting in the onset of isolated disturbances of language, gnosis, or praxis. Dementia may join these isolated syndromes with the development of new cortical infarctions caused by either thromboembolism or atherosclerosis of the medium and large vessels. It has been suggested that cerebral infarctions are caused by atherosclerosis of cerebral arteries in a small percentage of cases with a process of vascular dementia. Alzheimer (1904) described slow, progressive chronic ischemic changes that are produced by arteriosclerosis of small vessels and lead to cortical and subcortical atrophy and cerebral gliosis; such changes were not accounted for in these studies.

More recently, the idea that the development of cognitive impairments may be related not only to cerebral microinfarctions but also to general cerebral dysfunctions caused by general cerebral ischemia resulting from a reduction in blood supply to the brain has come to be recognized by researchers (Emory et al., 1994). According to the National Institute of Neurological and Communicative Disorders and Stroke (1975), abnormalities of general cerebral circulation may be related to various factors, including hypertension, hypotension, alterations in blood viscosity and coagulation, and abnormalities in blood gases, lipids, proteins, and glucose.

642

LOCALIZATION
OF CLINICAL
SYNDROMES IN
NEUROPSYCHOLOGY
AND NEUROSCIENCE

The introduction of head CT scans and, especially, MRI scans drew attention to the chronic ischemic changes in the cerebral white matter of elderly patients with dementia and other types of psychiatric symptoms. Such scans revealed that the chronic ischemic changes are manifested as white matter hyperintensity, either with or without cerebral microinfarctions. The role of cerebral arteriosclerosis of small vessels in the development of chronic ischemic changes in both the cortical gray matter and the subcortical white matter was once again brought to the attention of researchers. As a result of these studies, the term vascular dementia has been reintroduced and multi-infarct dementia has begun to be reconsidered as one of a number of vascular dementing processes, which also include general cerebral dysfunction, as well as arteriosclerosis of small cerebral arteries, resulting in chronic cerebral ischemia.

Some researchers have compared cognitive processing in subgroups of patients with different types of vascular disorders—focal cerebral dysfunction and general cerebral dysfunction. Emory et al. (1994) found no significant differences between the cognitive assessment scores of a subgroup of 14 patients with cerebral infarcts and a subgroup of 17 patients with generalized cerebral dysfunction and an absence of cerebral infarcts. Cognitive assessments included the Mini-Mental State Examination, the Dementia Rating Scale (Mattis, 1988), the Reitan Trail Making Test Parts A and B, the Wechsler Adult Intelligence Scale (Wechsler, 1955), the Western Aphasia Battery (Kertesz, 1982), and a series of other tests. The researchers explained the absence of differences between the two subgroups by a probable additional role of generalized cerebral dysfunction in the subgroup of patients with cerebral infarcts, since vascular abnormalities cross-cut both subgroups, including hypertension or hypotension, arteriosclerosis, ischemic heart disease, and abnormal EKGs. In future studies, it would be of interest to evaluate the role of chronic cerebral ischemia caused by arteriosclerosis of small cerebral vessels and resulting in cortical atrophy and white matter hyperintensity in both subgroups of patients.

Vascular Dementia and Alzheimer's Disease

The concomitant role of vascular pathology in the development of Alzheimer's-type dementia has begun to be evaluated by several groups of researchers. The measured size of the areas of infarction in the brain was used to determine cerebral vascular pathology. Blessed et al. (1968) stressed that ischemic lesions may be found in all groups of demented elderly patients, but that the clinical scores for dementia rise steeply when the total volume of ischemic lesions reaches more than 50 cc of infarcted tissue. Based on this assumption, the authors studied the correlation of dementia scores and a number of neuritique plaques in cases of dementia with less than 5 cc of infarcted cerebral tissue and found a high correlation between the number of plaques in the cerebral cortex and the severity of dementia.

This conclusion has recently begun to be challenged, and many researchers have shown that vascular pathology may play a significant role in the presence and severity of dementia in patients with Alzheimer's-type brain pathology. Snowdon et al. (1997) reported the results of a longitudinal study conducted with the participation of 678 nuns between the ages of 75 and 102, with a mean age of 83 years. All of the participants underwent a cognitive evaluation with a series of neuropsychological tests. By the end of 4 years, 161 of the participants had died, and a neuropathological evaluation was performed on 146 of the remaining participants. After excluding individuals whose brains showed signs of other diseases, and cases in which the level of education was lower than that of a bachelor's degree, 102 cases with brain autopsy were included in the final sample. The neuropathological criteria for Alzheimer's disease were met by 61 participants. Cognitive impairment was more prominent and dementia more severe in those with Alzheimer's disease who also had brain infarcts. The prevalence of dementia was 75% in a subgroup of the 61 participants with a large infarct in the lobes of the neocortex, and 57% in a subgroup of participants without such infarcts. Of the 57% in the subgroup of 61 cases with Alzheimer's disease and an absence of neocortical infarcts, the prevalence of dementia increased to 93% of cases with small lacunar infarcts in either basal ganglia, the thalamus, or deep white matter. These data support the role of cortical and, especially, subcortical infarcts in the development of dementia in cases with Alzheimer's disease. At the same time, dementia was present in only 3 participants from the group of 41 with brain infarctions and an absence of neuropathological signs of Alzheimer's disease. Researchers have recently reported that white matter hyperintensity, probably reflecting small-vessel ischemic disease, is frequently seen in patients with Alzheimer's disease (Tonkonogy, 2001).

Some authors have begun to describe cases of vascular dementia that are completely free of neuritique plaques and neurofibrillary tangles (Erkinjuntti, Haltia, Palo, Sulkava, & Paetau, 1988; Hulette et al., 1997). Such cases are rare, however, as are cases of Alzheimer's disease that are free of vascular pathology. Erkinjuntti et al. (1988) presented 15 autopsy-confirmed cases of dementia due to multiple cerebral infarctions that were completely free of senile plaques and neurofibrillary tangles. In 6 of 115 cases, the volume of infarcted tissue was less than 6 ml, which is in contrast to the 50 cc lower limits for vascular dementia that were used by Blessed et al. (1968). It is possible that ischemic cortical atrophy was not accounted for in a study published by Erkinjuntti

644

LOCALIZATION
OF CLINICAL
SYNDROMES IN
NEUROPSYCHOLOGY
AND NEUROSCIENCE

et al. (1988). Hulette et al. (1997) described 6 autopsied cases of multi-infarct dementia. In Case 2, however, the authors found neuropathological changes similar to those described by Alzheimer (1898, 1902, 1904) as they are related to the arteriosclerosis of small cortical arterioles. These changes included diffuse cortical atrophy with ischemic changes in the left frontal cortex and hippocampus, as well as neuronal loss and profound reactive astrogliosis. No infarction related to occlusive disease of the large vessels was found. Cognitive impairment and the clinical course of dementia were practically indistinguishable from Alzheimer's disease in 4 of the 6 cases described by Hulette et al. (1979).

Further studies are certainly needed to clarify the role of vascular changes in the expression of dementia in Alzheimer's disease, as well as to compare findings typical for Alzheimer's disease and vascular cortical and subcortical pathology in elderly patients with dementia.

Subcortical Dementia

The idea of subcortical dementia was first advanced by Naville (1922), and the term itself was coined by Von Stockert (1932). The concept of subcortical dementia, however, has been brought to attention as a distinctive entity for contemporary analysis by Albert, Feldman, and Willis (1974) and McHugh and Folstein (1975).

Subcortical Dementia as Bradyphrenia

Naville (1922) used the term *bradyphrenia* to describe a psychiatric syndrome of intellectual slowness in a patient with epidemic encephalitis. The syndrome consisted of a reduction in initiative, interest, and efforts. The capacity for work was also diminished, and mild, subjective memory problems were noted. Naville stressed that intellect is preserved in such cases and that the primary difficulties are the losses of initiative and the capacity for intellectual work. He found that this syndrome of mental retardation is pathognomic for few cases of classic parkinsonism.

The term *subcortical dementia* was first coined by Von Stockert (1932), who supported the concept of bradyphrenia. He described postencephalitic mental disturbances in a patient who had had no motor signs of parkinsonism. The disturbances included slowness, a memory disorder, and personality and affect changes, which von Stockert associated with bradyphrenia. (For a review, see Mandell & Albert, 1990.)

Stertz (1931) expanded the concept of bradyphrenia, considering a decrease in the general psychic level of energy as a cause of disturbances in all psychic performances. He related this decrease to the incomplete inactivation of the preserved cerebral cortical apparatus produced by the pathology in the subcortical structures. Stertz referred to this as *brain-stem dementia* (*Hirnstamdementz*), which he differentiated from *cortical dementia* (*Hirnmanteldemenz*). According to Stertz, brain-stem dementia results from a number of disorders, including tumors, multiple sclerosis, abscess, and hydrocephalus.

In the following years, mental disturbances caused by subcortical lesions continued to be considered as the results of a loss of initiative and a slowness of psychic activity. Hassler (1953) used the term *psychic akinesia* to describe dementia in patients with Parkinson's disease. Constantinidis, Tissot, and Ajuriaguerra (1970) noted the slowness of speech, reduced interest, and disturbances in practical efficiency in patients with progressive supranuclear palsy (PSP). They considered this to be a pseudodementia of PSP.

*Subcortical Dementia as Slowness of Mental Processing
Plus Memory and Executive Disturbances*

Albert et al. (1974) reintroduced the term subcortical dementia and considered a slowness of mental processing, or bradyphrenia, as an important manifestation of this type of dementia. Albert et al. (1974), however, also included in the description of subcortical dementia other symptoms usually described in cases of bradyphrenia: memory abnormalities, primarily consisting of forgetfulness; impaired manipulation of acquired knowledge, such as abstract abilities and calculation; and mood and personality changes marked by apathy and inertia with occasional irritability and brief bursts of rage. The authors did not directly connect these symptoms with bradyphrenia and a loss of psychic energy but instead considered them to be relatively independent, directly resulting from lesions of the various subcortical structures, primarily the striatum. Special attention was given to frontal disturbances, manifesting as difficulties in the executive functions of planning, organizing, and scheduling activities. The development of these difficulties was given a direct anatomical explanation as a result of a disruption of the fronto-subcortical connections, which are important for such activities. One possibility, which is not discussed by Albert et al. (1974), is that such development may be secondary to the inertia, apathy, and slowness of mental activity that is usually seen in patients with subcortical dementia.

Subcortical Dementia in Various Diseases

Progressive Supranuclear Palsy. Albert et al. (1974) introduced the term subcortical dementia after examining five patients with progressive PSP, as well as conducting a retrospective analysis of 42 previously published cases of PSP. The authors stressed the absence of aphasia, agnosia, and apraxia as a major difference between subcortical

646

LOCALIZATION
OF CLINICAL
SYNDROMES IN
NEUROPSYCHOLOGY
AND NEUROSCIENCE

dementia and cortical dementia. Subsequent studies of patients with PSP found evidence of dementia in 18 of 27 patients at the time of the first hospital referral, with 7 of the patients demonstrating difficulties in tests that were believed to be specific for frontal lobe function (Maher, Smith, & Lees, 1985). This is explained by the role of frontal-subcortical circuits in the functions of the frontal lobes (Cummings, 1990).

The neuropathological findings in PSP include marked nerve cell loss in a large number of brain stem structures with a predilection for the subthalamic nucleus, the globus pallidus, the substantia nigra, the periaqueductal gray matter, the superior colliculus, the locus coeruleus, and the dentate, pontine, and raphe nuclei. The cerebral cortex appeared to be spared according to the early anatomical and histopathological studies (Steele et al., 1964).

Later, several authors studied cognitive performance in patients with PSP and found performance difficulties on tests that were relatively specific for frontal lobe functions (Cambier, Masson, Viader, Limodin, & Strube, 1985; Maher et al., 1985; Pillon, Dubois, L'Hermitte, & Agid, 1986). The tests included tests of verbal fluency, Weigl's test, and a simplified version of the WCST. After reviewing the literature, Lees (1990) concluded that specific neuropsychological impairments in PSP included a "slowness of initiation and thought and a difficulty in generating and switching smoothly from one cognitive set to another" (p. 126). At the same time, Lees (1990) listed bradyphrenia as a frontal lobe symptom in patients with PSP. However, the author did not discuss the possibility that decreased speed of cognition, instead of a direct anatomical disruption of the frontal-subcortical circuit, may play a significant, if not major, role in the development of frontal lobe difficulties in patients with PSP.

Another possibility is a direct anatomical involvement of cortical areas, including the frontal lobes, as revealed by brain imaging in patients with PSP (for a review, see Lees, 1990). A number of CT scan studies found that atrophy of subcortical structures was accompanied by mild cortical atrophy in the prefrontal and temporal regions in patients with PSP (Haldeman, Goldman, Hyde, & Pribram, 1981; Masucci, Borts, Smirniotopoulos, & Kurtzke, 1985). Schonfield, Golbe, Sage, Safer, and Duvoisin (1987) reported CT findings of an increase in the severity of atrophy of the pons and midbrain with the progression of PSP and subsequent dilatation of the aqueduct and the third and fourth ventricles. While atrophy of the temporal lobes was observed at that advanced stage of PSP, cortical atrophy appeared to be variable and not pronounced. Lees (1990) also reviewed studies of brain glucose metabolism in PSP, which demonstrated a statistically significant decrease in mean glucose utilization in the frontal region of six patients with probable

PSP (D'Antona et al., 1985). Through his own research, Lees (1990) also found a global decrease in blood flow and oxygen utilization in five patients with PSP; this decrease was most marked in the frontal regions. No correlation was found between the decreases in blood flow and the participants' performance on psychological tests. Lees also presented a SPECT scan of a PSP patient, which demonstrated diminished activity in the frontal lobes, especially in the medial frontal region.

These neuropsychological and brain imaging data point to the need for further exploration of cognitive impairments and their anatomical backgrounds in PSP. It is not completely clear what role, if any, the cortical regions, especially the frontal and temporal areas, play in the development of relatively mild impairments of memory and executive functions in PSP, or if these cognitive problems are secondary to bradyphrenia, which is manifested as a decreased speed of cognitive processing and loss of initiation as produced by a subcortical lesion.

Huntington's Disease. McHugh and Folstein (1975) discussed the concept of subcortical dementia when describing their study of eight patients with Huntington's disease (HD). They stressed the dilapidation of all cognitive powers in such cases, including all aspects of thinking and memory functions, as well as a loss of initiative and the progressive development of apathy. In a review of their subsequent studies, Folstein, Brandt, and Folstein (1990) stressed that cognitive deficits in HD patients affect the ability to plan and organize, mental flexibility (changing sets), verbal fluency, attention and calculation, cognitive speed, and retrieval of memory. Folstein also found no evidence of the aphasia, apraxia, agnosia, and amnesia that are seen in patients with cortical dementia.

Despite a severely impaired ability to recall newly learned words, a patient with HD demonstrates a relatively normal ability to recognize verbal material that has been recently presented, in comparison to amnesic patients. The proposed explanation of this finding is based on the suggestion that HD patients are unable to initiate systematic search strategies for the retrieval of stored verbal information (Butters, 1978). The presence of mood and movement abnormalities is also included in the description of subcortical dementia in cases of HD.

As in research on patients with PSP, some authors have observed cognitive changes in cases of HD that are similar to those noted in patients with frontal lobe disease (Stuss & Benson, 1984). These changes include diminished verbal fluency (Butters, 1978), a loss of mental flexibility, and a reduction in the ability to alter one's perception of targets during a set (Bear & Fedio, 1977; Josiassen, Curry, & Mancall, 1983). This is explained by the fact that the caudate nuclei, which are most

648

LOCALIZATION
OF CLINICAL
SYNDROMES IN
NEUROPSYCHOLOGY
AND NEUROSCIENCE

severely affected in HD, receive their input from the prefrontal and parietal lobes.

Cortical atrophy, however, has also been noted in patients with HD (Starkstein, Robinson, & Price, 1988). In an attempt to stress the role of a caudate lesion in dementia as a result of HD, Starkstein, Robinson, and Price (1988) compared scores on cognitive tests and degrees of atrophy of the caudate nuclei and frontal lobes. The authors demonstrated a significant correlation between caudate atrophy, as measured by CT scans, and a decrease in scores on cognitive tests; no such correlation has been found to exist between CT scans and measures of cortical atrophy. Cortical atrophy is certainly quite prominent in advanced cases of HD, and its role in the development of cognitive impairments requires further study. It is also unclear to what extent apathy and the loss of initiative are involved in the formation of cognitive abnormalities in patients with HD.

J.M. was a patient of ours who was diagnosed with Huntington's disease. J.M. was a 50-year-old graduate of MIT who, with a fellow MIT graduate, had founded a successful software company. The patient was forced to resign, however, when he became unable to continue his work in the company as manager and programmer. After a period of unemployment, he got a job as a gardener on an estate and was able to perform his job in a satisfactory manner for more than a year. However, J.M. eventually developed difficulties in the ability to follow the instructions of his employers, became easily angered, and even physically assaulted his employer. He was brought in for a forensic psychiatric evaluation, as his behavior seemed to be strange and quite contradictory to his personal and professional history. During an interview upon his admission to the hospital, J.M. was found to be alert, cooperative, and unable to recall the incident of assaultive behavior. There was no mention of the patient's cognitive impairment in the accompanying medical record.

Once admitted, J.M. was found to have some symptoms pointing to possible cognitive impairments of conventional information processing that are typical of mild dementia. He demonstrated mild abnormalities in orientation in time, being unable to report the exact date. A mild anomia was manifested as an inability to recall relatively low-frequency words, such as *earlobe*. Memory of U.S. presidents, comprehension, and constructive praxis were completely preserved, as was demonstrated by his performance on the appropriate BNCE subtests of conventional information processing. Testing of unconventional information processing using the BNCE, however, revealed prominent disturbances, which apparently did not interfere with the patient's ability to live independently until his episode of assault (see Figure 12.3).

A neurological examination performed at the time J.M. was admitted revealed infrequent brisk choreic movements of the head and trunk,

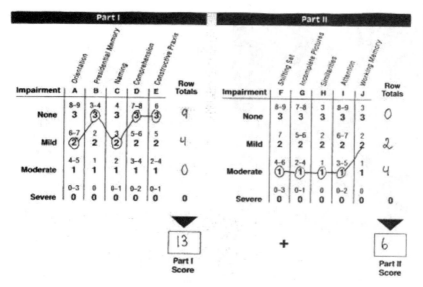

FIGURE 12.3 The Brief Neuropsychological Cognitive Examination (BNCE) profile of patient J.M., an individual with Huntington's disease. Note the relatively preserved conventional information processing (Part I), compared to low scores on the testing of unconventional information processing (Part II). J.M. was unable to recognize most of the incomplete drawings of objects (G), pointing to the presence of unconventional object agnosia. Agnosia of sequences was also apparent. The patient was unable to correctly copy sequences of shapes, which consisted of a repeated pattern of, for example, an open square and two triangles. J.M.'s working memory for those simple sequences was disturbed, even for a simple sequence of one open square followed by one open triangle (F, see also Figures 8.3 and 8.4). The cognitive disturbances observed in patient J.M. could underlie the impairments in gnosis of social actions, which is needed to continue successful occupational functioning. Disturbances of planning were also manifested as an inability to track the alternate connections of 12 numbers despite the correct understanding of instructions, as was demonstrated by the preserved ability to track a connection of six numbers (I). An impairment in semantic memory was manifested as a disturbance in explaining similarities (H). At the same time, working memory for words was only mildly disturbed (J). No clear signs of bradyphrenia or apathy were noted at that time.

positive snout, and Babinski's sign on the right. An MRI scan showed subcortical abnormalities compounded by mild frontoparietal atrophy (see Figure 12.4).

While the researchers eventually learned that a member of J.M.'s family had had Huntington's disease, the patient's mother had not shown any signs of Huntington's disease, and genetic testing had not been performed on J.M.'s family at that time. However, the Huntington's disease was considered as the highest on the list of possible diagnostic options for J.M.

The dilapidation of J.M.'s cognitive capabilities began with disturbances of occupational functioning, which may be considered as

650

LOCALIZATION
OF CLINICAL
SYNDROMES IN
NEUROPSYCHOLOGY
AND NEUROSCIENCE

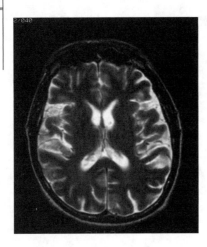

FIGURE 12.4 The T2-weighted MRI image of patient J.M., who had Huntington's disease, shows mild atrophy of the caudate nuclei with ex-vacuo enlargement of the anterior horns of the lateral ventriculi, as well as mild frontoparietal atrophy. Note also the moderate enlargement of the posterior horns and the third ventricle. These subcortical and partly cortical abnormalities are consistent with the patient's markedly low BNCE Part II scores (6/15) and relatively normal Part I scores (13/15).

signs of social agnosia and social apraxia accompanied by personality changes, as well as impairments in unconventional information processing in recognition and working memory, similar to those noted in cases of subcortical and cortical dementia. Evidence of atrophy of the caudate nuclei, as well as frontoparietal atrophy, was found via an MRI scan of J.M., supporting the role of both subcortical and cortical lesions in the development of dementia, at least in this particular patient.

Subcortical Lesions in Vascular Dementia. Special interest has been paid to the study of subcortical vascular dementia with localization of vascular lesions in the subcortical structures. Cummings (1987) and Stuss and Cummings (1990) described the profile of neuropsychological impairment in vascular dementia syndromes. These authors identified three types of small-vessel vascular dementia syndromes: lacunar state, Binswanger's disease, and thalamic dementia.

Lacunar state is characterized by multiple microinfarctions in the subcortical structures, the cerebral and cerebellar white matter, and the brain stem (Fisher, 1982). Dementia syndromes resulting from such pathology are known as multi-infarct dementia, or vascular dementia. The major manifestations of lacunar dementia are memory disturbances and frontal lobe types of deficits with social agnosia and social apraxia, and a relative sparing of the language function (Stuss & Cummings, 1990). Lacunes are usually multiple in nature and range in size from several millimeters to one or two centimeters in diameter. They result from the occlusion of small arterioles with fibrinoid necrosis of the walls and are related to hypertension and atherosclerosis.

However, the exclusive role of the lacunar state in relation to subcortical dementia has been questioned by data that demonstrate the weak association of both subcortical lacunar and nonlacunar ischemic changes with the cognitive performance of patients both with and without dementia (Mungas et al., 2001).

Binswanger's Disease, White Matter Hyperintensity. White matter hyperintensity (WMH), frequently revealed by MRI studies, is most likely the result of chronic cerebral ischemia in elderly patients and has been found to be implicated in the development of cognitive impairments, depression, and paranoid psychosis in these patients. Lacunar states are often accompanied by WMH, as observed via either MRI or head CT scans, though they are less distinct when viewed via the latter method. WMH may also be present without any symptoms of lacunar states in cases of Binswanger's disease; WMH is found primarily in the periventricular areas and the white matter of the cerebral hemisphere in such cases.

Binswanger (1894) described a condition that he named encephalitis subcorticalis chronica progressiva, a condition that consisted of a slowly developing dementia, gait ataxia, and dysarthria in eight cases of progressive pathology in the white matter of the cerebral hemispheres; interestingly, the cerebral cortex was remarkably spared in these cases. The term *subcortical arteriosclerotic encephalopathy* was introduced by Olszewski (1962), who conducted a literature review and presented the clinical and pathological descriptions of two cases. Similar cases were later described by Biemond (1970), Burger, Burch, and Kunze (1976), and Janota (1981). The disease has been considered as a result of ischemic injury to the periventricular areas and the cerebral white matter caused by a fibrous thickening of the walls of the small penetrating arteries to the subcortical gray substance and white matter, and it is supposedly a special form of cerebral arteriosclerosis associated with hypertension. The primary neuropathological feature of the disease is a diffuse and patchy loss of myelin in the cerebral hemisphere, which is then surrounded by areas of reactive gliosis (Janota, 1981; Olszewski, 1962). Binswanger's disease proved to be difficult to identify antemortem; fewer than 50 cases of Binswanger's disease have been described in the literature.

It became much easier to identify Binswanger's disease after the introduction of head CT and especially MRI scans, which revealed evidence of WMH in both the periventricular areas and the white matter of the cerebral hemispheres in patients with Binswanger's disease. These changes are reflected by periventricular lucencies and ragged margins of the lateral ventricles as seen via head CT scans and high signal intensities found in the same areas on T2-weighted MRI images. The neuropathological changes underlying WMH consist of local demyelination and a central microinfarct cavity, leading to an increase

652

LOCALIZATION
OF CLINICAL
SYNDROMES IN
NEUROPSYCHOLOGY
AND NEUROSCIENCE

in water collection in those areas as reflected by the signal hyperintensity on MRI scans and white matter lucencies on head CT films. The development of psychiatric and neurological abnormalities is usually accompanied by the presence of prominent and extensive WMH.

In addition to its association with cerebrovascular diseases, WMH may be caused by any one of a number of different pathologies, including multiple sclerosis, head trauma with a shearing injury, hypoxic encephalopathy, normal pressure hydrocephalus, and cerebral edema. Minimal and mild WMH may be noted in some elderly individuals who otherwise have no psychiatric or neurological abnormalities (Brant-Zawadzki et al., 1985; Fazekas, Chawluk, Alavi, Hurtig, & Zimmerman, 1987; Fisher et al., 1993; Rao, Mittenberg, Bernardin, Haughton, & Leo, 1989). It was suggested that WMH may be due to extracellular water surrounding extatic blood vessels, a condition that probably occurs with normal aging (e.g., Awad, Johnson, Spetzler, & Hodak 1986; Awad, Spetzler, et al., 1986). Thus, the presence of WMH may have varying clinical significance, representing both these changes as they occur in normal elderly subjects and the changes in white matter in various diseases. Tonkonogy (2001) also reported that prominent WMH may be observed at a rate that is several times more frequent in elderly patients with psychiatric disorders secondary to neurological illnesses such as Alzheimer's disease than in elderly subjects with early onset schizophrenia (Tonkonogy, 2001).

As in other cases of subcortical cognitive impairments, dementia in cases of Binswanger's disease is characterized by a slowness of mental processing and a loss of interest and spontaneity, which may be present along with memory deficits. Loizou, Kendall, and Marshall (1981) described 15 cases of subcortical arteriosclerotic encephalopathy in a group of individuals aged 50–70 with disturbances of gait, spastic dysarthria, and pseudobalbar palsy, as well as dementia with insidious memory loss progressing to a global intellectual impairment, a loss of interest, and a loss of drive. Head CT scans revealed bilateral decreased white matter attenuation, primarily in the frontal and parietal regions, along with either subcortical lacunes or cortical infarcts and mild to moderate cerebral atrophy. Gupta et al. (1988) studied the CT scan data of 43 patients with decreased attenuation in the periventricular white matter. Neuropsychological evaluations of the participants revealed symptoms typical for subcortical dementia, including slowness in memory tasks, difficulty in organizing the material to be learned, fluctuations in recall scores from trial to trial, and difficulties in recall following a 30-min delay unless cues were provided. Frontal lobe types of impairment were noted as well, including reduced spontaneity of thought and action, diminished concern, and blunting of affect; aphasia and apraxia were found to be absent.

Kinkel, Jacobs, Polachini, Bates, and Heffner (1985) described slow progressive dementia and gait disturbances in 8 of 23 patients with WMH. Another 8 patients were without any neurological deficits, while the remaining 7 had a history of stroke. Risk factors for arteriosclerosis were found in 18 of 27 patients. One case included an autopsy that revealed features characteristic of Binswanger's disease. The researchers stressed that a lack of neurological findings in elderly patients with WMH did not exclude a diagnosis of subclinical subcortical arteriosclerotic encephalopathy.

Late onset delusions and mood changes with manic and/or depressive symptoms are often observed in patients with prominent WMH (Coffey et al., 1988; Miller et al., 1989). These difficulties, however, may not lead to the development of a significant cognitive decline. For instance, evidence of moderate to severe WMH was noted in 7 out of 13 of our cases with late onset delusions, while testing via the BNCE revealed total scores of 26–28 (normal range is 28–30), which indicated either minimal or no disturbances (Tonkonogy & Geller, 1999).

Some more recent studies have shown a limited role of subcortical vascular pathology in the development of dementia. Mungas et al. (2001) compared the cognitive abilities and quantitative MRI measures of subcortical vascular disease and cortical and hippocampal atrophy in patients with subcortical ischemic vascular disease (SIVD) and Alzheimer's disease (AD). Independent variables included volumes of white matter lesions, lacunar subcortical infarcts, cortical gray matter, and the hippocampus. A series of neuropsychological tests included the evaluation of global cognitive function, memory, language, and executive function. The study showed that performance on these neuropsychological tests was most strongly correlated with the volume of cortical gray matter and the hippocampus. The volume of white matter lesions and subcortical lacunes is only weakly associated with a decline in cognitive performance.

These results point to the possible leading role of cortical vascular changes in the development of dementia. Another possibility is the coincidence of cortical changes of Alzheimer's disease types with the subcortical and cortical vascular changes that were observed in most of the cases. Alzheimer's disease, however, is not present in some such cases. Mungas et al. (2001) studied three cases via autopsy of dementia and ischemic vascular disease. The volumes of the cortical gray matter and the hippocampus were diminished in all three cases, and no neurofibrillary tangles were found in the neocortex. It may be suggested that cortical atrophy in patients with vascular dementia results from ischemic tissue changes that are similar to subcortical ischemic changes. Such an explanation was actually first promoted by Alzheimer (1904), who considered the role of cortical ischemic changes and perivascular

654

LOCALIZATION
OF CLINICAL
SYNDROMES IN
NEUROPSYCHOLOGY
AND NEUROSCIENCE

gliosis as a primary pathology underlying the development of vascular dementia. Another possibility was suggested by Mungas et al. (2001). They stressed that the structural changes in the cortical and hippocampal neurons are secondary to the damage to subcortical neurons and the demyelization of axons. Such a suggestion is at least useful to consider the presence of white matter ischemic lesions as markers of more extensive cortical ischemic changes, which are difficult to observe via conventional MRI scans.

At the same time, the role of subcortical ischemic changes in the development of dementia cannot be completely disregarded, since dementia in such cases may be less prominent and may be manifested, for instance, as changes in the speed of mental processing and memory capabilities, as was described in patients with Binswanger's subcortical arteriosclerotic encephalopathy. The possible role of subcortical ischemic changes may be reflected in impairments of unconventional information processing, while conventional information processing remains either completely intact or only mildly disturbed. Prominent WMH and subcortical microinfarctions may result in the development of mild cognitive impairments, which are limited to unconventional information processing. In such cases, especially in the early stages of progressive dementia, conventional information processing may be completely preserved, as demonstrated by Part I of the BNCE. Unconventional information processing as evaluated by Part II of the BNCE, however, is found to be prominently disturbed in such cases.

One of our patients, known as J.W., was a 66-year-old woman who, having no previous record of mental health or criminal problems, developed grandiose delusions, stopped paying her bills, and was observed wandering around outside her residence and trying to break into cars in the neighborhood. She was admitted to the hospital following an incident in which she waved a loaded gun at her neighbors. Upon admission, J.W. was alert and cooperative. She expressed grandiose delusions of being the daughter of a doctor, having graduated from college, and being the owner of the hospital to which she had been admitted. She demonstrated no recollection of the recent episodes of violence. Administration of the BNCE revealed cognitive disturbances for unconventional information processing (see Figure 12.5). An MRI scan performed on this patient supported the diagnosis of subcortical vascular dementia (see Figure 12.6).

It seems that the localization of subcortical ischemic pathology, for example, in the white matter of the frontal lobe, in the striatum, or in connections with memory circuits, may play an important role in the development of vascular dementia. In addition, neuropathological studies of Binswanger's disease are characterized by the development of dementia, which indicates subcortical ischemic changes and lacunes

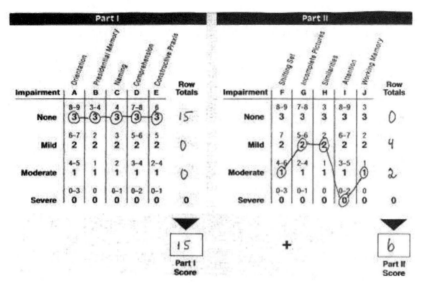

FIGURE 12.5 The BNCE profile of patient J.W., who had subcortical vascular pathology. The BNCE scores demonstrated a prominent discrepancy between the patient's ability to complete all of the subtests in Part I without difficulty in contrast to marked disturbances in performance on the subtests in Part II. Difficulties in test completion were especially prominent on the Shifting Set and Attention subtests, pointing to agnosia and apraxia of sequencing, and thus underscoring J.W.'s problems concerning recognition and social actions, as well as appropriate responses to social actions. Performance on the Working Memory subtest was also quite poor, demonstrating impairments of immediate memory.

FIGURE 12.6 The T2-weighted MRI image of patient J.W. The MRI revealed multiple microinfarctions in the semioval center, moderated periventricular white matter hyperintensity, and ventricular and sulcal dilatation. The types of cerebral lesions accompanied by the presence of diabetes mellitus and hypertension in the patient's medical history indicated that her mild dementia was of vascular origin. Normal scores for conventional information processing in this case point to the possible relative preservation of the cortex, while ischemia developed primarily in the subcortical white matter.

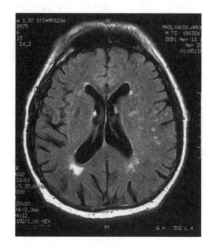

656

LOCALIZATION
OF CLINICAL
SYNDROMES IN
NEUROPSYCHOLOGY
AND NEUROSCIENCE

in the white matter of the frontal and parietal lobes and the periventricular area; the cortex is primarily preserved in such cases.

Thalamic Vascular Dementia. The thalamic syndrome of dementia is probably the most controversial concept, since it is manifested as inertia, apathy, and a decrease in information processing speed, as well as cognitive dilapidation, which may be secondary to the mental inertia and slowness. The development of thalamic vascular dementia is usually the product of bilateral thalamic infarctions (Castaigne et al., 1966; Chassagnon, Boucher, Tomassi, Bianchi, & Moene, 1969) and in most cases of additional lesions in the cortical and especially subcortical structures.

Parkinson's Disease. The absence of dementia was stressed in the original descriptions of Parkinson's disease (PD), a classical subcortical disorder. Cognitive impairments, however, were subsequently observed in a significant percentage of PD patients.

Dementia in PD patients has been characterized by features commonly observed in other subcortical diseases with dementia, especially PSP and HD. These features include a slowness of mental processing, a deficit in the free recall of words and visual material with a preserved ability to recognize visual and verbal stimuli, visuospatial disturbances, a mild disorder of retrograde memory, and a disturbance in the frontal lobe–type abilities of establishing, maintaining, and shifting focus and attention, as typically observed in patients with social agnosia and social apraxia (for a review, see Raskin, Borod, & Tweedy, 1990).

When dementia was originally observed in cases of PD, it was ascribed either to arteriosclerotic parkinsonism (Critchley, 1929), or as a sequela of epidemic encephalitis (Naville, 1922; von Economo, 1931). More recently, types of pathology that are typical for Alzheimer's disease (e.g., neurofibrillary tangles, senile plaques, and granulovacuolar degeneration) have been found in cases of PD with dementia (Boller, Mizutani, Roessmann, & Gambetti, 1980; Gaspar & Gray, 1984). Other studies reported a frequent lack of associations between Alzheimer's types of pathology and dementia in cases of PD (Ball, 1984; Perry et al., 1983). Parkinsonism has been found to be absent in 75% of such cases, and the dementia noted is marked by the presence of aphasia and apraxia, resembling the cognitive impairments observed in cases of Alzheimer's disease.

Though persistent neuropathological findings in PD include dopamine production cells from the pars compacta in the substantia nigra, the severity of dementia in PD does not lend itself to an association with the degree of cell loss in the substantia nigra (Gaspar & Gray, 1984). Lewy bodies, which are the eosinophylic cytoplasmic inclusions in the cells of the substantia nigra and the locus coeruleus, may be found in almost all cases of PD (Adams & Victor, 1985). However, Lewy bodies are considered to be major pathological findings in many cases that are marked by clinical manifestations characteristic of Alzheimer's disease, and the distribution of these inclusions in the cells may be observed not only in the brain stem but throughout the cerebral cortex as well. The terms Lewy body disease and Lewy body variant of Alzheimer's disease were suggested by the authors who described this new clinico-pathological entity (Kosaka et al., 1980; Kosaka, 1990).

Head CT and MRI scans often yield negative findings in patients with PD. In some such patients, cortical atrophy and ventricular enlargement may be observed via scans, but findings consistent with subcortical atrophy are associated with cognitive impairment (Inzelberg et al., 1987; Lichter et al., 1988; Starkstein & Leiguarda, 1993).

Since the depletion of dopamine production in the substantia nigra is a major cause of motor manifestations in PD, some researchers have used dopamine therapy to treat dementia in patients with PD (Meier & Martin, 1970; Mortimer, Pirozzolo, Hansch, & Webster, 1982). Some studies have demonstrated that the therapy partially reverses the intellectual loss that occurs in PD. This again raises the question concerning the role of mental slowness, which is in these cases secondary to dopamine depletion, as a primary cause of subcortical dementia, at least in cases of PD. It is also evident that the clinical manifestations of PD, including cognitive impairments, have a diverse pathological basis, which may account for differences in the presence, degree, and pattern of dementia in PD patients. It must also be stressed that cognitive impairments are minimal in many patients with PD, while mild and more severe cognitive impairments inevitably develop in all patients with HD and, though to a lesser extent, in those with PSP. This may be related to the more extended type of anatomical subcortical and, to some degree, cortical lesions in cases of HD and PSP compared to many cases of PD.

Dementia with Lewy Bodies.   Lewy bodies are characterized as neuronal eosinophylic inclusion bodies. They were first described by Friederich Lewy, who presented several cases of Parkinson's disease with unusual inclusions in the neurons of the substantia innominata (Lewy, 1912) and later published a detailed description of the clinical and neuropathological data on 43 cases of parkinsonism (Lewy, 1923). Dementia was found to be present in 21 of the 43 cases. In patients with parkinsonism, Lewy bodies may be found in the substantia nigra, the locus coeruleus, the substantia innominata, the nucleus basalis of Meinert, the dorsal vagal nucleus, and the hypothalamus; Lewy bodies are typically not found in the hippocampus (Gibb, Esiri, & Lees,

658

LOCALIZATION
OF CLINICAL
SYNDROMES IN
NEUROPSYCHOLOGY
AND NEUROSCIENCE

1985; Hansen & Galasko, 1992; Jellinger, 1986; Sandyk & Willis, 1992; for a review, see Cercy & Bylsma, 1997).

Cortical Lewy bodies were described as an underlying pathology for a distinct clinical syndrome characterized by the insidious onset of delusions and affective disorder with behavioral disturbances, and later by the development of memory disturbances and cognitive impairments (Hassler, 1938; Woodard, 1962). Cortical Lewy bodies are primarily concentrated in the frontal and temporal neocortex, the anterior cingulate gyrus, and the insula (Kosaka, 1990) and are usually accompanied by subcortical Lewy bodies. The term *diffuse Lewy bodies disease* was proposed for such cases (Kosaka, 1990). Interest in cortical Lewy bodies and dementia related to Lewy bodies disease began to increase in the 1980s (Burkhardt et al., 1988; Byrne, Lennox, Lowe, & Godwin-Austen, 1989; Gibb et al., 1985; Kosaka, 1990; Lenox & Lowe, 1996; Yoshimura, 1983). The diagnosis of Lewy body dementia requires the presence of many Lewy bodies throughout the neocortex and the limbic system (Mega et al., 1996).

Clinical manifestations of Lewy bodies dementia include fluctuating confusional states, which are similar to experiences of mild delirium, hallucinations, and delusions. Cognitive impairment in such cases usually develops later in the course of the disease and may be less prominent than in Alzheimer's disease (Cercy & Bylsma, 1997; Lennox & Lowe, 1996). Though Lewy bodies are observed in up to 20% of patients with Alzheimer's disease, their prevalence is much smaller compared to the high numbers found in cases of Lewy bodies disease; and the number of neuritic plaques is smaller in patients with Lewy bodies disease than in those with Alzheimer's disease (Hansen & Galasco, 1992; for a review, see Cercy & Bylsma, 1997). Prominent extrapyramidal signs are frequently noted in patients with Lewy bodies disease (Mega et al., 1996). Further studies of dementia in cases of Lewy bodies disease are needed.

Dementia in Other Brain Diseases
In addition to the disturbances already mentioned, dementia may also be associated with head injury, brain tumors, encephalitis, multiple sclerosis, and other brain diseases. The type of dementia that is experienced reflects the localization and extent of the brain lesion(s). The development of dementia in such cases is the result of particular acquired diseases. In neurodegenerative diseases dementia often appears without obvious, identifiable symptoms of a particular disease and thus remains itself the primary manifestation of the disease, which may be diagnosed with certainty via postmortem examination in many cases. Mild cognitive impairment with features of subcortical dementia has also been found in patients with multiple sclerosis (for a review, see

Rao, 1990), as well as in patients with the so-called AIDS dementia complex (Navia, 1990; Navia, Jordan, & Price, 1986).

Schizophrenia and Dementia

Emil Kraeplin first used the term *dementia praecox* in his seminal description of schizophrenia, to reflect progressive cognitive decline. Several recent studies have been directed toward the analysis of the neuropsychology of schizophrenia (for a review, see David & Cutting, 1994). However, the differentiation of cognitive impairments in elderly patients with early-onset schizophrenia and degenerative diseases, especially Alzheimer's disease and frontotemporal dementia, still remains difficult and often unreliable.

Winokur, Pfol, and Tsuang (1987) recognized severe cognitive deterioration in some elderly institutionalized patients with schizophrenia. Slow cognitive decline with a progression to severe dementia was also observed in a large, age-stratified cross-sectional study of institutionalized schizophrenics (Davidson et al., 1995; Tonkonogy, 1997).

Dunkley and Rogers (1994) studied cognitive impairment in severe psychiatric illness in 102 patients, 96 of whom had been diagnosed with schizophrenia. They found a positive correlation between the mean cognitive impairment score (CIS) and both age (r = 0.44; p = 0.0001) and length of current hospitalization (r = 0.5; p < 0.0001). The authors stressed that the cognitive deterioration observed in older patients was too pronounced to be simply an effect of aging. A suggested possibility was an interaction between the disease process and changes due to aging. The role of prolonged hospitalization or institutionalization was considered to be relatively small compared to the effect of the disease process (Goldberg et al., 1990; Johnston, Owens, Gold, Crow, & Macmillan, 1981; Mathai & Gopinath, 1986). Dunkley and Rogers (1994) also found a significant negative correlation (p < 0.01) between the mean CIS and the number of neuroleptic drugs the patient was taking at the time, as well as between the mean CIS and a history of previous ECT or insulin coma treatment (p > 0.8 and p < 0.9, respectively). Cognitive performance in patients with severe psychiatric illnesses may improve as a result of treatment with medications or ECT (Cassens, Inglis, Appelbaum, & Guthell, 1990; Devanand, Verma, Tirumalasetti, & Sackeim, 1991).

A substantial impairment in memory, especially semantic memory, has been observed in a number of patients with schizophrenia (McKenna et al., 1990; McKenna, Mortimer, & Hodges, 1994; Saykin et al., 1991). Tests directed toward the evaluation of disorders of language, gnosis, and motor praxis, however, showed the least impairment (Dunkley & Rogers, 1994; Tonkonogy, 1997). This pattern of cognitive deficits was originally considered to be compatible with the concept of subcortical dementia (Pantelis, Barnes, & Nelson, 1992). However,

660

LOCALIZATION
OF CLINICAL
SYNDROMES IN
NEUROPSYCHOLOGY
AND NEUROSCIENCE

the impairment of executive functions and memory seems to be much more pronounced in cases of schizophrenia than in cases of subcortical dementia.

Johnstone et al. (1989) found that patients with adolescent-onset schizophrenia received lower scores on remote memory tests than patients with adult-onset schizophrenia. Using extended neuropsychological batteries, Basso, Nasrallah, Olson, and Bornsteinn (1997) studied 44 patients with schizophrenia, 24 of whom had onset prior to the age of 21, and 20 of whom had onset at age 25 or older; a control group was composed of 20 individuals. The studied groups differed on nearly all of the neuropsychological tests, with the worst performance being demonstrated by the adolescent-onset group, and the best by the control group. The adolescent-onset group had substantially lower scores on measures of memory and executive functions, including visual and verbal memory, attention-concentration, complex abstract reasoning, and psychomotor problem solving. The mean performance on the Full-Scale IQ of the WAIS-R was 88.00 ± 12.14 for the adolescent-onset group, 100.70 ± 13.67 for the adult-onset group, and 103.75 ± 7.29 for the control group. For most of the neuropsychological tests that were used, no significant correlations were found between performance and the duration of illness, pointing to the role of severity rather than chronicity of illness in the development of more severe cognitive deficits, at least in the adolescent-onset group. These findings are consistent with brain-imaging data that show greater anatomical changes in adolescent-onset patients than in adult-onset patients, including greater sulcal enlargement (Mozley et al., 1994) and more prominent cytoarchitectonical abnormalities in the temporal lobes (Roberts, 1991).

Prominent cerebral atrophy markedly exceeding normal age-related changes was also noted in a group of 35 elderly patients with early-onset schizophrenia (PSCH; Tonkonogy & Geller, 1999). Moderate-to-severe enlargement of the lateral ventricle was seen in 28.6% of the patients, while no cases of moderate-to-severe ventricular enlargement were observed in a group of 13 patients with late-onset paranoid psychosis (LOPP). At the same time, the percentage of patients with lateral ventricles of a size that was either normal for their age or minimally enlarged was higher in the group of patients with LOPP (61.5%) than in the PSCH group (51.4%). The findings of more prominent ventricular enlargement in elderly patients with early-onset paranoid schizophrenia echo the findings that the ventricular: brain ratio increases without being noted during the visual inspection of MRI films in schizophrenic patients aged 20–40 years (Van Horn & McManus, 1992). It may be hypothesized that concomitant age-related changes and/or a natural progression of the underlying pathological process could amplify the ventricular atrophy in schizophrenia, making it visible via MRI films.

The degree and type of cognitive decline is not, however, reflected by cerebral atrophy revealed by head CT and brain MRI scans in patients with schizophrenia but is seen much more often in patients with neurologically defined diseases (Tonkonogy, 1997). For example, consider two of our patients: patient T.G., who had a long history of undifferentiated schizophrenia; and patient J.L., who suffered from the sequelae of severe head injury following a motor vehicle accident. Administration of the BNCE to each of the patients yielded scores at the level of moderate cognitive impairments, with a total score of 17 for patient T.G., and 16 for patient J.L. Brain imaging revealed a mild prominence of the ventricular system in T.G., the patient with schizophrenia, and prominent tissue loss at the base of the frontal lobes with an extension to the temporal lobe in J.L., the patient with a previous head injury (see Figure 12.7). For a more detailed description of patient J.L., see chapter 6, section titled "Social Apraxia."

The brain-imaging findings in these cases demonstrate that the moderate cognitive impairment noted in both cases is underlain by prominent frontotemporal tissue loss in patient J.L. and mild ventricular prominence in patient T.G. The discrepancy between the moderate cognitive impairment and minimal to mild MRI findings in patient

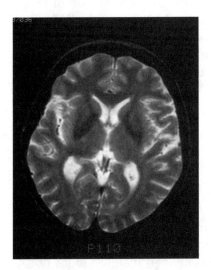 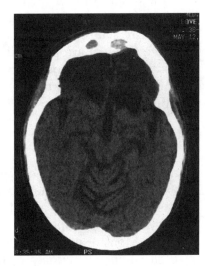

FIGURE 12.7   Left: The T2-weighted MRI image of 46-year-old patient T.G., who had undifferentiated schizophrenia, shows a mild prominence of the ventricular system. T.G.'s total score on the BNCE was 17/30, indicating a moderate level of cognitive impairment.

Right: The head CT scan of 28-year-old patient J.L., who had sustained a severe closed head injury, shows prominent tissue loss at the base of the right and left frontal lobes with an extension to the left temporal lobe. J.L.'s total score on the BNCE was 16/30, indicating a moderate level of cognitive impairment.

662

LOCALIZATION
OF CLINICAL
SYNDROMES IN
NEUROPSYCHOLOGY
AND NEUROSCIENCE

T.G. may be due to the presence of subtle but extended brain pathology, probably at the synaptic level, which is beyond the scope of MRI technique.

It must also be stressed that moderate-to-severe WMH, a symptom of demyelization of probable atherosclerotic origin, was recorded in only 14.3% of a group of 35 elderly patients with early-onset schizophrenia (Tonkonogy & Geller, 1999), while WMH may reach 70%–80% in patients with Alzheimer's disease. These differences may be used in the differentiation of dementia as a result of a progressive schizophrenic process from the Alzheimer's type of dementia.

In general, cognitive impairments in cases of schizophrenia often resemble frontotemporal dementia, especially during the first one or two decades of the disease progression. Personality and mood changes may dominate the clinical picture, and no prominent cognitive impairments may be noted or experienced. The patient appears to be functional, retaining his orientation in day-to-day living, but is also experiencing serious difficulties in occupational functioning and social relationships, which are symptoms typical for social agnosia and social apraxia and probably related to the personality and mood changes and loss of motivation that are often influenced by the delusional system and hallucinations. Cognitive impairments worsen with the progression of the disease through the years, often reaching the point of prominent dementia, which makes it difficult to differentiate schizophrenia from progressive degenerative diseases. However, cerebral atrophy as it is observed via head CT and brain MRI scans often does not reflect the degree and type of cognitive impairment, which can instead be exposed via testing in patients with schizophrenia.

Conclusions

1. Dementia syndromes are characterized by disturbances in occupational and social functioning, which are manifested in clinical syndromes of social agnosia and social apraxia and are amplified by specific multiple cognitive impairments. These impairments are extensive and may be produced not only by social agnosia and social apraxia but also by the combined manifestations of several clinical syndromes of agnosia and apraxia, including agnosia of space and time, object agnosia, motor apraxia, aphasia, and memory impairments. Though circumscribed local lesions usually lead to only one of these impairments, the development of multiple such disturbances would require extended pathology of cortical areas and often additional subcortical areas.

2. Social agnosia and social apraxia underlie the development of disturbances in occupational and social functioning and may be related to extensive cortical and subcortical pathology, though some specific lesions in specific regions are especially important. It is possible that extended frontal lobe pathology is manifested as primary social agnosia and apraxia, while pathology in the temporal and parietal lobes, leading to agnosia of time and space, underlie the development of secondary disturbances in social gnosis and praxis.

3. Various memory impairments that are typical for dementia may be related to pathology of the hippocampal, frontal lobe, and subcortical areas.

4. Involvement of the frontal lobe seems to be present in virtually every case of dementia, even in those cases in which initial pathology involves other cortical areas, for example, in patients with posterior cortical atrophy.

5. The destruction of brain tissue is extensive in cases of dementia, and in patients with degenerative diseases it is characterized by cortical and/or subcortical atrophy. The destruction of brain tissue is only partial, however, since cerebral and subcortical atrophy, or multiple microinfarctions in so-called multi-infarct dementia, do not result in the complete destruction of the brain tissue in particular areas. The partial destruction of brain tissue may result in clinical and neuropsychological manifestations that differ from the manifestations of circumscribed lesions, which completely destroy the brain tissue in particular areas and are caused by macroinfarctions, head tumors, or brain injury. Such injuries are usually described in patients with conventional aphasia, agnosia, and/or apraxia. This leads to the development of disturbances in language, gnosis, and praxis that differ from the classical syndromes of aphasia, agnosia, and apraxia, especially in the mild and moderate stages of dementia.

6. Language disorders in cases of dementia are characterized by anomia. Such disturbances are not accompanied by the comprehension disturbances that are observed in patients with transcortical sensory aphasia. Expressive speech in dementia becomes simplified, in what is known as poverty of speech, but is not accompanied by either the slow, laborious speech with the overprevalence of nouns typical of individuals with Broca's aphasia or the fluent garbled speech with the overprevalence of functional words typical of individuals with Wernicke's aphasia.

7. Conventional visual object agnosia does not usually develop in the mild and moderate stages of the majority of cases with

664

LOCALIZATION
OF CLINICAL
SYNDROMES IN
NEUROPSYCHOLOGY
AND NEUROSCIENCE

dementia and may be observed only in patients with dementia secondary to primarily posterior cortical atrophy. Unconventional object agnosia may be present in most dementia cases. Similarly, conventional prosopagnosia, or agnosia of faces, may be noted only in cases of advanced dementia and extends, in addition to impairments in the visual recognition of faces, to disturbances in the recognition of familiar voices. This is contrary to the more classic cases of prosopagnosia, in which impairments are limited to the visual recognition of faces and are the result of relatively circumscribed cortical lesions. At the same time, disturbances in the recognition of the faces of famous people in cases of dementia may be primarily related to anterograde and retrograde amnesia.

8. The patchy and incomplete but extended lesions may explain the predominance of disturbances of unconventional information processing as observed in cases of mild dementia, seen in the early stages of progressive dementing illnesses. At this stage, impairments may be predominantly manifested as unconventional disturbances in gnosis, praxis, and language. The development of incomplete patchy lesions may also explain why classical syndromes of particular lobe involvement are often not observed in patients with dementia. It is also possible that, in some types of dementia, such as frontotemporal dementia, the underlying patchy lesions are primarily located in the frontal lobes and the anterior parts of the temporal lobes, without the typical manifestations of posterior area disturbances as in Wernicke's aphasia.

9. The predominant localization of lesions, especially in the early stages of dementia progression, may also explain the specific manifestations of dementia syndromes in different types of dementia. Hippocampal lesions may result in the early development of memory disturbances during the course of senile-onset Alzheimer's disease. Frontal lobe involvement may be responsible for the early development of personality changes, loss of initiative, apathy, and mood disturbances in frontotemporal dementia. Since Alzheimer's original description of presenile dementia, the concentration of plaques and tangles in the temporoparietal cortex has been considered to be an important factor in the early manifestations of aphasia and agnosia in Alzheimer's disease of presenile onset. The early development of visual agnosia, Gerstman's syndrome, constructive apraxia, and alexia has been described in cases with dementia due to relatively isolated posterior cortical atrophy with prominent lesions in the parietal and occipital lobes.

10. Slowness of mental processing and memory disturbances have been described as the major manifestations of subcortical dementia. It is also important to note that Korsakoff's amnestic syndrome resulting from lesions in the mammillary bodies and thalamic nuclei is characterized by anterograde and retrograde amnesia with preserved immediate memory and the related functions of object and sequence recognition during the course of unconventional information processing; conventional information processing for language and constructive praxis is also preserved in such cases. At the same time, registration and working memory are prominently disturbed in cortical dementia, as in cases of Alzheimer's disease, underlying impairments in the recognition of objects and sequences during unconventional information processing, as noted via BNCE testing in such cases.

11. The development of hallucinations and delusions is facilitated by incomplete lesions. This is evidenced by the fact that relatively circumscribed cerebral infarctions underlying the development of the classical syndromes of aphasia, agnosia, and apraxia are only rarely accompanied by positive, or productive, psychiatric manifestations. It must also be stressed that hallucinations and delusions are two of the primary manifestations of schizophrenia and are characterized by the absence of large, anatomically verified cerebral lesions. In patients with dementia, delusions are simple and nonsystematized, and they eventually disappear, along with hallucinations, in the advanced stages of severe dementia. This is underlain by the progression of cortical atrophy and the confluence of a small patchy loss of brain tissue to larger areas of almost complete tissue loss. At this point, there is no longer enough functional tissue left to produce hallucinatory images or delusional beliefs.

12. Dementia syndromes usually include multiple cognitive impairments of social gnosis and social praxis. Various specific types of these impairments have been described by researchers relatively recently and include emotional agnosia, or aprosodia, which may be the result of a lesion of the right temporal lobe. Prosopagnosia, or agnosia of faces, may be defined as a type of social agnosia and is related to occipito-temporal lesions, primarily in the right hemisphere. Another syndrome is agnosia of social actions, which is described in this book and is probably related to frontal and temporal lesions. Disturbances in performance on theory of mind tests are another example of social agnosia of actions, while impairments in the planning and

666

LOCALIZATION
OF CLINICAL
SYNDROMES IN
NEUROPSYCHOLOGY
AND NEUROSCIENCE

execution of social actions represent a type of social apraxia related to frontal lobe lesions.

13. The isolated development of one or two clinical syndromes observed in cases of dementia is usually not sufficient to lead to the development of the generalized cognitive impairments typical of dementia. Agnosia of social actions as depicted via thematic pictures is frequently observed, for instance, in patients with either Broca's or Wernicke's aphasia due to local cortical lesions. These disturbances are, however, not accompanied by a dementia syndrome with its disturbances in the multiple areas of social gnosis and social praxis. Spatial agnosia is also usually listed as a sign of dementia but may also be present as a separate syndrome in nondemented patients with parietal lesions. The role of memory disturbances as a separate entity without significant generalized cognitive disturbances must also be considered, for instance, in cases of Korsakoff's amnestic syndrome due to limited lesions in the mammillary bodies and the thalamus.

14. Special interest is sparked by data concerning the role of disturbances of operations with nonsocial information in the development of social agnosia and apraxia. For instance, disturbances of executive functions have been widely recognized as signs of dementia, but the tests of executive functions are based on the categorization of nonsocial information, such as numbers, colors, and sizes of figures. It is possible that these higher-level operations involved in the formation and shifting of sequences are designed to process both social and nonsocial types of information. To the best of our knowledge, no such comparative studies have been conducted thus far. Some social information may be specifically processed separately: for example, disturbances in the recognition of an emotional state as expressed by the prosody of voice or facial expression were observed separately from impairments in language comprehension as well as from prosopagnosia. Special attention must be given to the studies of features, their categorization and sequences, and storage models at the different stages of social conventional and unconventional information processing and their disturbances in the various types of social agnosia and social apraxia in cases of dementia.

13

Neuropsychological Testing of Clinical Syndromes

NEUROPSYCHOLOGICAL TESTING AND BRAIN IMAGING

ADVANCES IN THE application of brain imaging and EEG techniques to the diagnostic evaluation of brain pathology seem to diminish the role of neuropsychological assessment as a diagnostic indicator of the type, localization, and extent of brain damage or dysfunction in patients with various psychiatric and neurological disturbances. This has allowed a "shift in the focus of neuropsychological assessment from the diagnosis of brain damage to a better understanding of specific brain-behavior relationships and the psychosocial consequences of brain damage" (Howieson & Lezak, 2002, p. 217). However, the correlation between clinical data and findings from brain images and EEGs remains weak in many cases, especially in patients with primary psychiatric illnesses such as schizophrenia and bipolar disorder.

Brain-imaging abnormalities are usually minimal and frequently either overlap with findings in normal control groups or are completely absent in patients with schizophrenia and bipolar disorder, and they are increasingly recognized to be the result of brain diseases. A weak correlation between the degree and type of cognitive decline and brain-imaging findings has also frequently been noted in patients with neurologically defined illnesses, such as the progressive degenerative dementia of Alzheimer's and Pick's diseases, vascular dementia, Huntington's disease, and brain injury. These make it important to return to the old goals

668

LOCALIZATION
OF CLINICAL
SYNDROMES IN
NEUROPSYCHOLOGY
AND NEUROSCIENCE

of neuropsychological testing as a way to obtain the diagnostic indicators of brain pathology. Neuropsychological diagnostic indicators may be used together with clinical data, brain images, and EEG data in the evaluation of the presence, the underlying type, the localization, and the extent of the lesions that result in particular clinical manifestations of cognitive disturbances.

The principles of the psychometric systems that have been employed for neuropsychological diagnostic assessment are systematized and described by Howieson and Lezak (2002). There are two major systems employed in this assessment: the psychometric system with normative data collected on a group of normal individuals, and the psychometric system based on clinical normative data.

PSYCHOMETRIC SYSTEM BASED ON NORMATIVE DATA OF NORMAL INDIVIDUALS

THIS PARTICULAR SYSTEM is based on the standardized statistical procedures that consider single scores as continuous variables forming a bell-shaped curve typical for the normal distribution of the performance of a large normative sample of individuals who have been stratified according to their demographic characteristics. The range of normal average performance falls in the middle of the curve, between –0.66 and +0.66 standard deviations, or between the 26th and 76th percentiles, while scores that are below average occupy the left end of the curve and are located more than 2 standard deviations from the mean, or between 0 and the 2nd percentile. Patients with mild and more severe degrees of cognitive impairments would fall into the extreme left end of the bell-shaped curve, at which 98% of a normative sample will achieve better scores than those in the affected population.

This system is principally based on the consideration of impaired range as a downward deviation from the performance of normal control groups. Most of the tests used in neuropsychological research and practice are constructed using this psychometric system. Their compilation is presented in manuals such as *A Compendium of Neuropsychological Tests* (Spreen & Strauss, 1998), which includes an overview of purpose, source, description, administration, scoring, comments, and normative data for numerous neuropsychological tests used in the course of a clinical evaluation. The tests may help to evaluate such signs and symptoms as general intellectual abilities that are affected, impaired memory, disorientation in time, visuospatial impairments, motor abnormalities, and speech and language disturbances (Howieson & Lezak, 2002).

WECHSLER ADULT INTELLIGENCE SCALE

AN EXAMPLE OF the successful use of one such approach is the Wechsler Adult Intelligence Scale–Revised (WAIS-R, 1981), WAIS III, and the upcoming WAIS IV, in which scores are considered to be continuous variables. The original scale (the Wechsler-Bellevue Scale) and its subsequent modifications, including WAIS III, cover a wide range and depth of information processing in their verbal and performance parts, enabling them to provide both an assessment of a patient's level of cognitive impairment and an evaluation of various aspects of cognitive functioning in nonimpaired individuals. The WAIS, as well as most similar types of neuropsychological assessment, may provide information needed for the evaluation of the presence and grade of cognitive impairments in patients with psychiatric and neurological disturbances, but it is difficult to employ for an evaluation of the clinical syndromes and brain pathology that underlie the abnormalities of intellectual functioning.

These tests, however, have not been specifically developed for the evaluation of the diagnostic indicators reflecting the size, localization, and type of brain lesion. With regard to memory disturbances, for example, testing based on the normative data of normal individuals has provided information that helps to assess the level of performance both of a particular normal individual and of patients engaging in particular tasks challenging either short-term or long-term memory. But the assessment of particular clinical syndromes and the brain pathology that underlies the abnormalities of intellectual functioning often remain beyond the scope of tests based on the normative data obtained from groups of normal individuals.

EXECUTIVE FUNCTIONS TESTING

THE TESTING OF executive functions is another example of the successful use of a psychometric system based on normative data collected via the testing of normal individuals. The term *executive functions* has been added to neuropsychological terminology only relatively recently (Lezak, 1982), and it defines higher-order cognitive processes such as planning, cognitive flexibility, and working memory. These are functions that may be impaired while conventional cognitive functioning remains relatively preserved (for a review, see Spreen & Strauss, 1998).

A series of special tests has been used in the evaluation of executive disturbances. These tests usually target the ability to sort cards according to sorting rules that reflect certain categories and use feedback as to whether a response was correct or incorrect as noted in the test procedure. The underlying category may be shifted to another category during the course of testing either with or without notification. This helps to evaluate cognitive flexibility and tendency toward perseveration. The most popular and widely used tests of this type are the Wisconsin Card Sorting Test (WCST; Berg, 1948; Grant & Berg, 1948; Heaton, Chelune, Talley, Kay, & Curtis, 1993) and the Category Test (Halstead, 1947) as included in the Halstead-Reitan Test Batteries (Reitan & Davison, 1974).

The Category Test includes several sets of items that should be interpreted based on certain principles, such as the number of objects, the ordinal position of an odd stimulus, and so forth. Subjects are required to recognize the principle underlying the set using feedback on correct versus incorrect responses. The WCST uses a set of 64 response cards that must be matched with four stimulus cards that differ by geometric form (triangles, stars, crosses, and circles), color (red, green, yellow, and blue), and number of objects on the card (one, two, three, and four). The feedback given to the subject consists of two responses—"right" and "wrong." The required sorting principle is shifted after 10 consecutive correct responses, from color to form, then to number, and then back to color.

Executive disturbances are also evaluated using tests that require the subject to overcome well-learned, automatic responses in order to achieve correct completion. For instance, the popular Stroop Test (Stroop, 1935) requires the subject to read the names of colors, ignoring the actual color of the print, which never corresponds to the color name (e.g., the words *blue, green,* and *red* will be printed in red, blue, and green ink, respectively, and so on). Thus, the subject is required to ignore his or her natural and automatic urge to read the word and instead must name the color of the ink, which provides for a usually difficult and frustrating couple of minutes. Another popular test, the Trail Making Test (TMT; Partington & Leiter, 1949) consists of two different parts—Part A and Part B. Part A requires the subject to use a pencil to "connect the dots" in sequence for the numbers 1 through 25 on a sheet of paper. In Part B, numbers are to be alternated with letters in the connection sequence, so that the subject connects the dots in the following manner: 1, A, 2, B, 3, C, 4, D, and so forth. Scoring for both parts is based on the speed of test performance. The TMT is actually based on the ability to plan construction of a sequence and execute it, which requires switching back and forth from one automated sequence to another.

The category tests actually target the ability to recognize a basic category, such as color, size, number of objects, and so on, in a series of objects or words, and to shift from one basic category to another during the course of testing. The various category tests may be considered as an evaluation of the ability to choose the simple feature that could be used for recognition. These features are usually employed in the recognition of well-known objects during information processing. The category tests require one to shift focus to unusual, unconventional uses of the features of a particular set of objects as artificially defined by the test procedure. Disturbances in an individual's performance on category tests may be considered as the manifestation of visual agnostic disturbances with impairments at the level of the perception of new category and feature selection via unconventional information processing. It would be of interest to compare these disturbances both with others that mimic the feature selection operations of the learning process in the recognition of novel objects and with unconventional agnostic disturbances, such as the recognition of partially occluded objects and of new objects by patients with difficulties in category test performance.

Such processing requires the participation of various operations in the visual recognition module for unconventional information processing, including either working or operational memory, hypothesis generation, cognitive flexibility, and planning. This is based on the use of operations performed in the areas of the anterior and posterior cortices. For example, the selection of common features such as color, number of objects, and shape may be processed in the occipito-temporal areas, which hold the locations of these features' temporary storage in the temporal region. Frontal lobe structures may provide the comparison and feedback that are necessary both for the recognition of a category and for a shift to another category.

Damage to one of these areas may result in disturbances in performance on the category tests, so that low scores could be caused not only by lesions in the prefrontal brain region, an area that has traditionally been considered as a lesion site producing executive disturbances, but also as a result of damage to the other brain regions, thus diminishing the localization value of such tests. It was, for instance, found that the WCST indices could not discriminate between neurological patients with lesions of the focal frontal lobes and those with lesions of the nonfrontal lobes (Anderson et al., 1991; Axelrod et al., 1996). Similar findings have also been reported for executive tests directed to the evaluation of the ability to shift from automated processing, including the Stroop Test and the TMT. The TMT, for instance, has been found to be sensitive to the presence of brain damage in patients with closed-head injury (DesRossiers & Kavanagh, 1987) and in HIV-positive patients (Di Sclafini et al., 1997), though no significant differences have been observed between groups of patients with various localizations of brain lesions (for a review, see Spreen & Strauss, 1998).

A substantial overlap was also observed between scores on executive tests in normal individuals at the lower edges of normative data and

672

LOCALIZATION
OF CLINICAL
SYNDROMES IN
NEUROPSYCHOLOGY
AND NEUROSCIENCE

patients with mild cognitive impairments. As a result, the executive tests may yield similar scores in patients with mild cognitive disturbances and some normal individuals, but they cannot be understood or completed correctly by patients with moderate and severe cognitive decline.

The further development of executive tests for clinical use requires them to be adjusted in such a way that the tests may produce low scores in patients with mild cognitive disturbances and remain within normal limits in normal individuals. The tests must be outlined more clearly in relation to the particular modules of brain information processing and the clinical manifestations of modules that malfunction in various different clinical syndromes, such as agnosia, apraxia, aphasia, and amnesia. This approach may be facilitated by the use of the psychometric neuropsychological system as described below.

PSYCHOMETRIC NEUROPSYCHOLOGICAL SYSTEM BASED ON CLINICAL NORMATIVE DATA

THIS SYSTEM, OFTEN referred to as the psychometric system, seems to be especially relevant to evaluation tasks concerning the localization, extent, and type of brain lesion in patients with cognitive disturbances. The role of normal control data is greatly minimized in this system, since special attention is given to the selection of tests that are easy for normal controls to perform but that reveal impairments specific to particular clinical syndromes. Normal individuals usually perform these types of tests without difficulty, so that the disturbances revealed by testing point to the specific clinical symptoms and underlying brain lesions related to the malfunctioning of particular modules and circuits, for example, anterograde and retrograde amnesia; anomia; agnosia for objects, scenes, and actions; constructional apraxia; motor apraxia; and so on. Normative data are usually collected using the results of neuropsychological tests that have been used to evaluate these disturbances in particular groups of patients, for instance, in patients with transcortical, cortical, or conduction aphasia, or in groups of patients with frontal, temporal, parietal, or occipital lesions. These types of neuropsychological tests based on the qualitative analysis of data were quite popular and widely used before the advances of the current psychometric approach with its reliance on normative data collected via the testing of large groups of normal individuals. One goal of the second psychometric system is that it tries to adjust the old qualitative neuropsychological tests and to develop new tests for quantitative and statistically based diagnostic decision making.

The latest type of test is usually directed to the evaluation of clinical syndromes resulting from various types of brain pathology. This divides the diagnostic process into two major stages. During the first stage, the diagnostic process is directed toward the recognition of a particular clinical pattern of disturbances, such as different types of aphasia, agnosia, apraxia, and amnesia. During the next stage, the findings may be used to evaluate the type, localization, and extent of the underlying lesions, as well as any indications of the patient's functional status.

The division of diagnostic decision making into two stages is similar to object recognition based on part decomposition and the structural description of the object (for more details, see chapter 2, section titled "Visual Object Agnosia"). The method is defined as the decomposition of an object into its generic parts, followed by a description of the object as a combination of its parts (Ullman, 1996). Instead of processing the common features at the level of the entire object, the decomposition method assumes that each object may be described as a combination of a smaller number of parts or components, such as clinical syndromes in dementia.

During the next step, these generic elements may be grouped in different ways to describe various objects (e.g., types of dementia) as combinations of parts. For instance, a face may be mentally decomposed and may be perceived as having a nose, eyes, ears, cheeks, and a mouth. Following the recognition of the parts, the entire face may be recognized as a combination of these generic parts. In case of dementia, the recognition of generic parts or clinical syndromes may also be used to point to the probable localization, extent, and type of lesion that underlies the development of particular clinical syndromes via different combinations that in this way define the various types of dementia. The role of such an approach is especially important since brain-imaging data, EEG data, and other clinical findings may be not sufficient for the correct assessment of underlying brain pathology, for example, in cases of schizophrenia, bipolar disorder, or degenerative dementia.

NEUROPSYCHOLOGICAL TESTING OF CLINICAL SYNDROMES

POPULAR EXAMPLES OF the clinical psychometric system used in the neuropsychological testing of clinical syndromes include simple signs tests and extended test batteries.

SIMPLE SIGNS TESTS

SOME TESTS ARE directed toward the evaluation of simple signs or symptoms of specific clinical syndromes. Visual object agnosia, for

674

LOCALIZATION
OF CLINICAL
SYNDROMES IN
NEUROPSYCHOLOGY
AND NEUROSCIENCE

example, is evaluated using the Hooper Visual Organization Test (Hooper, 1968) and the Facial Recognition Test (Benton & Van Allen, 1968); aphasia is evaluated via the Token Test (Boller & Vignolo, 1966; De Renzi & Vignolo, 1962) and the Boston Naming Test (Kaplan, Goodglass, & Weintraub, 1978).

The Token Test and the Facial Recognition Test are considered as good examples of simple signs tests and will now be explored in further detail.

TOKEN TEST

THE TOKEN TEST is directed toward the systematic assessment of verbal comprehension, which may be disturbed in various types of clinical syndromes, including aphasia syndromes and language disturbances in cases of dementia and schizophrenia. The administration of the test consists of presenting the subject with 20 plastic tokens in five different colors, two sizes, and two shapes. In the first part of the test, the subject is tested on the comprehension of one-, two-, and three-word commands. Specifically, the subject is asked to point to a single item in response to one-word commands (7 commands), then in response to two-word commands (5 commands), and finally in response to three-word commands (4 commands). During the next two subtests, each consisting of 4 commands, the subject must take two tokens in response to two-word commands, for example, "Take the red circle and the green square," or three-word commands, for example, "Take the large white circle and the small green square." The second part of the test is directed toward the evaluation of the subject's verbally mediated orientation in space and consists of 15 different commands. The commands primarily include the words *on, behind, away, in front of, beside,* and *between,* thus calling attention to the relative positions of two tokens in space, for example, "Put the white square behind the yellow circle."

Though the Token Test does not yield results that are sufficient for the evaluation of clinical syndromes such as aphasia, it does help to quantify the presence and degree of such signs as alienation of word meaning or disturbances in the comprehension of logico-grammatical structures. The main principles of the Token Test have, for obvious reasons, been used in many qualitative neuropsychological batteries (see Luria, 1966; Tonkonogy, 1973).

FACIAL RECOGNITION TEST

THE FACIAL RECOGNITION Test requires the subject to locate a single front-view photograph of a face in a display of either six photographs with three-quarter views of faces, three photographs of the same face and three photographs of other faces, or in a display with different lighting conditions. The test is considered as one of the first standardized tests to be developed for the evaluation of facial recognition. Its development led to the generation of a series of studies to compare the performance of various tests in localization of brain lesions. The test is not, however, directed toward the evaluation of prosopagnosia, which is clinically defined as agnosia of familiar faces. Instead, the test actually reflects the ability to recognize incomplete objects and requires comparison with the testing of the recognition of objects other than faces.

TESTING OF CLINICAL SYNDROMES

SEVERAL FIXED TEST batteries have been developed thus far for the direct testing of clinical syndromes. These batteries are often quite lengthy, often requiring 4–8 hours of testing. The shorter, briefer batteries have recently become widely popular since they require an administration time of only 20 or 30 min, making them much easier to use for the evaluation of psychiatric and neurological patients, many of whom often find it difficult to maintain the necessary levels of motivation and attention to complete a more lengthy test battery. These shorter batteries are also useful in everyday clinical practice, in which clinicians often find they have very limited time to meet with patients. Lengthier testing may certainly be used, however, for a more thorough and extensive evaluation of some of the disturbances that may be detected by the briefer tests.

EXTENDED TEST BATTERIES

THE STANDARD FIXED batteries that have been favored by many neuropsychologists for clinical neuropsychological examinations include the Luria-Nebraska Neuropsychological Battery and the Halstead-Reitan Test Batteries (Reitan & Davison, 1974).

LURIA-NEBRASKA NEUROPSYCHOLOGICAL BATTERY (LNNB)

THE LURIA-NEBRASKA NEUROPSYCHOLOGICAL Battery (LNNB) represents the quantification of a series of tests that were described by Luria and systematized by Cristensen (Freeland & Puente, 1984; Golden, Purish, & Hammeke, 1981; McKinzey, Roecker, Puente, & Rogers, 1998; Puente, 1998). The quantification is based on normative data from a population of normal individuals. The LNNB reflects Luria's popular

676

LOCALIZATION
OF CLINICAL
SYNDROMES IN
NEUROPSYCHOLOGY
AND NEUROSCIENCE

approach to the neuropsychological evaluation of local brain pathology, an approach that is based on the description of clinical syndromes as the result of underlying disturbances in particular functions of the local areas of the cortex. For example, acoustic agnosia and sensory aphasia are described as disturbances of higher cortical functions, especially phonemic analysis, with lesions of the cortical nucleus of the auditory analyzer. Such an approach helps to advance the understanding of the mechanisms underlying the development of particular clinical syndromes but in some sense departs from the important details of the clinical syndromes of sensory aphasia that cannot be explained by the impairments in phonemic analysis, such as expressive speech disturbances in cases of sensory aphasia. Quantification may somewhat amplify these difficulties, especially when based on normative data from a population of normal individuals. The usefulness of the LNNB for the practice of clinical neuropsychology may increase with its adjustment to the evaluation of particular clinico-anatomical syndromes based on the normative data collected by the testing of patients with these syndromes.

Halstead-Reitan Test Batteries

THE HALSTEAD-REITAN TEST Batteries (Reitan & Davison, 1974) also use normative data based on the testing of normal individuals, primarily helping to discriminate between normal individuals and patients with brain damage while not being normalized for the evaluation of specific clinical syndromes. The list of tests included in this battery does not emphasize the relationships of these tests to particular clinical syndromes. The Halstead-Reitan approach is based on older association psychology, which considered information processing in the brain to be composed of various relatively independent functions. At the same time, the neurobehavioral clinico-anatomical approach is actually underlain by an understanding that the brain is a structure designed to reach certain functional goals, such as recognition, action, and communication, by using special modules and circuits that may be damaged by pathological process, leading to the development of specific clinico-anatomical syndromes.

Boston Aphasia Diagnostic Examination

THE BOSTON APHASIA Diagnostic Examination (BDAE; Goodglass & Kaplan, 1983) is made up of a number of standardized clinical tests, which are closely related to the clinical syndromes of brain pathology. The BDAE is one such example. The important thing is that the test includes the evaluation of clinically important signs of aphasia syndromes, such as disturbances in expressive speech, auditory comprehension, reading, and writing. Expressive speech assessment, for instance, includes verbal agility; automated sequences; the repetition of words, phrases, and sentences; and various types of naming. Auditory comprehension is evaluated by subtests of word discrimination, body-part identification, and the following of commands. This allows the results of the BDAE to be used to diagnose particular clinical syndromes of aphasia, such as Broca's aphasia, Wernicke's aphasia, transcortical aphasias, and conduction aphasia, and to suggest with a relatively high level of accuracy the probable localization, extension, and type of possible brain lesions.

One large set of normative data was collected based on 232 patients, most of whom had developed aphasia following cerebro-vascular accidents. Further data collection will be useful when the normative data are broken down into data on relatively small groups with particular types of aphasia as well as being broken down in such a way as to evaluate the normative scores in patients with other than cerebrovascular diseases. The BDAE is also widely used in the process of rehabilitation of patients with aphasia. As for other neuropsychological tests, a short, but clinically targeted, version would be of special importance, especially to bring the test closer to the needs and reality of everyday clinical practice. In summary, the BDAE is probably the only neuropsychological test that has come even remotely close to the needs of clinical research and practice.

BRIEF TESTS

SEVERAL NEUROPSYCHOLOGICAL TESTS have been developed to assess the presence and degree of general cognitive decline within a rather short amount of in-office testing time. Examples of such tests are the Dementia Rating Scale; (Mattis, 1988), the Mini-Mental State Examination (Folstein et al., 1975), and the Brief Neuropsychological Cognitive Examination (Tonkonogy, 1997). These tests are based on consideration of cognitive decline as a clinical syndrome that is underlain by a combination of specific cognitive disturbances.

Dementia Rating Scale

The cognitive impairments tested in the Dementia Rating Scale (DRS; Mattis, 1988) include disturbances of attention, initiation, construction, conceptualization, and short-term memory. The scale actually consists of a set of easy items, including digit span for the evaluation of attention, alternating movements for the evaluation of initiation and perseveration, and copying of simple designs for construction,

678

LOCALIZATION
OF CLINICAL
SYNDROMES IN
NEUROPSYCHOLOGY
AND NEUROSCIENCE

which is especially relevant with regard to the assessment of severe dementia.

Mini-Mental State Examination (MMSE)

The Mini-Mental State Examination (MMSE; Folstein et al., 1975) consists of items that reflect the traditional clinical syndromes of aphasia, agnosia, apraxia, and amnesia as indicators of the presence and severity of general cognitive decline. This may explain the popularity of the test for the assessment of mental status in psychiatric and neurological clinical evaluations and research, as the test helps to uncover the symptoms of clinical syndromes that are well known to psychiatrists and neurologists. For example, 10 points out of the total possible 30 evaluate the symptoms of space and time agnosia via questions concerning verbally mediated orientation in time and place. An additional 8 points are allotted to items reflecting the language disturbances usually observed in cases of aphasia. These language items include naming (1 point), repetition (1 point), reading comprehension (1 point), sentence writing (1 point), and auditory comprehension (3 points). Auditory comprehension as it is used in the MMSE is a modification of Marie's well-known three pieces of paper test, which played a significant role in Marie's original findings of comprehension disturbances in cases of Broca's aphasia (Marie, 1906a).

The results of the Marie test correlate highly with the presence of disturbances in the comprehension of logico-grammatical structures. Such disturbances are revealed by confronting the patient with passive sentences, Head's hand–ear–eye test, or words that indicate spatial relations, such as *behind, in front of, above,* and so on (for more details, see chapter 7, section titled "Aphasia Syndromes and Other Language Disorders"). Constructional apraxia (worth 1 point) is tested by asking the subject to draw two intersecting pentagons, while a short-term memory test first requires the repetition of three words (worth 3 points); another 3 points are awarded if the subject is able to repeat those three words following a delay, during which attention and calculation are tested. During this time, the subject is asked to count in multiples of 7, beginning at 100 and counting backward by 7 for 5 subtractions (worth 5 points if performed correctly). In the case of inability or failure to complete the number-sequencing task, the subject is asked to spell the word *world* backward (also worth 5 points).

In summary, 60%–75% of the total possible 30 points on the MMSE are assigned to testing for space and time agnosia and language disturbances (23 points); short-term memory covers 6 points, or 20% of the total score. Therefore, a low total score on the MMSE often reflects the presence of a clinical syndrome of significant aphasia-like language disturbances, verbally mediated agnosia for time and space, and, although to a lesser extent, disturbances of short-term memory. These data may be used in the evaluation of a possible localization and evaluation of the extent of the underlying lesions, such as the major areas of cortical atrophy, that are found in cases of degenerative dementia.

The MMSE items primarily cover the disturbances of conventional information processing in space-time gnosis, language, memory, and constructional praxis, thus providing a quantitative assessment of the major cognitive signs of dementia, especially in its moderate and advanced stages. The signs of mild cognitive decline, however, remain beyond the scope of this particular test, since it does not specifically assess the disturbances of unconventional information processing, as in language, object and action recognition, or planning based on the recognition of unconventional sequences.

Brief Neuropsychological Cognitive Examination (BNCE)

The Brief Neuropsychological Cognitive Examination (BNCE; Tonkonogy, 1997) represents an attempt to use the clinical syndromological approach in the quantitative neuropsychological testing of cognitive impairments. The BNCE consists of two parts: Part I includes subtests for the clinical syndromes that are related to disturbances of conventional information processing; the subtests in Part II are directed toward the evaluation of clinical syndromes manifesting as impairments in unconventional information processing. Special attention is given to the testing of recognition and action involving the dynamic aspects of the world and the processing of incomplete information.

The BNCE includes five subtests, facilitating a comparison between the scores for Part I and Part II. The items in the subtests are simple and do not present much difficulty for normal individuals, regardless of age, gender, or cultural or educational background. This minimizes the overlap of results between the scores of impaired subjects and those of normal control groups, which is especially important for the evaluation of mild cognitive disturbances.

The results of the BNCE are presented in the form of raw scores—1 for correct responses and 0 for incorrect responses on the individual items. The raw scores are then transferred to adjusted scores as follows: 0—*poor*; 1—*moderate impairments*; 2—*mild impairments*; and 3—*normal performance*. The adjusted scores help to equalize the results of different subtests and to build a profile to facilitate a comparison between the results of the various subtests. This may be helpful in the evaluation of the presence and severity of particular types of disturbances, pointing to the possible localization and extension of underlying brain lesions, as well as to the dynamic of cognitive impairments over the course of disease progression, including any improvement of cognitive status.

680

LOCALIZATION
OF CLINICAL
SYNDROMES IN
NEUROPSYCHOLOGY
AND NEUROSCIENCE

Part I of the BNCE

Part I is similar to the MMSE and includes subtests that evaluate primarily disturbances of conventional information processing in the clinical syndromes of space-time agnosia, aphasia, amnesia, and constructional praxis.

Space-time agnosia is part of the Orientation subtest from Part I of the BNCE, and low scores on orientation indicate the presence of space-time agnosia. The items are derived from the conventional mental status examination used in clinical psychiatric and medical settings for the evaluation of dementia and confusion; they are limited to verbally encoded information about current time and place, and about the patient's age and date of birth. Visuospatial orientation is excluded from the subtest in order to narrow the target function assessed by the subtest. Orientation to time and place and knowledge of personal information may be preserved, while remote and recent memory may be prominently disturbed. Low scores on the Orientation subtest indicate prominent verbally mediated space-time agnosia, which is frequently observed in patients with dementia and relatively extended lesions of the fronto-subcortical circuits and the mesencephalic region, as well as in patients with acute confusion of various origins. Parietal and occipito-parietal lesions may also manifest in disturbances of orientation in space and time that usually include impairments of visuospatial orientation.

Aphasia is evaluated via the Comprehension and Naming subtests. The Comprehension subtest is a version of Head's hand–ear–eye test and has been a useful tool in the examination of comprehension deficits in cases of aphasia (Luria, 1966; Tonkonogy, 1973). The items on the Comprehension subtest are limited to the examination of a particular, narrowly defined function of spatial relationships in language with relatively minimal dependence on verbal memory, making the results easier to quantify and to compare to the scores on other subtests. Poor performance on this subtest points to the presence of aphasic types of disturbances, with possible localization of lesion in the areas around the Sylvian fissure of the dominant left hemisphere.

The Naming subtest is also designed to evaluate symptoms of aphasia. The subtest is limited to the ability to generate names for four body parts that are referred to relatively infrequently in everyday life—*earlobe, eyelashes, fingernails,* and *eyebrows.* This makes the subtest quite sensitive to mild disturbances in naming, which are often observed in patients with generalized cognitive impairments. As in cases with low scores on the Comprehension subtest, disorders of naming, or anomia, are often seen in patients with various types of aphasia resulting from lesions around the Sylvian fissure in the dominant hemisphere. Additionally, anomia and comprehension disturbances have recently been reported in cases with strokes involving the subcortical nuclei and thalamus of the dominant hemisphere. In most of these cases, the aphasia noted was moderate and transient.

Constructional Apraxia. The purpose of the Constructional Praxis subtest is to reveal signs of constructional apraxia. The items in the subtest minimize the effect of verbal encoding on performance. Low scores on this subtest point to the probable involvement of the parietal lobes, primarily in the left hemisphere.

Amnestic Syndrome and Long-Term Memory. The inclusion of the Presidential Memory subtest, which evaluates the symptoms of amnestic syndrome, serves to increase the sensitivity of Part I in comparison to the MMSE. The limitation of this remote memory subtest to the examination of memory for U.S. presidents who are cultural icons helps to minimize the influence of age, gender, ethnicity, and education on the results. These items reflect common knowledge that is usually overlearned, reliably recorded, and easy to retrieve for normal individuals. A disorder of presidential memory is a sign of an amnestic syndrome that may result from hippocampal and mesencephalic lesions and in some cases from involvement of the frontal lobe.

The BNCE is also enhanced in comparison to the MMSE by the addition of more difficult items in the language and constructive praxis subtests, for example, the naming of less frequently used words such as *earlobe* or *fingernail,* or the drawing of figures that cannot be mediated by verbal encoding. These two subtests may reveal signs of mild impairments that are missed by the MMSE.

Part II of the BNCE

A major advantage of the BNCE is the inclusion of Part II, which consists primarily of items directed toward the evaluation of unconventional information processing and is thus especially important for the detection of mild cognitive impairments. Two of the subtests are directed toward the detection of agnosia and apraxia of sequencing, which play an important role in the dynamic aspects of brain information processing, including the recognition of actions and their planning and execution.

Agnosia of Sequences. Agnosia of sequences is detected via the Shifting Set subtest in Part II, which focuses on the ability to recognize and copy simple novel sequences or to shift from an established pattern of responding. This may be considered a way to evaluate the agnosia of simple but unconventional actions formally represented by sequences. The test items are easy to perform for normal individuals, and impairments

682

LOCALIZATION
OF CLINICAL
SYNDROMES IN
NEUROPSYCHOLOGY
AND NEUROSCIENCE

in these items point to the presence of cognitive disturbances in unconventional information processing.

In the Shifting Set, for example, the Recurrent Figures item includes several repetitions of a simple sequence consisting of either a triangle and a square, or two triangles and one square. The item primarily evaluates the gnosis of sequences but also allows for the testing of working (operational) memory by asking the subject to copy the sequence after the sample has been removed from his or her visual field. In the Recurrent Figures item, the recognition of a sequence is based on its decomposition into its single parts—triangles and squares—as they are combined into generic elementary parts consisting, for instance, of one triangle and one square, or two triangles and one square. The repetition of these elementary parts reconstructs the sequence. The test is usually easy for normal individuals to complete, but errors are seen in patients with mild cognitive impairments, for example, in the relatively early stages of schizophrenia or Huntington's disease. A patient is usually able to perform the first stage of this process—the decomposition of the sequence into single parts, triangles and squares—but fails to perform the next stage, which consists of grouping them into generic parts, for example, two triangles and one square that are combined into a sequence by repetition.

Visual agnosia of sequences may be observed in patients with frontal lobe pathology. Lesions of the occipital and parietal lobes have also been observed in patients with visual agnosia of sequences, while agnosia of auditory sequences has been described in patients with circumscribed lesions in either the parietal or temporal lobes (for more details, see chapter 3, section titled "Agnosia of Action").

Apraxia of Simple Sequences. Apraxia of simple sequences is evaluated via the Attention item in the Number Tracking subtest. In this subtest, the examiner asks the subject to reverse the automatic recital of the months of the year, or to show one finger when the examiner shows two fingers and vice versa. Another, more difficult to perform, example of such reversal is the Tracking Test, which requires the subject to switch from the automatic recital of numbers (1, 2, 3 . . . 12) to an alternating forward and backward sequence (1, 12, 2, 11, 3, 10 . . .). The tracking is thus based on the construction of a new sequence by the combination of switching back and forth from automatic to backward recital in the range provided. As in the TMT, the correct sequence of numbers must be connected by a line, adding another component of motor praxis to the test, targeting the construction of action sequences, which may be considered an important part of praxis. The preservation of working (operational) memory is certainly required for the correct performance of this particular test.

Though difficulties in the performance of both the Number Tracking and Recurrent Figures items may be observed in the same patient, in some cases a gnosis of simple sequences in the Recurrent Figures may be impaired, while the construction of new sequences by overcoming automated responses in the Number Tracking items is preserved. This highlights some differences in the structure of the tests. The Recurrent Figures subtest is directed toward the evaluation of agnosia of sequences, while Number Tracking primarily targets the apraxia of sequences. Agnosia of sequences may reflect difficulties in the recognition of actions, while apraxia of sequences models the disturbances of planning and execution of actions. Agnosia and apraxia of sequences may be observed in patients with frontal and parietal lobe lesions.

Visual Agnosia of Partially Occluded Objects. The Incomplete Pictures subtest is designed to evaluate visual agnosia of partially occluded objects via the presentation of an incomplete set of information. The subtest requires the processing of incomplete information, which plays an important role in brain functioning. This may be considered as a type of executive function, or unconventional information processing. In cases of brain damage, the processing of conventional information processing, for example, the recognition of an unoccluded object, may be preserved, while disturbances may manifest in the recognition of partially occluded objects as represented by incomplete pictures.

The items in the Incomplete Pictures subtest are incomplete drawings of four relatively common objects. When a subject is unable to recognize some or all of these incomplete pictures, the complete pictures of all four objects are presented, and these are instantly recognized by both patients without severe visual object agnosia and normal individuals, who infrequently complain of an inability to recognize any of the four incomplete objects. This presentation of complete pictures helps to facilitate recognition by limiting the subject's choice of answers to a set of four known and complete objects. The incomplete pictures of the four objects are then presented again to the subject. In patients with unconventional visual object agnosia, the difficulties in the recognition of the incomplete drawings usually persist despite the attempted facilitation provided by the presentation of the complete images in the intermediate stage of testing.

Successful performance on the Incomplete Picture subtest requires a preserved ability to reconstruct the complete image of the object by using such features as proximity, co-linearity, symmetry, and so forth (for more details, see chapter 2, section titled "Visual Object Agnosia"). This ability may be disturbed in patients with unconventional visual object agnosia, while the recognition of complete, conventional presentations of objects is preserved, since it is performed with the use

684

LOCALIZATION
OF CLINICAL
SYNDROMES IN
NEUROPSYCHOLOGY
AND NEUROSCIENCE

of a well-learned set of features and does not require reconstruction during the course of recognition.

Lesions in patients with visual agnosia for partially occluded objects probably involve primarily the temporal lobe, especially the fusiform and the hippocampal gyri, and involve the frontal lobe in some cases.

Amnestic Syndrome. The long-term memory subtest in Part I is directed toward the examination of well-learned presidential, which is related to conventional information processing. The Working Memory subtest in Part II represents unconventional information processing, requiring the subject to memorize three words and then repeat them after a delay, during which the individual is tested for abilities in calculation. The results of this subtest may be influenced by lesions in a variety of areas, including the hippocampal and mesencephalic structures, as well as the frontal lobe and subcortical structures in some cases.

Disturbances of Categorization. The Similarities subtest is used to determine the presence of disturbances of categorization. Recognition of objects and actions, especially during unconventional information processing, may require the ability to categorize objects according to their functional property, as with fruits, tools, or representatives of law enforcement. The subtest evaluates this ability by asking subjects to define the common functional features of objects, for example, plums and cherries, or a hammer and a screwdriver, or the social features of a judge and a police officer. Poor performance on the Similarities subtest often indicates the presence of frontal lobe pathology.

Presence and Severity of Cognitive Impairment. The total score, which is the sum of all of the adjusted scores with a maximum score of 30, is used for the assessment of the presence and severity of cognitive disturbances, the severity of a cerebral lesion, functional status, and the course of disease progression. Individuals in nonclinical settings with no known cognitive impairment usually obtain a total score of 28–30. Mild impairments are indicated when the total score is between 22 and 27. Total scores between 10 and 21 point to moderate impairments, and severe cognitive impairments are indicated by a total score of 9 or below. The scores from Part I and Part II, each with a maximum of 15, allow for the evaluation of mild cognitive disturbances via the comparison of conventional and unconventional information cognitive processing, as well as the evaluation of functional status and disease progression.

Functional Status Assessment

The BNCE total score provides a highly accurate index of the functional status of patients with cognitive impairment. Patients with total scores of 28–30 are usually able to live independently at home, whereas patients with total scores of 21 and below, indicating moderate or severe impairments, usually require a living environment in which more support is available, such as group homes, nursing homes, or inpatient hospital units. Patients with mild impairments as indicated by total scores of 22–27 may be able to live independently in approximately 50% of cases.

*Clinical Syndromes Assessment: Comparison
with Brain-Imaging Results*

In addition to the general assessment of the presence and severity of cognitive impairments, as well as the functional status of the patients, the results of the BNCE may be used for the assessment of the specific clinical pattern and the underlying type and localization of brain pathology, especially when brain-imaging data are inconclusive. This may be achieved by taking into account the particular clinical syndromes that are revealed by the testing.

A typical example is a case of our own, known as J.H., who had inconclusive MRI data and demonstrated disturbances in the subtests of Part II, such as agnosia of sequences, apraxia of sequences, and agnosia for partly occluded objects; the patient's scores in Part I were minimally abnormal in some subtests and normal in the remaining subtests (Figure 13.1). Brain MRI images in this case demonstrated mild cerebral atrophy, which is difficult to differentiate from age-related changes, while the results of the BNCE clearly point to the presence and types of cognitive impairments (Figure 13.2).

The abnormalities revealed by the BNCE often involve either one or two subtests; for example, apraxia of sequencing appears in combination with agnosia of occluded objects without signs of agnosia of sequences. This points to the possible differences in pathological mechanisms and the localization of underlying lesions. In one of our cases with undifferentiated schizophrenia, for instance, the patient scored low on the Shifting (testing for agnosia of sequencing) and Incomplete Pictures (testing for visual agnosia for occluded objects) subtests, while the patient's scores were in the normal range for the Tracking Numbers subtest (apraxia of sequencing). Another patient with sequelae of severe head injury at the base of the frontal and temporal lobes showed no sign of agnosia of sequences, but scored rather low on the Shifting Set and Incomplete Pictures subtests.

Another example is a 21-year-old patient of ours with paranoid schizophrenia who dropped out of college after developing a loss of goal-directed, motivated behavior. The data obtained from brain MRI scans were found to be within normal limits. The BNCE, however, showed low scores in the subtests for agnosia of sequences and apraxia of sequencing, while other subtests were completed within

686

LOCALIZATION
OF CLINICAL
SYNDROMES IN
NEUROPSYCHOLOGY
AND NEUROSCIENCE

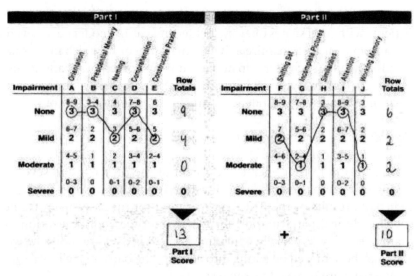

FIGURE 13.1 The Brief Neuropsychological Cognitive Examination (BNCE) profile of patient J.H., a 66-year-old male who had recently developed persecutory delusions and auditory hallucinations. His total score was 23, which put him at the lower level of mild cognitive impairment. J.H.'s score was primarily due to the low scores on the subtests of Part II, reflecting disturbances of unconventional information processing.

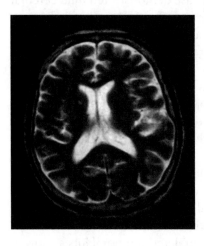

FIGURE 13.2 MRI findings with probable diagnosis of Alzheimer's disease in early stages. The T2-weighted images show a mild enlargement of the lateral ventriculi and mild cortical atrophy. Based on these MRI findings, age-related changes cannot be completely ruled out without using Brief Neuropsychological Cognitive Examination (BNCE) results to demonstrate mild cognitive impairments. These impairments, combined with clinical findings, allowed the researchers to make a probable diagnosis of Alzheimer's disease in its early stages.

normal levels and with normal scores. This pointed to possible frontal and temporal lobe involvement that was not visible on the MRI scan. The profile of the clinical syndrome provided by the BNCE may thus help to outline the possible sites of lesions in patients with schizophrenia, which are usually characterized by minimal findings on brain-imaging scans.

Though low scores on the Presidential Memory subtest, which evaluates remote memory, are in some cases accompanied by normal scores on the Orientation subtest, while disturbances in space-time orientation are not seen without prominent impairments in remote memory, also pointing to possible differences in the localization of underlying lesions in disturbances of space-time orientation in cases with or without accompanied remote memory impairment.

Further collection of neuropsychological, brain-imaging, EEG, and autopsy data is certainly needed to establish the typical profiles of clinical syndromes, their combinations in various types of dementing illnesses, and their relationships to the expected localization and types of lesions in particular cases. This collection of data may also clear the way for the use of diagnostic algorithms for diagnostic decision making based on the individual profiles of patients with dementia.

*BNCE in the Testing of Clinical Syndromes and the Assessment
of Dementia Progression*

The progression of dementia is usually manifested as a worsening of the agnosia and apraxia of sequencing that may underlay the progression of social agnosia and apraxia. Cognitive decline is also registered as the development of space-time agnosia and amnestic disturbances for remote memory as revealed by the Orientation and Presidential Memory subtests, respectively. The development of space-time disorientation is easily revealed during regular clinical evaluations, often representing the point in time at which the presence of dementia is fully recognized and confirmed. Signs of aphasia and constructional apraxia are usually not observed at the time of development of space-time disorientation in the course of dementia progression, pointing to the possible preservation of areas around the Sylvian fissure in the left hemisphere in such cases.

Brain MRI scans in such cases of Alzheimer's disease may show only generalized cortical and subcortical atrophy, not pointing to the visible progression of brain tissue loss and clinically relevant lesions. It is possible that more prominent frontal lobe involvement is responsible for this type of profile in cases of Alzheimer's disease.

In some cases, the signs of aphasia, especially anomia, appear at relatively early stages of dementia, for example, in early onset Alzheimer's disease. In most cases of progressive degenerative dementia, however, signs of aphasia and constructional apraxia develop later in the course of the disease. This development is traced by such tests as the BNCE, which is based on the evaluation of particular clinical syndromes in dementia, and points to the possible involvement of areas around the Sylvian fissure in the left hemisphere.

688

LOCALIZATION
OF CLINICAL
SYNDROMES IN
NEUROPSYCHOLOGY
AND NEUROSCIENCE

Differentiation of the Types of Dementia

The BNCE may be also helpful not only in evaluating the course of disease progression but also in analyzing the differences between various types of dementia. For instance, Korsakoff's amnestic syndrome is manifested by low scores on the subtest of long-term memory (Presidential Memory), while scores are normal for other subtests, for example, subtests for the evaluation of agnosia, apraxia, and aphasia. The score could also be normal for the Shifting Set and Working Memory subtests, which require the preservation of immediate memory. This points to the pattern typical of Korsakoff's amnestic syndrome, which is characterized by disturbances of long-term memory and the preservation of immediate memory for a length of time of about a few minutes, and a peculiar localization of lesion in the mammillary bodies, the thalamus, or the hippocampus.

USE OF DIAGNOSTIC ALGORITHMS IN NEUROPSYCHOLOGICAL TESTING OF CLINICAL SYNDROMES

PSYCHOMETRIC SYSTEMS BASED on normative data are primarily related to the assessment of test score percentiles within the range of a large sample of the population of normal individuals. Low total scores point to the presence and degree of general or particular cognitive impairments. The total scores are the sums of subtest scores, so that the weight of a score in a particular subtest reflects the individual's performance on that subtest. All of the subtests are considered to be equal for the purpose of the final decision, for example, for assessing the severity of impairments on the majority of the psychometric tests. The total scores in the neuropsychological testing of clinical syndromes are also based on the consideration of subtest scores as equal and necessary for diagnostic decision making.

The diagnostic assessment of particular clinical syndromes and their types, however, requires the weighting of a particular sign, which is reflected by subtests not only in relation to the severity of impairment but also to the overall significance of the sign in the targeted clinical syndrome. The authors of the tests are trying to solve these problems by using subscores, such as the verbal and performance quotient in the WAIS, or Parts I and II in the BNCE, for conventional and unconventional information processing. The number of items may also differ for the particular functions leading to the differences in their contribution to the total score. The MMSE, for example, has 10 items related to agnosia of space and time, 8 items related to aphasia, and only 3 items relating to memory disturbances, pointing to the leading roles of orientation and language disturbances in the assessment of the severity of dementia via the test. These preferences are not supported by corresponding diagnostic studies.

The use of diagnostic algorithms may help to minimize these problems in the neuropsychological testing of clinical cognitive syndromes. These algorithms are based on the assessment of the weight of a particular subtest in the diagnosis of a particular syndrome. For instance, the diagnostic algorithms of sequential statistical analysis (SSA) were developed by Wald (1947) as an application of Bayes's theorem of the differentiation of two classes. The diagnostic decision arrived at by the use of SSA methodology is based on the sequential summation of the diagnostic coefficients or weights of the items, which are ranged in order of decreasing validity in the differentiation between two diagnostic classes. A diagnostic coefficient is calculated as a logarithm of the relationship between the frequencies of particular subtests or features in the diagnostic Classes A and B, for example, two types of dementia. Summation is terminated when the sum exceeds certain limits, for example, +1 for Class A and –1 for Class B. If the sum remains between the two limits, the diagnosis is considered to be uncertain. Some additional neuropsychological testing, as well as brain imaging or EEG scans, may be suggested to aid and/or confirm the diagnosis. The results of the most recent testing may also be included in the algorithms for further processing.

We used SSA in the differentiation of anterior and posterior aphasia based on the results of neuropsychological testing (Frantsuz, Tonkonogy, & Levin, 1964; Tonkonogy & Armstrong, 1988). A comparison was made between anatomical data and results obtained via testing administered by experienced behavioral neurologists. The accuracy of the SSA diagnosis reached 88.5%. It is of interest that the use of linear discriminant analysis (LDA) and nonlinear discriminant analysis (NLDA) increases accuracy to 93.8% and 96.3%, respectively. LDA and NDLA differ from SSA in the use of a correlation between single items during the course of diagnostic decision making. We were able to reach 94.6% accuracy via SSA when some of the highly correlated pairs of items were combined into single features.

An analysis of diagnostic errors showed that there are similarities between traditional clinical thinking and the diagnostic algorithms of SSA. Despite high diagnostic accuracy, LDA and NLDA often led to diagnostic errors considered by physicians and neuropsychologists as "silly" or "strange." The incorrect diagnoses made via SSA were viewed as "understandable" and "reasonable," suggesting that physicians and neuropsychologists using the diagnostic procedure were probably less dependent on correlations between the items than in DLA and NDLA, and being similar to SSA.

690

LOCALIZATION
OF CLINICAL
SYNDROMES IN
NEUROPSYCHOLOGY
AND NEUROSCIENCE

The decision-making process employed by physicians and other health care providers seems to be more flexible and adjustable to the specific clinical manifestations in individual cases; this traditional diagnostic method may also be more efficient because correct assessment is often achieved by using a small number of signs and symptoms whose diagnostic validity is high. SSA offers similar advantages by making it possible to complete the diagnostic procedure, in many cases using several simple steps that require an assessment of not more than four or five signs, each with high diagnostic validity. This may also help significantly decrease the length of neuropsychological tests used in the diagnostic process. In our studies of the diagnostic decision making in aphasia, for example, we were able to use SSA to reduce the list of necessary items from 40 to 15, with the correct diagnosis of anterior or posterior aphasia being reached by the first four or five signs and with high diagnostic coefficients in 80% of cases.

Diagnostic algorithms like SSA may also be used to improve the use of numerous diagnostic scales employed in the assessment of psychiatric disturbances. The scales have become an important part of clinical research, especially in the process of evaluating new drugs. However, their use in everyday clinical practice has been quite limited, probably because of the unreliability of the results, which are often skewed by the equalization of diagnostically valuable and less valuable items included in the scales, for example, in various depression scales.

The diagnostic validity of such scales could be markedly improved by using diagnostic algorithms such as SSA to attach diagnostic coefficients to the items included in the scales and to make them more flexible by the procedure of sequential summation, which helps to reduce the length of the scale in particular cases and to contribute to improved organization, formalization, and reliability in the diagnostic process.

CONCLUSIONS AND FUTURE DEVELOPMENTS

1. The BNCE and similar tests may be considered as just a step on the way toward the development of fixed test batteries for the evaluation of clinical syndromes of cognitive disturbances. Whereas the most commonly used approach in clinical neuropsychology today appears to be the flexible approach, the correlation of fixed batteries to match clinical syndromes may be the next phase in the evolution of neuropsychological assessment. However, further development is required for the testing of disturbances of recognition and actions related to the dynamic aspects of the world, especially the social world.

2. Further data collected from the BNCE and similar test applications in cases with lesions that are relatively circumscribed and visible

via brain imaging may be classified and systematized as normative data. Such data may be used in the course of evaluation of localization and types of brain lesions underlying cognitive disturbances when brain-imaging data are inconclusive, as in patients with schizophrenia, as well as in cases with various types of dementia due to generalized cerebral atrophy and an absence of circumscribed local lesions.

3. Data collection is also needed to establish the typical profiles of clinical neuropsychological syndrome combinations in various types of dementing illnesses, and their relations to the expected localization and types of lesions in particular cases.

4. Such data collection may also open the way for the use of diagnostic algorithms in diagnostic decision making based on the individual profiles of patients. The use of these algorithms may help introduce into the diagnostic process the scores as they reflect the relative weight of a particular subtest, leading to a diagnostic evaluation of clinical syndromes.

5. The directions of development described above may lead to an increasing recognition of clinical neuropsychological tests as unique and important tools for the assessment of the localization, extent, and type of lesions underlying the development of cognitive disturbances in neurological and, especially, psychiatric patients.

6. The assessment of clinical syndromes as the essential parts of general cognitive disturbances may also be used in the analysis of existing tests and in the development of new types of neuropsychological cognitive tests. While the traditional neuropsychological tests based on normative data obtained from the normal population will certainly continue to be a major tool in neuropsychological examination, they will be supplemented and enriched by syndrome-oriented neuropsychological tests for the evaluation of underlying brain lesions, especially in cases with inconclusive brain-imaging data.

Appendix

TABLES OF MAIN SITES OF LESION LOCALIZATION IN NEUROPSYCHOLOGICAL SYNDROMES

The tables show the main sites of lesions and clinical syndromes of disturbances of the high level of brain information processing. The tables are based on a review of available clinical-anatomical data. The roles of the type of brain pathology, size of lesions, and other relevant findings are discussed in the text of the book. Further studies may help to clarify the localization, size, and type of brain pathology for disturbances of conventional versus unconventional brain information processing, and the role of subcortical pathology in a number of neurobehavioral and neuropsychiatric syndromes.

Abbreviations are as follows: L-left; R-right; O-occipital; T-temporal; P-parietal; F-frontal; B-bilateral; S-superior; I-inferior; M-Middle.

TABLE A.1 Neuropsychological Syndromes and Lesions Localizations
Recognition Disorders

Types of Disorders	Cortical Sites of Lesions			
	Frontal	**Occipital**	**Temporal**	**Parietal**
Visual Agnosia				
Object agnosia				
Apperceptive		LOI	LTI	
Associative			LTI	

(*Continued*)

TABLE A.1 Neuropsychological Syndromes and Lesions Localizations Recognition Disorders (*Continued*)

Types of Disorders	Cortical Sites of Lesions			
	Frontal	Occipital	Temporal	Parietal
Color agnosia				
Color agnosia, anomia		LOS+	LTI	LPI
Achromatopsia		ROI+ and R corpus callosum, genu		
Visuospatial disturbances				
Visual disorientation		ROI		RPI
Topographic agnosia		ROI	RTI	
Topographic apraxia				RPI
Auditory agnosia				
Apperceptive			LTS RTS + bilateral Heschl's gyri	
Associative			LTS	
Space			RTS	LPI
Tactile agnosia				
Apperceptive				RPI anterior
Associative				RPI posterior
Somatoagnosia				
Autotopagnosia				LPI anterior
Finger agnosia				LPI posterior
Anosognosia of aphasia			LTS posterior	
Pain				LPI
Blindness		BOI		
Left hemiplegia				RPI
Mental illnesses	BFI			
Agnosia of action				
Apperceptive		BOS		BPI
Associative	BFI		BTI	
Loss of visual imagery				
Objects		BOI	BTI	
Space		BOS		BPI

(*Continued*)

TABLE A.1   Neuropsychological Syndromes and Lesions Localizations
Recognition Disorders (*Continued*)

Types of Disorders	Cortical Sites of Lesions			
	Frontal	**Occipital**	**Temporal**	**Parietal**
Social agnosia of person				
Prosopagnosia		ROMI	RTI	
Emotional agnosia			RTSP	RP
Social agnosia of action				
Theory of mind tests	BFI and orbito-frontal		BTS and amygdala	
Disturbances of self-Image				
Depersonalization and derealization			BTS	
Disturbances of self-awareness	BFS and BFI		BTS	
Illusions				
Visual		BSO	BTS	
Auditory			BTS, Heschl's gyri	
Somatic				BPI
Hallucinations				
Visual elementary		LOI		
Visual complex			LTS	
Auditory elementary			BT Heschl's gyri	
Auditory complex			LTS	
Somatic				RPI anterior
Delusion				
Persecutory			RTS posterior	
Guilt			RTS middle	
Capgras syndrome	RFM posterior		RTS anterior	
Grandiose	BFI anterior			

(*Continued*)

TABLE A.1   Neuropsychological Syndromes and Lesions Localizations
Recognition Disorders (*Continued*)

Types of Apraxia	Motor and Social Apraxia			
	Frontal	**Occipital**	**Temporal**	**Parietal**
Motor apraxia				
Ideomotor				LPI anterior
Ideational				LPI posterior
Limbkinetic	LFI operculum			
Oral	LFI operculum			
Constructional				BPI posterior
Dressing				RPI posterior
Gate, Trunk	BFS			
Social apraxia				
Disorganization of social actions	BFI orbito-frontal			

Type of Disturbances	Communication Disorders			
	Frontal	**Occipital**	**Temporal**	**Parietal**
Anterior aphasia				
Broca's	LFI posterior, LCO			
Transcortical motor	LFI, LFM, LFS, posterior			
Articulation		LCO		
Posterior aphasia				
Wernicke's			LTS posterior	
Transcortical sensory			LTM, LTI, posterior	
Conduction			LTS, middle	
Word deafness			BTS, Heschl's gyri	

DISTURBANCES OF SUPPORTIVE AND REGULATORY FUNCTIONS

AMNESTIC DISORDER

Amnesia, anteroretrograde, primary_____BHippocampus,_____
_____Mammilary body_____Thalamus_, medio-dorsal nuclei_____
_____secondary to apathy_____BF
_____mild_____Fornix__Basal forebrain
Working memory disturbances_____BO_____BT_____BP_____BF

Transient global amnesia (TGA)   BF
_____Thalamus_____

Reduplicative paramnesia_____BF

ATTENTIONAL DISTURBANCES

Balint's syndrome_____RO_____RP

Neglect_____RP
_____Thalamus

Attention shifting disturbances_____BFS Premotor
_____Cingula, anterior

ASPONTANEITY

Abulia, Apathy_____BFS Premotor

_____Cingula, anterior_____Thalamus_____Globus pallidus

Akinetic mutism_____BFS Premotor
_____Cingula, anterior_____ Hypothalamus

Catatonia_____BFS Premotor
_____Globus pallidus Cingula, anterior_____Hypothalamus

MOOD DISTURBANCES

Secondary depression_____RT_____BFS Premotor
_____Caudate_____Mesencephalon

Secondary mania_____LT_____BFI, orbito-frontal
_____Thalamus_____Mesencephalon

Obsessive–compulsive disorder_____BFS Premotor
_____Cingula, anterior_____Caudate

Panic disorder_____Amygdala_____Hypothalamus

Aggression, Rage_____Amygdala_____Hypothalamus

TABLE A.2 Lesion Localizations and Neuropsychological Syndromes

A. RECOGNITION DISORDERS

OCCIPITAL

	Hemisphere		
	Left	Right	Bilateral
Inferior`	Apperceptive object agnosia	Achromatopsia Visual disorientation	Cortical blindness Loss of visual imagery for objects
	Hallucinations, visual elementary	Prosopagnosia	Topographic agnosia
Superior	Color agnosia		Apperceptive agnosia of action Loss of visual imagery for space Illusions, visual Anosognosia of blindness

TEMPORAL

	Left	Right	Bilateral
Inferior **Posterior**	Apperceptive object agnosia Associative object agnosia Color anomia Topographic agnosia		Associative agnosia of action Loss of visual imagery for objects
Amygdala and insula		Hallucinations, gustatory	Social agnosia of action
Uncus, olfactory bulb			Hallucinations, olfactory
Middle	Delusions of guilt		

(*Continued*)

TABLE A.2   Lesion Localizations and Neuropsychological Syndromes (*Continued*)

	Hemisphere		
	Left	**Right**	**Bilateral**
Superior			
Anterior		Capgras syndrome	Social agnosia of action
Posterior	Associative auditory agnosia	Auditory space agnosia Prosopagnosia, unconventional	Apperceptive auditory agnosia Hallucinations, auditory, elementary
	Auditory, complex anosognosia of aphasia	Delusions, persecutory nihilistic	auditory, complex verbal complex visual
Heschl's gyri			Apperceptive auditory agnosia Hallucinations, auditory, elementary
PARIETAL			
Inferior			
Anterior	Autotopagnosia	Apperceptive tactile agnosia Hallucinations, somatic	
Posterior	Color anomia Finger agnosia Anosognosia of pain	Visual disorientation Topographic agnosia Topographic apraxia Associative tactile agnosia Anosognosia of left hemiplegia	Apperceptive agnosia of action Loss of visual imagery for space Illusions, somatic Autoscopy Feeling of presence Anosognosia of pain
FRONTAL			
Inferior, orbito-frontal			Anosognosia of mental illnesses

(*Continued*)

TABLE A.2   Lesion Localization and Neuropsychological Syndromes (*Continued*)

	Hemisphere		
	Left	**Right**	**Bilateral**
			Disturbances of self-awareness Delusions, grandiose Social agnosia of action
Superior			Disturbances of self-awareness
Anterior			Delusions, Grandiose Nihilistic jealousy Capgras, impostor Anosognosia of mental illnesses Dementia Hallucinations

MESENCEPHALIC

Hallucinations, visual

B. DISTURBANCES OF ACTION

PARIETAL

	Hemisphere		
	Left	**Right**	**Bilateral**
Inferior			
Anterior	Apraxia, ideomotor		
Posterior	Apraxia, ideational	Apraxia, dressing	Apraxia, constructional
Frontal			
Inferior			
Orbito-frontal	Social apraxia		
Operculum	Apraxia, limbkinetic Apraxia, oral		
Superior	Apraxia of gait, trunk		

(*Continued*)

TABLE A.2 Lesion Localizations and Neuropsychological Syndromes (*Continued*)

C. COMMUNICATION DISTURBANCES

TEMPORAL

	Hemisphere		
	Left	**Right**	**Bilateral**
Superior			
Posterior	Wernicke's aphasia Surface dyslexia Sensory amusia	Emotional agnosia Sensory amusia	
Heschl's gyri			Word deafness
Middle	Conduction aphasia		
Inferior			
Posterior	Transcortical sensory aphasia Pure word blindness		
Middle			
Posterior	Transcortical sensory aphasia		

PARIETAL

Inferior			
Posterior	Alexia with agraphia, angular alexia Lexical (surface) agraphia Apraxic agraphia	Spatial agraphia (POT junction) Spelling agraphia	
Anterior	Phonological agraphia		

FRONTAL

Inferior			
Posterior	Broca's aphasia Deep dyslexia	Motor aprosodia	
Operculum	Broca's aphasia Articulation aphasia		
Middle			
Posterior	Transcortical motor Aphasia	Motor amusia Apraxic agraphia	
Superior			
Posterior	Transcortical motor aphasia		
Occipital			
Inferior	Pure word blindness		

(*Continued*)

TABLE A.2 Lesion Localization and Neuropsychological Syndromes (*Continued*)

D. DISTURBANCES OF SUPPORTIVE AND REGULATORY SYSTEMS

Abbreviations: WMD—Working memory disturbances; OCD—Obsessive-compulsive disorder; TGA—Transient global amnesia

	Hemisphere		
	Left	**Right**	**Bilateral**
Occipital	Neglect, rare	Balint's syndrome	WMD, visual
Parietal	Neglect	Balint's syndrome	WMD, visual and auditory
Temporal	Depression	Mania, rare	WMD, auditory
Temporal, medial		TGA	
Amygdala			Panic disorder Aggression, rage episode
Hippocampal formation			Amnesia, antero-retrograde Amnesia, anterograde
Frontal Prefrontal		TGA Reduplicative paramnesia Confabulation	
Superior, premotor		Neglect, rare	Attention shifting disturbances Catatonia Akinesia Akinetic mutism Abulia, depression Amnesia, antero-retrograde OCD WMD, space
Inferior, orbito-frontal			Mania Aggression WMD, objects

(*Continued*)

TABLE A.2 Lesion Localization and Neuropsychological Syndromes (*Continued*)

	Hemisphere		
	Left	**Right**	**Bilateral**
Cingula, anterior			Attention shifting disturbances OCD Abulia Catatonia Akinetic mutism
Subcortical and mesencephalic structures mesencephalon			Depression Mania
Hypothalamus			Panic disorder Aggression, rage episode Delusion, persecutory, autoscopic Catatonia Akinetic mutism
Mammillary bodies			Amnesia, antero-retrograde Confabulation
Thalamus			Neglect Abulia Mania TGA
Medial-dorsal nuclei			Amnesia, antero-retrograde Confabulation

BASAL GANGLIA

Globus pallidus			Abulia Catatonia Akinesia
Caudate			OCD Depression
Fornix			Amnesia, antero-retrograde
Basal forebrain			Amnesia, antero-grade

References

Abadi, R. V., Kulikowski, J. J., & Meudell, P. (1981). Visual performance in a case of visual agnosia. In M. W. van Hof & G. Mohn (Eds.), *Functional recovery from brain damage, developments in neuroscience 13* (pp. 275–286). North-Holland, Amsterdam, and Oxford: Elsevier.

Abrams, R., & Taylor, M. A. (1976). Catatonia: A prospective clinical study. *Archives of General Psychiatry, 33,* 579–581.

Abrams, R., Taylor, M. A., & Stoluarova, K. A. (1979). Catatonia and mania: Pattern of cerebral dysfunction. *Biological Psychiatry, 14,* 111–117.

Ackerley, S. (1937). Instinctive, emotional and mental changes following prefrontal lobe extirpation. *American Journal of Psychiatry, 92,* 717–729.

Adams, J. E., & Rutkin, B. B. (1970). Visual responses to subcortical stimulation in the visual and limbic systems. *Confinia Neurologica, 32,* 158–164.

Adams, R. D., & Victor, M. (1985). *Principles of neurology.* New York: McGraw-Hill.

Adler, A. (1944). Disintegration and restoration of optic recognition in visual agnosia. *Archives of Neurology. Psychiatry, 51,* 243–259.

Adolphs, R., Russel, J. A., & Tranel, D. (1994). A role for the human amygdala in recognizing emotional arousal from unpleasant stimuli. *Psychological Science, 10,* 167–171.

Aggleton, G. P., & Mishkin, M. (1983). Memory impairment following restricted medial thalamic lesions in monkeys. *Experimental Brain Research, 52,* 199–209.

Aggleton, G. P., & Mishkin, M. (1985). Mammillary-body lesion and visual recognition in monkeys. *Experimental Brain Research, 58,* 190–197.

Agostoni, E., Coletti, A., Orlando, G., & Fredici, C. (1983). Apraxia in deep cerebral lesions. *Journal of Neurology, Neurosurgery and Psychiatry, 46,* 804–808.

Ahlstrom, V., Blake, R., & Ahlstrom, U. (1997). Perception of biological motion. *Perception, 26,* 1539–1548.

Aigner, T. S., Mitchell, S., Aggleton, J., et al. (1984). Recognition deficit in monkeys following neurotoxic lesions of the basal forebrain. *Society of Neuroscience Abstracts, 10,* 386.

Aizenberg, D., Scwartz, B., & Modai, I. (1986). Musical hallucinations, acquired deafness, and depression. *Journal of Nervous and Mental Disease, 174,* 309–311.

Ajmone-Marsan, C., & Ralston, B. L. (1957). *The epileptic seizure.* Springfield, IL: Charles Thomas.

de Ajuriaguerra, J., & Hécaen, H. (1960). *Le cortex cerebral* (2nd ed.). Paris: Masson et Cie.

de Ajuriaguerra, J., Hécaen, H., & Angelergues, R. (1960). Les apraxies: varietes cliniques et lateralisation lesionnelle. *Revue Neurologique, 102,* 566–594.

Akelaitis, A. J. (1944). Atrophy of basal ganglia in Pick's disease. *Archives of Neurology and Psychiatry, 51,* 27–341.

Alajouanine, T., & Lhermitte, F. (1964). Les composantes phonemiques et semantiques de la jargonaphasie. *International Journal of Neurology, 4,* 277–286.

Alajouanine, T., Ombredane, T. A., & Durand, M. (1939). *Le syndrôme de désintegration phonétique dans l'aphasie.* Paris: Masson.

Alajouanine, T., Sabouraud, O., & DeRibaucourt, B. (1952). Le jargon des aphasics. Dèsintègration anosgnosique des valeurs sèmantiques du langage, I: Analyse des aspects principaux. *Journal de Psychologie, 45,* 168–180.

Albert, M. (1973). A simple test of visual neglect. *Neurology, 23,* 658–664.

Albert, M. L. (1979). Alexia. In K. M. Heilman & E. Valenstien (Eds.), *Clinical neuropsychology* (pp. 59–91). London: Oxford University Press.

Albert, M. L., & Bear, D. (1974). Time to understand: A case study of word deafness with reference to the role of time in auditory comprehension. *Brain, 97,* 383–394.

Albert, M., Cohen, C., & Koff, E. (1991). Perception of affect in patients with dementia of Alzheimer's type. *Archives of Neurology, 48,* 791–795.

Albert, M. L., Goodglass, H., Helm, N. A., Rubens, A. B., & Alexander, M. P. (1981). *Clinical aspects of dysphasia.* New York: Springer-Verlag.

Albert, M. L., & Obler, L. K. (1978). *The bilingual brain: Neurolinguistic and neuropsychological aspects of bilingualism.* New York: Academic Press.

Albert, M. L., Feldman, R. G., & Willis, L. A. (1974). The "subcortical dementia" of progressive supranuclear palsy. *Journal of Neurology, Neurosurgery and Psychiatry, 37,* 121–130.

Albert, M. L., Reches, A., & Silverberg, R. (1975). Hemianopic color blindness. *Journal of Neurology, Neurosurgery, and Psychiatry, 38,* 546–549.

Albright, T. D. (1984). Direction and orientation selectivity of neurons in visual area MT of the macaque. *Journal of Neurophysiology, 52,* 1106–1130.

Alexander, G. E., DeLong, M. R., & Strick, P. L. (1986). Parallel organization of functionally segregated circuits linking basal ganglia and cortex. *Annual Revue of Neuroscience, 9,* 357–381.

Alexander, M. C. (1926). Lilliputian hallucinations. *Journal of Mental Science, 72*, 187–191.

Alexander, M. P. (2002). Disorders of language after frontal lobe injury: Evidence for the neural mechanisms of assembling language. In D. T. Stass & R. T. Knight (Eds.), *Principle of frontal lobe function* (pp. 159–167). New York: Oxford University Press.

Alexander, M. P., Baker, E., Naeser, M. A., Kaplan, E., & Palumbo, C. (1992). Neuropsychological and neuroanatomical dimensions of ideomotor apraxia. *Brain, 115*, 87–107.

Alexander, M. P., Friedman, R. B., LoVerso, F., & Fischer, R. S. (1990). *Anatomical correlates of lexical agraphia.* Presented at the Academy of Aphasia, Baltimore, MD.

Alexander, M. P., & Schmitt, M. A. (1980). The aphasia syndrome of stroke in the left anterior cerebral artery territory. *Archives of Neurology, 37*, 97–100.

Alexander, P. M., & Albert, M. L. (1983). The anatomical basis of visual agnosia. In A. Kertesz (Ed.), *Localization in neuropsychology* (pp. 393–415). New York: Academic Press.

Alexopoulos, G. S. (1979). Lack of complaints in schizophrenics with tardive dyskinesia. *Journal of Nervous and Mental Disease, 167*, 125–127.

Ali-Cherif, A., Royere, M. L., Gosset, A., Poncet, M., Salamon, G., & Khalil, R. (1984). Troubles du comportemente et de l'activité mentale après intoxication oxycarboné. *Revue Neurologique, 140*, 401–405.

Allender, J., & Kazniak, A. (1989). Processing of emotional cues in patients with dementia of Alzheimer's type. *International Journal of Neuroscience, 46*, 147–155.

Alpers, B. J. (1937). Relation of the hypothalamus to disorders of personality. *Archives of Neurology and Psychiatry, 38*, 291–303.

Altshuler, L. L., Bartzokis, G., Grieder, T., Curran, J., & Mintz, J. (1998). Amygdala enlargement in bipolar disorder and hippocampal reduction in schizophrenia: An MRI study demonstrating neuroanatomic specificity. *Archives of General Psychiatry, 55*, 663–664.

Altshuler, L. L., Conrad, A., Hauser, P., Li, X., Guze, B. H., Denikoff, K., et al. (1991). Reduction of temporal lobe volume in bipolar disorder: A preliminary report of magnetic resonance imaging. *Archives of General Psychiatry, 48*, 482–483.

Altshuler, L. L., Curran, J. G., Hauser, P., Mintz, J., Denicoff, K., & Post, R. (1995). T2 hyperintensities in bipolar disorder: Magnetic resonance imaging comparison and literature meta-analysis. *American Journal of Psychiatry, 152*, 1139–1144.

Altshuler, L. L., Devinsky, O., Post, R. M., & Theodore, W. (1990). Depression, anxiety, and temporal lobe epilepsy. *Archives of Neurology, 47*, 284–288.

Altshuler, L., Raush, R., Delrahim, S., Kay, J., & Crandall, P. (1999). Temporal lobe epilepsy, temporal lobectomy, and major depression. *Journal of Neuropsychiatry and Clinical Neuroscience, 11*, 436–443.

Alzheimer, A. (1898). Neuere Artbeiten über die dementia senilis and die auf atheromatöser GefäBerberkrankung basierenden Gehirnkrankheiten. *Monatschrift für Psychiatrie und Neurologie, 3,* 101–115.

Alzheimer, A. (1902). Die Seelenstörungen auf ateriosclerotischer Grundlage. *Allgemeine Zeitshcrift für Psychiatrie, 59,* 695–711.

Alzheimer, A. (1904). *Histologische Studien zur Differential diagnose der progressiven paralyse: Habilitations schrift.* Munich: Ludwig-Maximilians-Universität.

Alzheimer, A. (1906). Über eine eigenartigen, schweren Erkrankungprocess der Hirnrinde. *Neurologischen Centralblat, 25,* 1134.

Alzheimer, A. (1911). Über eingartigen Krankheitsfalle des Spatern Alters. *Gesampte Neurologie und Psychiatrie, 4,* 356–385.

Amador, X. A., Flaum, M., Andreasen, N. C., Strauss, D. H., Yale, S. A., Clark, S. C., et al. (1994). Awareness in schizophrenia and schizoaffective and mood disorders. *Archives of General Psychiatry, 51,* 826–836.

American Psychiatric Association. (1994). *Diagnostic and statistical manual of mental disorders* (4th ed.). Washington, DC: Author.

American Psychiatric Association. (2000). *Diagnostic and statistical manual of mental disorders* (text revision). Washington, DC: Author.

Anderson, A. K., & Phelps, E. A. (2000). Expression without recognition: Contribution of the human amygdala to emotional communication. *Psychological Science, 11*(2), 106–111.

Andersen, R. A. (1997). Neural mechanisms of visual motion perception in primates. *Neuron, 18,* 865–872.

Anderson, S. W., Damasio, H., Jones, R. D., & Tranel, D. (1991). Wisconsin Card Sorting Test performance as a measure of frontal lobe damage. *Journal of Clinical and Experimental Neuropsychology, 13,* 909–922.

Andreasen, N. C. (1979). Thought, language, and communication disorders. 1. Clinical significance. *Archives of General Psychiatry, 36,* 1315–1321.

Andreasen, N. C. (1982). Negative symptoms in schizophrenia: Definition and reliability. *Archives of General Psychiatry, 39,* 784–788.

Andreasen, N. C., Olsen, S. A., Dennert, J. W., et al. (1982). Ventricular enlargement in schizophrenia: Relationship to positive and negative symptoms. *American Journal of Psychiatry, 139,* 297–302.

Andrews, E., Poser, C. M., & Kessler, M. (1982). Retrograde amnesia for forty years. *Cortex, 18,* 441–458.

Anton, G. (1898). Über Herderkrankungen des Gehirns, welche vom Patienten selbst nicht wahrgenommen werden. *Wiener klinische Wochenschrift, 11,* 227–229.

Anton, G. (1899). Über die selbst wharnehmoung der hrederkrankungen des gehirns durch den kranken der rindenblindheit und rindentaubheit. *Archiv für Psychiatrie und Nervenkrankheiten, 32,* 86–127.

Appel, J., Kertesz, A., & Fishman, M. (1982). A study of language functioning in Alzheimer patients. *Brain and Language, 17,* 73–91.

Arbib, M. A. (1981). Perceptual structures and distributed motor control. In V. B. Brooks (Ed.), *Handbook of physiology—the nervous system, II, Part I* (pp. 1449–1480). Bethesda, MD: American Physiological Society Press.

Ardila, A., Rosseli, M., Arvizu, L., & Kuljis, R. O. (1997). Alexia and agraphia in posterior cortical atrophy. *Neuropsychiatry, Neuropsychology, and Behavioral Neurology, 10,* 52–59.

Arena, R., & Gainotti, G. (1978). Constructional apraxia and visuo-perceptive disabilities in relation to laterality of cerebral lesions. *Cortex, 14,* 463–473.

Arendt, T., Bigl, V., Arendt, A., & Tennstedt, A. (1983). Loss of neurons in the nucleus basalis of Meynert in Alzheimer's disease, paralysis agitans, and Korsakoff's disease. *Acta Neuropathologica, 61*(2), 101–108.

Arseni, C., & Botez, M. I. (1961). Speech disturbances caused by tumors of the supplementary motor area. *Acta Psychiarica Scandinavica, 36,* 279–299.

Assal, G. (1969). Régression des troubles de la reconnaissance des physiognomies et de la mémoire topographique chez un malade opéré d'un hématome intracérébral parieto-temporal droit. *Revue Neurologique, 121,* 184–185.

Assal, G. (1973). Aphasie de Wernicke chez un pianiste. *Revue Neurologique, 129,* 251–255.

Assal, G., & Buttet, J. (1983). Agraphie et conservation l'écriture musical chez un professeur de piano bilingue. *Revue Neurologique, 139,* 569–574.

Assal, G., Buttet, J., & Jolivet, R. (1981). Dissociations in aphasia: A case report. *Brain and Language, 13,* 223–240.

Assal, G., Faure, C., & Anderes, J. P. (1984). Non-reconnaissance d'animaux familiers chez un paysan: zooagnosie ou prosopagnosie pour les animaux. *Revue Neurologique, 140,* 580–584.

Assal, G., Probst, A., Zander, E., & Rabinowicz, T. (1976). Syndrome amnesique par infiltration tumorale. *Archives Suisse de Neurologie, Neurochirurgie et de Psychiatrie, 119,* 317–324.

Auerbach, S. H., & Alexander, M. P. (1981). Pure agraphia and unilateral optic ataxia associated with a left superior parietal lobe lesion. *Journal of Neurology, Neurosurgery and Psychiatry, 44,* 430–432.

Auerbach, S. H., Allard, T., Naeser, M., Alexander, M. P., & Albert, M. L. (1982). Pure word deafness: Analysis of a case with bilateral lesions and a defect at the prephonemic level. *Brain, 105,* 271–300.

Awad, I. A., Johnson, P. C., Spetzler, R. F., & Hodak, J. (1986). Incidental subcortical lesions identified on magnetic resonance imaging in the elderly. II. Postmortem pathological correlations. *Stroke, 17,* 1090–1097.

Awad, I. A., Spetzler, R. F., Hodak, J. A., & Carey, R. (1986). Incidental subcortical lesions identified on magnetic resonance imaging in the elderly. 1. Correlation with age and cerebro-vascular risk factors. *Stroke, 17,* 1084–1089.

Axelrod, B. N., Goldman, R. S., Heaton, R. K., Lawless, G., Thompson, L. L., Chelune, G. J., et al. (1996). Discriminability of the Wisconsin Card

Sorting Test using the standardization sample. *Journal of Clinical and Experimental Neuropsychology, 18,* 338–342.

Babinski, J. (1914). Contribution à l'étude des troubles mentaux dans l'hemiplegie cerebrale (anosognosie). *Revue Neurologique, 27,* 845–847.

Bach, L. J., Happé, F., Fleminger, S., & Powell, J. (2000). Theory of mind: Independence of executive function and the role of the frontal cortex in acquired brain injury. *Cognitive Neuropsychiatry, 5*(3), 175–192.

Bachevalier, J. R., Saunders, R., & Mishkin, M. (1985). Visual recognition in monkeys: Effects of transection of fornix. *Experimental Brain Research, 57,* 547–553.

Bach-Y-Rita, G., Lion, J. R., Climent, C. I., & Ervin, F. R. (1971). Episodic dyscontrol: A study of 130 violent patients. *American Journal of Psychiatry, 127,* 1473–1478.

Baddeley, A. (1994). Working memory: The interface between memory and cognition. In D. L. Schachter & E. Tulving (Eds.), *Memory systems* (pp. 351–368). Cambridge, London: MIT Press.

Baddeley, A. (1998). The central executive: A concept and some misconceptions. *Journal of the International Neuropsychological Society, 4,* 523–526.

Baddeley, A. D., Della Sala, S., Papagno, C., & Spinnler, H. (1997). Dual task performance in dysexecutive and non-dysexecutive patients with a frontal lesion. *Neuropsychology, 11,* 187–194.

Baddeley, A. D., & Hitch, G. (1974). Working memory. In G. A. Bower (Ed.), *The psychology of learning and motivation* (Vol. 8, pp. 47–89). New York: Academic Press.

Baer, L. (1994). Factor analysis of symptom subtypes of obsessive-compulsive disorder and their relation to personality and tic disorders. *Journal of Clinical Psychiatry, 55*(Suppl.), 18–23.

Baer, L., Rauch, S. L., Ballantine, H. T., Jr., et al. (1995). Cingulotomy for intractable obsessive-compulsive disorder: Prospective long-term follow-up of 18 patients. *Archives of General Psychiatry, 52,* 384–392.

Bailey, P., Green, J. R., Amador, L., & Gibbs, F. A. (1953). Treatment of psychomotor states by anterior temporal lobectomy. *American Research in Nervous and Mental Diseases* [proceedings], *31,* 341.

Bajhin, E. F., Korneva, T. V., & Lomachenko, A. S. (1980). The ability of emotional perception in schizophrenic patients. In R. W. Rieber (Ed.), *Applied psycholinguistic and mental health* (pp. 78–79). New York: Plenum Press.

Bajhin, E. F., Meerson, Y. A., & Tonkonogy, J. M. (1973). Probability prediction in some of the psychopathological and neuropsychological syndromes [in Russian]. In V. M. Morozov & I. M. Feigenberg (Eds.), *Schizophrenia and probability prediction* (pp. 68–77). Moscow: Central Institute of CME Press.

Bajhin, E. F., Wasserman, L. I., & Tonkonogy, J. M. (1975). Auditory hallucinations and temporal lobe pathology. *Neuropsychologia, 13,* 481–487.

Bajin, Y. F., & Korneva, T. V. (1979). Auditory analysis as a method of examination of impressive actions [in Russian]. In M. M. Kabanov & J. M. Tonkonogy (Eds.), *Psychological methods of personality studies in clinical setting* (pp. 41–49). Leningrad: The Bechterev Institute Press.

Baldwin, M. A. (1960). Electrical stimulation of the mesial temporal region. In E. R. Ramey & D. S. O'Doherty (Eds.), *Electrical studies on the unanesthezide brain* (pp. 159–176). New York: Hoeber.

Balint, R. (1909). Die seelenlahmung des "Schauens." *Monatschrift für Psychiatrie und Neurologie, 1*(25), 51–81.

Ball, M. (1984). The morphological basis of dementia in Parkinson's disease. *Canadian Journal of Neurological Science, 11,* 180–184.

Balonov, L. Y., & Deglin, V. L. (1976). *Hearing and speech in the dominant and nondominant hemispheres* [in Russian]. Leningrad: Nauka.

Bar, M. (2003). A cortical mechanism for triggering top-down facilitation in visual object recognition. *Journal of Cognitive Neuroscience, 15*(4), 600–609.

Bar, M., Tootel, R., Schachter, D., Greve, D., Fishl, B., Mendola, B., et al. (2001). Cortical mechanisms of explicit visual object recognition. *Neuron, 29,* 529–235.

Barbur, J. L., Watson, J.D.G., Frackoviak, R.S.J., & Zeki, S. (1993). Conscious visual perception without V1. *Brain, 116,* 1293–1302.

Barcloiugh, B. M. (1987). The suicide rate of epilepsy. *Acta Psychiatrica Scandinavica, 76,* 339–345.

Barczak, P., Edmunds, E., & Betts, T. (1988). Hypomania following complex partial seizures. *British Journal of Psychiatry, 152,* 137–139.

Bard, P. A. (1928). Diencephalic mechanism for the expression of rage with special reference to the sympathetic nervous system. *American Journal of Physiology, 84,* 490–515.

Baron, J. C., Petit-Taboué, M. C., De Doze, F., Desgranges, B., Ravenel, L., & Marchal, G. (1994). Right frontal cortex hypometabolism in transient global amnesia: A PET study. *Brain, 117,* 545–552.

Baron-Cohen, S. (1995). *Mindblindness.* Cambridge, MA: MIT Press.

Baron-Cohen, S., Leslie, A., & Frith, U. (1985). Does the autistic child have a "theory of mind"? *Cognition, 21,* 37–46.

Baron-Cohen, S., O'Riordan, M., Stoen, V. E., Jones, R., & Plaisted, K. (1997). *Recognition of faux pas by normally developing children and children with Asperger's syndrome.* Unpublished manuscript, University of Cambridge.

Baron-Cohen, S., Ring, H., Moriarty, J., Schmitz, B., Costa, D., & Ell, P. (1994). Recognition of mental state terms: Clinical findings in children with autism and a functional neuroimaging study of normal adults. *British Journal of Psychiatry, 165,* 640–649.

Baron-Cohen, S., Ring, H. A., Wheelwright, S., Bullmore, E. T., Brammer, M. J., Simmons, A., et al. (1999). Social intelligence in the normal and autistic brain. *European Journal of Neuroscience, 11,* 1–8.

Barris, R. W., & Schuman, H. R. (1953). Bilateral anterior cingulate gyrus lesions. *Neurology, 3,* 44–52.

Barta, P. E., Pearlson, M. B., Powers, R. E., Richards, S. S., & Tune, L. E. (1990). Auditory hallucinations and smaller temporal lobe volume in schizophrenia. *American Journal of Psychiatry, 147,* 1457–1462.

Baru, A. V. (1966). On the role of temporal cortex in detection of sounds of different durations in the dog [in Russian]. *Journal of Higher Nervous Activity, 16,* 655–666.

Baru, A. V., Gershuni, G. V., & Tonkonogy, J. M. (1964). Detection of tone signals of various duration in diagnosis of the temporal lobe lesions [in Russian]. *The Korsakoff Journal of Neurology and Psychiatry, 11,* 1614–1619.

Baruk, H. (1926). *Les troubles mentaux dans les tumeurs cerebrales* (Vol. 1). Paris: G. Doin.

Basso, A. (1993). Amusia. In F. Boller & J. Grafman (Eds.), *Handbook of neuropsychology* (Vol. 8, pp. 391–409). Amsterdam: Elsevier Science.

Basso, A., Casati, G., & Vignolo, L. A. (1977). Phonemic identification defect in aphasia. *Cortex, 13,* 65–95.

Basso, A., Luzzatti, C., & Spinnler, H. (1980). Is ideomotor apraxia the outcome of damage to well-defined regions of the left hemisphere. *Journal of Neurology, Neurosurgery, and Psychiatry, 43,* 118–126.

Basso, L., & Capitani, E. (1985). Spared musical abilities in a conductor with global aphasia and ideomotor apraxia. *Journal of Neurology, Neurosurgery, and Psychiatry, 48,* 407–412.

Basso, M. R., Nasrallah, H. A., Olson, S. C., & Bornsteinn, R. A. (1997). Cognitive deficit distinguishes patients with adolescent- and adult-onset schizophrenia. *Neuropsychiatry, Neuropsychology, and Behavioral Neurology, 10,* 107–112.

Bastian, H. C. (1897). Some problems in connection with aphasia and other speech defects. *Lancet, 2,* 933–942, 1005–1017, 1132–1137, 1187–1194.

Baum, S. R., Blumstein, S. E., Naeser, M. A., & Palumbo, C. L. (1990). Temporal dimension of consonant and vowel production: An acoustic and CT scan analysis of aphasic speech. *Brain and Language, 39,* 33–56.

Baumann, B., Danos, P., Krell, D., Diekmann, S., Leschinger, A., Stauch, R., et al. (1999). Reduced volume of limbic system-affiliated basal ganglia in mood disorders: Preliminary data from a postmortem study. *Journal of Neuropsychiatry and Clinical Neuroscience, 11,* 71–78.

Bäumer, H. (1954). Veränderungen des thalamus bei schizophrenie. *Journal für Hirnforschung, 1,* 157–172.

Baxter, D. M., & Warrington, E. K. (1983). Neglect dysgraphia. *Journal of Neurology, Neurosurgery, and Psychiatry, 46,* 1073–1078.

Baxter, D. M., & Warrington, E. K. (1985) Category specific phonological dysgraphia. *Neuropsychologia, 23,* 653–666.

Baxter, D. M., & Warrington, E. K. (1986). Ideational agraphia: A single case study. *Journal of Neurology, Neurosurgery, and Psychiatry, 49,* 369–374.

Baxter, L. R., Phelps, M. E., Mazziotta, J. C., et al. (1987). Local glucose metabolic rates in obsessive-compulsive disorder: A comparison with rates in unipolar depression and normal controls. *Archives of General Psychiatry, 44,* 211–218.

Baxter, L. R., Phelps, M. E., Mazziota, J. C., Schwartz, J. M., Gerner, R. H., Selin, C. E., et al. (1985). Cerebral metabolic rates for glucose in mood disorders: Studies with positron emission tomography and fluorodeoxyglucose F 18. *Archives of General Psychiatry, 42,* 441–447.

Baxter, L. R., Schwartz, J. M., & Bergman, K. S. (1992). Caudate metabolic glucose rate changes with drug and behavior therapy for obsessive-compulsive disorder. *Archives of General Psychiatry, 49,* 681–689.

Baxter, L. R., Schwartz, J. M., Phelps, M. E., Guze, B. H., Selin, C. E., Gerner, R. H., et al. (1989). Reduction of prefrontal glucose metabolism common to three types of depression. *Archives of General Psychiatry, 46,* 243–250.

Baxter-Versi, D. M. (1987). *Acquired spelling disorders.* Unpublished doctoral dissertation, London University, London.

Bay, E. (1950). *Agnosie und Funktionswandel: Eine hirnpatologische Studie* (Monographien aus dem Gesamtgebiete der Neurologie und Psychiatrie, Vol. 73). Berlin: Springer.

Bay, E. (1953). Disturbances of visual perception and their examination. *Brain, 76,* 515–550.

Bay, E. (1957). Die corticale Dysarthrie und ihre Beziehungen zur sog: Motorische Aphasie. *Deutsche Zeitschrift für Nervenkrankheiten, 176,* 553–594.

Bay, E., Lauenstein, O., & Gibis, P. (1949). Ein Beitrag zur Frage der Seelenblinheit: Der Fall Schn. Von Gelb und Goldstein. *Psychiatrie, Neurologie, und Medical Psychologie* (Leipzig), *1,* 73–91.

Bayles, K. A., Tomoeda, C. K, & Rein, J. A. (1996). Phrase repetition in Alzheimer's disease: Effect of meaning and length. *Brain and Language, 54,* 246–261.

Bazemore, P. H., Tonkonogy, J., & Ananth, R. (1991). Dysphagia in psychiatric patients: Clinical and videofluroscopic study. *Dysphagia, 6,* 2–5.

Bazhin, E. F., Meerson, Y. A., & Tonkonogy, J. M. (1973). On distinguishing a visual signal from noise by patients with visual agnosia and visual hallucinations. *Neuropsychologia, 11,* 319–324.

Bear, D. (1979). Temporal lobe epilepsy—a syndrome of sensory-limbic hyperconnection. *Cortex, 15,* 357–384.

Bear, D. M., & Fedio, P. (1977). Quantitative analysis of interictal behavior in temporal lobe epilepsy. *Archives of Neurology, 34,* 454–467.

Bear, D. M., Levin, K., Blumer, D., Chetham, D., & Ryder, J. (1982). Interictal behavior in hospitalized temporal lobe epileptics: Relationship to idiopathic psychiatric syndromes. *Journal of Neurology, Neurosurgery, and Psychiatry, 45,* 481–488.

Beard, A. W. (1959). The association of hepatolenticular degeneration with schizophrenia. *Acta Psychiatrica et Neurologica Scandinavica, 34,* 411–428.

Beauclair, L., & Fontaine, R. (1986). Epileptiform abnormalities in panic disorder. Presented at the Society for Biological Psychiatry, 41st Annual Convention and Scientific Program, No. 96, 148.

Beauvois, M. F. (1982). Optic aphasia: A process of interaction between vision and language. *Philosophical Transactions of the Royal Society of London, Series B, 298,* 35–47.

Beauvois, M. F., & Dérouesné, J. (1979). Phonological alexia: Three dissociations. *Journal of Neurology, Neurosurgery, and Psychiatry, 42,* 1115–1124.

Beauvois, M. F., Saillant, B., Meninger, V., & Lhermitte, F. (1978). Bilateral tactile aphasia: A tacto-verbal dysfunction. *Brain, 101,* 381–401.

Becker, J. T., Huff, F. J., Nebes, R. D., Holland, A., & Boller, F. (1988). Neuropsychological functions in Alzheimer's disease: Pattern of impairment and rates of progression. *Archives of Neurology, 45,* 263–268.

Behar, D., Rapoport, J. L., Berg, C. J., et al. (1984). Computerized tomography and neuropsychological test measures in adolescents with obsessive-compulsive disorder. *American Journal of Psychiatry, 141,* 363–369.

Behrmann, M., Moscovitch, M., Black, S. E., & Mozer, M. (1990). Perceptual and conceptual factors in neglect dyslexia: Two contrasting case studies. *Brain, 113,* 1163–1183.

Belfer, M. L., & D'Autremont, C. C. (1971). Catatonia-like symptomatology: An interesting case. *Archives of General Psychiatry, 24,* 119–120.

Bender, B. G. (1973). Spatial interactions between the red- and green-sensitive color mechanisms of the human visual system. *Vision Research, 13,* 2205–2218.

Benes, F. M., Davidson, J., & Bird, E. D. (1984). Quantitative morphometric studies of schizophrenic cortex. In *Clinical neuropharmacology* (Vol. 7, Suppl. 1, p. S498). New York: Raven Press.

Benevento, L. A., & Yoshida, K. (1981). The afferent and efferent organization of the lateral geniculo-prestriate pathways in the macaque monkey. *Journal of Comparative Neurology, 203,* 455–474.

Benjamin, S. (1999). A neuropsychiatric approach to aggressive behavior. In F. Ovsiew (Ed.), *Neuropsychiatry and mental health services* (pp. 149–196). Washington, DC: American Psychiatric Press.

Benjamin, S., Kirsh, D., Vissher, T., Ozbayrak, K. R., & Weaver, J. P. (2000). Hypomania from left frontal AVM resection. *Neurology, 54,* 1389–1390.

Benkelfat, C., Nordahi, T. E., Semple, W. E., et al. (1990). Local cerebral glucose metabolic rates in obsessive-compulsive disorder: Patients treated with clomipramine. *Archives of General Psychiatry, 47,* 840–848.

Benson, D. (1988). Hypoglycemia and aggression: A review. *International Journal of Neuroscience, 41,* 163–168.

Benson, D. F. (1979). *Aphasia, alexia, agraphia.* New York: Elsevier.

Benson, D. F., Davis, J., & Snyder, B. D. (1988). Posterior cortical atrophy. *Archives of Neurology, 45,* 789–793.

Benson, D. F., & Geschwind, N. (1969). The alexias. In P. J. Vinken & G. W. Bruyn (Eds.), *Handbook of clinical neurology* (pp. 112–140). Amsterdam: North Holland Publishing Company.

Benson, D. F., & Greenberg, J. P. (1969). Visual form agnosia. *Archives of Neurology, 20*, 82–89.

Benson, D. F., Marsden, C. D., & Meadows, J. L. (1974). The amnesic syndrome of posterior cerebral artery occlusion. *Acta Neurologica Scandinavica, 50*, 133–145.

Benson, D. F., Marsden, C. D., & Meadows, J. C. (1976). Reduplicative paramnesia. *Neurology, 26*, 147–151.

Benson, D. F., Miller, B. L., & Signer, S. F. (1986). Dual personality associated with epilepsy. *Archives of Neurology, 43*, 471–474.

Benson, D. F., Sheramata, W. A., Bouchard, R., Segarra, J. M., Price, D., & Geschwind, N. (1973). Conduction aphasia: A clinicopathological study. *Archives of Neurology, 28*, 339–346.

Benton, A. L. (1961). The fiction of the "Gerstmann syndrome." *Journal of Neurology, Neurosurgery, and Psychiatry, 24*, 176–181.

Benton, A. L. (1980). The neuropsychology of face recognition. *American Psychologist, 35*, 176–186.

Benton, A. L., & Joynt, R. J. (1960). Early descriptions of aphasia. *Archives of Neurology, 3*, 205–221.

Benton, A. L., & Van Allen, M. W. (1968). Impairment in facial recognition in patients with cerebral disease. *Cortex, 4*, 344–358.

Benton, A. L., & Van Allen, M. W. (1972). Prosopagnosia and facial discrimination. *Journal of Neurological Science, 15*, 167–172.

Benton, A. L., Varney, N. R., & Hamsher, K. de S. (1978). Visuo-spatial judgment: A clinical test. *Archives of Neurology, 35*, 364–367.

Berg, E. A. (1948). A simple objective technique for measuring flexibility in thinking. *Journal of General Psychology, 39*, 15–22.

Berman, K. F., & Weinberger, D. R. (1991). Prefrontal dopamine and defect symptoms in schizophrenia. In J. F. Greden & R. Tandon (Eds.), *Negative schizophrenic symptoms: Pathophysiology and clinical implications* (pp. 83–95). Washington, DC: American Psychiatric Press.

Berman, K. F., Weinberger, D. R., Shelton, R. C., & Zec, R. F. (1987). A relationship between anatomical and physiological brain pathology in schizophrenia: Lateral cerebral ventricular size predicts cortical blood flow. *American Journal of Psychiatry, 144*, 127–128.

Berrington, W. P., Liddell, D. W., & Foulds, G. A. (1956). A reevaluation of the fugue. *Journal of Mental Science, 102*, 281–286.

Berrios, G. E., & Brook, P. (1985). Delusions and psychopathology of the elderly with dementia. *Acta Psychiatrica Scandinavica, 72*, 296–301.

Berthier, M. L., Leiguarda, R., Starkstein, S. E., Sevlever, G., & Taratuto, A. L. (1991). Alzheimer's disease with posterior cortical atrophy. *Journal of Neurology, Neurosurgery, and Psychiatry, 54*, 1110–1111.

Betts, T. A. (1981). Depression, anxiety and epilepsy. In E. H. Reynolds & M. R. Trimble (Eds.), *Epilepsy and psychiatry* (pp. 60–71). New York: Churchill Livingstone.

Bever, T. G., & Chiarello, R. J. (1974). Cerebral dominance in musicians and non-musicians. *Science, 185,* 137–139.

Beymer, D., & Poggio, T. (1996). Image representation for visual learning. *Science, 272,* 1905–1909.

Biederman, I. (1985). Human image understanding: Recent research and a theory. *Computer Vision, Graphics, and Image Processing, 32,* 29–73.

Biemond, A. (1970). On Binswanger's subcortical arteriosclerotic encephalopathy and the possibility of its clinical recognition. *Schweizer Archiv für Neurologie Neurochirurgie und Psychiatrie, 73,* 413–417.

Bingley, T. (1958). Mental symptoms in temporal lobe epilepsy and temporal lobe gliomas. *Acta Psychiatrica et Neurologica Scandinavica, 33*(120, Suppl.), 1–151.

Binkofski, F., & Block., R. A. (1996). Accelerate time experience after left frontal cortex lesion. *Neurocase, 2,* 485–493.

Binns, J. K., & Robertson, E. E. (1962). Pick's disease in old age. *Journal of Mental Science, 108,* 804–810.

Binswanger, O. (1894). Die Abrenzung der allgemeinen progressiven Paralyse. *Berlinische Klinische Wochenshrift, 31,* 1103–1105, 1137–1139; *32,* 1180–1186.

Bisiach, E., Capitani, E., Colombo, A., & Spinnler, H. (1976). Having a horizontal segment: A study on hemisphere damaged patients with focal lesions. *Archives Suisses de Neurologie, Neurochirurgie, et de Psychiatrie, 118,* 119–206.

Bisiach, E., Luzzatti, C., & Perani, D. (1979). Unilateral neglect, representational schema and consciousness. *Brain, 102,* 609–618.

Black, S. E., & Behrmann, M. (1994). Localization in alexia. In A. Kertesz (Ed.), *Localization and neuroimaging in neuropsychology* (pp. 331–376). San Diego, CA: Academic Press.

Blanchard, D. C., & Blanchard, R. J. (1972). Innate and conditioned reactions to threat in rats with amygdaloid lesions. *Journal of Comparative and Physiological Psychology, 81,* 281–290.

Blennow, K., Wallin, A., & Gottris, C. (1994). Clinical subgroups of Alzheimer's disease. In V. O. B. Emery & T. E. Oxman (Eds.), *Dementia, presentations, differential diagnosis, and nosology* (pp. 95–107). Baltimore, MD: Johns Hopkins University Press.

Blessed, G., Tomlinson, B. E., & Roth, M. (1968). The association between quantitative measures of dementia and of senile changes in the cerebral gray matter of elderly subjects. *British Journal of Psychiatry, 114,* 797–811.

Bleuler, E. P. (1951). Psychiatry of cerebral diseases. *British Medical Journal, 2,* 1233–1238.

Blumberg, H. P., Stern, E., Ricketts, S., et al. (1999). Rostral and orbital prefrontal cortex dysfunction in the manic state of bipolar disorder. *American Journal of Psychiatry, 156,* 1986–1988.

Blumer, D., & Benson, D. F. (1975). Personality changes with frontal and temporal lobe lesions. In E. D. Benson and D. Blumer (Eds.), *Psychiatric aspects of neurologic disease* (pp. 151–170). New York: Grune & Stratton.

Blumstein, J. E., Baker, E., & Goodglass, H. (1977). Phonological factors in auditory comprehension. *Neuropsychologia, 15,* 19–30.

Blumstein, S. E. (1995). The neurobiology of sound structure of language. In M. S. Gazzaniga (Ed.), *The cognitive neurosciences* (pp. 915–930). Cambridge, MA: MIT Press.

Bocca, E., Calearo, C., Cassinori, V., & Migliavocca, F. (1955). Testing "cortical" hearing in temporal lobe tumours. *Acta Oto-laryngologica, 45,* 289–304.

Bodamer, J. (1947). Die Prosopagnosie. *Archiv für Psychiatrie und Nervenkrankheiten, 179,* 6–54.

Bogen, J. E. (1993). The callosal syndrome. In K. M. Heilman & E. Valenstein (Eds.), *Clinical neuropsychology* (3rd ed., pp. 337–407). New York: Oxford University Press.

Bogerts, B., Meertz, E., & Schönfeldt-Bausch, R. (1985). Basal ganglia and limbic system pathology in schizophrenia. *Archives of General Psychiatry, 42,* 784.

Bogousslavsky, J., Ferrazzini, M., Regli, F., et al. (1988). Manic delirium and frontal-like syndrome with paramedian infarction of the right thalamus. *Journal of Neurology, Neurosurgery, and Psychiatry, 51,* 116–119.

Bogousslavsky, J., Regli, F., & Assal, G. (1988). Acute transcortical mixed aphasia: A carotid occlusion syndrome with pial and watershed infarcts. *Brain, 11,* 631–641.

Boiten, J., & Lodder, J. (1989). An unusual sequela of a frequently occurring neurological disorder: Delirium caused by brain infarct. *Nederlands Tijdschrift voor Geneeskunde, 133,* 617–620.

Boller, F. (1973). Destruction of Wernicke's area without language disturbance: A fresh look at crossed aphasia. *Neuropsychologia, 11,* 243–246.

Boller, F., Kim, Y., & Mack, J. L. (1977). Auditory comprehension in aphasia. In H. Whitaker & H. A. Whitaker (Eds.), *Studies in neurolinguistics* (Vol. 3, pp. 1–63). New York: Academic Press.

Boller, F., Mizutani, T., Roessmann, U., & Gambetti, P. (1980). Parkinson disease, dementia, and Alzheimer disease: Clinicopathological correlations. *Annals of Neurology, 7,* 329–335.

Boller, F., & Vignolo, L. (1966). Latent sensory aphasia in hemisphere-damaged patients: An experimental study with Token Test. *Brain, 89,* 815–831.

Bolles, R. C., & Cain, R. A. (1982). Recognizing and locationing partially visible objects: The local-feature-focus method. *International Journal of Robotics Research, 1*(3), 57–82.

Bonda, E., Petrides, M., Ostry, D., & Evans, A. (1996). Specific involvements of human parietal systems and the amigdala in the perception of biological motion. *Journal of Neuroscience, 16*, 3737–3744.

Bonnet, C. (1769). *Essay analytique sur les facultés de l'âme* (Vol. 2, 2nd ed.). Copenhagen and Geneva.

Bonvicini, G. (1905). Subcorticale sensorische Aphasie. *Journal of Psychiatry and Neurology, 26*, 126–229.

Borchgrevink, H. M. (1980). Cerebral lateralization of speech and singing after intracarotid amytal injection. In M. Y. Sarno & O. Hook (Eds.), *Aphasia, assessment and treatment*. Stockholm: Almqvist and Wiksell.

Bornstein, B. (1963). Prosopagnosia. In L. Halpern (Ed.), *Problems of dynamic neurology* (pp. 283–318). Jerusalem: Hadasseh Medical Organization.

Botez, M. I., & Wertheim, N. (1959). Expressive aphasia and amusia following right frontal lesion in a right-handed man. *Brain, 82*, 186–203.

Boudouresques, J., Pocet, M., Cherif, A., & Balzamo, M. (1979). L'agnosie de visage: Un temoin de la desorganisation fonctionnelle d'un certain type de connaissance des elements du monde exterieur. *Bulletin de l'Academie Nationale de Medicine, 163*, 695–702.

Bouillaud, J. (1825). Recherches cliniques propres à démontrer que la perte de la parole correspond à la lésion des lobules anterieurs de cerveau et à confirmer l'opinion de M. Gall sur le siege de l'organe du langage articulé. *Archives Géneralés de Médicine, 8*, 25–45.

Boussaud, D., Ungerleider, L. C., & Desimone, R. (1990). Pathways for motion analysis: Cortical connection of the medial superior temporal and fundus of the superior temporal visual areas in the macaque. *Journal of Comparative Neurology, 296*, 462–495.

Bowen, D. M., Najlerahim, A., Procter, A. W., et al. (1989). Circumscribed changes of the cerebral cortex in neuropsychiatric disorders of later life. *Proceeding of the National Academy of Science, 86*, 9504–9508.

Bowers, D., Coslett, H. B., Bauer, R. M., Speedie, L. J., & Heilman, K. M. (1987). Comprehension of emotional prosody following unilateral hemispheric lesions: Processing defect vs distraction defect. *Neuropsychologia, 25*, 317–328.

Boyko, O. B., Alston, S. R., & Burger, P. C. (1989). Neuropathologic and postmortem MR imaging correlation of confluent periventricular white matter changes in the aging brain [Abstract]. *Radiology, 173*(P), 86.

Brain, R. (1941). Visual disorientation with special reference to the lesions of the right cerebral hemisphere. *Brain, 64*, 244–272.

Brain, R. (1965). *Speech disorders* (2nd ed.). London: Butterworths.

Brandt, J., Seidman, L. J., & Kohl, D. (1985). Personality characteristics of epileptic patients: A controlled study of generalized and temoral lobe cases. *Journal of Clinical and Experimental Neuropsychology, 7*, 25–38.

Brant-Zawadzki, M., Fein, G., Van Dyke, C., et al. (1985). MR imaging of aging brain: Patchy white matter lesions and dementia. *American Journal of Noninvasive Radiology, 6*, 675–682.

Braun, A. R., Balkin, T. J., Wesensten, N. J., Carson, R. E., Varga, M., Baldwin, P., et al. (1997). Regional cerebral blood flow throughout the sleep-wake cycle. *Brain, 120*, 1173–1197.

Braun, A. R., Balkin, T. J., Wesensten, N. J., Gwadry, F., Carson, R. E., Varga, M., et al. (1998). Dissociated pattern of activity in visual cortices and their projections during human rapid-eye-movement sleep. *Science, 279*, 91–95.

Breiter, H. C., Etcoff, N. L., Whalen, P. J., Kennedy, W. A., Rauch, S. L., Buckner, R. L., et al. (1996). Response and habituation of the human amygdala during visual processing of facial expression. *Neuron, 17*, 885–887.

Bremner, J. D., Narayan, M., Anderson, E. R., Staib, L. H., Miller, H. L., & Charney, D. S. (2000). Hippocampal volume reduction in major depression. *American Journal of Psychiatry, 157*, 115–117.

Brickner, R. M. (1936). *The intellectual functions of the frontal lobes*. New York: Macmillan.

Brickner, R. M., Rosner, A. A., & Munro, R. (1940). Physiological aspects of the obsessive state. *Psychosomatic Medicine, 11*, 369–383.

Brickner, R. M., & Stein, A. (1942). Intellectual symptoms in temporal lobe lesions including "déjà pense." *Journal of Mount Sinai Hospital, 9*, 344–348.

Brierley, J. B. (1966). The neuropathology of amnesic states. In C. W. N. Whitty & O. L. Zangwill (Eds.), *Amnesia* (pp. 150–180). London: Butterworths.

Brierley, J. B., Corsellis, J. A. N., Hierons, R., & Nelvin, S. (1960). Subacute encephalitis of later adult life mainly affecting the limbic area. *Brain, 83*, 357–368.

Brion, S., & Jedynak, C. P. (1972). Troubles du transfert interhémisphéric. A propos de trois observations de tumeurs du corps calleux. Le signe de la main êtrangère. *Revue Neurologique, 126*, 257–266.

Brion, S., & Mikol, J. (1978). Atteinte du noyau lateral dorsal du thalamus et syndrome de Korsakoff alcoolique. *Journal of Neurological Science, 38*, 249–261.

Broca, P. (1861a). Perte de la parole, ramolissement chronique et destruction partielle du lobe antérieur gauche du cerveaux. *Bulletin de la Société d' Anthropologie, 2*, 235–237.

Broca, P. (1861b). Remarques sur le siège de la faculté articulé suives d'une observation d'aphémie. *Bulletin de la Société d'Anthropologie, 2*, 330–357.

Broca, P. (1878). Anatomie comparée des circonvolutions cérébrales: Le grand lobe limbique et la scissure limbique dans la série mammifères. *Revue d'Anthropologie, ser. 21*, 384–498.

Brodal, A. (1969). *Neurological anatomy in relation to clinical medicine*. New York: Oxford University Press.

Bromberg, W. (1930). Mental state in chronic encephalitis. *Psychiatric Quarterly, 4*, 537–566.

Brooks, R. (1981). Symbolic reasoning among 3-dimensional models and 2-dimensional images. *Artificial Intelligence, 17*, 285–349.

Brouwers, P., Cox, D., Martin, A., et al. (1984). Differential perceptual-spatial impairment in Huntington's and Alzheimer's dementias. *Archives of Neurology, 41,* 1073–1076.

Brown, R. G., MacCarthy, B., Gotham, A. M., Der, G. J., & Marsden, C. D. (1988). Depression and disability in Parkinson's disease: A follow-up study of 132 cases. *Psychological Medicine, 18,* 49–55.

Bruce, C., Desimone, R., & Gross, C. G. (1981). Visual properties of neurons in a polysensory area in superior temporal sulcus of the macaque. *Journal of Neurophysiology, 46,* 369–384.

Bruder, G., Rabinowicz, E., Towey, J., et al. (1995). Smaller right ear (left hemisphere) advantage for dichotic fused words in patients with schizophrenia. *American Journal of Psychiatry, 152,* 932–935.

Brugge, J. F., & Merzenich, M. M. (1973). Patterns of activity of single neurons of the auditory cortex in monkey. In A. R. Moller (Ed.), *Basic mechanisms of hearing* (pp. 745–766). New York: Academic Press.

Brugger, P., Regard, M., & Landis, T. (1996). Unilaterally felt "presence": The neuropsychiatry of one's invisible doppelgänger. *Neuropsychiatry, Neuropsychology, and Behavioral Neurology, 9,* 114–122.

Brun, A. (1987). Frontal lobe degeneration of non-Alzheimer type, I: Neuropathology. *Archives of Gerontology and Geriatrics, 6,* 193–208.

Brun, A. (1993). Frontal lobe dementia of the non-Alzheimer type revisited. *Dementia, 4,* 126–131.

Brun, A., & Gustafson, L. (1978). Limbic lobe involvement in presenile dementia. *Archiv für Psychiatrie und Nervenkrankheiten, 226,* 79–93.

Brust, J. (1980). Music and language: Musical alexia and agraphia. *Brain, 103,* 367–392.

Bruyer, R., Laterre, C., Seron, X., Feyereisne, P., Strypstein, E., Pierard, E., et al. (1983). A case of prosopagnosia with some preserved covert remembrance of familiar faces. *Brain and Cognition, 2,* 257–284.

Bub, D., & Kertesz, A. (1982). Deep agraphia. *Brain and Language, 17,* 146–165.

Büchel, C., Morris, J., Dolan, R. J., & Friston, K. J. (1998). Brain systems mediating aversive conditioning: An event-related MRI study. *Neuron, 20,* 947–957.

Buchsbaum, M. S., DeLisi, L. E., Holcomb, H. H., et al. (1984). Antero-posterior gradients in cerebral glucose use in schizophrenia and affective disorders. *Archives of General Psychiatry, 41,* 1159–1166.

Buchsbaum, M. S., Gillin, J. C., Wu, J., Hazlett, E., Siicotte, M., Dupont, R. M., et al. (1989). Regional cerebral glucose metabolic rate assessed by positron emission tomography. *Life Science, 45,* 1349–1356.

Buchsbaum, M. S., Ingvar, D., Kessler, R., et al. (1982). Cerebral glucography with positron tomography. *Archives of General Psychiatry, 39,* 251–259.

Buchsbaum, M. S., Wu, J., DeLisi, L. E., et al. (1986). Frontal cortex and basal ganglia metabolic rates assessed by positron emission tomography with

[18 F] 2-deoxyglucose in affective illness. *Journal of Affective Disorder, 10,* 137–152.

Burger, P. C., Burch, J. G., & Kunze, U. (1976). Subcortical arteriosclerotic encephalopathy (Binswanger disease). *Stroke, 7,* 626–631.

Burkhardt, C. R., Filley, C. M., Kleinschmidt-DeMasters, B. K., de la Monte, S., Norenberg, M. D., & Schneck, S. A. (1988). Diffuse Lewy body disease and progressive dementia. *Neurology, 38,* 1520–1528.

Burns, A., Jacoby, R., & Levy, R. (1990). Psychiatric phenomena in Alzheimer's disease. I: Disorders of thought content. *British Journal of Psychiatry, 157,* 72–76.

Burns, S. B., & Burns, J. L. (1998). The strange case of Phineas Gage. *Neurology Review, 6*(2), 6.

Burton, H., Videen, T. O., & Raichle, M. E. (1993). Tactile-vibration-activated foci in insular and parietal-opercular cortex studies with positron emission tomography: Mapping the second somatosensory area in humans. *Somatosensory and Motor Research, 3,* 297–308.

Bush, E. (1940). Psychical symptoms in neurological disease. *Acta Psychiatrica et Neurologica Scandinavica, 15,* 257–290.

Butler, P. B., Harkavy-Freedman, J. M., Amador, X. F., & Gorman, J. M. (1996). Backward masking in schizophrenia: Relationship to medication status, neuropsychological functioning, and dopamine metabolism. *Biological Psychiatry, 40,* 295–298.

Butters, N. (1978). Comparison of the neuropsychological deficits associated with early and advanced stages of Huntington's disease. *Archives of Neurology, 35,* 585–589.

Butterworth, B. (1979). Hesitation and the production of verbal paraphasias and neologisms in jargon aphasia. *Brain and Language, 8,* 133–161.

Bylsma, F. W., Folstein, F. M., Devanant, D. P., Richards, M., Bello, J., Albert, M.,et al. (1994). Delusions and pattern of cognitive impairment in Alzheimer's disease. *Neuropsychiatry, Neuropsychology, and Behavioral Neurology, 7,* 98–103.

Byrne, E. J., Lennox, G., Lowe, J., & Godwin-Austen, R. B. (1989). Diffuse Lewy body disease: Clinical feature in 15 cases. *Journal of Neurology, Neurosurgery, and Psychiatry, 52,* 709–717.

Cadieux, N. L., & Greve, K. W. (1997). Emotion processing in Alzheimer's disease. *Journal of International Neuropsychological Society, 3,* 411–419.

Caffarra, P., & Venneri, A. (1996). Isolated degenerative amnesia without dementia: An 8-year longitudinal study. *Neurocase, 2,* 99–106.

Cahill, L., Haier, R. J., Fallon, J., Alkire, M. T., Tang, C., Keator, D., et al. (1996). Amygdala activity at encoding correlated with long-term, free recall of emotional information. *Proceedings of the National Academy of Sciences, USA, 93,* 8016–8021.

Caine, E. D., & Shoulson, I. (1983). Psychiatric syndromes in Huntington's disease. *American Journal of Psychiatry, 140,* 728–733.

Cairns, H., Oldfield, R. C., Pennybacker, J. B., & Whitteridge, D. (1941). Akinetic mutism with an epidermoid cyst of the third ventricle. *Brain, 64,* 273–290.

Calder, A. J., Young, A. W., Rowland, D., Perrett, D. I., Hodges, J. R., & Etcoff, N. L. (1996). Facial emotion recognition after bilateral amygdala damage: Differentially severe impairment of fear. *Cognitive Neuropsychology, 13,* 699–745.

Cambier, J., Masson, M., Viader, F., Limodin, J., & Strube, L. (1985). Le syndrome frontal de la paralysie supranucleaire progressive. *Revue Neurologique, 141,* 528–536.

Campion, J., & Latto, R. (1985). Apperceptive agnosia due to carbon monoxide poisoning: An interpretation based on critical band masking from disseminated lesions. *Behavioral Brain Research, 15,* 227–240.

Cancelliere, A. E. B., & Kertesz, A. (1990). Lesion localization in acquired deficits of emotional expressions and comprehension. *Brain and Cognition, 13,* 133–147.

Caplan, D. (1996). Language and neuropsychiatry. In B. S. Fogel, R. B. Schiffer, & S. M. Rao (Eds.), *Neuropsychiatry* (pp. 723–755). Baltimore, MD: Williams and Wilkins.

Caplan, D., & Waters, G. (1999). Verbal working memory and sentence comprehension. *Behavior and Brain Sciences, 22,* 77–126.

Caramazza, A., & Zurif, E. B. (1976). Dissociation of algorithmic and heuristic processes in language comprehension: Evidence from aphasia. *Brain and Language, 3,* 572–582.

Carson, A. J., MacHale, S., Allen, K., et al. (2000). Depression after stroke and lesion location: A systematic review. *Lancet, 356,* 122–126.

Cascino, G. D., & Adams, R. D. (1986). Brainstem auditory hallucinosis. *Neurology, 36,* 1042–1047.

Caselli, R. J. (1991). Rediscovering tactile agnosia. *Mayo Clinic Proceedings, 66,* 129–142.

Casseday, J. H., & Covey, E. (1992). Frequency tuning properties of neurons in the inferior colliculus of an FM bat. *Journal of Comparative Physiology, 319,* 34–50.

Cassens, G., Inglis, A. K., Appelbaum, P. S., & Guthell, T. G. (1990). Neuroleptics: Effects in neuropsychological function in chronic schizophrenic patients. *Schizophrenia Bulletin, 16,* 477–499.

Castaigne, P., Buge, A., Cambier, J., Escourolle, R., Brunet, P., & Degos, J. D. (1966). Demence thalamique d'origine vasculaire par ramollissement bilateral, limite au territoire du pedicule retro-mamillaire: A propos de deux observations anatomo-cliniques. *Revue Neurologique, 114,* 89–107.

Castaigne, P., Lhermitte, F., Buge, A., Escourolle, R., Hauw, J. J., & Lyon-Caen, O. (1981). Paramedian thalamic and midbrain infarcts: Clinical and neuropathological study. *Annals of Neurology, 10,* 127–148.

Castaigne, P., Lhermitte, F., Signoret, J. L., & Albanet, R. (1980). Description et étude scannographique du cervaux de Leborgne: La découverte de Broca. *Revue Neurologique, 136,* 563–683.

Cercy, S. P., & Bylsma, F. W. (1997). Lewy bodies and progressive dementia: A critical review and meta-analysis. *Journal of the International Neuropsychological Society, 3,* 179–194.

Chaffe, M. V., & Goldman-Rakic, P. S. (1998). Matching patterns of activity in primate prefrontal area 8a and parietal area 7ip neurons during spatial working memory task. *Journal of Neurophysiology, 79,* 2919–2940.

Chapanis, N. P., Utmatsu, S., Konigsmark, B., & Walker, A. E. (1972). Central phosphenes in man: A report of three cases. *Neuropsychologia, 10,* 27–42.

Charcot, J. M. (1883). Un cas de suppression brusque et isollé de la vision mentale des signes et des objets (formes et couleurs). *Progress Medicale, 11,* 568–571.

Charcot, J., & Marie, P. (1892). On hystero-epilepsy. In D. H. Tuke (Ed.), *A dictionary of psychological medicine* (Vol. 1, pp. 627–641). Philadelphia: Blakiston, Son, and Co.

Chassagnon, C., Boucher, M., Tomassi, M., Bianchi, G.-S., & Moene, Y. (1969). Demence thalamique d'origine vaculaire observation anatomo-clinique. *Journal de Medicine, Lion, 50,* 1153–1166.

Chen, E. Y. H., & Berrious, G. E. (1998). The nature of delusions: A hierarchical neural network approach. In D. J. Stein & J. Ludik (Eds.), *Neural network and psychopathology: Connectionist models in practice and research* (pp. 167–188). Cambridge: Cambridge University Press.

Chocolle, R., Chedru, F., Botte, M. C., Chain, F., & L'hermitte, F. (1975). Etude psychoacoustique d'un cas de "surdite corticale." *Neuropsychologia, 2*(13), 163–172.

Chow, K. L. (1951). Effects of partial extirpations of the posterior associative cortex on visually mediated behavior in monkeys. *Comparative psychology monographs, 20,* pp. 187–217. Berkeley and Los Angeles: University of California Press.

Christodoulou, G. N. (1978). Syndrome of subjective doubles. *American Journal of Psychiatry, 135,* 249–251.

Christodoulou, G. N. (1991). The delusional misidentification syndrome. *British Journal of Psychiatry, 159,* 65–69.

Chui, H. C. (1989). Dementia: A review emphasizing clinicopathologic correlation and brain behavior relationships. *Archives of Neurology, 46,* 806–814.

Chusid, G. J., de Gutierrez-Mahoney, C. G., & Margules-Lavergne, M. P. (1954). Speech disturbances in association with parasaggital frontal lesions. *Journal of Neurosurgery, 11,* 193–204.

Cipolotti, L., & Warrington, E. K. (1995). Semantic memory and reading ability: A case report. *Journal of the International Neuropsychological Society, 1,* 104–110.

Cleghorn, J. M., Franco, S., Szechtman, B., Kaplan, R. D., Szechtman, H., Brown, G. M., et al. (1992). Toward a brain map of auditory hallucinations. *American Journal of Psychiatry, 149*, 1062–1069.

Cleghorn, J. M., Garnett, E. S., & Nahmias, C. (1989). Increased frontal and reduced parietal glucose metabolism in acute untreated schizophrenia. *Psychiatry Research, 28*, 119–133.

Cloning, I., Cloning, K., & Hoff, H. (1968). *Neuropsychological symptoms and syndromes in lesions of the occipital lobe and the adjacent areas*. Paris: Gauthier-Villars.

Cocozza, J. J., & Stedman, H. J. (1976). The failure of psychiatric predictors of dangerousness: Clear and convincing evidence. *Rutgers Law Review, 29*, 1084–1101.

Coffey, C. E., Figiel, G. S., Djang, W. T., Cress, M., Saunders, B., & Weiner, R. D. (1988). Leukoencephalopathy in elderly depressed patients referred for ECT. *Biological Psychiatry, 24*, 143–161.

Coffey, C. E., Wilkinson, W. E., Weiner, R. D., et al. (1993). Quantitative cerebral anatomy in depression: A controlled magnetic resonance imaging study. *Archives of General Psychiatry, 50*, 7–16.

Cogan, D. G. (1973). Visual hallucinations as release phenomena. *Albrecht V Graefe Archives of Clinical and Experimental Ophalmology, 188*, 139–150.

Cohen, M. R., & Niska, R. W. (1980). Localized right hemisphere dysfunction and recurrent mania. *American Journal of Psychiatry, 137*, 847–848.

Cohen, N. J., & Squire, L. R. (1980). Preserved learning and retention of pattern analyzing skill in amnesia: Dissociation of knowing how and knowing that. *Science, 210*, 207–209.

Cohn, H. (1874). Über hemianopie bei Hirnleiden. *Klinische Monatsblätt für Augenheilkunde, 12*, 203.

Colombo, A., De Renzi, E., & Faglioni, P. (1976). The occurrence of visual neglect in patients with unilateral cerebral disease. *Cortex, 12*, 221–231.

Conrad, K. (1953). Un cas singular de "fantôme spéculaire." Phénomène héeautoscopique comme état permanent dans une tumuer de l'hypophyse. *L'Encéphale, 42*, 338–351.

Constantinidis, J., Tissot, R., & de Ajuriaguerra, J. (1970). Dystonie oculo-facio-cervicale ou paralysie progressive supranucléaire de Steele-Richardson-Olszewski. *Revue Neurologique, 122*, 249–262.

Convit, A., Jaeger, J. J., Lin, S. P., Meisuer, M., & Volavka, J. (1988). Predicting assaultiveness in psychiatric patients: A pilot study. *Hospital and Community Psychiatry, 39*, 429–434.

Corcoran, R., Cahill, C., & Frith, C. D. (1997). The appreciation of visual jokes in people with schizophrenia: A study of "mentalizing" ability. *Schizophrenia Research, 24*, 319–327.

Corcoran, R., Mercer, G., & Frith, C. D. (1995). Schizophrenic, symptomatology and social inference: Investigating "theory of mind" in people with schizophrenia. *Schizophrenia Research, 17*, 5–13.

Corkin, S. (1978). The role of different cerebral structures on somesthetic perception. In C. E. Carterette & M. P. Friedman (Eds.), *Handbook of perception* (Vol. 6B, pp. 105–155). New York: Academic Press.

Corkin, S. (1984). Lasting consequences of bilateral medial temporal excision: Clinical course and experimental findings in H.M. *Seminar in Neurology, 4,* 249–259.

Cornblatt, B. A., & Keilp, J. G. (1994). Impaired attention, genetic, and the pathophysiology of schizophrenia. *Schizophrenia Bulletin, 20,* 31–46.

Cornette, L., Dupont, P., Salmon, E., & Orban, G. A. (2001). The neural substrate of orientation working memory. *Journal of Cognitive Neuroscience, 13*(6), 813–828.

Corsellis, J. A. N. (1976). Aging and the dementias. In W. Blackwood & J. A. N. Corsellis (Eds.), *Greenfield's neuropathology* (pp. 796–848). Year Book Medical Publishers.

Cotard, J. (1882). Nihilistic delusions. In S. C. R. Hirsch & M. Shepherd (Eds.), *Themes and variations in European psychiatry* (M. Rohde, Trans.) (pp. 353–374). 1974. Bristol: John Wright.

Courbon, P., & Fail, G. (1927). Illusion de Frégoli. *Bulletin de la Societe/Clinique de Medicine Mental, 15,* 121–124.

Courbon, P., & Tusques, J. (1932). Illusion d'intermetamorphose et de charme. *Annales Medico-psychologiques, 90,* 401–405.

Courtney, S. M., Petit, L., Maisog, J. M., Ungerleider, L. G., & Haxby, J. V. (1998). An area specialized for spatial working memory in human frontal cortex. *Science, 279,* 1347–1351.

Courtney, S. M., Ungerleider, L. G., Keil, K., & Haxby, J. V. (1997). Transient and sustained activity in the distributed neural system for human working memory. *Nature, 386,* 608–611.

Courville, C. B. (1928). Auditory hallucinations provoked by intracranial tumors. *Journal of Nervous and Mental Diseases, 67,* 265–274.

Courville, C. B. (1955). *The effect of alcohol on the nervous system of man.* Los Angeles, CA: San Lucas Press.

Coyle, J. T., Price, D. L. & DeLong, M. R. (1983). Alzheimer's disease: A disorder of cortical cholinergic innervation. *Science, 219,* 1184–1190.

Craig, A. H., Cummings, J. L., Fairbanks, L., et al. (1996). Cerebral blood flow correlates of apathy in Alzheimer's disease. *Archives of Neurology, 53,* 1116–1120.

Cramon, D. Y., von Markowitsch, H. J., & Shuri, U. (1993). The possible contribution of the septal region to memory. *Neuropsychologia, 31,* 1159–1180.

Crary, M. A., & Heilman, K. M. (1988). Letter imagery deficits in a case of pure apraxic agraphia. *Brain and Language, 34,* 147–156.

Cravioto, A., Silverman, J., & Fergini, I. (1960). A clinical and pathological study of akinetic mutism. *Neurology, 10,* 10–21.

Critchley, M. (1929). Arteriosclerotic parkinsonism. *Brain, 52,* 23–83.

Critchley, M. (1950). The body image in neurology. *Lancet,* 335–340.

Critchley, M. (1953). *The parietal lobes*. London: E. Arnold and Co.

Croisile, B., Trillet, M., Hibert, O., et al. (1991). Désordres visuo-constructifs et alexie-agraphie associés à une atrophie corticale postérieure. *Revue Neurologique, 147,* 138–143.

Crow, T. J. (1980a). Molecular pathology of schizophrenia: More than one disease process? *British Medical Journal, 280,* 66–68.

Crow, T. J. (1980b). Positive and negative schizophrenic symptoms and the role of dopamine. *British Journal of Psychiatry, 137,* 383–386.

Cummings, J. (1985a). Organic delusions: Phenomenology, anatomical correlations, and review. *British Journal of Psychiatry, 146,* 184–197.

Cummings, J. (1985b). *Clinical neuropsychiatry*. Orlando, FL: Grune and Stratton.

Cummings, J. (1986). *Behavior and mood disorders in focal brain lesions*. Cambridge: Cambridge University Press.

Cummings, J. (1987). Multi-infarct dementia: Diagnosis and management. *Psychosomatics, 28,* 117–126.

Cummings, J. (1990). Introduction. In J. Cummings (Ed.), *Subcortical dementia* (pp. 3–16). New York: Oxford University Press.

Cummings, J. (1992). Depression and Parkinson's disease: A review. *American Journal of Psychiatry, 149,* 443–454.

Cummings, J. (1993). Frontal-subcortical circuits and human behavior. *Archives of Neurology, 50,* 873–880.

Cummings, J. (1994). Depression in neurologic diseases. *Psychiatric Annals, 24,* 525–539.

Cummings, J., Benson, D. F., Hill, M. A., et al. (1985). Aphasia in dementia of Alzheimer type. *Neurology, 35,* 394–397.

Cummings, J., & Duchen, L. W. (1981). The Kluver-Bucy syndrome in Pick disease. *Neurology, 31,* 1415–1422.

Cummings, J., Gosenfeld, L. F., Hooulihan, J. P., & Mccaffrey, T. (1983). Neuropsychiatric disturbances associated with idiopathic calcification of the basal ganglia. *Biological Psychiatry, 18,* 591–601.

Cummings, J., Hebben, N. A., Obler, L., & Leonard, P. (1980). Nonaphasic misnaming and other neurobehavioral features of an unusual toxic encephalopathy: Case study. *Cortex, 16,* 315–323.

Cummings, J., Miller, B., Hill, M. A., & Neshkes, R. (1987). Neuropsychiatric aspects of multi-infarct dementia and dementia of the Alzheimer type. *Archives of Neurology, 44,* 389–393.

Cummings, J., Syndulko, K., Goldberg, Z., & Treiman, D. M. (1982). Palinopsia reconsidered. *Neurology, 32,* 444–447.

Curran, F. J., & Schilder, P. (1935). Paraphasic signs in diffuse lesions of the brain. *Journal of Nervous and Mental Diseases, 82,* 613–636.

Currie, S., Heathfield, K. W. G., Henson, R. A., & Scott, D. F. (1971). Clinical course and prognosis of temporal lobe epilepsy: A survey of 666 cases. *Brain, 94,* 173–190.

Cutting, J. (1987). The phenomenology of acute organic psychosis: Comparison with acute schizophrenia. *British Journal of Psychiatry, 151,* 324–332.

Daly, D. D., & Love, J. G. (1958). Akinetic mutism. *Neurology, 8,* 238–242.

Damasio, A. R. (1985). Disorders of complex visual processing: Agnosia, achromatopsia, Balint's syndrome, and related difficulties in orientation and construction. In M. M. Mesulam (Ed.), *Principles of behavioral neurology* (pp. 259–288). Philadelphia: F. A. Davis.

Damasio, A. R. (1994). *Descarte's error: Emotion, reason and human brain.* New York: Grosset/Putnam.

Damasio, A. R., & Damasio, H. (1983). The anatomic basis of pure alexia. *Neurology, 33,* 1573–1583.

Damasio, A. R., Damasio, H., & Chang, C. H. (1980). Neglect following damage to frontal lobe or basal ganglia. *Neuropsychologia, 18,* 123–132.

Damasio, A. R., Damasio, H., Rizzo, M., Varney, N., & Gersh, F. (1982). Aphasia with non-hemorrhagic lesions in the basal ganglia and internal capsule. *Archives of Neurology, 39,* 15–20.

Damasio, A. R., Damasio, H., & Van Hoesen, G. W. (1982). Prosopagnosia: Anatomic basis and behavioral mechanisms. *Neurology, 32,* 331–341.

Damasio, A. R., Eslinger, P. J., Damasio, H., Van Hoesen, G. W., & Cornell, S. (1985). Multimodal amnesia syndrome following bilateral temporal and basal forebrain damage. *Archives of Neurology, 42,* 252–259.

Damasio, A. R., Graff-Radford, N. R., Eslinger, P. J., Damasio, H., & Kassel, N. (1985). Amnesia following basal forebrain lesions. *Archives of Neurology, 42,* 263–271.

Damasio, A. R., Tranel, D., & Damasio, H. C. (1991). Somatic markers and the guidance of behavior: Theory and preliminary testing. In H. S. Levin, H. M. Eisenberg, & A. L. Benton (Eds.), *Frontal lobe function and dysfunction* (pp. 217–229). New York: Oxford University Press.

Damasio, A. R., & Van Hoesen, G. W. (1983). Emotional disturbances associated with focal lesions of the limbic frontal lobe. In K. M. Heilman & P. Satz (Eds.), *Neuropsychology of human emotion* (pp. 85–110). New York: Guilford Press.

Damasio, H., Grabovski, T., Frank, R., Galaburda, A. M., & Damasio, A. R. (1994). The return of Phineas Gage: Clues about the brain from the skull of a famous patient. *Science, 264,* 1053–1224.

Damas-Mora, J. M. R., Jenner, M. A., & Eacott, S. E. (1980). On heautoscopy or the phenomenon of double: Case presentation and review of literature. *British Journal of Medical Psychology, 53,* 75–83.

Danielczyk, W. (1983). Various mental behavioral disorders in Parkinson's disease, primary degenerative senile dementia, and multiple infarction dementia. *Journal of Neural Transmissions, 56,* 161–176.

D'Antona, R., Baron, J. C., Samson, Y., Serdaru, M., Viader, F., Agid, Y., et al. (1985). Subcortical dementia: frontal cortex hypometabolism detected by positron tomography in patients with progressive supranuclear palsy. *Brain, 108,* 785–799.

Darby, D. G. (1993). Sensory aprosodia: A clinical clue to lesions of the inferior division of the right middle cerebral artery. *Neurology, 43,* 567–572.

David, A. (2001). Language and thought in schizophrenia. *Twelfth Annual Meeting of the American Neuropsychiatric Association,* Fort Meyers, FL.

David, A. S. (1990). Insight and psychosis. *British Journal of Psychiatry, 156,* 798–808.

David, A. S., & Cutting, J. C. (1994). *The neuropsychology of schizophrenia.* Hove, UK: Lawrence Erlbaum Associates.

Davidenkoff, S. N. (1912). Note sur la surdité verbale chromatoptique. *L'Encéphale, 2,* 127–140.

Davidenkov, S. N. (1956). *Clinical lectures on nervous illnesses* [in Russian]. Leningrad: Meditsina.

Davidenkova-Kulkova, E. F. (1959). *Diencephalic epilepsy* [in Russian]. Leningrad: Meditsina.

Davidson, M., Harvey, P. D., Powchik, P., et al. (1995). Severity of symptoms in chronically institutionalized geriatric schizophrenic patients. *American Journal of Psychiatry, 152,* 197–207.

Davies, J. M., Davies, K. R., Kleinman, G. M., Kirchner, H. S., & Taveras, J. M. (1978). Computer tomography of herpes simplex encephalitis with clinico-pathological correlation. *Radiology, 129,* 409–417.

Davis, M. (1986). Pharmacological and anatomical analysis of fear conditioning using the fear-potentiated startle paradigm. *Behavioral Neuroscience, 100,* 814–824.

Dax, M. (1865). Lesions de la moitie gauche de l'encephale coincidant avec trouble des signs de la penseé (lu a Montpellier nel 1836). *Gazette Hebdomadaire de Medécine et de Chirurgie, 17*(2ieme serie, 2), 259–260.

Déjerine, J. (1907). A propos de l'agnosie tactile. *Revue Neurologique, 15,* 781–784.

Déjerine, J. (1914). *Semiologie des affections du systeme nerveux.* Paris: Masson et Cie.

DeJong, R. N., Itabashi, H. H., & Olson, J. R. (1969). Memory loss due to hippocampal lesions: Report of a case. *Archives of Neurology, 20,* 339–348.

DeKosky, S. T., Heilman, K. M., Bowers, K. M., & Valenstein, E. (1980). Recognition and discrimination of emotional faces and pictures. *Brain and Language, 9,* 206–214.

Delay, J. (1935). *Les astereognosies: Pathologie de toucher.* Paris: Masson et Cie.

Delay, J., Brion, S., & Derouesné, J. (1964). Syndrome de Korsakoff et étiologie tumorale. *Revue Neurologique, 3,* 97–133.

Delay, J., Brion, S., & Ellissalde, B. (1958). Corpus mammilaires et syndrome de Korsakoff: Etude anatomique de huit cas de syndrome Korsakoff d'origine alcoholique sans alteration significative du cortex cerebrale. *Press Medicale, 66,* 1849–1852.

Delgado-Escueta, A. V., Mattson, R. H., King, L., et al. (1981). The nature of aggression during epileptic seizures. Special report. *New England Journal of Medicine, 305,* 711–716.

DeLisi, L. E., Buchsbaum, M. S., Holcomb, H. H., et al. (1985). Clinical correlates of decreased anteroposterior gradients in positron emission tomography (PET) of schizophrenic patients. *American Journal of Psychiatry, 142,* 78–81.

Della Salla, S., Laiacona, M., Spinnler, H., & Trivelli, C. (1993). Autobiographical recollection and frontal damage. *Neuropsychologia, 31,* 823–839.

Della Salla, S., Lucchelli, F., & Spinner, H. (1987). Ideomotor apraxia in patients with dementia of Alzheimer type. *Journal of Neurology, 234,* 91–93.

Della Salla, S., Muggia, S., Spinner, H., & Zuffi, M. (1995). Cognitive modeling of face procession: Evidence from Alzheimer patients. *Neuropsychologia, 33,* 675–687.

Della Sala, S., & Spinnler, H. (1999). Slowly progressive isolated cognitive deficits. In G. Denes & L. Pizzamiglio (Eds.), *Handbook of clinical and experimental neuropsychology* (pp. 775–807). Hove, UK: Psychology Press.

DeLuca, J., & Cicerone, K. D. (1991). Confabulation following the aneurysm of the anterior communicating artery. *Cortex, 27,* 417–423.

DeLuca, J., & Diamond, B. J. (1995). Aneurysm of the anterior communicating artery: A review of neuroanatomical and neuropsychological sequelae. *Journal of Clinical and Experimental Psychology, 17,* 100–121. ‘

Denes, G., Cipolotti, L., & Zorgi, M. (1999). Acquired dyslexias and dysgraphias. In G. Denes & L. Pizzamiglio (Eds.), *Handbook of clinical and experimental neuropsychology* (pp. 289–317). Hove, UK: Psychology Press.

Denny-Brown, D. (1958). The nature of apraxia. *Journal of Nervous and Mental Disease, 1,* 9–33.

De Morsier, G. (1938). Les hallucinations visuelles dans les lésions du diencéphale (section 2). *Revue Neuro-Oto-Ophtalmologie, 16,* 244–352.

De Poorter, M. C., Pasquier, F., & Petit, H. (1991). Akinésie psychique et troubles mnésiques après intoxication oxycarbonée. *Acta Neurologica Belgica, 91,* 271–279.

De Renzi, E. (1983). *Disorders of space exploration and cognition.* Chichester, UK: Wiley.

De Renzi, E. (1986). Prosopagnosia in two patients with CT scan evidence of damage confined to the right hemisphere. *Neuropsychologia, 24,* 385–389.

De Renzi, E. (1999). Agnosia. In G. Denes & L. Pizzamiglio (Eds.), *Handbook of clinical and experimental neuropsychology* (pp. 371–407). Hove, UK: Psychology Press.

De Renzi, E., & Faglioni, P. (1963). L'autotopagnosia. *Archiv di Psicologia, Neurologia e Psichiatria, 24,* 1–34.

De Renzi, E., & Faglioni, P. (1967). The relationship between visuo-spatial impairment and constructional apraxia. *Cortex, 3,* 327–342.

De Renzi, E., Faglioni, P., & Scotti, G. (1970). Hemisphere contribution to exploration of space through the visual and tactile modality. *Cortex, 6,* 191–203.

De Renzi, E., & Lucchelli, F. (1988). Ideational apraxia. *Brain, 11,* 1173–1185.

De Renzi, E., & Lucchelli, F. (1993). Dense retrograde amnesia, intact learning capability and abnormal forgetting rate: A consolidation deficit. *Cortex, 29,* 449–466.

De Renzi, E., Motti, F., & Nichelli, P. (1980). Imitating gestures: A quantitative approach to ideomotor apraxia. *Archive of Neurology, 37,* 6–10.

De Renzi, E., Pieczuro, A., & Vignolo, L. A. (1966). Oral apraxia and aphasia. *Cortex, 2,* 50–73.

De Renzi, E., Scotti, G., & Spinnler, H. (1969). Perceptual and associative disorders of visual recognition: Relationship to the side of cerebral lesion. *Neurology, 19,* 634–642.

De Renzi, E., & Spinnler, H. (1966). Facial recognition in brain-damaged patients: An experimental approach. *Neurology, 16,* 145–152.

De Renzi, E., & Vignolo, L. (1962). The Token Test: A sensitive test to detect receptive disturbances in aphasics. *Brain, 85,* 665–678.

De Renzi, E., Zambolin, A., & Grisi, G. (1987). The pattern of neuropsychological impairment associated with left posterior cerebral artery infarcts. *Brain, 110,* 1099–1116.

Deshimaru, M., Miyakawa, T., & Suzuki, T. (1977). An autopsy case of head injury with a manic depressive state. *Brain Nerve (Tokyo), 29,* 787–790.

Desimone, R., Albright, T. D., Cross, C. G., & Bruce, C. J. (1984). Stimulus-selective properties of inferior temporal neurons in the macaque. *Journal of Neuroscience, 8,* 2051–2068.

Desimone, R., & Underleider, L. G. (1989). Neural mechanisms of visual processing in monkeys. In F. Boller & F. Grafman (Eds.), *Handbook of neuropsychology.* Amsterdam: Elsevier.

D'Esposito, M., Verfaellie, M., Alexander, M. P., & Katz, D. I. (1995). Amnesia following bilateral fornix transection. *Neurology, 45,* 1546–1550.

DesRossiers, G., & Kavanagh, D. (1987). Cognitive assessments in closed head injury: Stability, validity and parallel forms for two neuropsychological measures of recovery. *International Journal of Clinical Neuropsychology, 9,* 162–173.

Deutsch, G., & Eisenberg, H. M. (1997). Frontal blood flow changes in recovery from coma. *Journal of Cerebral Blood Flow Metabolism, 7,* 29–34.

Devanand, D. P., Verma, A. K., Tirumalasetti, F., & Sackeim, H. A. (1991). Absence of cognitive impairment after more than 100 lifetime ECT treatments. *American Journal of Psychiatry, 148,* 929–932.

Devinsky, O., & Bear, D. (1984). Varieties of aggressive behavior in temporal lobe epilepsy. *American Journal of Psychiatry, 141,* 651–665.

Devinsky, O., Kelley, K., Porter, R. J., & Theodore, W. H. (1988). Clinical and electroencephalographic features of simple partial seizures. *Neurology, 38,* 1347–1352.

Devinsky, O., Putnam, F., Graftman, J., Bromfield, E., & Theodor, W. H. (1989). Dissociative states and epilepsy. *Neurology, 39,* 835–840.

Devous, M. D., Rush, A. J., Schlesser, M. A., et al. (1984). Single-photon tomographic determination of cerebral blood flow in psychiatric disorders. *Journal of Nuclear Medicine, 25,* 57.

Dewhurst, K., Oliver, J., Trick, K. L. K., & McKnight, A. L. (1969). Neuro-psychiatric aspects of Huntington's disease. *Confina Neurologica, 31,* 258–268.

DeWitt, L., Grek, A., Kisler, J. P., Levine, D. N., Davis, K., Brady, T. J., et al. (1984). Nuclear magnetic resonance imaging and neurobehavioral syndromes: Five illustrative cases. *Neurology, 34,* 88–188.

Di Sclafini, V., MacKay, R. D. S., Meyerhoff, D. J., Norman, D., Weiner, M. W., & Fein, G. (1997). Brain atrophy in HIV infection is more strongly associated with CDC clinical stage than with cognitive impairment. *Journal of the International Neuropsychological Society, 3,* 276–287.

Dobelle, W. N., & Mladejorsky, M. G. (1974). Phosphenes produced by electrical stimulation of human occipital cortex, and their application to the development of a prosthesis for the blind. *Journal of Physiology, 2,* 553–576.

Doehring, D. G., & Reitan, R. M. (1962). Concept attainment of human adults with lateralized cerebral lesions. *Journal of Nervous and Mental Disease, 161,* 185–190.

Dominian, J., Serafetinides, E. A., & Dewhurst, M. (1963). A follow-up study of late onset epilepsy. *British Medical Journal, 1,* 431–435.

Donaldson, A. A. (1979). CT scan in Alzheimer pre-senile dementia. In A. I. M. Glen & L. J. Whalley (Eds.), *Alzheimer's disease: Early recognition of potentially reversible deficit* (pp. 97–101). New York: Churchill Livingstone.

Dongier, S. (1959/1960). Statistical study of clinical and electroencephalographic manifestations of 536 psychotic episodes occurring in 516 epileptics between clinical seizures. *Epilepsia, 1,* 117–142.

Doniger, J. M., Silipo, G., Rabinowicz, E., Snodgrass, J. G., & Javitt, D. C. (2002). Impaired sensory processing as a basis for object recognition deficits in schizophrenia. *American Journal of Psychiatry, 158,* 1818–1826.

Donovan, N. J., & Barry, J. J. (1994). Compulsive symptoms associated with frontal lobe injury. *American Journal of Psychiatry, 151,* 618.

Doody, R. S., & Jankovic, J. (1992). The alien hand and related signs. *Journal of Neurology, Neurosurgery and Psychiatry, 55,* 806–810.

Dooneief, G., Mirabello, E., Bell, K., et al. (1992). An estimate of the incidence of depression in idiopathic Parkinson's disease. *Archives of Neurology, 49,* 305–307.

D'Orban, P. T., & Dalton, J. (1989). Violent crime and the menstrual cycle. *Psychological Medicine, 10,* 353–359.

Dorofeeva, S. A. (1967). Study of auditory perception in local lesions of cerebral hemispheres [in Russian]. In J. M. Tonkonogy (Ed.), *Psychological clinical studies* (pp. 145–149). Leningrad: Bechterev Institute Press.

Dorofeeva, S. A. (1970). *Study of the peculiarities of auditory perception in sensory aphasia in relation to the goals of speech rehabilitation* [in Russian]. Leningrad: Bechterev Institute Press.

Dorofeeva, S. A., & Kaidanova, S. I. (1969). On disorders of memory traces in auditory analyzer in sensory aphasia [in Russian]. In J. M. Tonkonogy (Ed.), *Psychological experiment in neurological and psychiatric clinic* (pp. 185–199). Leningrad: Bechterev Institute Press.

Drachman, D. A., & Adams, R. D. (1962). Herpes simplex and acute inclusion-body encephalitis. *Archives of Neurology, 7,* 45–63.

Drachman, D. A., & Arbit, J. (1966). Memory and the hippocampal complex. II. Is memory a multiple process? *Archives of Neurology, 15,* 52–61.

Drake, M. E. (1988). Cotard's syndrome and temporal lobe epilepsy. *Psychiatry Journal of University of Ottawa, 13,* 36–39.

Drevets, W. C., & Rubin, E. H. (1989). Psychotic symptoms and the longitudinal course in senile dementia of the Alzheimer type. *Biological Psychiatry, 25,* 39–48.

Drevets, W. C., Videen, T. O., Price, J. L., Preskorn, S. H., Carmichael, S. T., & Raichle, M. E. (1992). A functional anatomical study of unipolar depression. *Journal of Neuroscience, 12,* 3628–3641.

Dugas, L., & Moutier, F. (1911). *La dépersonalisation.* Paris: Félix Alcan.

Dunkley, G., & Rogers, D. (1994). The cognitive impairment of severe psychiatric illness. In eds

Dupont, R. M., Jernigan, T. L., Gillin, J. C., et al. (1987). Subcortical signal hyperintensities in bipolar patients detected by MRI. *Psychiatry Research, 21,* 357–358.

Duyckaerts, C., Derouesne, C., Signoret, J. L., Gray, F., Escourolle, R., & Castaigne, P. (1985). Bilateral and limited amygdalohippocampal lesions causing a pure amnestic syndrome. *Annals of Neurology, 18,* 314–319.

Early, T. S. (1990). Assymetric metabolism over basal ganglia in catatonia. *Biological Psychiatry, 28,* 177–179.

Early, T. S., Relman, E. M., Raichle, M. E., & Spitzmagel, E. L. (1987). Left globus pallidus abnormality in newly medicated patients with schizophrenia. *Proceeding of the National Academy of Science USA, 84,* 561–563.

Eastwood, M. R., Rifat, S. L., Nobbs, H., et al. (1989). Mood disorder following cerebrovascular accident. *British Journal of Psychiatry, 154,* 195–200.

Ebert, D., Feistel, H., Barocka, A., et al. (1994). Increase limbic flow in total sleep deprivation in major depression with melancholia. *Psychiatric Research, 55,* 101–109.

Efron, R. (1963). Temporal perception, aphasia and *déjà vu. Brain, 86,* 403–424.

Efron, R. (1968). What is perception? *Boston Studies in Philosophy of Science, 4,* 137–173.

Egger, M. D., & Flynn, J. P. (1981). Effects of electrical stimulation of the amygdala on hypothalomically elicited attack behavior in cats. *Journal of Neurophysiology, 26,* 705–720.

Elithorn, A. (1964). Intelligence, perceptual integration and the minor hemisphere syndrome. *Neuropsychologia, 2,* 327–332.

Elkis, H., Freedman, L., Wise, A., & Meltzer, H. Y. (1995). Meta-analyses of studies of ventricular enlargement and cortical sulcal prominence in mood disorders. *Archives of General Psychiatry, 52,* 735–745.

Elliot, F. A. (1976). The neurology of explosive rage: The dyscontrol syndrome. *Practitioner, 217,* 51–60.

Elliot, F. A. (1977). Propranolol for the control of dangerous behavior following acute brain damage. *Annals of Neurology, 1,* 489–491.

Elliot, F. A. (1982). Neurological findings of an adult minimal brain dysfunction and the dyscontrol syndrome. *Journal of Nervous and Mental Diseases, 170,* 680–687.

Elliot, F. A. (1992). Violence: The neurologic contribution: An overview. *Archives of Neurology, 49,* 595–603.

Elman, J. L., Bates, E., Johnson, M. H., Karmiloff-Smith, A., Parisi, D., & Plunkett, K. (1996). *Rethinking innateness: A connectionist perspective on development.* Cambridge, MA: MIT Press.

Emey, V. O. B., Gillie, E., & Ramdev, P. T. (1994). Vascular dementia redefined. In V. O. B. Emery & T. E. Oxman (Eds.), *Dementia, presentation, differential diagnosis, nosology* (pp. 162–194). Baltimore, MD: Johns Hopkins University Press.

Endo, K., Makishita, H., Yangisawa, N., & Sugishita, M. (1992). Tactile agnosia and tactile aphasia: Symptomatological and anatomical differences. *Cortex, 28,* 445–449.

Engel, G., & Aring, C. (1945). Hypothalamic attacks with thalamic lesion. I. Physiologic and psychologic considerations. *Archives of Neurology and Psychiatry, 54,* 37–43.

Engel, G. L., & Romano, J. (1959). Delirium: A syndrome of cerebral insufficiency. *Journal of Chronic Diseases, 9,* 260–277.

Erkinjuntti, T., Haltia, M., Palo, J., Sulkava, R., & Paetau, A. (1988). Accuracy of the clinical diagnosis of vascular dementia: A prospective clinical and postmortem neuropathological study. *Journal of Neurology, Neurosurgery, and Psychiatry, 51,* 1037–1044.

Escueta, A. V., Boxley, J., Stubbs, N., Waddel, G., & Wilson, W. A. (1974). Prolonged twilight state and automatisms: A case report. *Neurology, 24,* 331–339.

Eslinger, P. J., & Damasio, A. R. (1985). Severe disturbances in higher cognition after bilateral frontal lobe ablation: Patient EVR. *Neurology, 35,* 1731–1741.

Esquirol, J. E. D. (1814). *Les Maladies Mentales.* Paris, Ballières. [*Mental Malady* (1965). New York: Hafner Press.]

Ettlinger, G. (1956). Sensory deficit in visual agnosia. *Journal of Neurology, Neurosurgery and Psychiatry, 19,* 297–308.

Evans, J., Wilson, B., Wraight, E. P., & Hodges, J. R. (1993). Neuropsychological and SPECT scan findings during and after transient global amnesia: Evidence for the differential impairment of remote episodic memory. *Journal of Neurology, Neurosurgery, and Psychiatry, 56,* 1227–1230.

Exner, S. (1881). *Untersuchungen über die Lokalisation der Funktionen in der Grosshirnrinde des Menschen.* Vienna: Braumuller.

Faglioni, P., Spinnler, H., & Vignolo, L. A. (1969). Contrasting behaviour of right and left hemisphere damaged patients on a discriminative and semantic task of auditory recognition. *Cortex, 5,* 366–389.

Fairweather, D. (1947). Psychiatric aspects of post-encephalitic syndrome. *Journal of Mental Science, 93,* 201–254.

Farah, M. (1989). The neural basis of mental imagery. *Trends in Neuroscience, 12,* 395–399.

Farah, M. J. (1990). *Visual agnosia.* Cambridge, MA: MIT Press.

Farah, M. J. (1995). The neural bases of mental imagery. In M. S. Gazzaniga (Ed.), *The cognitive neuroscience* (pp. 963–975). Cambridge, MA: MIT Press.

Farah, M. J., Hammond, K. L., Levine, D. N., & Calvanio, R. (1988). Visual and spatial mental imagery: Dissociable system of representation. *Cognitive Psychology, 20,* 439–462.

Farkas, T., Reivich, M., Alavi, A., et al. (1980). The application of 18-fluoro-2-deoxyglucose and positron emission tomography in the study of psychiatric conditions. In J. V. Assoneau, R. A. Hawkins, W. D. Lest, & F. A. Welch (Eds.), *Cerebral metabolism and neural function* (pp. 403–411). Baltimore, MD: Williams and Wilkins.

Farnsworth, D. (1957). *Farnsworth-Munsell 100-hue test for color vision.* Baltimore, MD: Munsell Color Company.

Farrell, M. J. (1996). Topographical disorientation. *Neurocase, 2,* 509–520.

Faust, C. (1955). *Die zerebralen herdstorungen bein hinterhaupverletzungen und ihre beuteilung.* Stuttgart: G. Thieme Verlag.

Faust, G. (1960). Die psychischen Storungen nach Hirntraumen: Akute traumatische Psychosen und psychische Spatfolgen nach Hirnverletzungen. In H. W. Gruhle, B. R. Jung, W. Mayer-gross, & M. Muller (Eds.), *Psychiatrie der Gegenwart* (Vol. 2, pp. 552–646). Berlin: Springer.

Fay, T., & Scott, M. (1939). Auditory and formed visual hallucinations in a case of meningioma of the brain. *Archives of Neurology and Psychiatry, 41,* 859–860.

Fazekas, F., Chawluk, J. B., Alavi, A., Hurtig, H. I., & Zimmerman, R. A. (1987). MR signal abnormalities at 1.5 T in Alzheimer's dementia and normal aging. *American Journal of Neuroradiology, 8,* 421–426.

Feinberg, T. E. (2001). *Altered ego: How the brain creates the self.* Oxford: Oxford University Press.

Feinberg, W. M., & Rapcsak, S. Z. (1989). "Peduncular hallucinosis" following paramedian thalamic infarction. *Neurology, 39,* 1535–1536.

Felleman, D. J., & Van Essen, C. (1991). Distributed hierarchical processing in the primate cerebral cortex. *Cerebral Cortex, 1,* 1–47.

Féré, M. Ch. (1891). Note sur les hallucinations autoscpoiques ou spéculaires et sur les hallucinations altruits. *Comptes Rendue des Séances de la Société du Biologie, 3,* 1–453.

Ferro, J. M., & Santos, M. E. (1984). Associative visual agnosia: A case study. *Cortex, 20,* 121–134.

Feuchtwanger, E. (1923). *Die Funktionen des Stirnhirns: Ihre Pathologie und Psychologie.* Berlin: Springer.

Feuchtwanger, E. (1930). *Amusie, Studien zur pathologischen Psychologie der acustischen Warnehmung und Vorstellung und ihrer Struktugebiete in Musik und Sprache*. Berlin: J. Springer.

Ffytche, D. H., Guy, C. N., & Zeki, S. (1996). Motion specific responses from a blind hemifield. *Brain, 119,* 1971–1982.

Figiel, G. S., Hassen, M. A., Zorumski, C., et al. (1991). ECT-induced delirium in depressed patients with Parkinson's disease. *Journal of Neuropsychiatry and Clinical Neuroscience, 3,* 405–411.

Figiel, G. S., Krishnan, K. R., Breitner, J. C., et al. (1989). Radiologic correlates of anti-depressants-induced delirium: The possible significance of basal ganglia lesion. *Journal of Neuropsychiatry and Clinical Neuroscience, 1,* 188–190.

Figiel, G. S., Krishnan, K. R. R., Doraiswamy, P. M., et al. (1990). Brain MRI subcortical structural changes in late age onset depression. *Biological Psychiatry, 27,* 61.

Figiel, G. S., Krishnan, K. R., Doraiswamy, P. M., Rao, V. P., Nemeroff, C. B., & Boyko, O. B. (1991). Subcortical hyperintensities on brain magnetic imaging: A comparison between late age onset and early onset elderly depressed subjects. *Neurobiology of Aging, 12,* 245–247.

Finkelnburg, F. C. (1870). Vortrag in der Niederrheinischen Geselschaft in Bonn: Medicinische Section. *Berliner klinishen Wochenschrift, 187,* 449–450, 460–461.

Fires, W. (1981). The projection from the lateral geniculate nucleus to the prestriate cortex of the macaque monkey. *Proceeding of the Royal Society of London, B, 213,* 73–80.

Fish, F. (1967). *Clinical psychopathology*. Bristol: John Wright.

Fish, F. (1985). *Fish's clinical psychopathology* (M. Hamilton, Ed.). Bristol, UK: Wright.

Fisher, C. M. (1982). Disorientation for place. *Archives of Neurology, 30,* 33–36.

Fisher, M., Brant-Zzawadzki, M., Ameriso, S., et al. (1993). Subcortical magnetic resonance imaging changes in a healthy elderly population. *Journal of Neuroimaging, 3,* 28–32.

Fisher, S. (1961). Psychiatric considerations of cerebral vascular disease. *American Journal of Cardiology, 7,* 379.

Fitzgerald, R. G. (1971). Visual phenomenology in recent blind adult. *American Journal of Psychiatry, 127,* 1533–1539.

Fleming, G. W. T. H. (1923). A case of Lilliputian hallucinations with a subsequent single macroscopic hallucination. *Journal of Mental Science, 69,* 86–89.

Fletcher, P. C., Happé, F., Frith, U., Baker, S. C., Dolan, R. J., Frakowiak, R. S., et al. (1995). Other minds in the brain: A functional imaging study of "theory of mind" in story comprehension. *Cognition, 57,* 109–128.

Flor-Henry, P. (1969). Psychosis and temporal lobe epilepsy: A controlled investigation. *Epilepsia, 10,* 363–395.

Flourens, M. J. P. (1842). *Examen de phrénologie*. Paris: Hachette.

Flourens, M. J. P. (1824). *Recherches expérimentales sur les propriétés et les fonctions du système nerveux dans les animaux vertébrés*. Paris: Crovost.

Flynn, F. C., Cummings, J. L., & Tomiyasu, U. (1989). Altered behavior associated with damage to the ventro-medial hypothalamus. *Behavioural Neurology, 1*, 49–58.

Fodor, J. A. (1983). *Modularity and mind*. Cambridge, MA: MIT Press.

Foerster, O. (1931). The cerebral cortex in man. *Lancet, 2*, 309–312.

Foerster, O. (1936). Sensible cortical felder. In O. Bumke & O. Foerster (Eds.), *Bumke Foerster Handbuch der Neurologie* (Vol. 6, pp. 1–448). Berlin: Springer.

Foix, C. (1916). Contribution a l'étude de l'apraxie ideomotrice. *Revue Neurologique, 1*, 285–298.

Foix, C. (1922). Sur une varieté de troubles bilateraux de la sensibilité par lesion unilaterale du cerveau. *Revue Neurologique, 29*, 322–331.

Folstein, M. F., Folstein, S. E., & McHugh, P. R. (1975). "Mini-mental state": A practical method for grading thru cognitive state of patients for the clinician. *Journal of Psychiatric Research, 12*, 189–198.

Folstein, M. F., Maiberger, R., & McHugh, P. R. (1977). Mood disorder as a specific complication of stroke. *Journal of Neurology, Neurosurgery, and Psychiatry, 40*, 1018–1020.

Folstein, S. E. (1989). *Huntington's disease: A disorder of families*. Baltimore, MD: Johns Hopkins University Press.

Folstein, S. E., Brandt, J., & Folstein, M. (1990). Huntington's disease. In J. L. Cummings (Ed.), *Subcortical dementia* (pp. 87–107). New York: Oxford University Press.

Folstein, S. F., Folstein, M. F., & McHugh, P. R. (1979). Psychiatric syndromes in Huntington's disease. *Advances in Neurology, 23*, 281–289.

Folstein, S. F., Franz, M. L., Jensen, B. A., et al. (1983) Conduct disorder and affective disorder among the offspring of patients with Huntington's disease. *Psychological Medicine, 13*, 45–52.

Fontaine, R., & Breton, G. (1990). Temporal lobe abnormalities in panic disorder: An MRI study. *Biological Psychiatry, 27*, 304–310.

Forster, R. (1890). Ueber Rinden blindheit. *Graefe's Archiv für Ophtalmologie, 36*, 94–108.

Förstl, H., Howard, R., & Levy, R. (1992). Mental disturbances of arteriosclerotic origin: A. Alzheimer. *Neuropsychiatry, Neuropsychology, and Behavioral Neurology, 5*, 1–6.

Foster, N. L., Chase, T. N., Fedio, P., Patronas, N. J., Brooks, R. A., & DiChiro, G. (1983). Alzheimer's disease: Focal cortical changes shown by positron emission tomography. *Neurology, 33*, 961–965.

Foster, N. L., Wilhelmsen, K., Sima, A. A., Jones, M. Z., D'Amato, C. J., & Gilman, S. (1997). Frontotemporal dementia and parkinsonism linked to chromosome 17: A consensus conference. *Annals of Neurology, 41*, 706–715.

Fox, J. H., Topel, J. L., & Huckman, M. S. (1975). Use of computerized tomography in senile dementia. *Journal of Neurology, Neurosurgery, and Psychiatry, 38,* 948–953.

Frances, A. (1979). Familial basal ganglia calcification and schizophreniform psychosis. *British Journal of Psychiatry, 135,* 360–362.

Frantsuz, A. G., Tonkonogy, J. M., & Levin, I. Y. (1964). Computer application in differential diagnosis of aphasia [in Russian]. *The Korsakoff Journal of Neurology and Psychiatry, 64,* 1759–1765.

Fredricks, J. A. M. (1969). Disorders of body schema. In P. J. Vinken & G. W. Bruyn (Eds.), *Handbook of clinical neurology* (Vol. 4, pp. 207–240). Amsterdam: North Holland Publishing Company.

Freedman, D. J., Riesenhuber, M., Poggio, T., & Miller, E. K. (2001). Categorical representation of visual stimuli in the primate prefrontal cortex. *Science, 291,* 312–316.

Freedman, M., Alexander, M. P., & Naeser, M. A. (1984). Anatomical basis of transcortical motor aphasia. *Neurology, 34,* 409–417.

Freedman, M., Black, S., Ebert, P., & Bimms, M. (1998). Orbitofrontal function: Object alternation and perseveration. *Cerebral Cortex, 8*(1), 18–27.

Freeland, J., & Puente, A. E. (1984). Discrimination of schizophrenics and brain-damaged patients with the Luria-Nebraska Neuropsychological Battery and the WAIS. *International Journal of Clinical Neuropsychology, 6,* 261–263.

Freeman, F. S. (1959). *Theory and practice of neuropsychological testing.* New York: Henry Holt.

Freeman, W., & Watts, J. W. (1942). *Psychosurgery.* Springfield, IL: Carles C. Thomas.

Freeman, W., & Watts, J. W. (1943). Prefrontal lobotomy. *American Journal of Psychiatry, 99,* 798–806.

Freidenberg, D. L., & Cummings, J. L. (1989). Parkinson's disease, depression, and the on-off phenomenon. *Psychosomatics, 30,* 94–99.

Freud, S. (1891). *Zur Auffassung der Aphasien: Eine kritische Studie, Leupzig & Wien, Deuticke [On aphasia: A critical study by E. Stengel]* (E. Stengel, Trans.). (1953). New York: International Universities Press.

Freund, C. S. (1889). Über optische Aphasie and Seelenblindheit. *Archiv für Psychiatrie und. Nervenkrrankheiten, 20,* 276–297, 371–416.

Fried, I., MacDonald, K. A., & Wilson, C. L. (1997). Single neuron activity in human hippocampus and amygdala during recognition of objects and faces. *Neuron, 18,* 753–765.

Friedland, R. P., Budinger, T. F., Ganz, E., et al. (1983). Regional cerebral metabolic alterations in dementia of Alzheimer type: Positron emission tomography with [18F]fluorodeoxyglucose. *Journal of Computer Assisted Tomography, 7,* 590–598.

Friedlander, W. J., & Feinstern, G. H. (1956). Petit mal status. *Neurology (Minneapolis), 6,* 357–364.

Friedman, J. H. (1985). Syndrome of diffuse encephalopathy due to nondominant thalamic infarction. *Neurology, 35,* 1524–1526.

Fries, W., & Swihart, A. (1990). Disturbance of rhythm sense following right hemisphere damage. *Neuropsychologia, 28,* 1137–1323.

Frith, C., Stevens, M., Johnstone, E., Deaken, J., Lawler, P. & Crow, T. (1983). Effect of ECT and depression on various aspects of memory. *British Journal of Psychiatry, 142,* 610–617.

Frith, C. D., & Corcoran, R. (1996). Exploring "theory of mind" in people with schizophrenia. *Psychological Medicine, 26,* 521–530.

Fröshaug, H., & Ytrehus, A. (1956). A study of general paresis with special reference to the reason for the admission of these patients to hospital. *Acta Psychiatrica and Neurologica Scandinavica, 31,* 35–60.

Fujii, K., Sadoshima, S., Ishitsuka, T., Kusuda, K., Kuwabara, Y., Ichiya, Y., et al. (1989). Regional cerebral blood flow and cerebral metabolism in patients with transient global amnesia: A positron emission tomography study. *Journal of Neurology, Neurosurgery, and Psychiatry, 52,* 622–630.

Fujita, I., Tanaka, K., Ito, M., & Cheng, K. (1992). Columns for visual features of objects in monkey inferotemporal cortex. *Nature, 360,* 343–346.

Funahashi, S., Bruce, C. J., & Goldman-Rakic, P. S. (1989). Mnemonic coding of visual space in the monkey's dorsal prefrontal cortex. *Journal of Neurophysiology, 61,* 331–349.

Funnel, E. (1983). Phonological processing in reading: New evidence from acquired dyslexia. *British Journal of Psychology, 74,* 159–180.

Fuster, J. M. (1989). *The prefrontal cortex: Anatomy, physiology, and neuropsychology of the frontal lobe.* New York: Raven Press.

Gade, A. (1982). Amnesia after operation on aneurysm of the anterior communicating artery. *Archives of Neurology, 18,* 46–49.

Gaffan, D., & Gaffan, E. A. (1991). Amnesia in man following transection of the fornix: A review. *Brain, 114,* 2611–2618.

Gainotti, G. (1968). Les manifestation de negligence et d'inattention pour l'hemiespace. *Cortex, 4,* 64–91.

Gainotti, G., Caltagirone, C., & Ibba, A. (1975). Semantic and phonemic aspects of auditory language comprehension in aphasia. *Linguistics, 154/155,* 15–30.

Gainotti, G., Caltagirone, C., Masullo, C., et al. (1980). Patterns of neuropsychologic impairment in various diagnostic groups of dementia. In L. Amaducci, A. N. Davison, & P. Anuono (Eds.), *Aging of the brain and dementia* (pp. 245–250). New York: Raven Press.

Gainotti, G., D'Erme, P., Montelone, D., & Silveri, M. C. (1986). Mechanisms of lateral spatial neglect in relation to laterality of cerebral lesion. *Brain, 109,* 599–612.

Gainotti, G., Messerli, P., & Tissot, R. (1972). Qualitative analysis of unilateral spatial neglect in relation to laterality of cerebral lesion. *Journal of Neurology, Neurosurgery, and Psychiatry, 35,* 545–550.

Gainotti, G., & Tiacci, C. (1970). Patterns of drawing disability in right and left hemispheric patients. *Neuropsychologia, 8,* 379–384.

Gainotti, G. (1972). Emotional behavior and hemispheric side of the lesion. *Cortex, 8,* 41–55.

Gal, P. (1958). Mental symptoms in cases of tumor of temporal lobe. *American Journal of Psychiatry, 115,* 157–160.

Gall, F. J., & Spurzheim, H. (1810–1819). *Anatomie et physiologie du systèm nerveaux en général et du cerveau en particulier* (4 vol.). Paris: F. Schoell.

Gallagher, M., Graham, P. W., & Holland, P. (1990). The amygdala central nucleus and appetitive Pavlovian conditioning: Lesions impair one class of conditioned behavior. *Journal of Neuroscience, 10,* 1906–1911.

Gallese, V., Fadiga, L., Fogassi, L., Luppino, G., & Murata, A. (1997). A parietal-frontal circuit for hand grasping movements in the monkey: Evidence from reversible inactivation experiments. In P. Their & H.-O. Karnath (Eds.), *Parietal lobe contribution to orientation in 3D space.* Experimental Brain Research Series (Vol. 25, pp. 225–270). Berlin, Springer.

Gallese, V., Fadiga, L., Fogassi, L., & Rizzolatti, G. (1996). Action recognition in the premotor cortex. *Brain, 119,* 593–609.

Gallese, V., Murata, A., Kaseda, M., Niki, N., & Sakata, H. (1994). Deficit of hand preshaping after muscimol injection in monkey parietal cortex. *Neuroreport, 5,* 1525–1529.

Gallistel, C. R. (1990). *The organization of learning.* Cambridge, MA: MIT Press.

Gamper, E. (1928). Zur frague der poliencephalitis haemorrhagica der chronischen alkoholiker: Befund beim alkoholishcen Korsakow and ihre beziehungen zum klinischen bild. *Deutsche Zeitschrift für Nervenkrankheiten, 102,* 122–129.

Gandour, J., & Dandarananda, R. (1984) Voice onset time in aphasia: Thai II. Production. *Brain and Language, 23,* 177–205.

Garcha, H. S., & Ettlinger, G. (1978). The effects of unilateral and bilateral removals of the second somatosensory cortex (area SII): A profound tactile disorder in monkeys. *Cortex, 14,* 319–326.

Garcha, H. S., & Ettlinger, G. (1980). Tactile discrimination learning in monkeys: The effect of unilateral and bilateral removals of the second somatosensory cortex (SII). *Cortex, 16,* 397–412.

Garcia-Bengochea, F., de la Torre, O., Esquivel, O., et al. (1954). The section of the fornix in the surgical treatment of certain epilepsies. *Transactions of American Neurological Association, 79,* 176–178.

Gardner, H., Siverman, J., Denes, F., Semenza, C., & Rosentiel, A. (1977). Sensitivity to musical denotation and connotation in organic patients. *Cortex, 13,* 242–256.

Gaspar, P., & Gray, F. (1984). Dementia in idiopathic Parkinson's disease. *Acta Neuropathologica, 64,* 43–52.

Gastaut, H., Roger, J., & Roger, A. (1956). Sur la signification de certaines fugues épileptic clouded state: A propos d'une observation electro-clinique de "état de mal temporal." *Revue Neurologique, 94,* 298–301.

Gauthier, I., & Tarr, M. J. (1997). Orientation priming of novel shapes in the context of viewpoint-dependent recognition. *Perception, 26,* 51–73.

Gazzaniga, M. S., Bogen, J. E., & Sperry, R. W. (1962). Some functional effects of sectioning the comissures in man. *Proceeding of the National Academy of Sciences of the U.S.A., 48,* 1765–1769.

Gazzaniga, M., Bogen, J., & Sperry, R. (1967). Dyspraxia following division of the cerebral commisures. *Archives of Neurology (Chicago), 16,* 606–612.

Gazzaniga, M. S., & Freedman, H. (1973). Observations on visual processes after posterior callosal section. *Neurology, 23,* 1126–1130.

Gelb, A. (1926). Die psychologische Bedeutung pathologischer Störungen der Raumwahrnehmung. In K. Bühler (Ed.), *Bericht über den 9. Kongress für experimentelle Psychologie in München 1925* (pp. 23–80). Jena: Fisher.

Gelb, A., & Goldstein, K. (1924). Über Farbenamnesie. *Psychologische Forschung, 6,* 128–186.

Gelenberg, A. J. (1976, June 19). The catatonic syndrome. *Lancet, 2,* 1339–1341.

Geller, T. J., & Bellur, S. N. (1987). Peduncular hallucinosis: Magnetic resonance imaging confirmation of mesencephalic infarction during life. *Annals of Neurology, 21,* 602–604.

Gentilucci, M., & Rizzolatti, G. (1990). Cortical motor control of arm and hand movements. In M. A. Goodale (Ed.), *Vision and action: The control of grasping* (pp. 147–162). Norwood, NJ: Ablex.

George, A. E., de Leon, M., Gentes, C., Miller, J., London, E., Budzilovich, G., et al. (1986). Leukoenecephalopathy in normal and pathologic aging: 1. CT of brain luicencues. *American Journal of Neuroradiology, 7,* 561–566.

George, M. S., Ketter, T. A., Gill, D. S., et al. (1993). Blunted CBF with emotion recognition in depression [Abstract]. American Psychiatric Association New research abstracts, 114-NR #88.

George, M. S., Ketter, T. A., Parekh, P. J., et al. (1994). Spatial ability in affective illness: Differences in regional brain activation during a spatial matching task (H2 15 PET). *Neuropsychiatry, Neuropsychology, and Behavioral Neurology, 7,* 143–153.

George, M. S., Ketter, T. A., Parekh, P. I. et al. (1995). Brain activity during transient sadness and happiness in healthy women. *American Journal of Psychiatry, 152,* 341–351.

George, M. S., Ketter, T. A., Parekh, P. I., Rosinski, N., Ring, H. A., Pazzaglia, P. J., et al. (1997). Blunted left cingular activation in mood disorder subjects during a response interference task (the Stroop). *Journal of Neuropsychiatry and Clinical Neuroscience, 9,* 55–63.

Gershuni, G. V., Bary, A. V., Karaseva, T. A., & Tonkonogy, J. M. (1971). Effects of temporal lobe lesions on perception of sounds of short duration. In G. V. Gershuni & J. Roze (Eds.), *Sensory processes at the neuronal and behavioral levels* (pp. 287–300). New York, London: Academic Press.

Gerstmann, J. (1918). Reine taktile agnosie. *Monatschrift für Psychiatrie und Neurologie, 44,* 329–343.

Gerstmann, J. (1924). Fingeragnosie: Eineum schriebene Storung der Orientierung am eigenen Korper. *Wienner Medical Wohenschrift, 37,* 1010–1012.

Gerstmann, J. (1927). Fingeragnosie and isolierte Agraphie, ein neuen Syndrom. *Zeitschrift für Neurologiq und Psychiatrie, 18,* 152–177.

Gerstmann, J. (1930). Zur symptomatologie der hirnlasionem im über gangsgebiet der unteren parietal and mitteren occipital windung. *Nervenartz, 3,* 691–695.

Gerstmann, J. (1942). Problems of imperception of disease and of impaired body territories with organic lesions: Relations to body scheme and its disorder. *Archives of Neurology and Psychiatry, 48,* 890–913.

Geschwind, D. G., Iacoboni, M., Mega, M. S., Zaidel, D. W., Cloughesy, T., & Zaidel, F. (1995). Alien hand syndrome: Interhemispheric motoric disconnection due to lesion in the midbody of the corpus callosum. *Neurology, 435,* 802–808.

Geschwind, N. (1964). Non-aphasic disorders of speech. *International Journal of Neurology, 4,* 207–214.

Geschwind, N. (1965). Disconnection syndromes in animals and man. Part I and Part II. *Brain 88,* 273–294, 585–645.

Geschwind, N. (1973). The brain and language. In G. A. Miller (Ed.), *Communication, language, and meaning* (pp. 61–72). New York: Basic Books.

Geschwind, N. (1975). The apraxias: Neural mechanisms of disorders of learned movements. *American Scientist, 63,* 188–195.

Geschwind, N., & Kaplan, E. (1962). A human cerebral disconnection syndrome. *Neurology, 12,* 675–685.

Ghaemi, N. (1997). Insight and psychiatric disorders: A review of the literature, with a focus on its clinical relevance for bipolar disorder. *Psychiatric Annals, 27,* 782–790.

Ghaemi, S. N., Stoll, A. L., & Pope, H. G. (1995). Lack of insight in bipolar disorder. *Journal of Nervous and Mental Diseases, 183,* 464–467.

Gibb, W. R. G., Esiri, M. M., & Lees, A. J. (1985). Clinical and pathological features of diffuse cortical Lewy body disease (Lewy body dementia). *Brain, 110,* 1131–1153.

Gibbs, F. A. (1932). Frequency with which tumors in various parts of the brain produce certain symptoms. *Archives of Neurology and Psychiatry, 28,* 969–989.

Gibson, J. J. (1979). *The ecological approach to visual perception.* Boston: Houghton Mifflin.

Gillig, P., Sackellares, S., & Greenberg, H. S. (1988). Right hemisphere partial complex seizures: Mania, hallucinations, and speech disturbances during ictal events. *Epilepsia, 29,* 26–29.

Girotti, F., Milanese, C., Casazza, M., Allegranza, A., Corridori, F., & Avanzini, G. (1982). Oculomotor disturbances in Balint's syndrome: Anatomoclinical findings and electrooculographic analysis in a case. *Cortex, 18,* 603–614.

Glaser, G. H. (1964). The problem of psychosis in psychomotor temporal lobe epileptics. *Epilepsia, 5,* 271–278.

Glees, P., & Griffith, H. B. (1952). Bilateral destruction of the hippocampus (cornus ammonis) in a case of dementia. *Monatschrift für Psychiatrie und Neurologie, 123,* 193–204.

Gloning, I., Gloning, K., & Hoff, H. (1955). Die Störung von Zey und Raum in der Hirnpathologie. *Wiener Zeitshrift für Nervenheilkunde und deren Grenzgebiete, 10,* 346–377.

Gloning, I., Gloning, K., & Hoff, H. (1968). *Neuropsychological symptoms and syndromes in lesions of the occipital lobe and adjacent areas.* Paris: Gauthier-Villars.

Gloning, K., & Quatember, R. (1966). Metodishcer Beitrag zur Untersuchung der prosopagnosie. *Neurospychologia, 4,* 133–141.

Gloor, P., Olivier, A., Quesney, L. F., Andermann, F., & Horowitz, S. (1982). The role of the limbic system in experiential phenomena of temporal lobe epilepsy. *Annals of Neurology, 12,* 129–144.

Glosser, G., Kohn, S. E., Friedman, R. B., Sands, L., & Grugan, P. (1997). Repetition of single words and nonwords in Alzheimer's disease. *Cortex, 23,* 653–666.

Gluck, M. A., & Bower, G. H. (1988). From conditioning to category learning: An adaptive network model. *Journal of Experimental Psychology: General, 117,* 227–247.

Godwin-Austen, R. B. (1965). A case of visual disorientation. *Journal of Neurology, Neurosurgery, and Psychiatry, 28,* 453–458.

Goebel, R., Khorram-Sefat, D., Muckli, L., Haccker, H., & Singer, W. (1998). The constructive nature of vision: Direct evidence from functional magnetic resonance imaging studies of apparent motion and motion imagery. *European Journal of Neuroscience, 10,* 1563–1573.

Goel, V., Grafman, J., Sadato., N., & Hallen, M. (1995). Modeling other minds. *Neuroreport: An International Journal for the Rapid Communication of Research in Neuroscience, 6,* 1741–1746.

Golant, R. Y. (1935). *About disorders of memory* [in Russian]. Leningrad: Meditsina.

Gold, T. W., Goodwin, F. K., & Chrousos, G. P. (1981). Clinical and biochemical manifestation of depression. *New England Journal of Medicine, 319,* 348–353, 413–420.

Goldberg, E., Antin, S. P., Hughes, J. E. O., & Mattis, S. (1981). Retrograde amnesia: Possible role of mesencephalic reticular activation in long-term memory. *Science, 213,* 1392–1394.

Goldberg, G. (1985). Supplementary motor area structure and function: Review and hypotheses. *The Behavioral and Brain Sciences, 8,* 567–616.

Goldberg, G., Mayer, M. H., & Toglis, J. U. (1981). Medial frontal cortex infarction and the alien hand syndrome. *Archives of Neurology, 38,* 683–686.

Goldberg, T. E., Ragland, J. D., Torrey, E. F., Gold, J. M., Bigelow, L. B., & Weinberger, D. R. (1990). Neuropsychological assessment of monzygotic twins discordant for schizophrenia. *Archives of General Psychiatry, 47,* 1066–1072.

Golden, C. J., Purish, A. D., & Hammeke, T. A. (1981). *Luiria-Nebraska Neuropsychological Battery: Manual*. Los Angeles, CA: Western Psychological Services.

Goldenberg, G. (1992). Loss of visual imagery and loss of visual knowledge: A case study. *Neuropsychologia, 30,* 1081–1099.

Goldenberg, G., Müllbacker, W., & Novak, A. (1995). Imagery without perception—a case study of anosognosia for cortical blindness. *Neuropsychologia, 33,* 1373–1382.

Goldenberg, G., Wimmer, A., & Maly, J. (1983). Amnesic syndrome with unilateral thalamic lesion: A case report. *Journal of Neurology, 229,* 79–86.

Goldin, S. (1955). Lilliputian hallucinations. *Journal of Mental Science, 101,* 569–576.

Goldman-Rakic, P. S. (1987). Circuitry of primate prefrontal cortex and regulation of behavior by representational knowledge. In F. Plum & V. B. Mountcastle (Eds.), *Handbook of physiology* (Vol. 5, pp. 373–417). Rockville Park, MD: American Physiological Society.

Goldman-Rakic, P. S., & Porino, L. J. (1985). The primate mediodorsal nucleus (MD) and its projections to the frontal lobe. *Journal of Comparative Neurology, 242,* 535–560.

Goldman-Rakic, P. S., O'Scalaidhe, S. P., & Chafee, M. V. (2000). Domain specificity in cognitive systems. In M. S. Gazzaniga (Ed.), *The New Cognitive Neurosciences* (pp. 733–742). Cambridge, MA: MIT Press.

Goldstein, K. (1909). Der makroskopische Hirndefund in einen Falle von linkseitiger motorisher Apraxie. *Neurologische Centralblatt, 28,* 898–906.

Goldstein, K. (1916). Über kortikale Sensibilitatstorungen. *Neurologische Centralblatt, 19,* 825–827.

Goldstein, K. (1934). *De Aujbau des Organismus*. Hague, Holland: Nijhoff.

Goldstein, K. (1948). *Language and language disturbances*. New York: Grune and Stratton.

Goldstein, K., & Gelb, A. (1918). Pyschologische Analysen Hirnpathologischer Fälle auf Grund von Untersuchungen Hirnverletzter. *Zeitschrift für die gesamte Neurologie und Psychiatrie, 41,* 1–142.

Goldstein, L. H., Bernard, S., Fenwick, P. B. C., Burgess, P. W., & McNeil, J. (1993). Unilateral frontal lobectomy can produce strategy application disorder. *Journal of Neurology, Neurosurgery, and Psychiatry, 56,* 274–276.

Goldstein, P. C., Brown, G. G., Welch, K. M. A., et al. (1985). Age-related decline of rCBF in schizophrenia and major affective disorder. *Journal of Cerebral Blood Flow Metabolism, 5*(suppl. 1), 203–204.

Gollin, E. S. (1960). Developmental studies of visual recognition of incomplete objects. *Perceptual and Motor Skills 2,* 289–298.

Goltz, F. (1876–1884). Über die Verrichtungen des Grosshirn. *Pfluger's Archiv Gesamte Physiology, 13, 14, 20, 26.*

Goodglass, H., & Kaplan, E. (1963). Disturbance of gesture and pantomime in aphasia. *Brain, 86,* 703–720.

Goodglass, H., & Kaplan, E. (1983). *Boston Diagnostic Aphasia Examination.* Philadelphia: Lee and Fabiger.

Goodglass, H., Klein, B., Carey, P., & Jones, K. J. (1966). Specific semantic categories in aphasia. *Cortex, 2,* 74–89.

Goodglass, H., & Quadfasel, F. (1954). Language laterality in left-handed aphasics. *Brain, 77,* 521–548.

Gordon, H. W., & Bogen, J. E. (1974). Hemispheric lateralization of singing after intracarotid sodium amylobarbitone. *Journal of Neurology, Neurosurgery, and Psychiatry, 37,* 727–738.

Gordon, P. C., Hendrick, R., & Levine, W. (2002). Memory-load interference in syntactic processing. *Psychological Science, 13*(5), 425–430.

Gotham, A. M., Brown, R. G., & Marsden, C. D. (1986). Depression in Parkinson's disease: A quantitative and qualitative analysis. *Journal of Neurology, Neurosurgery, and Psychiatry, 49,* 381–389.

Grady, C. L., McIntosh, A. R., Horowitz, B., Maisog, J. M., Ungerleider, L. G., Menits, M. J., et al. (1995). Age-related reductions in human recognition memory due to impaired encoding. *Science, 269,* 218–221.

Graff-Radford, N., Damasio, H., Yamada, T., Eslinger, P. J., & Damasio, A. R. (1985). Nonhaemorrhagic thalamic infarction. *Brain, 108,* 485–516.

Graff-Radford, N. R., Welsh, K., & Godersky, J. (1987). Callosal apraxia. *Neurology, 37,* 100–105.

Grafman, J., Vance, S. C., Swingartner, H., et al. (1986). The effects of lateralized frontal lesions on mood regulation. *Brain, 109,* 1127–1148.

Grant, D. A., & Berg, E. A. (1948). A behavioral analysis of degree of impairment and ease of shifting to new responses in a Weigl-type card sorting problem. *Journal of Experimental Psychology, 39,* 404–411.

Green, E., & Howes, D. H. (1977). The nature of conduction aphasia: A study of anatomic and clinical features and of underlying mechanisms. In H. Whitaker & H. A. Whitaker (Eds.), *Studies in neurolinguistics* (pp. 123–156). New York: Academic Press.

Green, G. L., & Lessel, S. (1977). Acquired cerebral dyschromatopsia. *Archives of Ophthalmology, 95,* 121–128.

Greenblatt, M., & Solomon, H. C. (1966). Studies of lobotomy. *Proceedings of Association for Research of Nervous and Mental Diseases, 36,* 19–34.

Greenblatt, S. H. (1983). Localization of lesions in alexia. In A. Kertesz (Ed.), *Localization in neuropsychology* (pp. 323–356). New York: Academic Press.

Greenblatt, S. H., Saunders, R. L., Culver, C. M., & Bogdanowicz, W. (1980). Normal interhemispheric visual transfer with incomplete section of the splenium. *Archives of Neurology (Chicago), 37,* 567–571.

Griesinger, W. (1845). *Die Pathologie und Therapie der Psychischen Krankheiten.* Stuttgart: Aerzte und Studirende.

Groot, J. C. de, Leeuw, F. de, Oudkerk, M., Hofman, A., Jolles, J., & Breteler, M. M. B. (2000). Cerebral white matter lesions and depressive symptoms in elderly adults. *Archives of General Psychiatry, 57,* 1071–1076.

Gros, B. L., Blake, R., & Haris, E. (1998). Anisotrophies in visual motion perception: A fresh look. *Journal of the Optical Society of America, A, 15*, 2003-2011.

Gross, C. G. (1992). Representation of visual stimuli in inferior temporal cortex. *Philosophical Transactions of the Royal Society, London, B, 335*, 3-10.

Grossberg, S. (1976). Adaptive pattern classification and parallel recording, II: Feedback, expectation, olfaction, and illusions. *Biological Cybernetics, 23*, 187-202.

Grossberg, S. (1980). How does the brain build a cognitive code? *Psychological Review, 87*, 1-51.

Grossi, D. A., Orsini, A., & Modafferi, A. (1986). Visuoimaginal constructive apraxia: On a case of selective deficit of imagery. *Brain and Cognition, 5*, 255-267.

Grossman, E., Donnelly, M., Price, R., Pickens, D., Morgan, V., Neighbor, G., et al. (2000). Brain areas involved in perception of biological motions. *Journal of Cognitive Neuroscience, 12*(5), 711-720.

Grunbaum, A. A. (1930). Aphasie and Motorik. *Zeitschrift für gesamte Neurologie und Psychiatrie, 130*, 385-412.

Gruner, J. E. (1956). Sur la pathologie des encéphalopathies alcooliques. *Revue Neurolgique, 94*, 682-689.

Grüntal, E. (1939). Ueber das corpus mammillare and den Korsakowschen symptomen complex. *Confinia Neurologica, 2*, 64-95.

Grush, R. (1997). The architecture of representation. *Philosophical Psychology, 10*, 5-25.

Grüsser, O. J., & Landis, T. (1991). *Visual agnosias and other disturbances of visual perception and cognition.* London: Macmillan Press.

Guberman, A., & Stuss, D. (1983). The syndrome of bilateral paramedian thalamic infarction. *Neurology, 33*, 540-546.

Guillan, J., & Bize, P. R. (1932). Astreognsie pure par lesion corticale parietal traumatique. *Revue Neurologique, 39*, 502-509.

Gumpert, J., Hansotia, P., & Upton, A. (1970). Gelastic epilepsy. *Journal of Neurology, Neurosurgery, and Psychiatry, 33*, 479-483.

Gupta, S. R., Naheedy, M., Young, J. C., Ghobrial, M., Rubino, F. A., & Hindo, W. (1988). Periventricular white matter changes and dementia: Clinical, neuropsychological, radiological, and pathological correlation. *Archives of Neurology, 45*, 637-641.

Gur, R. E., Skolnick, B. E., Gur, R. C., et al. (1984). Brain function in psychiatric disorders: II. Regional cerebral blood flow in medicated unipolar depressives. *Archives of General Psychiatry, 41*, 695-699.

Gustafson, I., & Nilsson, L. (1982). Differential diagnosis of presenile dementia on clinical grounds. *Acta Psychiatrica Scandinavica, 65*, 194-207.

Gustafson, L. (1993). Clinical picture of frontal lobe degeneration of non-Alzheimer type. *Dementia, 4*, 143-148.

Gustafson, L., Hagberg, B., & Ingvar, D. H. (1978). Speech disturbances in presenile dementia related to local cerebral blood flow abnormalities in the dominant hemisphere. *Brain and Language, 5*, 103-118.

Guttman, E., & Herrmann, K. (1932). Ueben psychisce Storungen beihiris Stanimerkrakungen und des Automatosesyndrome. *Zeitschrift für Gesamte Neurologie und Psychologie, 140*, 439–472.

Habib, M., & Ponset, M. (1988). Perte de l'élan vital, de l'intérét et de l'affectivité (syndrome athymhomique) au courd de lésions lacunaires des corps striés. *Revue Neurologique, 144*, 571–577.

Hachinski, V. C., Lassen, L. A., & Marshall, J. (1974). Multi-infarct dementia: A cause of mental deterioration in elderly. *Lancet, ii*, 207–210.

Hahn, E. (1895). Pathologish-anatomische Untersuchung des Lissauer'schen Falles von Seelenblindheit. *Arbeiten aus der psychiatrische Klinik Breslau, 2*, 105–119.

Hahn, R. D., Webster, D., Weickhardt, G., et al. (1959). Penicillin treatment of general paresis (dementia paralytica). *Archives of Neurology and Psychiatry, 81*, 557–590.

Haldeman, S., Goldman, J. W., Hyde, J., & Pribram, H. F. W. (1981). Progressive supranucalear palsy: Computed tomography and response to antiparkinsonian drugs. *Neurology, 31*, 442–445.

Halgren, E., Babb, T. L., & Crandall, P. H. (1978). Activity of human hippocampal formation and amygdala neurons during memory tests. *Electroencephalography and Clinical Neurophysiology, 45*, 585–601.

Halstead, W. C. (1947). *Brain and intelligence. A quantitative study of the frontal lobes*. Chicago: Chicago University Press.

Hamann, S. B., Stefanacci, L., Squire, R. L., Adolphs, R., Tranel, D., Damasio, H., et al. (1996). Recognizing facial emotion. *Nature, 379*, 497.

Hamann, S. B., & Squire, L. R. (1997). Intact perceptual memory in the absence of conscious memory. *Behavioral Neuroscience, 11*, 850–854.

Hamilton, M. (Ed.). (1985). *Fish's clinical psychopathology* (2nd ed.). Bristol, UK: John Wright and Sons.

Hammeke, T. A., Mcquillen, M. P., & Cohen, B. A. Musical hallucinations associated with acquired deafness. *Journal of Neurology, Neurosurgery, and Psychiatry, 46*, 570–572.

Hansch, E. C., & Pirozzollo, F. J. (1980). Task relevant effects on the assessment of cerebral specialization for facial emotions. *Brain and Language, 10*, 51–59.

Hansen, L. A., & Galasko, D. (1992). Lewy body disease. *Current Opinion in Neurology and Neurosurgery, 5*, 889–894.

Happé, F. G. E. (1994). An advanced test of theory of mind: Understanding of story character's thoughts and feelings by able autistic, mentally handicapped, and normal children and adults. *Journal of Autism and Developmental Disorder, 24*, 129–154.

Happé, F., Brownell, H., & Wimmer, E. (1999). Acquired "theory of mind" impairments following stroke. *Cognition, 70*, 211–240.

Hare, E. H. (1959). The origin and spread of Dementia Paralytica. *Journal of Mental Science, 105*, 594–626.

Harlow, J. M. (1868). Recovery after severe injury to the head. *Publications of Massachusetts Medical Society, 2*, 327–346.

Hartmann, F. (1907). Beitrage zur Apraxielehre. *Monatsschrift für Psychiatrie und Neurologie, 21,* 97–118, 248–270.

Hassler, R. (1938). Zur pathologie der paralysis agitatis und des postenecephalitischen parkinsonismus. *Journal of Psychology and Neurology (Leipzig), 48,* 387–476.

Hassler, R. (1979). Striatal reputation of adverting and attention directing induced by pallidal stimulation. *Applied Neurophysiology, 42,* 98–102.

Hauser, P., Altshuler, L. L., Berrettini, W., et al. (1989). Temporal lobe measurement in primary affective disorder by magnetic resonance imaging. *Journal of Neuropsychiatry and Clinical Neuroscience, 1,* 128–134.

Hawton, K., Feagg, J., & Marsack, P. (1980). Association between epilepsy and attempted suicide. *Journal of Neurology, Neurosurgery, and Psychiatry, 43,* 168–170.

Haxby, J. V., Grady, C. L., Horwitz, B., Salerno, J., Ungerleider, L. G., Mishkin, M., et al. (1993). Dissociation of object and spatial visual processing pathways in human extrastriate cortex. In B. Gulays, D. Ottoson, & P. E. Roland (Eds.), *Organization of the human visual cortex* (pp. 329–340). New York: Pergamon Press.

Haxby, J. V., Grady, C. L., Horwitz, B., Ungerleider, L. G., Mishkin, M., Carson, R. E., et al. (1991). Dissociation of objects and visual spatial processing pathways in human extrastriate cortex. *Proceedings of the National Academy of Science U.S.A., 88,* 1621–1625.

Haxby, J. V., Horwitz, B., Ungerleider, L. G., Maisog, J. M., Pietrini, P., & Grady, C. L. (1994). The functional organization of human extrastriate cortex: A PETrCBF study of selective attention to faces and location. *Journal of Neuroscience, 14,* 6336–6353.

Haxby, J. V., Raffaele, K., Gillette, J., Schapiro, M. B., & Rapoport, S. I. (1992). Individual trajectories of cognitive decline in patients with dementia of Alzheimer type. *Journal of Clinical and Experimental Neuropsychology, 14,* 575–592.

Hays, P., Krikler, B., Sutcliffe W. L., et al. (1966). Psychological changes following surgical treatment of parkinsonism. *American Journal of Psychiatry, 123,* 657–663.

Head, H. (1926). *Aphasia and kindred disorders of speech.* London: Cambridge University Press.

Head, H., & Holmes, G. (1911). Sensory disturbances from cerebral lesions. *Brain, 34,* 102–254.

Heath, R. G. (1971). Depth recording and stimulation studies in patients. In A. Winter (Ed.), *The surgical control of behavior* (pp. 21–37). Springfield, IL: Charles C. Thomas.

Heath, R. G. (1980). The neural basis for violent behavior: Physiology and anatomy. In I. Valzelli & I. Margese (Eds.), *Aggression and violence: A psycho/ biological and clinical approach* (pp. 176–194). Milan, Italy: Edizioni Saint Vincent.

Heaton, R. K., Chelune, G. J., Talley, J. L., Kay, G. G., & Curtis, G. (1993). *Wisconsin Card Sorting Test (WSCT) manual revised and expanded*. Odessa, FL: Psychological Assessment Resources.

Hebb, D. O., & Penfield, W. (1940). Human behavior after extensive bilateral removal from the frontal lobes. *Archives of Neurology and Psychiatry, 44,* 421–438.

Hécaen, H. (1962). Clinical symptomology in right and left hemisphere lesions. In V. B. Mountcastle (Ed.), *Interhemisphere relations and cerebral dominance* (pp. 215–243). Baltimore, MD: Johns Hopkins University Press.

Hécaen, H. (1964). Mental symptoms associated with tumors of the frontal lobe. In J. M. Warren & K. Akert (Eds.), *The frontal granular cortex and behavior* (pp. 335–352). New York: McGraw-Hill.

Hécaen, H. (1972). *Introduction a la neuropsychologie*. Paris: Larousse.

Hécaen, H., & de Ajuriaguerra, J. (1942–1945). L'apraxie d'habillage, ses rapports avec la planotopkinesie et les troubles de la somatognosie. *L'E/ncephale, 35,* 113–114.

Hécaen, H., & de Ajuriaguerra, J. (1950). Asymbolie a la douleur, étude anatomo-clinique. *Revue Neurologique, 83,* 300–302.

Hécaen, H., & de Ajuriaguerra, J. (1952). *Méconnaissances et hallucinations corporelles*. Paris: Masson et Cie.

Hécaen, H., & de Ajuriaguerra, J. (1954). Balint's syndrome (Psychic paralysis of visual fixation and its minor forms). *Brain, 77,* 373–400.

Hécaen, H., & de Ajuriaguerra, J. (1956). *Les troubles mentaux au course du tumeurs intacraniennes*. Paris: Masson et Cie.

Hécaen, H., de Ajuriaguerra, J., David, M., Rouques, M. B., & Dell, R. (1950). Paralysie psychique du regard de Balint au cours de l'evolution d'une leuco-encephalite type Balo. *Revue Neurologique, 83,* 81–104.

Hécaen, H., de Ajuriaguerra, J., & Massonet, J. (1951). Les troubles visuoconstructifs par lésions pariéto-occipitales droites: Rôle of perturbations vestibulaires. *L'Encéphale, 1,* 122–179.

Hécaen, H., & Albert, M. (1978). *Human neuropsychology*. New York: John Wiley & Sons.

Hécaen, H., & Angelergues, R. (1963). *La Cécité Psychique*. Paris: Masson et Cie.

Hécaen, H., Angelergues, R., Bernhardt, C., & Chiarelli, J. (1957). Essai de distinction des modalités cliniques de l'agnosie des physiognomies. *Revue Neurologique, 96,* 125–144.

Hécaen, H., & Assal, G. A. (1972). comparison of constructive deficits following right and left hemispheric lesions. *Neuropsychologia, 8,* 289–303.

Hécaen, H., & Consoli, J. (1973). Analyse des troubles du langage au cours des lésions de l'aire de Broca. *Neuropsychologia, 2,* 377–388.

Hécaen, H., & David, M. (1945). Syndrome parietal traumatique: Asymbolie tactile et hemisomatognosie paroxystique et douloureuse. *Revue Neurologique, 77,* 113–123.

Hécaen, H., & Gimeno, A. (1960). L'apraxie idémotrice unilateral gauche. *Revue Neurologique, 102,* 648–653.

Hécaen, H., Goldblum, M. C., Masure, M. C., & Ramier, A. M. (1974). A new case of object agnosia: A deficit in association or categorization specific for the visual modality. *Neuropsychologia, 12,* 447–464.

Hécaen, H., & Green, A. (1957). Sur L'héautoscopie. *L'Encephale, 46,* 581–594.

Hécaen, H., Penfield, W., Bertrand, C., & Malmo, R. (1956). The syndrome of apractognosia due to lesions of the minor cerebral hemisphere. *Archives of Neurology and Psychiatry, 75,* 400–434.

Hécaen, H., Tzortis, C., & Rondot, P. (1980). Loss of topographic memory with learning deficits. *Cortex, 16,* 525–542.

Heffner, H. E., & Heffner, R. S. (1990). Effect of bilateral auditory cortex lesion on sound localization in Japanese mackaques. *Journal of Neurophysiology, 64,* 915–931.

Heilbronner, K. (1910). Die aphasischen, apraktischen und agnostischen Störungen. In M. Lewandowski (Ed.), *Handbuch der neurologie* (pp. 982–1002). Berlin: Springer.

Heilman, K. M. (1996). Ideational apraxia: A re-definition. *Brain, 96,* 861–864.

Heilman, K. M., Bowers, D., Speedie, L., & Coslett, H. B. (1984). Comprehension of affective and nonaffective speech. *Neurology, 34,* 917–921.

Heilman, K. M., Rothi, L. J. G., & Kertesz, A. (1983). Localization of apraxia-producing lesions. In A. Kertesz (Ed.), *Localization in Neuropsychology* (pp. 371–392). New York: Academic Press.

Heilman, K. M., Scholes, R., Watson, R. T. (1975). Auditory affective agnosia: Disturbed comprehension of affective speech. *Journal of Neurology, Neurosurgery, and Psychiatry, 38,* 69–72.

Heilman, K. M., & Sypert, G. W. (1977). Korsakoff syndrome resulting from bilateral fornix lesions. *Neurology, 3,* 490–493.

Heilman, K. M., & Valenstein, E. (1979). Mechanisms underlying hemispatial neglect. *Annals of Neurology, 5,* 166–170.

Heimburger, R. F., Whillock, C. C., & Kalsbeck, J. E. (1966). Stereotaxic amygdalotomy for epilepsy with aggressive behavior. *Journal of the American Medical Association, 198,* 741–745.

Heindel, W. C., Butters, N., & Salmon, D. P. (1988). Impaired learning of motor skill in patients with Huntington's disease. *Behavioral Neuroscience, 103,* 141–147.

Heindel, W. C., Salmon, D. P., Shults, C. W., Walicke, P. A., & Butters, N. (1989). Neuropsychological evidence for multiple implicit memory systems: A comparison of Alzheimer's, Huntington's, and Parkinson's disease patients. *Journal of Neuroscience, 9,* 582–587.

Hellerstein, D., Frosh, W., & Koenisberg, H. W. (1987). The clinical significance of command hallucinations. *American Journal of Psychiatry, 144,* 219–221.

Helmchen, H. (1976). Reversible psychic disorders in epileptic patients. In W. Birkenmayer (Ed.), *Epileptic Seizures-Behavior-Pain*. Bern, Switzerland: Huber.

Hemmingsen, R., Vorstrup, S., Clemmesen, L., et al. (1988). Cerebral blood flow during delirium tremens and related clinical states studied with Xenon-133 inhalation tomography. *American Journal of Psychiatry, 145*, 1384–1390.

Henschen, S. E. (1920–1922). *Klinische und anatomische Beiträge zur Pathologie des Gehirns*. Stockholm: Nordiska Bokhandlin.

Hermann, B. P., & Riel, P. (1981). Interictal personality and behaviour traits in temporal lobe and generalized epilepsy. *Cortex, 17*, 125–128.

Hermann, B. P., & Wyler, A. R. (1989). Depression, locus of control, and the effects of epilepsy surgery. *Epilepsia, 30*, 332–338.

Hermann, B. P., Wyler, A. R., Blumer, D., & Richey, E. T. (1992). Ictal fear: Lateralizing significance and implications for understanding the neurobiology of pathological fear states. *Neuropsychiatry, Neuropsychology, and Behavioral Neurology, 5*(3), 205–210.

Herrman, G., & Pötzl, O. (1926). *Über die Agraphie und ihre lokaldiagnostischen Beziehungen*. Berlin: S. Karger.

Herrmann, G., & Pötzl, O. (1928). *Die optische alaesthesie*. Berlin: Karger.

Heywood, C. A., Cadotti, A., & Cowey, A. (1992). Cortical area V4 and its role on perception of colour. *Journal of Neuroscience, 12*, 4056–4065.

Heywood, C. A., & Cowey, A. (1987). On the role of cortical area V4 in the discrimination of hue and pattern in macaque monkeys. *Journal of Neuroscience, 7*, 2602–2617.

Hikosaka, O., Sakai, K., Nakahar, H., Lu, X., Miyachi, S., Nakamura, K., et al. (2000). Neural mechanisms for learning of sequential procedures. In M. S. Gazzaniga (Ed.), *The new cognitive neurosciences* (pp. 553–572). Cambridge, MA: MIT Press.

Hill, D., & Mitchell, W. (1953). Epileptic amnesias. *Folia Psychiatry, 56*, 718–725.

Hill, D., & Pond, D. A. (1952). Reflection on one hundred capital cases submitted to electroencephalography. *Journal of Mental Science, 98*, 23–43.

Hillbom, E. (1960). After-effects of brain injuries. *Acta Psychiatrica et Neurologica, 35* (Suppl. 142), 1–135.

Hirono, N., Mori, E., Ishii, K., Ikejiri, Y., Imamura, T., Shimomura, T., et al. (1998). Frontal lobe hypometabolism and depression in Alzheimer's disease. *Neurology, 50*, 380–383.

Hobson, J. A., Pace-Schott, E. F., & Stickgold, R. (1998). The neuropsychology of REM sleep dreaming. *NeuroReport, 9*, R1–R14.

Hobson, J. A., Pace-Schott, E. F., & Stickgold, R. (2000). Consciousness: Its vicissitudes in waking and sleep. In M. S. Gazzaniga (Ed.), *The New Cognitive Neuroscience* (pp. 1341–1354). Cambridge, MA: MIT Press.

Hodges, J. R. (1994). Semantic memory and frontal executive function during transient global amnesia. *Journal of Neurology, Neurosurgery, and Psychiatry, 57*, 605–608.

Hodges, J. R., & Carpenter, K. (1991). Anterograde amnesia with fornix damage following removal of IIIrd ventricle colloid cyst. *Journal of Neurology, Neurosurgery, and Psychiatry, 54*, 633–638.

Hodgkiss, A. D., Malizia, A. L., Bartlett, J. R., & Bridges, P. K. (1995). Outcome after psychosurgical operation of stereotactic subcaudate tractotomy. *Journal of Neuropsychiatry and Clinical Neuroscience, 7*(2), 230–234.

Hoehn, M. M., & Yahr, M. D. (1967). Parkinsonism: Onset, progression, and mortality. *Neurology, 17*, 427–442.

Hoff, H., & Pötzl, O. (1934). Über eine Zeitrafferwirkung bei homonymer linksseitiger Hemianopsie. *Zeitschrift für die Gesamte Neurologie und Psychiatrie, 151*, 599–641.

Hoff, H., & Pötzl, O. (1935). Über ein neues parieto-occipitaler syndrom (Seelenlahmung des Schauens Storung des korperschemas Wegfall der zentralen Schens). *Jahrbuch für Psychiatrie und Neurologie, 52*, 173–218.

Hoff, H., & Pötzl, O. (1937). Über eine optisch-agnostishe Störung des "Physiognomie-Gedächtnisses." *Zeitschrift für Gesamte Neurologie und Psychiatrie, 159*, 367–395.

Hoff, H., & Pötzl, O. (1938). Anatomischer befund eines Falles mit Zeitrafferphänomenon. *Deutsche Zeitschrift für Nervenhielkunde, 145*, 150–178.

Hoffman, D., & Richards, W. (1984). Parts of recognition. *Cognition, 18*, 65–96.

Hoffman, H. (1885). Stereognostische Versuche, angestlelf zur Ermi Helangder Elemente des Gefahisinnes, aus denen die Vorstellungen des Korps vin Raume gebildet warden. *Deutsche Archiv für klinische Medicin, 36*, 398–426.

Hofle, N., Paus, T., Reutens, D., Fiset, P., Gotman, J., Evans, A. C., et al. (1997). Regional cerebral blood flow changes as function of delta and spindle activity during slow wave sleep in humans. *Journal of Neuroscience, 17*, 4800–4808.

Holland, A. L., McBurney, D. H., Moossy, J., & Reinmuth, O. M. (1985). The dissolution of language in Pick's disease with neurofibrillary tangles: A case study. *Brain and Language, 24*, 36–58.

Holmes, G. (1918). Disturbances of visual orientation. *British Journal of Opthalmology, 2*, 449–468, 506–516.

Holmes, G., & Horrax, G. (1919). Disturbances of spatial orientation and visual attention with loss of stereoscopic vision. *Archives of Neurology and Psychiatry, 1*, 385–407.

Holroyd, S., Rabins, P. V., Finkelstein, D., Nicholson, M. C., Chase, G. A., & Wisniewskiy, S. C. (1992). Visual hallucinations in patients with macular degeneration. *American Journal of Psychiatry, 149*, 1701–1706.

Homa, Y., Takahashi, H., Takeda, S., & Ikuta, F. (1987). An autopsy case of progressive supranuclear palsy showing "pure akinesia" without rigidity and tremor and with no effect by L-dopa therapy (Imai). *No To Shinkei, 39*, 183–187.

Homan, B. L., Johnson, K. A., Gerada, B., Carvalho, P. A., & Satlin, A. (1992). The scintigraphic appearance of Alzheimer's disease: A prospective study using technecium-99m HMPAO SPECT. *Journal of Nuclear Medicine, 33,* 181–185.

Honer, W. G., Hurwitz, T., Li, D. K. B., et al. (1987). Temporal lobe involvement in multiple sclerosis patients with psychiatric disorders. *Archives of Neurology, 44,* 187–190.

Hooper, H. E. (1968). *The Hooper Visual Organization Test, Manual.* Beverly Hills, CA: Western Psychological Services.

Hopf, A. Z. (1957). Architektonische Untersuchungen um sensorischen Aphasien. *Journal für Hirnforschung, 3,* 276–530.

Horenstein, S., Chamberlain, W., & Conomy, J. (1967). Infarctions in the fusiform and calcarine regions with agitated delirium and hemianopsia. *Transactions of Amerian Neurological Association, 92,* 85–89.

Horowitz, M. J., Adams, J. E., & Rutkin, B. B. (1968). Visual imagery on brain simulation. *Archives of General Psychiatry, 19,* 469–486.

Horton, P., & Miller, D. (1972). The etiology of multiple personality. *Comparative Psychiatry, 13,* 151–159.

Howard, J. R., Almeida, O., Levy, R., Graves, P., & Graves, M. (1994). Qualitative magnetic resonance imaging volumetry distinguishes delusional disorder from late-onset schizophrenia. *British Journal of Psychiatry, 165,* 474–480.

Howard, R. J., Brammer, M., Wright, I., Woodruff, P. W., Bullmore, E. T., & Zeki, S. (1996). A direct demonstration of functional specialization within motion-related visual and auditory cortex in the human brain. *Current Biology, 6,* 1015–1019.

Howieson, D. B., & Lezak, M. D. (2002). The neuropsychological evaluation. In S. C. Yudofsky & R. E. Hales (Eds.), *Neuropsychiatry and Clinical Neurosciences* (4th ed., pp. 217–244). Washington, DC: American Psychiatric Publishing.

Hubel, D. H., & Wiesel, T. N. (1959). Receptive fields of single neurons in cat's striate cortex. *Journal of Physiology, 148,* 574–591.

Hubel, D. H., & Wiesel, T. N. (1968). Receptive fields and functional architecture of monkey striate cortex. *Journal of Psychology, 195,* 215–243.

Huber, S. J., Paulson, G. W., & Shuttleworth, E. C. (1988). Depression in Parkinson's disease. *Neuropsychiatry, Neuropsychology, and Behavioral Neurology, 1,* 47–51.

Hughes, W. (1970). Alzheimer's disease. *Gerontological Clinic, 12,* 129–148.

Huiette, C. M., & Crain, B. J. (1992). Lobar atrophy without Pick body. *Clinical Neuropathology, 11,* 151–156.

Hulette, C., Nochlin, D., McKeel, D., Morris, J. C., Mirra, S. S., Sumi, S. M., et al. (1997). Clinical-neuropathologic findings in multi-infarct dementia: A report of six autopsied cases. *Neurology, 48,* 668–672.

Humphreys, G. W., & Riddoch, M. J. (1984). Routes to objects constancy: Implications from neurological impairments of object constancy. *Quarterly Journal of Experimental Psychology, 36A,* 385–415.

Humphreys, G. W., & Riddoch, M. J. (1985). Author's correction to "Routes to object constancy." *Quarterly Journal of Experimental Psychology, 377A,* 493–495.

Humphreys, G. W., Riddoch, M. J., & Quinlan, P. T. (1988). Cascade processes in picture identification. *Cognitive Neuropsychology 5,* 67–103.

Hutto, B. (1999). The symptoms of depression in endocrine disorders. *CNS Spectrums, 4*(4), 51–61.

Ingvar, D. H., & Frazen, G. (1974). Abnormalities of cerebral flow distribution in patients with chronic schizophrenia. *Acta Psychiatrica Scandinavica, 50,* 425–462.

Inzelberg, R., Treves, T., Reider, I., et al. (1987). Computed tomography brain changes in Parkinson's disease. *Neuroradiology, 29,* 535–539.

Irigaray, L. (1973). *Le language des déments.* The Hague: Mouton.

Irle, E., Peper, M., Wovra, B., & Kunze, S. (1994). Mood changes after surgery for tumors of the cerebral cortex. *Archives of Neurology, 51,* 164–174.

Irwin, W., Davidson, R. J., Lowe, M. J., Mock, B. J., Sorenson, J. A., & Tuski, P. A. (1996). Human amygdala activation detected with echoplanar functional magnetic resonance imaging. *NeuroReport, 7,* 1765–1769.

Ishai, A., & Sagi, D. (1997). Visual imagery facilitates visual perception: Psychophysical evidence. *Journal of Cognitive Neuroscience, 9,* 476–489.

Ishihara, S. (1983). *Ishihara's Test for Color Blindness.* Toyko: Kanehara.

Jackendoff, R. (1992). *Languages of the mind: Essays of mental representation.* Cambridge, MA: MIT Press.

Jackobson, R., Fant,G., & Jerrier, H. (2000). EEG in delirium. *Seminars in Clinical Neuropsychiatry, 5,* 86–92.

Jackson, H. J. (1988). On a particular variety of epilepsy ("intellectual aura"), one case of organic brain disease. *Brain, 11,* 179–207.

Jackson, J. H. (1869). *On localization: Selected writings* (Vol. 2). Reprinted 1958 in J. Taylor (Ed.), New York: Basic Books.

Jackson, J. H. (1875). On temporary mental disorders after epileptic paroxisms. *West Riding Lunatic Asylum Report, 5,* 105–129.

Jackson, J. H. (1876.) Case of large cerebral tumour without optic neuritis and with left hemiplegia and imperception. Reprinted 1958 in J. Taylor (Ed.), *Selected Writings of John Hughlings Jackson* (pp. 146–152). New York: Basic Books.

Jackson, J. H. (1884). *Evolution and dissolution of the nervous system: Selected Writings* (Vol. 2). Reprinted 1958 in J.Taylor (Ed.), New York: Basic Books.

Jacobsen, C. F. (1935). Functions of the frontal association in primates. *Archives of Neurology and Psychiatry, 33,* 558–569.

Jacobsen, C. F. (1936). Studies of cerebral function in primates. *Comparative Psychology Monograffes, 13,* 1–60.

Jacoby, R. J., & Levy, R. (1980). Computed tomography in elderly, 3: Affective disorder. *British Journal of Psychiatry, 136,* 270–275.

Jacoby, R. J., Levy, R., & Bird, J. M. (1981). Computer tomography and the outcome of affective disorder: A follow-up study of elderly persons. *British Journal of Psychiatry, 139,* 288–292.

Jaffe, R., & Bender, M. B. (1966). EEG studies in the syndrome of isolated episodes of confusion with amnesia, "transient global amnesia." *Journal of Neurology, Neurosurgery, and Psychiatry, 29,* 472.

Jagust, W. J., Budinger, T. F., & Reed, B. R. (1987). The diagnosis of dementia with single photon emission computed tomography. *Archives of Neurology, 44,* 258–262.

Jagust, W. J., Davies, P., Tiller-Borcich, J. K., & Reed, B. R. (1990). Focal Alzheimer's disease. *Neurology, 40,* 14–19.

Jagust, W. J., Reed, B. R., Scab, J. P., Kramer, J. H., & Budinger, T. F. (1989). Clinical-physiologic correlates of Alzheimer's disease and frontal lobe dementia. *American Journal of Physiological Imaging, 4,* 89–96.

Jampala, V. C., & Abrams, R. (1983). Mania secondary to left and right hemisphere damage. *American Journal of Psychiatry, 140,* 1197–1199.

Janer, K. W., & Pardo, J. V. (1991). Deficits in selective attention following bilateral anterior cingulotomy. *Journal of Cognitive Neuroscience, 3,* 231–241.

Jankowiak, J., & Albert, M. L. (1994). Lesion localization in visual agnosia. In A. Kertesz (Ed.), *Localization and neuroimaging in neuropsychology* (pp. 429–472). San Diego, CA: Academic Press.

Janota, I. (1981). Dementia, deep white matter damage and hypertension. *Psychological Medicine, 11,* 39–48.

Jasper, K. (1963). *General psychopathology.* J. Hoening & M. W. Hamilton translated from the German's 7th ed., Manchester, UK: Manchester University Press. First edition in German in 1959.

Jastrowitz, M. (1888). Bieträrage zur Localisation im Grosshirn und über deren praktishce Verwerthung. *Deutsche Medzinische Wochenschrift, 14,* 81–83.

Jeannerod, M. (1984). The timing of natural prehension movements. *Journal of Motor Behavior, 16,* 235–254.

Jellinger, K. (1986). Overview of morphological changes in Parkinson's disease. *Advances in Neurology, 45,* 1–18.

Jenike, M. A., Breiter, H. C., Baer, L., et al. (1996). Cerebral structural abnormalities in obsessive-compulsive disorder: A quantitative morphometric magnetic resonance imaging study. *Archives of General Psychiatry, 53,* 625–632.

Jenkins, W. M., & Masterton, R. B. (1982). Sound localization: Effects of unilateral lesions in central auditory system. *Journal of Neurophysiology, 4,* 987–1016.

Jerger, J. (1964). Auditory test for disorder of central auditory mechanisms. In W. J. Fields & B. R. Alfordi (Eds.), *Neurological aspects of auditory and vestibular disorders* (pp. 77–86). Springfield, IL: Charles C. Thomas.

Jervis, G. A. (1937). Alzheimer's disease. *Psychiatric Quaterly, 11*, 5–18.

Jervis, G. A. (1971). Pick's disease. In J. Minkler (Ed.), *Pathology of the nervous system* (Vol. 2, pp. 1385–1395). New York: McGraw-Hill.

Johansen, A., Gustafson, L., & Risberg, J. (1985). Psychological evaluation in dementia and depression. *Danish Medical Bulletin, 32* (Suppl. 1), 60–62.

Johanson, A., & Hagberg, B. (1989). Psychometric characteristics in patients with frontal lobe degeneration of non-Alzheimer type. *Archives of Gerontology and Geriatrics, 8*, 129–137.

Johnson, C. N., & Wellman, H. M. (1980). Children's developing understanding of mental verbs: Remember, know and guess. *Child Development, 51*, 1095–1102.

Johnson, J. (1993). Catatonia: The tension insanity. *British Journal of Psychiatry, 162*, 733–738.

Johnston, E. C., Owens, D. G. C., Gold, A., Crow, T. T. J., & Macmillan, J. F. (1981). Institutionalization and the defects of schizophrenia. *British Journal of Psychiatry, 139*, 195–203.

Johnstone, E. C., Crow, T. J., Frith, D. C., Husband, J., & Krel, L. (1976). Cerebral ventricular size and cognitive impairment in schizophrenia. *Lancet, 2*, 924–926.

Johnstone, E. C., Owens, D. G. C., Bydder, G. M., et al. (1989). The spectrum of structural brain changes in schizophrenia: Age of onset as a predictor of cognitive and clinical impairment and their cerebral correlates. *Psychological Medicine, 19*, 91–103.

Johnstone, P. A., Rundell, J. R., & Esposito, M. (1990). Mental status changes of Addison's disease. *Psychosomatics, 31*, 103–107.

Jorge, R. E., Robinson, R. G., Starkstein, S. E., et al. (1993). Manic syndromes following traumatic brain injury. *American Journal of Psychiatry, 150*, 916–921.

Joseph, A. B. (1986). Cotard's syndrome in patient with coexistent Capgras' syndrome, syndrome of subjective doubles, and palinopsia. *Journal of Clinical Psychiatry, 47*, 605.

Joseph, A. B., Anderson, W. A., & O'Leary, D. H. (1985). Brainstem and vermis atrophy in schizophrenia. *American Journal of Psychiatry, 142*, 352–354.

Joseph, A. B., & O'Leary, D. H. (1986). Brain atrophy and interhemispheric fissure enlargement in Cotard's syndrome. *Journal of Clinical Psychiatry, 47*, 518–520.

Joseph, A. B., O'Leary, D. H., & Wheeler, H. G. (1990). Bilateral atrophy of frontal and temporal lobes in schizophrenic patients with Capgras syndrome: A case-control study using computed tomography. *Journal of Clinical Psychiatry, 51*, 322–325.

Joseph, R. (1990). *Neuropsychology, neuropsychiatry, and behavioral neurology*. New York, London: Plenum Press.

Josiassen, R. C., Curry, L. M., & Mancall, E. L. (1983). Development of neuropsychological deficits in Huntington's disease. *Archives of Neurology, 40*, 791–796.

Julesz, B. (1971a). Experiments in visual perception of texture. *Scientific American, 232*, 34–43.

Julesz, B. (1971b). *Foundations of cyclopean perception.* Chicago: Chicago University Press.

Jung, C. (1949). Über eine Nachuntersuchung des Falles Schn. von Goldstein und Gelb. *Psychiatrie, Neurologie, und Medizinische Psychologie, 1*, 353–362.

Just, M. A., & Carpenter, P. A. (1992). A capacity theory of comprehension: Individual difference in working memory. *Psychological Review, 99*, 122–149.

Just, M. A., Carpenter, P. A., & Keller, T. A. (1996). The capacity theory of comprehension: New frontier of evidence and arguments. *Psychological Review, 103*, 773–780.

Kabelyanskaya, L. G. (1957). Function of the auditory analyzer in sensory aphasia [in Russian]. *The Korsakoff Journal of Neuropathology and Psychiatry, 57*(6), 712–716.

Kahlbaum, K. L. (1973). *Catatonia* (Levij Y. & Pridau, T.) Trans. Baltimore: Johns Hopkins University Press. (original work published 1874)

Kahn, E. A. A., & Crosby, E. C. (1972). Korsakoff's syndrome associated with surgical lesion involving the mammilary bodies. *Neurology, 22*, 117–125.

Kaidanova, S. I., & Meerson, Y. A. (1961). About peculiarities of function of auditory analyzer in aphasia [in Russian]. *Journal of Higher Nervous Activity, 11*, 185–199.

Kaidanova, S. I., Meerson, Y. A., & Smirnoff, V. M. (1963). The Bechterev Institute Press, 32; 21:

Kaidanova, S. I., Meerson, Y. A., & Tonkonogy, J. M. (1965). Disorders of sound localization in patients with local brain lesions [in Russian]. *Vestnik Otorinolaringologii, 2*, 39–43.

Kamo, H., McGeer, P. L., Harrop, R., et al. (1987). Positron emission tomography and histopathology in Pick's disease. *Neurology, 37*, 439–445.

Kantimulina, N. V. (1961). Local adaptation and visual afterimages in patients with different cerebral localization of lesions [in Russian]. In G. B. Abramovich & G. Z. Levin (Eds.), *Problems of localization in psychiatry and neurology, Vol. 21*, (pp. 93–100). Leningrad: The Bechterev Institute Press.

Kanwal, J. S., Ohlemiller, K. K., & Suga, N. (1993). Communication sounds of mustached bats: Classification and multidimensional analyses of cell structure. *Association Research in Otolaryngology, Abstracts, 11*, 442.

Kanwisher, N., Chun, M. M., McDermott, J., & Ledden, P. J. (1996). Functional imaging of human visual recognition. *Cognitive Brain Research 5*, 55–67.

Kaplan, E. F., Goodglass, H., & Weintraub, S. (1978). *The Boston Naming Test* [Experimental edition]. Philadelphia: Lee and Fabiger.

Kapp, B. S., Frisinger, R. C., Gallagher, M., & Haselton, J. (1979). Amygdal central nucleus lesions: Effects on heart rate conditioning in the rabbit. *Physiology and Behavior, 23*, 1109–1117.

Kapur, N., & Coughlan, A. K. (1980). Confabulation and frontal lobe dysfunction. *Journal of Neurology, Neurosurgery, and Psychiatry, 43,* 461–463.

Kapur, N., Turner, A., & King, C. (1988). Reduplicative paramnesias: Possible anatomical and neuropsychological mechanisms. *Journal of Neurology, Neurosurgery, and Psychiatry, 51,* 579–581.

Kapur, N., Young, A., Bateman, D., & Kennedy, P. (1989). Focal retrograde amnesia: A long term and clinical neuropsychological follow-up. *Cortex, 25,* 387–402.

Kapur, S., Craik, F. I. M., Tulving, E., Wilson, E. E., Houle, S., & Brown, G. (1994). Neuroanatomical correlates of encoding in episodic memory: Levels of processing effect. *Proceedings of the National Academy of Sciences U.S.A., 91,* 2008–2011.

Karaseva, T. A. (1972). The role of temporal lobe in human auditory perception. *Neuropsychologia, 10,* 227–231.

Karmiloff-Smith, A. (1992). *Beyond modularity: A developmental perspective on cognitive science.* Cambridge, MA: MIT Press.

Karmiloff-Smith, A., Klima, E., Bellugi, U., Grant, J., & Baron-Cohen, S. (1995). Is there a social module? Language, face processing, and theory of mind in individuals with Williams syndrome. *Journal of Cognitive Neuroscience, 7,* 196–208.

Karp, E., Belmont, I., & Birch, H. G. (1969). Unilateral hearing loss in hemiplegic patients. *Journal of Nervous and Mental Diseases, 148,* 83–86.

Karpov, B. A., Meerson, Y. A., & Tonkonogy, J. M. (1979). On some peculiarities of the visuomotor system in visual agnosia. *Neuropsychologia, 17,* 281–294.

Kartsounis, L. D., Rudge, P., & Stevens, J. M. (1995). Bilateral lesions of CA1 and CA2 fields of the hippocampus are sufficient to cause a severe amnesic syndrome in humans. *Journal of Neurology, Neurosurgery, and Psychiatry, 59,* 95–98.

Kartsounis, L. D., & Warrington, E. K. (1989). Unilateral visual neglect overcome by cues implicit in stimulus arrays. *Journal of Neurology, Neurosurgery, and Psychiatry, 52,* 1253–1259.

Kase, C. S., Troncoso, J. F., Court, J. E., Tapia, F. J., & Mohr, J. P. (1977). Global spatial disorientation. *Journal of Neurological Science, 34,* 267–278.

Katz, D. I., Alexander, M. P., & Mandell, A. M. (1987). Dementia following stroke in the mesencephalon and diencephalon. *Archives of Neurology, 44,* 1127–1133.

Kaufer, D., Mendez, M. F., Mishel, P. S., Verity, M. A., & Benson, D. F. (1996). Alien hand syndrome in adult onset orthochromatic leukodystrophy: Disconnection of a limb from supplementary motor areas. *Behavioral Neurology, 9,* 5–10.

Kaushall, P. I., Zetin, M., & Squire, L. R. (1981). A psychological study of chronic, circumscribed amnesia. *Journal of Neurology, Neurosurgery, and Psychiatry, 169,* 383–389.

Kawamura, M., & Takahashi, N. (1995). Prosopagnosia and facial discrimination. *Advances in Neurological Sciences, 39,* 674–682.

Kay, S. R., Wolkenfeld, F., & Murrill, L. M. (1988). Profiles of aggression among psychiatric patients. II. Covariates and predictors. *Journal of Nervous and Mental Diseases, 176,* 547–557.

Kazui, H., Tanabe, H., Ikeda, M., Hashimoto, H., Yamada, N., Okuda, J., et al. (1996). Retrograde amnesia during transient global amnesia. *Neurocase, 2,* 127–133.

Kazui, H., Tanabe, H., Ikeda, M., Nakagawa, Y., Shiraishi, J., & Hashikawa, K. (1995). Memory and cerebral blood flow in cases of transient global amnesia during and after the attack. *Behavioural Neurology, 8,* 93–101.

Keane, M. M., Gabrieli, J. D. E., Mapstone, H. C., Johnson, K. A., & Gorkin, S. (1995). Normal perceptual priming of orthographically illegal nonwords in amnesia. *Brain, 1,* 425–433.

Kelley, W. M., Miezin, F. M., McDermott, K. B., et al. (1988). *CT scanning in panic disorder* [Abstract 37A]. Presented at the American Psychiatric Association, Montreal, Canada.

Kelly, W. F. (1996). Psychiatric aspects of Cushing's syndrome. *QJM, 89,* 543–551.

Kellner, C. H., & Uhde, T. W. (1988). *CT scanning in panic disorder* [Abstract 37A]. Presented at the American Psychiatric Association, Montreal, Canada.

Kelsoe, J. R., Cadet, J. L., Pickar, D., et al. (1988). Quantitative neuroanatomy in schizophrenia: A controlled magnetic resonance imaging study. *Archives of General Psychiatry, 45,* 533–541.

Kenna, J. C., & Sedman, G. (1965). Depersonalization in temporal lobe epilepsy and organic psychosis. *British Journal of Psychiatry, 11,* 293–299.

Kennard, M. A., Bueding, E., & Wortis, W. B. (1945). Some biochemical and electroencephalographic changes in delirium tremens. *Quarterly Journal of Studies on Alcohol, 6,* 4–14.

Kennedy, A. (1959). Psychological factors in confusional states in the elderly. *Gerontological Clinic, 1,* 71–82.

Kertesz, A. (1979). *Aphasia and associated disorders: Taxonomy, localization, and recovery.* New York: Grune and Stratton.

Kertesz, A. (1982). *The Western Aphasia Battery.* New York: Grune and Stratton.

Kertesz, A. (1983). Localization of lesions in Wernicke's aphasia. In A. Kertesz (Ed.), *Localization in neuropsychology* (pp. 209–230). New York: Academic Press.

Kertesz, A. (1985). Apraxia and aphasia: Anatomical and clinical relationship. In E. A. Roy (Ed.), *Neuropsychological studies of apraxia and related disorders* (pp. 163–178). Amsterdam: Elsevier Science Publishers.

Kertesz, A. (1987). The clinical spectrum and localization of visual agnosia. In J. W. Humphreys & M. J. Riddoch (Eds.), *Visual object processing: A cognitive neuropsychological approach.* London: Lawrence Erlbaum Associates.

Kertesz, A. (1994). Language deterioration in dementia. In V. O. B. Emery & T. E. Oxman (Eds.), *Dementia: Presentation, differential diagnosis, and nosology* (pp. 123–138). Baltimore, MD: Johns Hopkins University Press.

Kertesz, A. (1982). *Varieties of reading disorders*. Presented at the Winter Conference on Brain Research, Steamboat Springs, Colorado.

Kertesz, A., & Ferro, J. M. (1984). Lesion size and location in ideomotor apraxia. *Brain, 107*, 921–933.

Keschner, M., Bender, M., & Strauss, I. (1936). Mental symptoms in cases of tumor of temporal lobe. *Archives of Neurology and Psychiatry, 35*, 572–593.

Keshavan, M. S., Brar, J., & Kahn, M. (1988). Musical hallucinations following removal of a frontal lobe meningioma. *Journal of Neurology, Neurosurgery, and Psychiatry, 51*, 1235–1236.

Keshavan, M. S., David, A. S., Steingard, S., & Lishman, W. A. (1992). Musical hallucinations: A review and synthesis. *Neuropsychiatry, Neuropsychology, and Behavioral Neurology, 5*, 211–223.

Ketter, T. A., Andreasen, P. J., George, M. S., et al. (1993). Blunted CBF response to procaine in mood disorders [Abstract]. American Psychiatric Association, new research abstracts; 134-NR#297.

Ketter, T. A., Andreasen, P. J., George, M.S., et al. (1996). Paralimbic rCBF increases during procaine-induced psychosensory and emotional experiences. *Archives of General Psychiatry, 53*, 59–69.

Kettl, P. A., & Marks, I. M. (1986). Neurological factors in obsessive compulsive disorder: Two case reports and review of the literature. *British Journal of Psychiatry, 149*, 315–319.

Killefer, F. A., & Stern, W. E. (1970). Chronic effect of hypothalamic injury. *Archives of Neurology, 22*, 419–429.

Kiloh, R. S., Gye, R. S., Rusworth, R. G., et al. (1974). Stereotaxic amygdalotomy for aggressive behavior. *Journal of Neurology, Neurosurgery, and Psychiatry, 37*, 437–444.

Kim, K. W., & Lee, D. Y. (2002). Obsessive-compulsive disorder associated with a left orbitofrontal infarct. *Journal of Neuropsychiatry and Clinical Neuroscience, 14*, 88–89.

Kimberg, D. Y., D'Eposito, M., & Farah, M. J. (1998). Cognitive functions in prefrontal cortex-working memory and executive control. *Journal of the American Psychological Society, 6*, 185–192.

Kimura, D. (1963). Right temporal lobe damage: Perception of unfamiliar stimuli after damage. *Archives of Neurology (Chicago), 8*, 264–271.

Kimura, D. (1977). Acquisition of a motor skill after left hemisphere damage. *Brain, 100*, 527–542.

Kimura, D. (1982). Left hemisphere control of oral and brachial movements and their relationship to communication. *Philosophical Transactions of the Royal Society of London*, Series B, *298*, 135–149.

Kimura, D., & Archibald, Y. (1974). Motor functions of the left hemisphere. *Brain, 97*, 337–350.

King, A. J., & Carlile, S. (1995). Neural coding for auditory space. In M. Gazzaniga (Ed.), *The cognitive neurosciences* (pp. 279–293). Cambridge, MA: MIT Press.

King, D. W., & Ajmone-Marsan, C. A. (1977). Clinical features and ictal patterns in epileptic patients with EEG temporal lobe foci. *Annals of Neurology, 2*, 138–147.

King, F. L., & Kimura, D. (1972). Left-ear superiority in dichotic perception of vocal nonverbal sounds. *Canadian Journal of Psychology, 26*, 111–116.

Kinkel, W. R., Jacobs, L., Polachini, I., Bates, V., & Heffner, R. R. (1985). Subcortical arteriosclerotic encephalopathy (Binswanger's disease). *Archives of Neurology, 42*, 951–959.

Kinsbourne, M. (1977). Hemi-neglect and hemisphere rivalry. In E. N. Weinstein & R. P. Fridland (Eds.), *Advances in neurology* (pp. 41–49). New York: Raven Press.

Kinsbourne, M., & Rosenfeld, D. B. (1974). Agraphia selective for written spelling: An experimental case study. *Brain and Language, 1*, 215–225.

Kinsbourne, M., & Warrington, E. K. (1962). A disorder of simultaneous form perception. *Brain, 85*, 461–486.

Kinsbourne, M., & Warrington, E. K. (1963). A study of visual perseveration. *Journal of Neurology, Neurosurgery, and Psychiatry, 26*, 468–475.

Kinsbourne, M., & Warrington, E. K. (1965). A case of showing selectively impaired oral spelling. *Journal of Neurology, Neurosurgey, and Psychiatry, 28*, 563–567.

Kinsella, G., Moran, C., Ford, B., & Ponsford, J. (1988). Emotional disorder and its assessment within the severe head injured population. *Psychological Medicine, 18*, 1857–1863.

Kirby, G. H. (1913). The catatonic syndrome and its relation to manic-depressive insanity. *Journal of Nervous and Mental Diseases, 40*, 694–740.

Kirch, D. G., & Weinberger, D. R. (1986). Anatomical neuropathology in schizophrenia: Post-mortem findings. In H. A. Nasrallah & D. R. Weinberger (Eds.), *The neurology of schizophrenia* (pp. 325–348). Amsterdam: Elsevier Science.

Kirk, A., & Kertesz, A. (1989). Hemispheric contribution to drawing. *Neuropsychologia, 27*, 881–886.

Kirk, A., & Kertesz, A. (1994). Localization of lesions in constructional impairment. In A. Kertesz (Ed.), *Localization and neuroimaging in neuropsychology* (pp. 525–544). New York: Academic Press.

Kirshner, H. S., Webb, W. G., Kelly, M. P., & Wells, C. E. (1984). Language disturbance: An initial symptom of cortical degeneration and dementia. *Archives of Neurology, 41*, 491–496.

Kishimoto, H., Kuwahar, H., Ohno, S., et al. (1987). Three subtypes of chronic schizophrenia identified using 11C-glucose positron emission tomography. *Psychiatry Research, 21*, 285–292.

Klages, W. (1954). Zur psychopatologies der Pickshen und Alzheimerschen Krankheit. *Archiv für Psychiatrie und Neurologie, 191*, 508–522.

Klee, A. (1961). Akinetic mutism: Review of the literature and report of a case. *Journal of Nervous and Mental Diseases, 133*, 536–553.

Klein, R., & Harper, J. (1956). The problem of aphasia in the light of a case of pure word deafness. *Journal of Mental Science, 102,* 112–120.

Kleist, K. (1912). Der gang und der gegenwurtige Stand der Apraxie-forschung. *Ergebniss für Neurologie and Psichiatrie, 1,* 342–352.

Kleist, K. (1934). *Gehirnpathologie.* Leipzig: Burth.

Klingon, G. H., & Bontecou, D. C. (1966). Localization in auditory space. *Neurology, 16,* 879–886.

Klüver, H., & Bucy, P. (1937). Psychic blindness and other symptoms following bilateral temporal lobectomy in Rhesus monkeys. *American Journal of Physiology, 119,* 352–353.

Klüver H., & Bucy, P. (1939). Preliminary analysis of functions of the temporal lobe in monkeys. *Archives of Neurology and Psychiatry, 42,* 979–1000.

Knecht, S., Kunesh, E., & Schnitzler, A. (1996). Parallel and serial processing of haptic information in man: Effects of parietal lesions on sensorimotor hand function. *Neuropsychologia, 7,* 669–687.

Knight, G. (1965). Stereotactic tractotomy in the surgical treatment for mental illness. *Journal of Neurology, Neurosurgery, and Psychiatry, 28,* 304–310.

Knopman, D. S., & Nissen, M. J. (1991). Procedural learning is impaired in Huntington's disease: Evidence from the serial reaction time test. *Neuropsychologia, 29,* 245–254.

Knopman, D. S., Selnes, O. A., Niccum, N., & Rubens, A. B. (1984). Recovery of naming in aphasia: Relationship to fluency comprehension and CT findings. *Neurology, 34,* 1461–1470.

Köhler, S., Kapur, S., Moscovitch, M., Vinocur, G., & Houle, S. (1995). Dissociation of pathways for object and spatial vision: A PET study in human. *Neuroreport, 6,* 1865–1868.

Kohonen, T. (1989). *Self-organization and associative memory* (3rd ed.). Berlin: Springer-Verlag.

Kok, E. P. (1967). *Visual agnosias* [in Russian]. Leningrad: Meditsina.

Kolb, B., & Milner, B. (1981). Performance of complex arm and facial movements after focal brain lesions. *Neuropsychologia, 19,* 491–503.

Kölmel, H. W. (1988). Pure homonimous hemiachromatopsia: Findings with neuro-ophatlmologicala examination and imaging procedures. *Europian Archives of Psychiatric and Neurological Science 237,* 237–243.

Kolodny, A. (1929). Symptomatology of tumors of the frontal lobe. *Archives of Neurology and Psychiatry, 21,* 1107–1127.

Komori, T. (1999). Tau-positive glial inclusions in progressive supranuclear palsy, corticobasal degeneration and Pick's disease. *Brain Pathology, 9,* 663–679.

Konorski, J. (1967). *Integrative activity of the brain: An interdisciplinary approach.* Chicago: University of Chicago Press.

Koponen, H., Partanen, J., Paakkonen, A., et al. (1989). EEG spectral analysis in delirium. *Journal of Neurology, Neurosurgery, and Psychiatry, 52,* 980–985.

Korsakoff, S. S. (1887). Disturbance of psychic function in alcoholic paralysis and its relation to the disturbance of the psychic sphere in multiple neuritis of non-alcoholic origin [in Russian]. *Vestnik Psychiatrii, 4*(2), 1–10.

Korst, L. O. (1964). *Tumors of the parietal lobes of the brain* [in Russian]. Moscow: Meditsina.

Kosaka, K. (1976). On aphasia of Pick's disease: A review of our own three cases and 49 autopsy cases in Japan. *Seishin Igaku, 18,* 1181–1189.

Kosaka, K. (1990). Diffuse Lewy body disease in Japan. *Journal of Neurology, 237,* 197–204.

Kosaka, K., Ikeda, K., Matsushita, M., & Iizuka, R. (1986). A combination of Alzheimer's disease and Binswager's disease—a clinicopathologic study of four cases. *Japanese Journal of Psychiatry and Neurology, 40,* 685–692.

Kosaka, K., Matsushita, M., Oyanagi, S., et al. (1980). A clinicopathological study of the "Lewy body disease." *Seishin Shinkeigaku Zasshi (Pschiatria et neurolica Japonica), 82,* 292–311.

Kosslyn, S. M., Alpert, N. M., Thompson, W. L., Chabris, C. F., Rauch, S. L., & Anderson, A. K. (1994). Identifying objects seen from different viewpoints: A PET investigation. *Brain, 117,* 1055–1071.

Kosslyn, S. M., Flynn, R. A., Amsterdam, J. B., & Wang, G. (1990). Components of high-level vision: A cognitive neuroscience analysis and accounts for neurological syndromes. *Cognition, 34,* 203–207.

Kostic, V. S., Djuricic, B. M., Covickovic-Sternic, N., Bumbasirevic, L., Nicolic, M., & Mrsulja, B. B. (1987). Depression and Parkinson's disease: Possible role of serotoninergic mechanisms. *Journal of Neurology, 234,* 94–96.

Kotrla, K. J., Chacko, R. C., Harper, R. G., Jihnran, S., & Doody, R. (1995). SPECT findings on psychosis in Alzheimer's disease. *American Journal of Psychiatry, 152,* 1470–1475.

Kovacs, M., Mukerk, P., Drash, A., et al. (1995). Biomedical and psychiatric risk factors for retinopathy among children with IDDM. *Diabetes Care, 18,* 1592–1599.

Kraepelin, E. (1917). *Lectures on clinical psychiatry* (T. Johnston, Trans.). New York: W. Wood. (original work published 1905)

Kraepelin, E. (1913). *Psychiatrie* (8th ed., Vol. 3). Leipzig: Johann Ambrosius Barth.

Kraepelin, E. (1919). Dementia praecox and paraphrenia. In G. M. Robertson (Ed.) & R. M. Barclay (Trans.), *Textbook of psychiatry* (Vol. 3, part 2, section endogenious dementias, pp.). Edinburgh: Livingston.

Kramer, J. H., Delis, D. C., & Nakada, T. (1985). Buccofacial apraxia without aphasia due to right parietal lesion. *Annals of Neurology, 18,* 512–514.

Kremin, H. (1987). Is there more than ah-oh-oh? Alternative strategies for writing and repeating lexically. In M. Coltheart, R. Sartori, & R. Job (Eds.), *The cognitive neuropsychology of language* (pp. 295–335). London: Erlbaum.

Kretchmer, E. (1949). Die Irbital hitn und Zwischenhirnsyndrome nach Schadelbasisfrakturen. *Archiv für Psychiatrie, 182,* 452–477.

Krishaber, H. (1873). *La Névropathie Cérébro-Cardiaque*. Paris: Masson.

Krishnan, K. R., McDonald, W. M., Escalona, P. R., et al. (1992). Magnetic resonance imaging of depression: Preliminary observations. *Archives of General Psychiatry, 49*, 553–557.

Kritchevsky, M., Graff-Redfford, N. R., & Damasio, A. R. (1987). Normal memory after damage to medial thalamus. *Archives of Neurology, 44*, 959–962.

Kritchevsky, M., & Squire, L. R. (1993). Permanent global amnesia with unknown etiology. *Neurology, 43*, 326–332.

Kroll, L., & Drummond, I. M. (1993). Temporal lobe epilepsy and obsessive-compulsive symptoms. *Journal of Nervous and Mental Diseases, 181*, 457–458.

Kroll, M. B. (1910). Beiträge zum Studium der Apraxia. *Zeitschrift für Gesamte Neurologie und Psychiatrie, 2*, 315–325.

Kroll, M. B. (1933). *Neurological syndromes* [in Russian]. Kharkiv, Kiev: Meditsina.

Kroll, M. B. (1934). *Progress in the study of aphasia, agnosia, apraxia* [in Russian]. Moscow: Meditsina.

Kroth, N. (1967). Status with psychomotor attacks. *Electroencephalography and Clinical Neurophysioogy, 23*, 183–184.

Kullberg, G. (1977). Differences in effects of capsulotomy and cingulotomy. In W. H. Sweet, W. S. Obrador, & J. G. Martin-Rodriguez (Eds.), *Neurological treatment in psychiatry, pain and epilepsy* (pp. 301–308). Baltimore, MD: University Park Press.

Kumar, A., & Gottlieb, G. (1993). Frontotemporal dementia: A new clinical syndrome? *The American Journal of Geriatric Psychiatry, 1*, 95–106.

Kumar, A., Koss, E., Metzler, D., et al. (1988). Behavioral symptomatology in dementia of the Alzheimer type. *Alzheimer's Disease and Associated Disorders, 2*, 363–365.

Kurachi, M., Yamaguchi, N., Inasaka, T., & Torii, H. (1979). Recovery from alexia without agraphia: Report of an autopsy. *Cortex, 15*, 297–312.

Kurth, W. (1941). Pseudohalluzination bei organischen Krankheiten. *Archiv für Psychiatrie und Nervenkrankheiten, 112*, 90–100.

Kussmaul, A. (1877). *Die Störungen der Sprache*. Leipzig: Vogel.

Kuypers, H. G. J. M. (1978). The general organization of the thalamo-cortical connections in the rhesus monkey. In J. E. Desmedt (Ed.), *Cerebral motor control in man* (pp. 10–20). Basel: Karger.

LaBar, K. S., Gatenby, J. C., Gore, J. C., LeDoux, J. E., & Phelps, E. A. (1998). Human amygdala activation during conditioned fear acqustion and extinction: a mixed-trial fMRI study. *Neuron, 20*, 937–945.

Lackner, J. R., & Teuber, H. L. (1973). Alterations in auditory fusion thresholds after cerebral injury in man. *Neuropsychologia, 11*, 409–415.

Ladavas, E., Umilta, C., & Ricci-Bitti, P. E. (1980). Evidence for sex differences in right hemisphere dominance for emotions. *Neuropsychologia, 18*, 361–366.

Laignel-Lavastine, M., Alajouanine, T. (1921). Un cas d'agnosie auditive. *Revue Neurologique, 37*, 194–198.

Lamy, M. (1907). Amnésie musical chez un aphasique sensoriele. *Revue Neuro-logique, 15*, 688–693.

Landis, T., Cummings, J. L., Christen, L., Bogen, J. E., & Imhof, H. G. (1986). Are unilateral posterior cerebral lesions sufficient to cause prosopagnosia? Clinical and radiological findings in six additional patients. *Cortex, 22*, 243–252.

Landis, T., Graves, R., Benson, F., & Hebben, N. (1982). Visual recognition through kinaesthetic mediation. *Psychological Medicine, 12*, 515–531.

Landis, T., & Regard, M. (1988). Two cases of prosopagnosia and alexia. Part I: Neuropsychological findings. In M. Bjic (Ed.), *Neuron, brain and behavior, advances in biosciences: Vol. 80* (pp. 89–95). Oxford: Pergamon Press.

Lando, M., & Edelman, S. (1995). Receptive field spaces and class-based generalization from a single view in face recognition. *Network, 6*, 551–576.

Landolt, H. (1958). Serial EEG investigations during psychotic episodes in epileptic patients and during schizophrenic attacks. In L. De Haas (Ed.), *Lectures on Epilepsy* (pp. 91–133). Amsterdam: Elsevier.

Landolt, H. (1963). Die Daemmer und Verstimmungszustaende bei Epilepsie and ihre EEG. *Deutsche Zeitschfrift Für Nervenheikunde, 185*, 411–430.

Lange, J. (1930). Fingeragnosie und Agraphie (ein psychopathologische Studie). *Monatschrift für Psychiatrie und Neurologie, 76*, 129–188.

Lange, J. (1936). Agnosien and Apraxien. In O. Bumke & O. Foerster (Eds.), *Handbuch der Neurologie* (pp. 807–960). Berlin: Springer.

Lanska, D. J., Lanska, M. J., & Mendez, M. (1987). Brainstem auditory hallucinosis. *Neurology, 37*, 1685.

Laplane, D., Baulac, M., Widlocher, D., & Dubois, B. (1984). Pure psychic akinesia with bilateral lesions of basal ganglia. *Journal of Neurology, Neurosurgery, and Psychiatry, 47*, 377–385.

Laplane, D., Levasseur, M., Pillon, B., et al. (1989). Obsessive-compulsive and other behavioural changes with bilateral basal ganglia lesions. *Brain, 112*, 699–725.

Laplane, D., Widlocher, D., Pillon, B., Baulac, M., & Binoux, F. (1981). Comportement compulsif d'allure obsessionelle par necrose circonscrite bilaterale pallido-striatale: enecephalopathie par piqure de guepe. *Revue Neurologique, 137*, 269–276.

Larsson, T., Sjoegren, T., & Jacobson, G. (1963). Senile dementia: a clinical, sociomedical, and genetic study. *Acta Psysciatrica Scandinavica, 167* (Suppl.), 1–259.

Lashley, K. S. (1929). *Brain mechanisms and behavior.* Chicago: University of Chicago Press.

Latto, R., & Cowey, A. (1971). Visual field defects after frontal eye-field lesions in monkeys. *Brain Research, 30*, 1–24.

Lauterbach, E. C., Jackson, J. G., Wilson, A. N., Dever, G. E. A., & Kirsh, A. D. (1997). Major depression after left posterior globus pallidus lesions. *Neurposychiatry, Neuropsyhology, and Behavioral Neurology, 10*, 9–16.

Lavenue, I., Pasquier, F., Leben, F., et al. (1999). Perceptions of emotion in frontotemporal dementia and Alzheimer's disease. *Alzheimer Disease and Associated Disorders, 13,* 96–101.

Lavy, S. (1959). Akinetic mutism in a case of craniopharyngioma. *Fortschrite der Neurologie, Psychiatrie und ihrer Grenzgebiete, 138,* 369–374.

Leckman, J. F., Grice, D. E., Boardman, J., et al. (1997). Symptoms of obsessive-compulsive disorder. *American Journal of Psychiatry, 154,* 911–917.

LeCours, A. R., & L'hermitte, F. (1976). The "pure" form of phonetique disintegration syndrome (pure anarthria); Anatomical-clinical report of a historical case. *Brain and Language, 3,* 88–113.

LeDoux, J. E. (1995). In search of an emotional system in the brain: Leaping from fear to emotion and consciousness. In M. S. Gazzaniga (Ed.), *The cognitive neuroscience* (pp. 1049–1061). Cambridge, MA: MIT Press.

LeDoux, J. E., Ciccetti, P., Xagoraris, A., & Romanski, L. M. (1990). The lateral amygdaloid nucleus: sensory interface of the amygdala in fear conditioning. *Journal of Neuroscience, 10,* 1062–1069.

Lee, H. W., Hong, S. D., Seo, D. W., Tae, W. S., & Hong, S. C. (2000). Mapping of functional organization in human visual cortex. *Neurology, 54,* 849–854.

Lees, A. J. (1990). Progressive supranuclear palsy. In J. L. Cummings (Ed.), *Subcortical dementia* (pp. 123–131). New York: Oxford University Press.

Leishner, A. (1961). Die autoscopischen Halluzinationen (Hautoscopie). *Fortschritte der Neurologie, Psychiatrie, und ihrer Grenzgebiete, 29,* 550–584.

Lemoyne, J., & Mahoudeau, D. (1959). A propos d'un cas d'agnosieauditive pure avec surdité cortical associée àune dysphonie fonctionelle. Observation anatomo-clinique. *Annals of Oto-Laryngology, 4,* 293–310.

Lennox, W. G. (1945). The petit mal epilepsies, their treatment with tridione. *Journal of American Medical Association, 129,* 1069–1074.

Lenox, G. G., & Lowe, J. S. (1996). The nosological status of Lewy body dementia. In R. H. Perry, I. G. McKeith, & E. K. Perry (Eds.), *Dementia with Lewy bodies* (pp. 9–20). Cambridge, UK: Cambridge University Press.

Lepola, U., Nousiainen, U., Riekkinen, P., & Rimón, R. (1990). EEG and CT findings in patients with panic disorder. *Biological Psychiatry, 28,* 721–727.

Leslie, A. M. (1990). Pretence, autism, and the basis of "theory of mind." *British Psychology Society, 3,* 120–123.

Lespérance, F., Frasure-Smith, N., & Talajic, M. (1996). Major depression before and after myocardial infarction. Its nature and consequences. *Psychosomatic Medicine, 58,* 99–110.

Lesser, I. M., Mena, I., Boone, K. B., Miller, B. L., Mehringe, C. M., & Wohl, M. (1994). Reduction in cerebral blood flow in older depressed patients. *Archives of General Psychiatry, 51,* 677–686.

Levin, B. E., Llabre, M. M., & Weiner, W. J. (1988). Parkinson's disease and depression: Psychometric properties of Back Depression Inventory. *Journal of Neurology, Neurosurgery, and Psychiatry, 51,* 1401–1404.

Levin, G. Z., Povorinsky, Y. A., & Tonkonogy, J. M. (1961). Analysis of the case with agnosia of faces developed after air embolism of cerebral vessels [in Russian]. In G. B. Abramovich & G. Z. Levin (Eds.), *Problems of Localization and Focal Diagnostic in Neurology and Psychiatry* (pp. 111–123), Leningrad: Bechterev Institute Press.

Levine, D., & Calvanio, R. (1978). A study of the visual defect in verbal alexia-simultanagnosia. *Brain, 101,* 65–81.

Levine, D. N., & Finkelstein, S. (1982). Delayed psychosis after right temporoparietal stroke or trauma: relation to epilepsy. *Neurology, 32,* 267–273.

Levine, D. N., Lee, J. M., & Fisher, C. M. (1993). The visual variant of Alzheimer's disease. *Neurology, 43,* 305–313.

Levine, D. N., Warach, J., & Farah, M. J. (1985). Two visual systems in mental imagery; Dissociation of "what" and "where" in imagery disorders due to bilateral posterior cerebral lesions. *Neurology, 35,* 1010–1018.

Lewandowsky, M. (1908). Uber abspaltung des Farbensinnes. *Monatschrift für Psychiatrie, 23,* 488–510.

Lewis, D. J. (1961). Lilliputian hallucinations in the functional psychoses. *Canadian Psychiatric Association Journal, 6,* 177–201.

Lewis, D. O., Pincus, J. H., Feldman, M., Jackson, L., & Brad, B. (1986). Psychiatric, neurological, and psychoeducational characteristics of 15 death row inmates in the United States. *American Journal of Psychiatry, 143,* 838–845.

Lewis, D. O., Pincus, T. H., Shanok, S. S., & Glaser, D. H. (1982). Psychomotor epilepsy and violence in a group of incarcerated adolescent boys. *American Journal of Psychiatry, 139,* 882–887.

Lewis, R. I. (1996). Interference in short-term memory: Magic number two (or three) in sentence processing. *Journal of Psycholinguistic Research, 25,* 93–115.

Lewis, S. W. (1987). Brain imaging in a case of Capgras syndrome. *British Journal of Psychiatry, 150,* 117–121.

Lewy, F. H. (1912). Paralysis agitans. In M. Lewandowsky (Ed.), *Handbuch der Neurologie* (Vol. 3/II, pp. 920–933). Berlin: Julius Springer.

Lewy, F. H. (1923). *Die Lehre vom Tonus and Bewegung.* Berlin: Springer.

Ley, R. G., & Bryden, M. P. (1981). Consciousness, emotion and right hemisphere. In G. Underwood & R. Stevens (Eds.), *Aspects of consciousness* (Vol. 2, pp. 216–239). Orlando: Academic Press.

Ley, R. G., & Bryden, M. P. (1982). Hemispheric differences in processing emotions and faces. *Brain and Language, 7,* 127–138.

Lezak, M. D. (1982). The problem of assessing executive functions. *International Journal of Psychology, 17,* 281–297.

Lhermitte, F., & Beauvois, M. F. (1973). A visual-speech disconnection syndrome: report of a case with optic aphasia, agnostic alexia, and colour agnosia. *Brain, 96,* 695–714.

Lhermitte, F., Chain, F., Escourorolle, A., Ducarne, B., Pillon, B., & Chedru, F. (1971). Etude des troubles perceptifs auditifs dans les lésions temporales bilatérales. *Revue Neurologique, 124,* 329–351.

Lhermitte, F., & Pillon, B. (1975). La prosopagnosie. Rôle de l'émisphère droit dans la perception visuelle. *Revue Neurologique, 131,* 791–812.

L'Hermitte, J. (1922). Syndrome dela callotte du pédoncle cérébral. Les troubles psycho-sensorieles dans les lésions du mesencéphale. *Revue Neurologique, 38,* 1359–1365.

L'Hermitte, J., & de Ajuriaguerra, J. (1938). Asymbolie tactile et hallucinations du toucher. Etude anatomoclinique. *Revue Neurologique, 70,* 492–495.

L'Hermitte, J., Levy, G., & Trelles, J. (1932). L'hallucinose pédonculaire (étude anatomique d'un cas). *Revue Neurologique, 48,* 382–388.

Liberman, A. M., Delattre, P. C., Gerstman, L. J., & Cooper, F. S. (1956). Tempo of frequency change as a cue for distinguishing classes of speech sounds. *Journal of Experimental Psychology, 52,* 127–137.

Lichter, D. G., Corbett, A. J., Fitzgibbon, G. E., et al. (1988). Cognitive and motor dysfunction in Parkinson's disease. *Archives of Neurology, 45,* 854–860.

Lichtheim, L. (1884). Uber aphasie. *Deutsche Archiv für Klinische Medizine, 36,* 204–208.

Lichtheim, L. (1885). On aphasia. *Brain, 7,* 433–484.

Liepmann, H. (1900). Das Krankheitshild der Apraxie (motorischen Asymbolie). *Monatschrift für Pyschiatrie, 8,* 15–44, 102–132, 182–197.

Liepmann, H. (1905). Die linke Hemisphare und das Handeln. *Munchen Medizinische Wochenschrift, 49,* 2375–2378.

Liepmann, H. (1906). Der weiterer Kranksheirverlauf bei den einseitig Apraktischen und der gehirnbefund auf Grund von Schnittserien. *Monatsschrift für Psychiatrie und Neurolologie, 17,* 289–311.

Liepmann, H. (1908). *Drei Aufsatze aus dem Apraxiegebiet* (Vol. 1). Berlin: Krager.

Liepmann, H. (1920). Apraxie. *Ergebnisse bei Gesamter Medizine, 1,* 515–543.

Liepmann, H., & Maas, O. (1907). Fall von Liksseitiguer Agraphie und Apraxie bei rechtsseitiger Laehmung. *Zeitschrift für Psychologie und Neurologie, 10,* 214–227.

Liepmann, H., & Pappenheim, M. (1914). Uber einen Fall von Sogennanter Leitungsaphasie mit anatomischen Befund. *Zeitschrift für gesamte Neurolgie und Psychiatrie, 27,* 1–41.

Lilly, R., Cummings, J. L., Benson, D. F., et al. (1983). The human Kluver-Bucy syndrome. *Neurology, 33,* 1141–1145.

Lin, K. N., Liu, R. S., Yeh, T. P., Wang, S. J., & Liu, H. S. (1993). Posterior ischemia during an attack of transient global amnesia. *Stroke, 103,* 161–178.

Lindqvist, G., & Norlen, G. (1966). Korsakoff's syndrome after operation of ruptured aneurismy of the anterior communicating artery. *Acta Psychiatrica Scandinavica, 42,* 24–34.

Lipowski, Z. J. (1967). Delirium, clouding of consciousness and confusion. *Journal of Mental and Nervous Diseases, 145,* 227–255.

Lipowski, Z. J. (1980). *Delirium: Acute brain failure in man.* Springfield, IL: Charles C. Thomas.

Lipowski, Z. J. (1983). Transient cognitive disorders (delirium, acute confusional states) in the elderly. *American Journal of Psychiatry, 140,* 1426–1436.

Lippa, C. F. R., Cohen, R., Smith, T. W., & Drachman, D. A. (1991). primary progressive aphasia with focal neuronal achromatopsia. *Neurology, 41,* 882–886.

Lishman, W. A. (1966). Psychiatric disability after head injury: The significance of brain damage. *Proceeding of the Royal Society of Medicine, 59,* 261–266.

Lishman, W. A. (1968). Brain damage in relation to psychiatric disability after head injury. *British Journal of Psychiatry, 114,* 373–410.

Lishman, W. A. (1978). *Organic psychiatry. The psychological consequences of cerebral disorder.* Oxford, England: Blackwell Scientific Publications.

Lisovski, F., Koskas, P., Dubard, T., Dassarts, I., Dehen, H., & Cambier, J. (1993). Left tuberothalamic artery territory infarction: Neuropsychological and MRI features. *European Neurology, 33,* 181–184.

Lissauer, H. (1890). Ein Fall von Seelinblindheit nebst einem Beitrag zur Theorie derselben. *Archiv für Psychiatrie und Nervenkrankheiten, 21,* 222–270.

Litvan, I., Grimes, D. A., Lang, A. E., et al. (1999). Clinical features differentiating patients with postmortem confirmed progressive supranuclear palsy and corticobasal degeneration. *Journal of Neurology, 246* (Suppl. 2), II1–II5.

Logothetis, N. K., Pauls, J., & Poggio, T. (1995). Shape representation in the inferior temporal cortex of monkeys. *Current Biology, 5*(5), 552–563.

Loizou, L. A., Kendall, B. E., & Marshall, J. (1981). Subcortical arteriosclerotic encephalopathy: a clinical and radiological investigation. *Journal of Neurology, Neurosurgery, and Psychiatry, 44,* 294–304.

Lombroso, C. (1911). *Crime: Its cause and remedies.* Boston: Little and Brown.

Louiseau, P., Cahadon, F., & Cahadon, S. (1971). Gelastic epilepsy. *Epilepsia, 12,* 313–323.

Lowenberg, K. (1936). Pick's disease. A clinicopathologic contribution. *Archive of Neurology and Psychiatry, 36,* 768–789.

Lucchelli, F., De Renzi, E., Perani, D., & Fazio, F. (1994). Primary amnesia of insidious onset with subsequent stabilization. *Journal of Neurology, Neurosurgery, and Psychiatry, 57,* 1366–1370.

Luchins, D. J., Metz, J. T., Marks, R. C., & Cooper, M. D. (1989). Basal ganglia regional glucose metabolism asymmetry during a catatonic episode. *Biological Psychiatry, 26,* 725–728.

Lugaresi, A., Montagna, P., Morreale, A., & Gallassi, R. (1990). "Psychic akinesia" following carbon monoxide poisoning. *European Neurology, 30,* 167–169.

Lugaresi, E., Pazzaglia, P., & Tassinari, C. A. (1971). Differentiation of "absence status" and "temporal lobe status." *Epilepsia, 12,* 77–87.

Lukianowicz, N. (1958). Autoscopic phenomena. *Archives of Neurology and Psychiatry, 80,* 190–220.

Luria, A. R. (1959). Disorders of "simultaneous perception" in a case of bilateral occipitoparietal brain injury. *Brain, 83,* 437–449.

Luria, A. R. (1966). *Higher cortical functions in man.* New York: Basic Books.

Luria, A. R. (1970). *Traumatic aphasia* (2nd ed.). The Hague: Mouton.

Luria, A. R., Pravdina-Vinarskaya, E. N., & Yarbuss, A. L. (1963). Disorders of ocular movement in a case of simultanagnosia. *Brain, 86,* 219–228.

Luria, A. R., Tsvetkova, L. S., & Futer, J. C. (1965). Aphasia in a composer. *Journal of Neurological Science, 2,* 250–262.

Lynch, M. J. G. (1960). Brain lesions in chronic alcoholism. *Archives of Pathology* (Chicago), *69,* 242–252.

Mackie, J., Ebmeier, K. P., & O'Carroll, R. E. (1994). An MRI, SPECT and neuropsychological study of a patient presenting with Capgras syndrome. *Behavioural Neurology, 7,* 211–215.

MacLean, P. D. (1952). Some psychiatric implications of physiological studies on the frontotemporal portion of the limbic system (visceral brain). *Electorencephalography and Clinical Neurophysiology, 4,* 407–418.

Maher, E. R., Smith, E. M., & Lees, A. J. (1985). Cognitive defects in the Steele-Richardson-Olszewski syndrome (progressive supranuclear palsy). *Journal of Neurology, Neurosurgery, and Psychiatry, 48,* 1234–1239.

Mahoudeau, D., Lemoyne, J., Foncin, J. F., & Dubrisay, J. (1958). Considérations sur l'agnosie auditive (àpropos d'un cas anatomoclinique). *Revue Neurologique, 99,* 454–471.

Mahut, H., Zola-Morgan, S., & Moss, M. (1982). Hippocampal resections impair associative learning and recognition memory in the monkey. *Journal of Neurscience, 2,* 1214–1229.

Malamud, N. (1967). Psychiatric disorder with intracranial tumors of limbic system. *Archives of Neurology, 17,* 113–123.

Malamud, N., & Skillicorn, S. A. (1956). Relationship between the Wernicke and Korsakoff syndrome. *Archives of Neurology and Psychiatry, 76,* 585–596.

Malloy, P., Cimino, C., & Westlake, R. (1992). Differential diagnosis of primary and secondary Capgras delusions. *Neuropsychiatry, Neuropsychology, and Behavioral Neurology, 5,* 83–96.

Malloy, P. F., & Richardson, E. D. (1994). The frontal lobe and content-specific delusions. *Journal of Neuropsyhiatry and Clinical Neuroscience, 6,* 455–466.

Mandell, A. M., & Albert, M. L. (1990). History of subcortical dementia. In J. L. Cummings (Ed.), *Subcortical dementia* (pp. 17–30). New York: Oxford University Press.

Mandell, A. M., Alexander, M. P., & Carpenter, S. (1989). Creutzfeldt-Jacob disease presenting as isolated aphasia. *Neurology, 39,* 55–58.

Mann, S. C., & Caroff, S. N. (1987). Lethal catatonia and neuroleptic malignant syndrome. *American Journal of Psychiatry, 144,* 1106–1107.

Mann, S. C., Caroff, S. N., & Bleiler, H. R. (1986). Lethal catatonia. *American Journal of Psychiatry, 143,* 1374–1381.

Maquet, P., Degueldre, D., Delfiore, G., et al. (1997). Functional neuroanatomy of human slow wave sleep. *Journal of Neuroscience, 17,* 2807–2812.

Marcuse, H. (1904). Apraktische Symptome bei einem Fall von senile Demenz. *Zentralblatt für Nervenheilkunde und Psychiatrie, 27,* 737–751.

Marg, E., & Dierssen, G. (1965). Reported visual percepts from stimulation of human brain during therapeutic surgery. *Comparative Neurology, 26,* 57–75.

Marie, P. (1906a). Revision de la question de l'aphasia: La troisième convolution frontale gauche ne joue aucun róle spécial dans la fonction du language. *Semaine Médicale, 26,* 241–247.

Marie, P. (1906b). Revision de la question de l'aphasie: Que faut-il penser des aphasies sous-corticales (aphasies pures)? *Semaine Médicale, 46,* 493–500.

Marie, P., & Foix, C. (1917). Les aphasies de guerre. *Revue Neurologique, 24,* 53–87.

Marin, O. S. M. (1980). CAT scans of five deep dyslexic patients. In M. Coltheart, K. Patterson, & J. C. Marshall (Eds.), *Deep dyslexia* (pp. 452–453). London: Routledge and Kegan Paul.

Marin, R. S. (1996). Apathy and related disorders of diminished motivation. In I. J. Dickstein, M. B. Riba, & J. M. Oldham (Eds.), *American psychiatric press review of psychiatry,* Vol. 15 (pp. 304–314), Washington, DC: American Psychiatric Press.

Mark, V. H., & Ervin, F. R. (1970). *Violence and brain.* New York: Harper and Row.

Markowitsch, H. J., Calabrese, P., Haupts, M., Durwen, H. F., Liess, J., & Gehlen, W. (1993). Searching for the anatomical basis of retrograde amnesia. *Journal of Clinical Experimental Neuropsychology, 15,* 947–967.

Marr, D. (1982). *Vision: A computational investigation into human representation and processing of visual information.* San Francisco: Freeman.

Marshall, J. C., & Newcombe, F. (1966). Syntactic and semantic errors in paralexia. *Neuropsychologia, 4,* 169–176.

Marshall, J. C., & Newcombe, F. (1973). Patterns of paralexia: A psycholinguistic approach. *Journal of Psycholinguistic Research, 2,* 175–199.

Marshall, V. G., Bradley, W. G., & Marshall, C. E., et al. (1988). Deep white matter infarction: Correlation of MRI imaging and histopathological findings. *Radiology, 16,* 517–522.

Martinot, J. L., Hardy, P., Feline, A., et al. (1990). Left prefrontal glucose hypometabolism in the depressed state: A confirmation. *American Journal of Psychiatry, 147,* 1313–1317.

Masdeu, J. C., Schoene, W. C., & Funkenstien, H. (1978). Aphasia following infarction of the left supplementary motor area. *Neurology, 28,* 1220–1223.

Master, D. R., Toone, B. K., & Scott, D. F. (1984). Interictal behavoir in TLE. In R. Porter (Ed.) *Advances in Epileptology: 15th Epilepsy International Symposium* (pp. 557–565). New York: Raven Press.

Masucci, E. F., Borts, F. T., Smirniotopoulos, J. G., & Kurtzke, J. F. (1985). Thin section CT of midbrain abnormalities in progressive supranuclear palsy. *American Journal of Neuroradiology, 6,* 767–772.

Matelli, M., & Luppino, G. (1997). Functional anatomy of human motor cortical areas. In F. Boller & J. Grafman (Eds.), *Handbook of neuropsychology, Volume XI* (pp. 9–26). Amsterdam: Elesvier.

Mathai, J. P., & Gopinath, P. S. (1986). Deficits of chronic schizophrenia in relation to long-term hospitalization. *British Journal of Psychiatry, 148,* 59–516.

Matsuo, H., Takashima, H., Kumamoto, T., et al. (1991). Pure akinesia: An atypical manifestation of progressive supranuclear palsy. *Journal of Neurology, Neurosurgery, and Psychiatry, 54,* 397–400.

Matthew, R. G., Meyer, J. S., Francis, D. J., et al. (1980). Cerebral blood flow in depression. *American Journal of Psychiatry, 137,* 1449–1450.

Mattis, S. (1976). Mental status examination for organic mental syndrome in the elderly patient. In L. Bellak & T. B. Larasu (Eds.), *Geriatric psychiatry* (pp. 77–121). New York: Grune and Stratton.

Mattis, S. (1988). *Dementia Rating Scale: Professional manual.* Odessa, FL: Psychological Assessment Resources.

Maturanath, P. S., Xuereb, J. H., Bak, T., et al. (2000). Corticobasal ganglionic degeneration and/or frontotemporal dementia? A report of two overlap cases and review of literature. *Journal of Neurology, Neurosurgery, and Psychiatry, 68,* 304–312.

Maunsell, J. H. R., & Newsome, W. T. (1987). Visual processing in monkey extrastriate cortex. *Annual Review of Neuroscience, 10,* 363–402.

Maunsell, J. H. R., & Van Essen, D. C. (1983). The connections of the middle temporal visual area (MT) and their relationship to a cortical hierarchy in the macaque monkey. *Journal of Neuroscience, 3,* 2563–2586.

Mavlov, L. (1980). Amusia due to rhythm agnosia in a musician with left hemisphere damage: A non auditory supramodel defect. *Cortex, 16,* 321–338.

Mayberg, H. S, Starstein, S. E., Peyser, C. E., Brandt, J., Dannals, R. F., & Folstein, S. E. (1992). Paralimbic frontal lobe hypometabolism in depression associated with Hungtington's disease. *Neurology, 42,* 1791–1797.

Mayberg, H. S, Starstein, S. E., Sadzot, B., et al. (1990). Selective hypometabolism in the inferior frontal lobe in depressed patients with Parkinson's disease. *Annals of Neurology, 28,* 57–64.

Mayer-Gross, W. (1935). On depersonalization. *British Journal of Medical Psychology, 15,* 103–122.

Mayer-Gross, W. (1936). Further observations on apraxia. *Journal of Mental Science, 82,* 744–762.

Mayer-Gross, W., Critchley, M., Greenfield, J. G., & Meyer, A. (1937–1938). Discussion on the presenile dementias: Symptomathology, pathology, and differential diagnosis. *Proceeding of the Royal Society of Medicine, 31,* 1433–1454.

Mayer-Gross, W., Slater, E., & Roth, M. (1960). *Clinical Psychiatry* (2nd ed.). London: Bailliere, Tindall, and Cassel.

Mayeux, R., Stern, Y., Cote, C., & Williams, J. B. (1984). Altered serotonin metabolism in depressed patients with Parkinson's disease. *Neurology, 34,* 642–646.

Mayeux, R., Stern, Y., Rosen, J., et al. (1983). Is "subcortical dementia" a recognizeable clinical entity? *Annals of Neurology, 14,* 278–283.

Mazzocchi, F., & Vignolo, L. A. (1979). Localization of lesions in aphasia: Clinical-CT scan correlation in stroke patients. *Cortex, 15,* 227–254.

McCarthy, R. A., Evans, J. J., & Hodges, G. R. (1996). Topographic amnesia: spatial memory disorder, perceptual dysfunction, or category specific semantic memory impairment? *Journal of Neurology, Neurosurgery, and Psychiatry, 60,* 318–325.

McCarthy, R. A., & Warrington, E. K. (1986). Visual associative agnosia: A clinico-anatomical study of a single case. *Journal of Neurology, Neurosurgery, and Psychiatry, 49,* 1233–1240.

McCarthy, M. A., & Warrington, E. K. (1988). Evidence for modality specific meaning systems in the brain. *Nature (London), 334,* 428–430.

McCarthy, R. A., & Warrington, E. K. (1990). *Cognitive neuropsychology, a clinical introduction.* San Diego: Academic Press.

McClelland, J. L., & Rumelhart, D. E. (1986). Amnesia and distributed memory. In J. L. McClelland & D. E. Rumelhat (Eds.), *Parallel distributed processing* (pp. 503-528). Cambridge, MA: MIT Press.

McEntee, W. J., Biber, M. P., Perl, D. P., & Benson, F. D. (1976). Diencephalic amnesia: A reappraisal. *Journal of Neurology, Neurosurgery, and Psychiatry, 39,* 436–441.

McEnvoy, J. P., Apperson, L. J., Appelbaum, P. S., et al. (1989). Insight in schizophrenia: Its relationship to acute psychopathology. *Journal of Nervous and Mental Diseases, 177,* 43–47.

McFarland, H. R., & Fortin, D. (1982). Amusia due to right temporoparietal infarct. *Archives of Neurology, 39,* 725–726.

McFee, J., & Zangwill, O. L. (1960). Visual-constructive disabilities associated with lesions of the left cerebral hemisphere. *Brain, 82,* 243–259.

McFie, J., Piercy, M. F., & Zangwill, O. L. (1950). Visual spatial agnosia associated with lesions of the right cerebral hemisphere. *Brain, 73,* 167–190.

McGeachie, R. E., Fleming, J. O., Sharer, L. R., & Hyman, R. A. (1979). Diagnosis of Pick's disease by computed tomography. *Journal of Computer Assisted Tomography, 3,* 113–115.

McGlynn, S. M., & Kazniak, A. W. (1991). Unawareness of deficit in dementia and schizophrenia. In G. P. Prigatano & D. L. Schacter (Eds.), *Awareness of deficit after brain injury: Clinical and theoretical issues* (pp. 84–110). New York: Oxford University Press.

McGlynn, S. M., & Schacter, D. L. (1997). The neuropsychology of insight: Impaired awareness of deficits in a psychiatric context. *Psychiatric Annals, 27,* 806–811.

McHugh, P. R., & Folstein, M. F. (1975). Psychiatric syndromes of Hungtington's chorea: A clinical and pharmacological study. In D. F. Benson & D. Blumer (Eds.), *Psychiatric aspects of neurologic disease* (pp. 267–285). New York: Grune and Stratton.

McKee, A. C., Levine, D., Kowall, N. W., Resell, H., & Richardson, E. P. (1988). Peduncular hallucinosis due to the bilateral infarction of media substantia nigra pars reticularis: a serial section, postmortem analysis [abstract]. *Annals of Neurology, 124,* 125–126.

McKeefry, D. J., & Zeki, S. (1997). The position and topography of the human colour centre as revealed by functional magnetic resonance imaging. *Brain, 120,* 2229–2242.

McKenna, P. J. (1984). Disorders with overvalued ideas. *British Journal of Psychiatry, 121,* 4.

McKenna, P. J., Mortimer, A. M., & Hodges, J. R. (1994). Semantic memory and schizophrenia. In A. S. David & J. C. Cutting (Eds.), *The neuropsychology of schizophrenia* (pp. 163–178). Hove, UK: Hillsdale.

McKenna, P. J., Tamlyn, D., Lund, C. E., Mortimer, A., Hummond, S., & Baddeley, A. D. (1990). Amnesic syndrome in schizophrenia. *Psychological Medicine, 20,* 967–972.

McKinlay, W. W., Brooks, D. N., Bonds, M. R., et al. (1981). The short-term outcome of severe blunt head injury as reported by relatives of the head injury person. *Journal of Neurology, Neurosurgery, and Psychiatry, 44,* 527–533.

McKinzey, R. K., Roecker, C. E., Puente, A. E., & Rogers, E. B. (1998). Performance of normal adults on Luria-Nebraska Neuropsychological Battery. *Archives of Clinical Neuropsychology, 13,* 397–413.

Meadows, J. C. (1974). Disturbed perception of color associated with localized cerebral lesions. *Brain, 97,* 615–632.

Meadows, J. C., & Munro, S. S. F. (1977). Palinopsia. *Journal of Neurology, Neurosurgery, and Psychiatry, 40,* 5–8.

Meager, D. J., & Trepacz, P. T. (2000). Motoric subtypes of delirium. *Seminars in Clinical Neuropsychiatry, 5,* 76–85.

Medina, J. L., Chokroverty, S., & Rubino, F. A. (1977). Syndrome of agitated delirium and visual impairment: A manifestation of medial temporo-occipital infarction. *Journal of Neurology, Neurosurgery, and Psychiatry, 40,* 861–864.

Medina, J. L., Rubino, F. A., & Ross, E. (1974). Agitated delirium caused by infarctions of the hippocampal formation and fusiform and lingual gyri: A case report. *Neurology, 24,* 1181–1183.

Meerson, Y. A. (1977). About participation of the anterior parts of the left and right temporal lobes in the high visual functions [in Russian]. *Physiology of Man, 3,* 266–275.

Meerson, Y. A. (1986). *Higher visual functions. Visual gnosis* [in Russian]. Leningrad: Nauka.

Mega, M. S., Cummings, J. L., Salloway, S., & Malloy, P. (1997). The limbic system: An anatomic, phylogenetic, and clinical perspective. In S. Salloway, P. Malloy, & J. L. Cummings (Eds.), *The neuropsychiatry of limbic and subcortical disorders* (pp. 3–18). Washington, DC: American Psychiatric Press.

Mega, M. S., Masterman, D. L., Benson, F., Vinters, H. V., Tomiyasu, U., Craig, A. H., et al. (1996). Dementia with Lewy bodies: reliability and validity of clinical and pathologic criteria. *Neurology, 47,* 1403–1409.

Mehler, M. F. (1988). Mixed transcortical aphasia in nonfamilial dysphasic dementia. *Cortex, 24,* 545–554.

Mehta, Z., Newcombe, F., & DeHaan, E. (1992). Selective loss of imagery in a case of visual agnosia. *Neuropsychologia, 30,* 645–655.

Meier, M. G., & Martin, W. E. (1970). Intellectual changes associated with levodopa therapy. *Journal of American Medical Association, 213,* 465–466.

Mendez, M. F., Cherrier, M., Perryman, K. M., Pachana, N., Miller, B. L., & Cummings, J. (1996). Frontotemporal dementia versus Alzheimer's disease: Differential cognitive features. *Neurology, 47,* 1189–1194.

Mendez, M. F., Cummings, J. L., & Benson, F. (1986). Depression in epilepsy: Significance and phenomenology. *Archives of Neurology, 43,* 766–770.

Mendez, M. F., Martin, R. J., Smyth, K. A., & Whitehouse, P. J. (1990). Psychiatric symptoms associated with Alzheimer's disease. *Journal of Neuropsychiatry and Clinical Neuroscience, 2,* 28–33.

Menninger-Lerchental, E. (1935). *Das Truggebilde der Eigenen Gestalt* (Haeutoscopie, Doppelgaenger). Berlin: Karger.

Merigan, W. H., Nealey, T. A., & Maunsell, H. R. (1993). Visual effects of lesions of cortical area V2 in macaques. *Journal of Neuroscience, 13*(7), 3180–3191.

Merigan, W. H., & Pham, H. A. (1998). V4 lesions in macaques affect both single and multiple view-point shape. Discriminations. *Visual Neuroscience, 13,* 51–60.

Mesulam, M. M. (1981). Dissociative states with abnormal temporal EEG. *Archives of Neurology, 38,* 176–181.

Mesulam, M. M. (1982). Slowly progressive aphasia without generalized dementia. *Annals of Neurology, 11,* 592–597.

Mesulam, M. M., Waxman, S. C., Geschwind, N., & Sabin, T. D. (1976). Acute confusional state with right middle cerebral artery infarctions. *Journal of Neurology, Neurosurgery, and Psychiatry, 39,* 84–89.

Metter, E. J., Kempler, D., Jackson, C., Hanson, W. R., Mazziota, J. C., & Phelps, M. E. (1987). Cerebellar glucose metabolism in chronic aphasia. *Neurology, 37,* 1599–1606.

Mettler, F. A. (1955). Perpetual capacity, functions of the corpus striatum, and schizophrenia. *Psychiatric Quarterly, 29,* 89–111.

Metzinger, T. (2000). The *subjectivity* of subjective experience: A representationalist analysis of the first-person perspective. In T. Metzinger (Ed.), *Neural correlates of consciousness, empirical and conceptual questions* (pp. 285–306). Cambridge, MA: MIT Press.

Meyer, J. C., & Barron, D. W. (1960). Apraxia of gait: A clinicophysiological study. *Brain, 83,* 261–284.

Meyer, O. (1900). Ein-und doppelseitige homonyme Hemianopsie mit Orientirungsstorungen. *Monatschrift für Psychiatrie und Neurologie, 8,* 440–456.

Meyerson, R. A., Richard, I. H., & Kastenberg, J. S. (1997). Mood disorders secondary to demyelinating and movement disorders. *Seminars in Clinical Neuropsychiatry, 2,* 252–264.

Miceli, G., & Caramazza, A. (1993). The assignment of word stress in oral reading: Evidence from a case of acquired dyslexia. *Cognitive Neuropsychology, 10,* 273–296.

Miceli, G., Silvery, M. C., & Caramazza, A. (1985). Cognitive analysis of a case of pure agraphia. *Brain and Language, 25,* 187–212.

Michalakeas, A., Skoutas, C., Charalambous, A., Peristeris, A., Marinos, V., Keramari, E., et al. (1994). Insight in schizophrenia and mood disorders and its relation to psychopathology. *Acta Psychiatrica Scandinavica, 90,* 46–49.

Michel, F., Perenin, M. T., & Sieroff, E. (1986). Prosopagnosie sans hemianopsie apres lesion unilaterale occipito-temporal droite. *Revue Neurologic, 142,* 542–549.

Michel, F., Poncet, M., & Signoret, J. L. (1989). Les lesions responsables de la prosopagnoise sont-elles toujours bilaterales? *Revue Neurologique, 145,* 764–770.

Michon, A., Deweer, B., Pillon, B., Agid, Y., & Dubois, B. (1994). Relation of anosognosia to frontal lobe dysfunction in Alzheimer's disease. *Journal of Neurology, Neurosurgery, and Psychiatry, 57,* 805–809.

Middlebrooks, J. C. (1999). Cortical representation of auditory space. In M. Gazzaniga (Ed.), *The new cognitive neurosciences* (pp. 425–436). Cambridge, MA: MIT Press.

Migliorelli, R., Starkstein, S. E., Teson, A., et al. (1993). SPECT findings in patients with mania. *Journal of Neuropsychiatry and Clinical Neuroscience, 5,* 379–383.

Mignone, R. J., Donnely, E. F., & Sadowsky, D. (1970). Psychological and neurological comparisons of psychomotor and non-psychomotor epileptic patients. *Epilepsia, 11,* 345–359.

Mikorey, M. (1952). *Phantome and Doppelgaenger.* Munich: Lehmann.

Miller, B. L., Cummings, J. L., Villanueva-Meyer, D., et al. (1991). Frontal lobe degeneration: clinical, neuropsychological, and SPECT characteristics. *Neurology, 41,* 1374–1382.

Miller, B. L., Lesser, I. M., Boone, K., Goldberg, M., Hill, E., Miller, M. H., et al. (1989). Brain white-matter lesions and psychosis. *British Journal of Psychiatry, 155,* 73–78.

Miller, B. L., Lesser, I. M., Boone, K. B., Mill, E., Mehringer, C. M., & Wong, K. (1991). Brain lesions and cognitive functions in late-life psychosis. *British Journal of Psychiatry, 158,* 76–82.

Miller, T. C., & Crosby, T. W. (1979). Musical hallucinations in a deaf elderly patient. *Annals of Neurology, 5,* 301–302.

Mills, R. P., & Swanson, P. D. (1978). Verticular oculomotor apraxia and memory loss. *Annals of Neurology, 4,* 149–153.

Milner, A. D., & Goodale, M. A. (1993). Visual pathways to perception. *Progress in Brain Research, 95,* 317–337.

Milner, A. D., Perrett, D. I., Johnston, R. S., Baenson, P. J., Jordan, T. R., Heeley, D. W., et al. (1991). Perception and action in "visual form agnosia." *Brain, 114,* 405–428.

Milner, B. (1958). Visual recognition and recall after right temporal lobe excision in man. *Neuropsychologia, 6,* 191–210.

Milner, B. (1962). Laterality effect in audition. In V. B. Mountcastle (Ed.), *Interhemispheric relations and cerebral dominance* (pp. 111–145). Baltimore: Johns Hopkins Univesity Press.

Milner, B. (1963). Effects of different brain lesions on card sorting: The role of the frontal lobe. *Archives of Neurology, 9,* 90–100.

Milner, B. (1965). Visually guided maze learning in man: Effects of bilateral hippocampal, bilateral frontal, and unilateral cerebral lesions. *Neuropsychologia, 3,* 317–338.

Milner, B. (1967). Brain mechanisms suggested by studies of temporal lobes. In F. L. Darley (Ed.), *Brain mechanisms underlying speech and language* (pp. 122–145). New York: Grune and Stratton.

Milner, B. (1968). Visual recognition and recall after rigtht temporal lobe excision in man. *Neuropsychologia, 6,* 191–209.

Milner, B. (1971). Interhemispheric differences in the localization of pathological processes in man. *British Medical Bulletin, 27,* 272–277.

Milner, B., & Teuber, H. L. (1968). Alteration of perception and memory in man. In L. Weiskrantz (Ed.), *Analysis of behavioral changes* (pp. 268–235). New York: Harper and Row.

Milner, P. M. (1974). A model for visual shape recognition. *Psychological Review, 81*(6), 521–535.

Minden, S. L., Orav, J., & Reich, P. (1989). Characteristics and predictors of depression in multiple sclerosis. In K. Jensen, L. Knudsen, & E. Stenager (Eds.), *Mental disorders and cognitive deficit in multiple sclerosis* (pp. 129–139). London: John Libbey.

Minden, S. L., & Shiffer, R. B. (1990). Affective disorders in multiple sclerosis: Review and recommendations for clinical research. *Archives of Neurology, 47,* 98–104.

Mishkin, M. (1966). Visual functions beyond striate cortex. In R. W. Russel (Ed.), *Frontiers of psychological psychology.* New York: Academic Press.

Mishkin, M. (1978). Memory in monkeys severely impaired by combined but not separate removal of amygdala and hippocampus. *Nature, 273,* 297–298.

Mishkin, M., & Manning, F. J. (1978). Non-spatial memory after selective prefrontal lesions in monkeys. *Brain Research, 143,* 313–323.

Mishkin, M., & Pribram, K. (1954). Visual discrimination performance following partial ablation of the temporal lobe. *Journal of Comparative Physiology and Psychology, 47*, 14–20.

Mitchell, S. L. (1817). Case report: Miss Mary Reynolds. *Medical Repository, 3*, 185–186.

Mitchell-Heggs, N., Kelly, D., & Richardson, A. (1976). Stereotactic limbic leucotomy: A follow-up at 16 months. *British Journal of Psychiatry, 128*, 226–240.

Miyachi, S., Hikosaka, O., Miyashita, K., Karadi, Z., & Rand, M. K. (1997). Differential roles of monkey striatum in learning of sequential hand movement. *Experimental Brain Research, 115*, 1–5.

Mizusawa, H., Mochizuki, A., Ohkoshi, N., Yosizawa, K., Kanazawa, I., & Imai, H. (1993). Progressive supranuclear palsy presenting with pure akinesia. *Advances in Neurology, 60*, 618–621.

Mohr, J. P., Leicester, J., Stoddard, I. T., & Sidman, M. (1971). Right hemianopia with memory and color deficits in circumscribed left posterior cerebral artery territory infarction. *Neurology, 21*, 1104–1111.

Mohr, J. P., Pessin, M. J., Finkelstein, J., Funkenstein, S. S., Duncan, G. W., et al. (1978). Broca's aphasia: pathologic and clinical. *Neurology, 4*, 311–324.

Monakow, C. von. (1904). Uber den gegenwaertigen Stand der Frage nach der Lokalisation im groshirn, VII, Frontale Rindenfelder. *Ergebniss Physiologie, 3*, 100–122.

Monrad-Krohn, G. H. (1947). Dysprosody or altered "melody of language." *Brain, 70*, 405–415.

Morlaas, J. (1928). *Contribution a l'etude de l'apraxia.* Paris: Amedée Legrand.

Morris, J. S., Frith, C. D., Perrett, D. I., et al. (1996). A differential neural response in the human amygdala to fearful and happy facial expressions. *Nature, 383*, 812–815.

Morris, M. K., Bowers, D., Chaterjee, A., & Heilman, K. M. (1992). Amnesia following a discrete forebrain lesion. *Brain, 115*, 1827–1847.

Morse, R. M., & Litin, E. M. (1971). The anatomy of delirium. *American Journal of Psychiatry, 128*, 111–115.

Mortimer, J. A., Pirozzolo, F. J., Hansch, E. C., Webster, D. D. (1982). Relationship of motor symptoms to intellectual deficit in Parkinson's disease. *Neurology, 32*, 133–137.

Moutier, F. (1908). *L'Aphasie de Broca.* Paris: Steinheil.

Mozley, P. D., Gur, R. E., Resnick, S. M., et al. (1994). Magnetic resonance imaging in schizophrenia: Relationship with clinical measures. *Schizophrenia Research, 12*, 195–203.

Mulder, D. W. (1953). Paroxysmal psychiatric symptoms observed in epilepsy. *Staff Meeting MAYO Clinic, 28*, 31–35.

Mullan, S., & Penfield, W. (1959). Illusions of comparative interpretation and emotions: production by electrical discharge and by electrical stimulation in the temporal cortex. *AMA Archives of Neurology and Psychiatry, 81*, 269–284.

Muller, B., & Reinhardt, J. (1991). *Neural networks: An introduction*. Berlin: Springer-Verlag.

Mungas, D. (1982). Interictal behavior abnormalities in TLE. *Archives of General Psychiatry, 39*, 108–111.

Mungas, D., Jagust, W. J., Reed, B. R., Kramer, J. H., Weiner, M. W., Schuuff, N., et al. (2001). MRI predictor of cognition in subcortical ischemic vascular disease and Alzheimer's disease. *Neurology, 57*, 2229–2235.

Munk, H. (1881). *Uber die Functionen der Grosshirnrinde. Gesamte Mittheilungenaus der Jahren, 1877–1880*. Berlin: Hirschwald.

Murata, S., Naritomi, H., & Sawada, T. (1994). Musical auditory hallucinations caused by a brainstem lesion. *Neurology, 44*, 154–158.

Murrell, J. R., Koller, D., Foroud, T., et al. (1997). Familial multiple system tauopathy with presenile dementia is localized to chromosome 17. *American Journal of Human Genetics, 61*, 1131–1138.

Murphy, D., & Cutting, J. (1990). Prosodic comprehension and expression in schizophrenia. *Journal of Neurology, Neurosurgery, and Psychiatry, 53*, 727–730.

Naguib, M., & Levy, R. (1982). Prediction of outcome in senile dementia: A computed tomography study. *British Journal of Psychiatry, 140*, 263–267.

Naguib, M., & Levy, R. (1987). Late paraphrenia: Neuropsychological impairment and structural brain abnormalities on computed tomography. *International Journal of Geriatric Psychiatry, 2*, 83–90.

Nakamura, K., Sakai, K., & Hikosaka, O. (1998). Neuronal activity in medial frontal cortex during learning of sequential procedures. *Journal of Neurophysiology, 80*, 2671–2687.

Narabayashi, H., Nagao, T., Saito, Y., et al. (1963). Stereotaxic amygdalotomy for behavior disorders. *Archives of Neurology, 9*, 1–16.

Nasrallah, H. A., Fowler, R. C., & Judd, L. L. (1981). Schizophrenia-like illness following head injury. *Psychosomatics, 22*, 359–361.

Nasrallah, H. A., Jacoby, C. G., McCalley-Whitters, M., et al. (1982). Cerebral ventricular enlargement in schizophrenia and mania. *Lancet, 1*, 1102.

Nasrallah, H. A., Kuperman, S., Hamra, B. J., et al. (1983). Clinical differences between schizophrenic patients with and without large cerebral ventricles. *Journal of Clinical Psychiatry, 44*, 407–409.

Nathan, P. W. (1947). Facial apraxia and apraxic dysarthria. *Brain, 70*, 449–478.

National Institute of Neurological and Communicative Disorders and Stroke. (1975). *A Classification and Outline of Cerebrovascular Disease, II Stroke, 6*, 564–616.

Nauta, W. J. H. & Feirtag, M. (1986). Fundamental neuroanatomy. New York: W. H. Freeman and Company.

Navia, B. A. (1990). The AIDS dementia complex. In J. L. Cummings (Ed.), *Subcortical dementia* (pp. 181–198). New York: Oxford University Press.

Navia, B. A., Jordan, B. D., & Price, R. W. (1986). The AIDS dementia complex. 1. Clinical features. *Annals of Neurology, 19*, 517–524.

Naville, F. (1922). Etudes sur les complications et les séquelles mentales de l'ecéphalite épidémique. La bradyphrénie. *L'Encéphale, 17,* 369–375, 423–436.

Neary, D., Snowden, J. S., & Mann, D. M. A. (1993). The clinical pathological correlates of lobar atrophy. *Dementia, 4,* 154–159.

Neary, D., Snowden, J. S., Norsen, B., & Goulding, P. (1988). Dementia of the frontal lobe type. *Journal of Neurology, Neurosurgery, and Psychiatry, 51,* 353–361.

Neuberger, K. T. (1957). The changing neuropathological picture of chronic alcoholism. *Archives of Pathology, 63,* 1–6.

Neumann, M. A. (1949). Pick's disease. *Journal of Neropathology and Experimental Neurology, 8,* 255–282.

Neumann, M. A., & Cohn, R. (1967). Progressive subcortical gliosis; a rare form of presenile dementia. *Brain, 90,* 405–418.

Newcombe, F. (1969). *Missile wounds of the brain.* London: Oxford University Press.

Newcombe, F. (1979). The processing of visual information in prosopagnosia and acquired dyslexia: Functional versus physiological interpretation. In D. J. Oborne, M. M. Gruneberg, & J. R. Eiser (Eds.), *Research in psychology and medicine* (pp. 315–322). London: Academic Press.

Newcombe, F., & Marshall, J. C. (1980). Transcoding and lexical stabilization in deep dyslexia. In M. Coltheart, K. E. Patterson, & J. C. Marshall (Eds.), *Deep dyslexia* (pp. 160–175). London: Routledge & Kegan Paul.

Newcombe, F., Young, A. W., & De Haan, E. H. F. (1989). Prosopagnosia and object agnosia without covert recognition. *Neuropsychologia, 27,* 179–191.

Newman, P. J., & Sweet, J. J. (1992). Depressive disorders. In A. E. Puente & R. J. McCaffrey (Eds.), *Handbook of neuropsychological assessment: A biopsychosocial perspective* (pp. 263–307). New York: Plenum Press.

Niedermeyer, E., & Khalifeh, R. (1965). Petit mal status ("spike wave stupro"). An electro-clinical appraisal. *Epilepsia, 6,* 250–262.

Nielsen, J. M. (1937). Unilateral cerebral dominance as related to mind blindness. *Archives of Neurology and Psychiatry, 38,* 108–135.

Nielsen, J. M. (1939). The unsolved problems in aphasia. II. Alexia resulting from a temporal lesion. *Bulletin of the Los Angeles Neurological Societies, 4,* 168–183.

Nielsen, J. M. (1946). *Agnosia, apraxia, aphasia: Their value in cerebral localization.* New York: Hoeber.

Nielsen, J. M., & Jacobs, L. I. (1951). Bilateral lesions of the *anterior cingulate gyri.* Report of a case. *Bulletin of the Los Angeles Neurological Society, 16,* 231–234.

Nightingale, S. (1982). Somatoparaphrenia: A case report. *Cortex, 18,* 463–467.

Nishijo, H., Ono, T., Nakamura, K., Kawabata, M., & Yamatani, K. (1986). Neuronal activity in and adjacent to the dorsal amygdala of monkey during operant feeding behavior. *Brain Research Bulletin, 17,* 847–854.

Nishijo, H., Ono, T., & Nishino, H. (1988). Single neuron responses in amygdala of alert monkey during complex sensory stimulation with affective significance. *Journal of Neuroscience, 8,* 3570–3583.

Nissen, M. J., & Bullemer, P. (1987). Attentional requirement of learning: Evidence from performance measures. *Cognitiva Psychology, 19,* 1–32.

Nissenbaum, H., Quinn, N. P., Brown, R. G., Toone, B., Gotham, A. M., & Marsden, C. D. (1987). Mood swings associated with the "on-off" phenomenon in Parkinson's disease. *Psychological Medicine, 17,* 899–904.

Nobler, M. S., Sackeim, H. A., Prohovnik, I., et al. (1994). Regional cerebral blood flow in mood disorders. III: Treatment and clinical response. *Archives of General Psychiatry, 51,* 884–897.

Nofzinger, E. A., Mintun, M. A., Wiseman, M. B., Kupfer, D. J., & Moore, R. Y. (1997). Forebrain activation in REM sleep: An FDG PET study. *Brain Research, 770,* 192–201.

Noguchi, H., & Moore, J. W. (1913). A demonstration of treponema pallidum in the brain in cases of general paralysis. *Journal of Experimental Medicine, 17,* 232–238.

Nolan, K. A., & Carramazza, A. (1982). Modality independent impairments in word processing in a deep dyslexic patient. *Brain and Language, 16,* 237–264.

Norman, D. A., & Shallice, T. (1986). Attention to action: Willed and automatic control of behavior. In R. J. Davidson, J. E. Schwartz, & D. Shapiro (Eds.), *Consciousness and self-regulation* (pp. 1–18). New York: Plenum Press.

Ochipa, C., Rothi, L. J., & Heilman, K. M. (1992). Conceptual apraxia in Alzheimer's disease. *Brain, 115,* 1061–1071.

O'Connor, M., Butter, N., Miliotis, P., & Eslinger, P. (1992). The dissociation of retrograde and anterograde amnesia in a patient with herpes encephalitis. *Journal of Clinical and Experimental Neuropsychology, 14,* 159–178.

O'Craven, K. M., & Konvisker, N. (2000). Mental imagery of faces and places activates corresponding stimulus-specific brain regions. *Journal of Cognitive Neuroscience, 126,* 1013–1023.

Ogden, J. A. (1985). Autotopagnosia: Occurrence in a patient without nominal aphasia and with intact ability to point to parts of animals and objects. *Brain, 108,* 1009–1022.

Ogden, J. A. (1987). The "neglected" left hemisphere and its contribution to visuospatial neglect. In M. Jeannerod (Ed.), *Neurophysiological and neuropsychological aspects of spatial neglect* (pp. 215–233). Amsterdam: Elsevier-Nort-Holland.

Ogrocki, P. K., Hills, A. C., & Strauss, M. E. (2000). Visual exploration of facial emotion by healthy older adults and patients with Alzheimear's disease. *Neuropsychiatry, Neuropsychology, and Behavioral Neurology, 13*(4), 271–278.

Ojemann, G. A., & Whitaker, H. (1978). Language localization and variability. *Brain and Language, 6,* 239–260.

Okasha, A., Sadek, A., & Moneim, S.A. (1975). Psychosocial and electroencephalographic studies of Egyptian murderers. *British Journal of Psychiatry, 126,* 34–40.

Olson, S. C., Nasrallah, H. A., Coffman, J. A., Schwarzkopf, S. B. (1991). CT and MRI abnormalities in schizophrenia: relationship with negative symptoms. In J. F. Greden & R. Tandon (Eds.), *Negative schizophrenic symptoms: Pathophysiology and clinical implications* (pp. 145–160). Washington, DC: American Psychiatric Press.

Olszewski, J. (1962). Subcortical arteriosclerotic encephalopathy. *World Neurology, 3,* 359–375.

Olton, D. S., & Wenk, G. L. (1987). Dementia: Animal model of the cognitive impairment produced by degeneration of the basal forebrain cholinergic system. In H. Y. Meltzer (Ed.), *Psychopharmacology: The thrid generation of progress* (pp. 941–953). Ney York: Raven Press.

Ombredane, A. (1951). *L'aphasie et l'élaborationde la pensée explicite.* Paris: Presse Universitaire.

Ono, T., & Nishijo, H. (2000). Neurophysiological basis of emotion in primates: Neuronal responses in the monkey amygdala and anterior cingular cortex. In M. S. Gazzaniga (Ed.), *The new cognitive neuroscience* (pp. 1099–1114). Cambridge, MA: MIT Press.

Oppenheim, H. (1989). Zur Pathologie der Grooshirngeschwulste. *Archiv für Psychiatrie und Nervenkrankheiten, 21,* 560–587.

Oppler, W. (1950). Manic psychosis in case of parasaggital meningioma. *Archives of Neurology and Psychiatry, 64,* 417–430.

Orsillo, S. M., & McCaffrey, R. J. (1992). Anxiety disorder. In A. E. Puente & R. J. McCaffrey (Eds.), *Handbook of neuropsychological assessment: A biopsychosocial perspective* (pp. 215–261). New York: Plenum Press.

O'Scalaidhe, S. P., Wilson, F. A. W., & Goldman-Rakic, P. S. (1997). A real segregation of face-processing neurons in prefrontal cortex. *Science, 278,* 1135–1138.

O'Sullivan, B. T., Roland, P. E., & Kawashima, R. (1994). A PET study of somatosensory discrimination in man: Microgeometry vs. macrogeometry. *European Journal of Neuroscience, 6,* 137–148.

Owens, D. G. C., Johnstone, E. C., Crow, T. J., et al. (1985). Lateral ventricular size in schizophrenia: Relationship to the disease process and its clinical manifestations. *Psychological Medicine, 15,* 27–41.

Oxbury, J. M., Oxbury, S. M., & Humphrey, N. K. (1969). Varieties of color anomia. *Brain, 92,* 847–860.

Ozonoff, S., Pennington, B. F., & Rogers, S. J. (1991). Executive function deficits in high-functioning autistic individuals: Relationship to theory of mind. *Journal of Child Psychology and Psychiatry and Allied Disciplines, 32,* 1081–1105.

Pachana, N. A., Boone, K. B., Miller, B. L., Cummings, L., & Berman, N. (1996). Comparison of neuropsychological functioning in Alzheimer's disease and frontotemporal dementia. *Journal of International Neuropsychological Society, 2*, 505–510.

Paillas, J. E., Bourdouresques, J., Bonnal, J., & Provansal, J. (1950). Tumeurs frontales. Considérations anatomo-cliniques ápropos de 72 tumeurs opérées. *Revue Neurologique, 83*, 470–473.

Paillas, C. A. (1955). Impaired identification of faces and places with agnosia for colours. Report of a case due to cerebral embolism. *Journal of Neurology, Neurosurgery, and Psychiatry, 18*, 218–224.

Pandurangi, A. K., Bilder, R. M., Rieder, R. O., et al. (1988). Schizophrenic symptoms and deterioration: Relation to computed tomography findings. *Journal of Nervous and Mental Diseases, 176*, 200–206.

Pandya, D. N., & Kuypers, H. J. G. M. (1969). Cortico-cortical connections in the resus monkey. *Brain Research, 13*, 13–36.

Pantelis, C., Barnes, T. R. E., Nelson, H. E. (1992). Is the concept of frontal-subcortical dementia relevant to schizophrenia? *British Journal of Psychiatry, 160*, 442–460.

Pantev, C. M., Hoke, M., Lehnertz, K., & Lutkenhoner, B. (1989). Neuromagnetic evidence of an amplitopic organization of the human auditory cortex. *Encephalography and Clinical Neurophysiology, 72*, 225–231.

Papez, J. W. (1937). A proposed mechanism of emotion. *Archive of Neurology and Psychiatry, 38*, 725–733.

Parasuraman, R. (1998). The attentive brain: Issues and prospects. In R. Parasurama (Ed.), *The attentive brain* (pp. 3–15). Cambridge, MA: MIT Press.

Pardo, J. V., Pardo, P. J., Raichie, M. E. (1993). Neural correlates of self-induced dysphoria. *American Journal of Psychiatry, 150*, 713–719.

Parekh, P. I., Spencer, J. W., George, M. S., et al. (1995). Procaine-induced increases in limbic rCBF correlate positively with increases in occipital and temporal EEG fast activity. *Brain Topography, 7*, 209–216.

Parker, A. J., Cummings, B. G., Johnston, E. B., & Hurlbert, A. C. (1995). Multiple cues for three-dimensional shape. In M. S. Gazzaniga (Ed.), *The cognitive neurosciences* (pp. 351–364). Cambridge, MA: MIT Press.

Parkin, A. J. (1984). Amnestic syndrome: A lesion specific disorder? *Cortex, 20*, 479–508.

Parkin, A. J. (1998). The central executive does not exist. *Journal of International Neuropsychological Society, 4*, 518–522.

Parkinson, J. (1817). *An essay on the shaking palsy*. London: Neely and Jones.

Partington, J. E., & Leiter, R. G. (1949). Partington's Pathway Test. *The Psychological Service Center Bulletin, 1*, 9–20.

Passingham, R. E. (1975). Delayed matching after selective prefrontal lesions in monkeys (Macaca mulatta). *Brain Research, 92*, 89–102.

Paterson, A., & Zangwill, O. L. (1944). Disorders of visual space perception associated with lesions of the right cerebral hemisphere. *Brain, 67*, 331–358.

Paterson, A., & Zangwill, O. L. (1945). A case of topographical disorientation associated with a unilateral cerebral lesion. *Brain, 68,* 188–211.

Patterson, K. E., & Hodges, J. (1992). Deterioration of word meaning: Implications for reading. *Cognitive Neuropsychology, 30,* 1025–1040.

Patterson, K. E., Marshall, J. C., & Coltheart, M. (1985). *Surface dyslexia: Neuropsychological and cognitive studies of phonological reading.* London: Erlbaum.

Patterson, K. E., & Wilson, B. (1990). A rose is a rose or a nose: A deficit in initial letter identification. *Cognitive Neuropsychology, 7,* 447–477.

Pause, M., Kunesh, E., Binkofski, F., & Freund, H. J. (1989). Sensorimotor disturbances in patients with lesions of the parietal cortex. *Brain, 112,* 1599–1625.

Payk, T. R. (1977). Storungen des Zeiterlebens bei den endogenen Psychosen. *Schweizer Arciv für Neurologie, Neurochirurgie und Psychiatrie, 121,* 277–285.

Pearlson, G. D., Barta, P. E., Powers, R. E., Menon, R. R., Richard, S. S., Ayward, E. H., et al. (1997). Medial and superior temporal gyral volumes and cerebral asymmetry in schizophrenia versus bipolar disorder. *Biological Psychiatry, 41,* 1–14.

Penfield, W. (1929). Diencephalic autonomic epilepsy. *Archives of Neurology and Psychiatry, 22,* 358–374.

Penfield, W., & Erickson, T. C. (1941). *Epilepsy and cerebral localization.* Springfield, IL: Thomas.

Penfield, W. & Evans, J. (1934). Functional defects caused by cerebral lobectomies. *Publication Association of Research of Nervous and Mental Diseases, 13,* 352–377.

Penfield, W., & Evans, J. (1935). The frontal lobe in man: A clinical study of maximum removals. *Brain, 58,* 115–133.

Penfield, W., & Jasper, H. (1954). *Epilepsy and functional anatomy of the human brain.* Boston: Little, Brown.

Penfield, W., & Mathieson, G. (1974). Memory; autopsy findings and comments on the role of hippocampus in experiential recall. *Archives of Neurology, 31,* 145–154.

Penfield, W., & Milner, B. (1958). Memory deficit produced by bilateral lesions in the hippocampal zone. *Archives of Neurology and Psychiatry, 79,* 475–497.

Penfield, W., & Perot, P. (1963). The brain's record of auditory and visual experience. *Brain, 86,* 595–696.

Penfield, W., & Rassmussen, T. (1950). *The cerebral cortex of man.* New York: MacMillan.

Penfield, W., & Roberts, L. (1959). *Speech and brain mechanisms.* Princeton, NJ: Princeton University Press.

Perani, D., Colombo, C., Bressi, S., et al. (1995). (18F)-FDG PET study in obsessive-compulsive disorder: A clinical metabolic correlation study after treatment. *British Journal of Psychiatry, 166,* 244–250.

Peretz, A. (1990). Processing of local and global musical information in unilateral brain-damaged patients. *Brain, 113,* 1185–1205.

Perini, G. I., Tosin, C., Carraro, C., et al. (1996). Interictal mood and personality disorders in temporal lobe epilepsy. *Journal of Neurology, Neurosurgery, and Psychiatry, 61,* 601–605.

Perner, J., Leekam, S. R., & Wimmer, H. (1987). Three-years old's difficulty with false belief: The case for a conceptual deficit. *British Journal of Developmental Psychology, 5,* 125–137.

Perner, J., & Wimmer, H. (1985). "John thinks that Mary thinks that....": Attribution of second-order false belief by 5- to 10-year-old children. *Journal of Experimental and Child Psychology, 39,* 437–471.

Péron, N., Droguet, P., & Granier, M. (1946). Agnosie visuelle avec perte élective de la reconnaissance topographique: hémianopsie homonyme gauche. *Revue Neurologique, 78,* 596–597.

Peroutka, S. J., Sohmer, B., Kumar, A. J., Folstein, M., & Robinson, R. G. (1982). Hallucinations and dellusions following a right temporoparietooccipital infarction. *The Johns Hopkins Medical Journal, 151,* 181–185.

Perrett, D. I., Harries, M. H., Bevan, R., Thomas, S., Benson, A. J., Mistlin A. J., et al. (1989). Frameworks of analysis for the neural representation of animal objects and actions. *Journal of Experimental Biology, 146,* 87–113.

Perrett, D. I., Mistlin, A. J., Harries, M. H., & Chitty, A. J. (1990). Understanding of the visual appearance and consequence of hand actions. In M. A. Goodale (Ed.), *Vision and action: The control of grasping* (pp. 163–180). Norwood, NJ: Ablex.

Perrett, D. I., Rolls, E. T., & Caan, W. (1982). Visual neurons responsive to faces in the monkey temporal cortex. *Experimental Brain Research, 47,* 329–342.

Perry, R. H., Tomlinson, B. E., Candy, J. M., et al. (1983). Cholinergic deficit in mentally impaired parkinsonian patients. *Lancet, 2,* 789–790.

Petit-Dutaillis, D., Guiot, G., Meising, R., & Bourdillon, C. (1954). A propos d'une aphémie par attente de la zone motrice supplémentaire de Penfield, au cours de l'évolution d'un anevrisme artério-veineux. *Revue Neurologique, 2,* 95–106.

Phillips, D. P., & Orman, S. S. (1984). Responses of single neurons in posterior field of cat auditory cortex to tonal stimuli. *Journal of Neurophysiology, 51,* 147–163.

Pia, H. W. (1953). Klinik und ssyndrome der schlaffenlappengerchwulste. *Fortschritte der Neurologie und Psychiatrie, 21*(12), 555–595.

Picard, N., & Strick, P. L. (1996). Motor areas of the medial wall: A review of their location and functional activation. *Cerebral Cortex, 6,* 342–353.

Pichler, E. (1943). Uber Storungen des Raum-und Zeiterlebens bei Verletzungen des Hinterhauptlappens. *Zeitschrift für die Gesamte Neurologie und Psychiatrie, 176,* 434–464.

Pick, A. (1892). Uber die beziehungen der senilen Hirnatrophie zur Aphasie. *Prager Medizinische Wochenshrift, 17,* 165–167.

Pick, A. (1903). On reduplicative paramnesias. *Brain, 26,* 242–267.

Pick, A. (1905). *Studien uber motorische Apraxie and ihr nahestehenden Erschei-nungen.* Leipzig: Deuticke.

Pick, A. (1906). Uber einen weiteren Symptomenkomplex in Rahmen der Dementia senilis bedingt durch imschriebane staerkere Hirnatrophie (ge-mischte Apraxie). *Monatsschrift für Psychiatrie und Neurologie, 19,* 97–108.

Pick, A. (1908). *Uber Storungen derorientirierung am eigenen korper. Arbeiten aux der deutschen Psychiatrischen Universitat-klinik in Prag.* Berlin: Karger.

Pick, A. (1922). Storung der orientierung am eigenen korper. Beitrag zur Lehre von Bewusstein des eiginen korpers. *Psychologie Forschung, 1,* 303–318.

Pieczuro, A. C., & Vignolo, L. A. (1967). Studio sperimentale sulla aprassia ideo-motoria. *Sistema Nervoso, 19,* 131–143.

Pillon, B., Dubois, B., L'Hermitte, F., & Agid, Y. (1986). Heterogeneity of intellec-tual impairment in progressive supranulear palsy, Parkinson's disease and Alzheimer's disease. *Neurology, 36,* 1179–1185.

Pinel, P. (1809). *A treatise of insanity,* D. Davis (Trans.). Washington: University Publications America.

Platz, T. (1996). Tactile agnosia: Casuistic evidence and theoretical remarks on modality-specific meaning representation and sensorimotor integra-tion. *Brain, 119,* 1565–1574.

Poeck, K. (1984). Neuropsychological demonstration of splenial interhemispheric disconnection in a case of optic anomia. *Neuropsychologia, 22,* 707–713.

Poeck, K., & Lehmkuhl, G. (1980). Das Syndrom der ideatirischen Apraxie und zeine Localization. *Nervenarzt, 51,* 217–225.

Poeck, K., & Luzzatti, C. (1988). Slowly progressive aphasia in three patients: The problem of accompanying neuropsychological deficit. *Brain, 111,* 151–168.

Poetzl, O. (1924). Uber die Storungen der Selbst wahrnehmung bey linksetiger hemiplegie. *Zeitschrift für Neurologie und Psychiatrie, 93,* 117–168.

Poetzl, O. (1928). *Die aphasielehre fom Standpunkte der klinischen Psychiatrie. Erster Band: Die optisch-agnostischen Storungen.* In G. Aschaffenburg (Ed.), *Handbuch der Psychiatrue.* Leipzig-Wien: F. Deuticke.

Poetzl, O. (1937). Zur pathologie der amusie. *Wiener klinische Wochenschrsift, 50,* 770–775.

Poetzl, O. (1951). Weiteres ueber das Zeitraffer-Erlebnis. *Wiener Zeitschrift für Nervenheilkunde und der en Grenzgebiete, 4,* 9–39.

Pogacar, S., & Williams, R. S. (1984). Alzheimer's disease presenting as slowly progressive aphasia. *RI Medical Journal, 67,* 181–185.

Poggio, T., & Edelman, S. (1990). A network that learns to recognize three-dimensional objects. *Nature, 343,* 263–266.

Pollen, D. A. (1999). On the neural correlates of visual perception. *Cerebral Cortex, 9,* 4–19.

Pollock, D. C. (1987). Model for understanding the antagonism between seizures and psychosis. *Progress of Neuropsychopharmacology, Biological Psychiatry, 11,* 483–504.

Popkin, M. K., & Andrews, J. E. (1997). Mood disorders secondary to systemic medical conditions. *Seminars in Clinical Neuropsychiatry, 2,* 296–306.

Popkin, M. K., & Tucker, G. J. (1992). "Secondary" and drug-induced mood, anxiety, psychotic, catatonic, and personality disorder: A review of the literature. *Journal of Neuropsychiatry and Clinical Neuroscience, 24,* 369–385.

Poppelreuter, W. (1917). Die psychischen Shadigungen durch Kopfschuss im Kriege 1914/1916 (Vol. 1). *Die Storungen der niederen and hoheren Schleistungen durch Verletzungen des Okzipitalhirns.* Leipzig: Voss.

Poppelreuter, W. (1923). Zur Psychologie and Pathologie der optischen Wahrnehmung. *Zeitschrift für die gesamte Neurologie und Psychiatrie, 83,* 26–152.

Posner, M. I., & DiGirolamo, J. (1998). Executive attention: Conflict, target detection, and cognitive control. In R. Parasuraman (Ed.), *The attentive brain* (pp. 401–424). Cambridge, MA: MIT Press.

Posner, M. I., & DiGirolamo, J. (2000). Attention in cognitive neuroscience: An overview. In M. S. Gazzaniga (Ed.), *The new cognitive neurosciences* (pp. 623–632). Cambridge, MA: MIT Press.

Posner, M. I., & Peterson, S. E. (1990). The attention system of the human brain. *Annual Revue of Neuroscience, 13,* 25–42.

Posner, M. I., Walker, J. A., Friedrich, F. J., & Rafal, R. D. (1984). Effects of parietal injury on covert orienting of attention. *Journal of Neuroscience, 4,* 1863–1874.

Post, R. M., DeLisi, L. E., Holcomb, H. H., Uhde, T. W., Cohen, R., & Buchsbaum, M. S. (1987). Glucose utilization in the temporal cortex of affectively ill patients: Positron emission tomography. *Biological Psychiatry, 22,* 545–553.

Poyton, A. M., Kartsounis, L. D., & Bridges, P. K. (1995). A prospective clinical study of stereotactic subcaudate tractotomy. *Pyschological Medicine, 25,* 763–770.

Premack, D., & Woodruff, G. (1978). Does the chimpanzee have a theory of mind? *Behavioral and Brain Sciences, 1,* 515–526.

Pribram, K. H. (1974). How is it in sensing so much we can do so little? In F. O. Shmitt & F. G. Worden (Eds., pp. 217–263), *The neurosciences: Third study program.* Cambridge, MA: MIT Press.

Pribram, K. H., & Mishkin, M. (1956). Analysis of the effects of frontal lesions in monkey: III. Object alternation. *Journal of Comparative Physiology and Psychology, 49,* 42–45.

Pribram, K. H., Mishkin, N., Rosvold, H. E., & Kaplan, S. J. (1952). Effects on delayed response performance of lesions of dorsolateral and ventromedical frontal cortex of baboons. *Journal of Comparative Physiology and Psychology, 45,* 565–575.

Pribram, K. H., & Tubbs, W. E. (1967). Short-term memory, parsing, and the primate frontal cortex. *Science, 156,* 1765–1767.

Price, B. H., Gurvit, H., Weintraub, S., Geula, C., Leimkuhler, E., & Mesulam, M. (1993). Neuropsychological patterns and language deficits in 20 consecutive cases of autopsy-confirmed Alzheimer's disease. *Archives of Neurology, 50,* 931–937.

Price, C. J., Wise, R. J. S., & Frackowiak, R. S. J. (1996). Demonstrating the implicit processing of visually presented words and pseudowords. *Cerebal Cortex, 6,* 62–69.

Prisko, L. (1963). *Short term memory in focal cerebral damage.* Unpublished doctoral thesis, McGill University, Canada. Quoted from Milner, B., & Teuber, H. L. (1968). Alteration of perception and memory in man. In L. Weiscrantz (Ed.), *Analysis of behavioral changes* (pp. 268–375). New York: Harper and Row.

Pro, J. D., & Wells, C. E. (1977). The use of electroencephalogram in the diagnosis of delirium. *Diseases of the Nervous System, 38,* 804–808.

Proust, A. (1872). De l'aphasie. *Archives Générale dé Médicine, 1,* 147–166, 303–318, 653–685.

Puce, A., Allison, T., Bentin, S., Gor, J. C., & McCarthy, G. (1998). Temporal cortex activation in humans viewing eye and mouth movements. *Journal of Neuroscience, 18,* 2188–2199.

Puce, A., Allison, T., Gore, J. C., & McCarthy, G. (1995). Face-sensitive regions in human extrastriate cortex studied by functional MRI. *Journal of Neurophysiology, 74,* 1192–1199.

Puchelt, F. (1844). Uber partielle Empfindungs lahmung. *Heidelberg Medizine Annalen, 10,* 485.

Puente, A. E. (1998). The application of Luria's approach in North Amearica. In E. D. Homskaya & T. V. Akhutina (Eds.), *Proceeding of the First International Luria Memorial Conference* (p. 122). Moscow: Russian Psychological Association.

Quaglino, A. (1867). Emiplegia sinstra con amaurosi-Guarigione-perdita totale della percezione dei colori e della memoria della configurazione degli oggetti. *Giornale D'Oftalmologia Italiane, 10,* 106–117.

Quensel, P., & Pfeiffer, R. A. (1923). Über reine sensorische amusie. *Zeitschrift für Neurologie und Psychiatrie, 81,* 311–330.

Rabins, P. V., Starstein, S. E., & Robinson, G. R. (1991). Risk factors of developing atypical (schizophreniform) psychosis following stroke. *Journal of Neuropsychiatry and Clinical Neuroscience, 3,* 6–9.

Raine, A., Lencz, T., Reynolds, G., Harrison, G., Sheared, C., Medley, I., et al. (1992). An evaluation of structural and functional prefrontal deficits in schizophrenia: MRI and neuropsychological measures. *Psychiatry Research, 45,* 123–137.

Rainer, G., & Miller, E. K. (2000). Effects of visual experience on the representation of objects in the prefrontal cortex. *Neuron, 27,* 179–189.

Rajaram, S. (1997). Basal forebrain amnesia. *Neurocase, 3,* 405–415.

Ramachandran, V. S., & Rogers-Ramachandran, D. (1996). Synaesthesia in phantom limbs induced with mirror. *Proceeding of the Royal Society, London, B, 263,* 377–386.

Rao, S. M. (1990). Multiple sclerosis. In J. L. Cummings (Ed.), *Subcortical dementia* (pp. 164–180). New York: Oxford University Press.

Rao, S. M., Mittenberg, W., Bernardin, L., Haughton, V., Leo, G. J. (1989). Neuropsychological test findings in subjects with leukoaraiosis. *Archives of Neurology, 46,* 40–44.

Rapcsak, S. Z., Galper, S. R., Comer, J. F., Reminger, M. A., Nieslen, M. A., Kazniak, L. W., et al. (2000). Fear recognition deficits after focal brain damage. *Neurology, 54,* 575–581.

Rapcsak, S. Z., Krupp, L. B., Rubens, A. B., & Reim, J. (1990). Mixed transcortical aphasia without anatomical isolation of the speech area. *Stroke, 21,* 953–956.

Rapcsak, S. Z., Rothi, L. J. G., Heilman, K. M. (1987). Apraxia in a patient with atypical cerebral dominance. *Brain and Cognition, 6,* 450–463.

Rapcsak, S. Z., & Rubens, A. B. (1994). Localization of lesions in transcortical aphasia. In A. Kertesz (Ed.), *Localization and neuroimaging in neuropsychology* (pp. 297–329). San Diego: Academic Press.

Raskin, S. A., Borod, J. C., & Tweedy, J. (1990). Neuropsychological aspects of Parkinson's disease. *Neuropsychological Review, 1,* 185–221.

Rasmussen, S., Greenberg, B., Mindus, P., Friehs, G., & Noren, G. (2000). Neurosurgical approaches to intractable obsessive-compulsive disorder. *CNS Spectrum, 5*(11), 23–34.

Raush, R., Lee, M., Kramer, S., et al. (1998). Long term changes in self-reported mood of patients with epilepsy following temporal lobe surgery [Abstract]. *Epilepsia, 39,* 67.

Rawlings, E. (1920). The histopathologic findings in dementia praecox. *American Journal of Insanity, 76,* 265–282.

Raymond, R., & Egger, M. (1906). Un cas d'aphasie tactile. *Revue Neurologique, 14,* 371–375.

Reber, A. S. (1989). Implicit learning and tacit knowledge. *Journal of Experimental Psychology, 118,* 219–235.

Reed, C. L., & Caselli, R. J. (1994). The nature of tactile agnosia: A case study. *Neuropsychologia, 32,* 527–539.

Reed, C. L., Caselli, R. J., & Farat, M. J. (1996). Tactile agnosia: Underlying impairment and implications for normal tactile object recognition. *Brain, 119,* 875–888.

Reeves, A. G., & Plum, F. (1969). Hyperphagia, rage and dementia accompanying a ventromedial hypothalamic neoplasm. *Archives of Neurology, 20,* 616–624.

Redlich, F., & Dorsey, J. F. (1945). Denial of blindness by patients with cerebral diseases. *Archives of Neurology and Psychiatry, 53,* 407–417.

Regard, M., & Landis, T. (1984). Transient global amnesia: Neuropsychological dysfunction during attack and recovery in two "pure" cases. *Journal of Neurology, Neurosurgery, and Psychiatry, 44,* 668–672.

Reiman, E. M., Raichle, M. E., Butler, F. K., Herscovitch, P., & Robins, E. (1984). A focal brain abnormality in panic disorder, a severe form of anxiety. *Nature, 310,* 683–685.

Reiman, E. M., Raichle, M. E., Robins, E., et al. (1986). The application of positron emission tomography to the study of panic disorder. *American Journal of Psychiatry, 143,* 469–477.

Reisberg, B., Borenstein, J., Salob, S., et al. (1987). Behavioural symptoms in Alzheimer's diseases: Phenomenology and treatment. *Journal of Clinical Psychiatry, 48*(Suppl. 3), 9–15.

Reisberg, B., Gordon, B., McCarthy, M., & Ferris, S. H. (1985). Clinical symptoms accompanying progressive cognitive decline in Alzheimer's disease. In V. L. Melnick & N. N. Dubler (Eds.), *Alzheimer's dementia* (pp. 19–39). Clifton, NJ: Humana Press.

Reitan, R. M., & Davison, L. A. (1974). *Clinical neuropsychology: Current status and applications.* Washington, DC: Winston.

Reitan, R. M., & Wolfson, D. (1985). *The Halstead-Reitan neuropsychological test battery.* Tucson, AZ: Neuropsychology Press.

Rempel-Clower, N. L., Zola-Morgan, S., & Squire, R. L. (1994). Damage to the hippocampal region in human amnesia: neuropsychological and neuro-anatomical findings. *Society of Neuroscience Abstracts, 24, 1975.*

Rempel-Clower, N. L., Zola-Morgan, S., & Squire, R. L. (1995). Importance of the hippocampal region and enthorinal cortex in human memory. *Society of Neuroscience Abstracts, 25,* 1493.

Remy, M. (1942). Contribution a l'étude de la maladue de Korsakow. *Monatsschrft für Psychiatrie und Neurologie, 106,* 128–144.

Renner, J., Morris, J., Storandt, M., La Barge, E. (1992). Progressive posterior cortical dysfunction predicts global dementia. *Neurology, 42,* (Suppl. 3),

Rennick, P. H. M., Perez-Borja, C., & Rodin, E. A. (1969). Transient mental deficit associated with reccurent prolonged epileptic clouded state. *Epilepsia, 10,* 397–405.

Rennik, P., Nolan, D., Baver, R., et al. (1973). Neuropsychological and neurological follow up after herpes hominis encephalitis. *Neurology, 23,* 42–47.

Rhodes, G., Byatt, G., Michie, P. T., & Puce, A. (2004). Is the fusiform face area specialized for faces, individuation, or expert individuation? *Journal of Cognitive Neuroscience, 16*(2), 189–203.

Richardson, E. D., Malloy, P. F., & Grace, J. (1991). Othello syndrome secondary to righ cerebro-vascular infarction. *Journal of Geriatric Psychiatry and Neurology, 4,* 160–165.

Riddoch, G. (1935). Visual disorientation in homonymous half-fields. *Brain, 58,* 376–382.

Riddoch, M. J. (1990). Loss of visual imagery: A generation deficit. *Cognitive Neuropsychology, 7,* 149–273.

Riddoch, M. J., & Humphreys, G. W. (1987). A case of integrative visual agnosia. *Brain, 110,* 1431–1462.

Riddoch, M. J., Humphreys, G. W., Cleton, P., & Fery, P. (1990). Interaction of attentional and lexical processes in neglect dyslexia. *Cognitive Neuropsychology, 7*(5/6), 479–517.

Riley, D. E., Fogt, N., & Leigh, R. J. (1994). The syndrome of "pure akinesia" and its relationship to progressive supranuclear palsy. *Neurology, 44,* 1025–1029.

Risberg, J., Passant, U., Warkentin, S., et al. (1993). Regional cerebral blood flow in frontal lobe dementia of non-Alzheimer type. *Dementia, 4,* 186–187.

Rizzolatti, G., & Arbib, M. A. (1998). Language within our grasp. *Trends in Neuroscience, 21,* 188–194.

Rizzolatti, G., Faddiga, L., Fogassi, L., & Gallese, V. (1996). Premotor cortex and the recognition of motor actions. *Cognitive Brain Research, 3,* 131–141.

Rizzolatti, G., Fogassi, L., & Gallese, V. (2000). Cortical mechanisms subserving object grasping and action recognition: A new view on the cortical motor functions. In M. S. Gazzaniga (Ed.), *The new cognitive neurosciences* (pp. 539–552). Cambridge, MA: MIT Press.

Rizzolatti, G., & Gentilucci, M. (1988). Motor and visual-motor functions of the premotor cortex. In P. Rakic & W. Singer (Eds.), *Neurobiology of neocortex* (pp. 269–284). Chichester: Wiley.

Roberts, G. W. (1991). Schizophrenia: a neuropathological perspective. *British Journal of Psychiatry, 158,* 8–17.

Roberts, V., Ingram, S. M., Lamar, M., & Green, R. C. (1996). Prosody impairment and associated affective and behavioral diturbances in Alzheimer's disease. *Neurology, 47,* 1482–1488.

Robertson, E. E., Le Roux, A., & Brown, J. H. (1958). The clinical differentiation of Pick's disease. *Journal of Mental Science, 104,* 1000–1024.

Robertson, M. M., & Trimble, M. R. (1983). Depressive illness in patients with epilepsy: A review. *Epilepsia, 24*(Suppl 2.), S190–S196.

Robinson, R. G., & Benson, D. F. (1981). Depression in aphasic patients: Frequency, severity, and clinical pathological correlations. *Brain and Language, 14,* 282–291.

Robinson, R. G., Bolduc, P. L., & Price, T. R. (1987). Two-year longitudinal study of poststroke mood disorders: Diagnosis and outcome at one and two years. *Stroke, 18,* 837–843.

Robinson, R. G., & Jorge, R. (1994). Mood disorders. In J. M. Silver, S. C. Yudofsky, & R. E. Hales (Eds.), *Neuropsychiatry of traumatic brain injury* (pp. 219–250). Washington, DC: American Psychiatric Press.

Robinson, R. G., Kubos, K. L., Starr, L. B., Rao, K., & Price, T. R. (1984). Mood disorder in stroke patients: Importance of location of lesion. *Brain, 107,* 81–93.

Robinson, D., Wu, H., Munne, R. A., et al. (1995). Reduced caudate nucleus volume in obsessive-compulsive disorder. *Archives of General Psychiatry, 52,* 393–398.

Rockland, K. S., & Pandia, D. N. (1979). Laminar origin and terminations of cortical connections of the occipital lobe in the rhesus monkeys. *Brain Research, 179,* 3–20.

Rodin, E., & Schmaltz, S. (1984). The Bear-Fedio Personality Inventory. *Neurology, 34,* 591–596.

Roeltgen, D. (1983). Proposed anatomic substrates for phonological and surface dyslexia. *Academy of Aphasia* [Abstract].

Roeltgen, D. P., & Heilman, K. M. (1984). Lexical agraphia: Further support for the two strategy hypothesis of linguistic agraphia. *Brain, 107,* 811–827.

Roeltgen, D. P., Sevuch, S., & Heilman, K. M. (1983). Phonological agraphia: Writing by the lexical-semantic route. *Neurology, 33,* 755–765.

Rogelet, P., Delafosse, A., & Destee, A. (1996). Posterior cortical atrophy: Unusual feature of Alzheimer's disease. *Neurocase, 2,* 495–501.

Roger, J., Grangeon, H., Guey, J., & Lob, H. (1968). Incidence psychiatriques et psychologiques du traitement par l'éthosuccimide chez les épileptiques. *L'éncephale, 57,* 407–438.

Roland, P. E. (1976). Astereognosis. *Archives of Neurology, 33,* 543–550.

Roland, P. E., O'Sullivan, B. T., & Kawashima, R. (1998). Shape and roughness activate different somatosensory areas in human brain. *Proceedings of the National Academy of Sciences USA, 95,* 3295–3300.

Romano, J., & Engel, G. L. (1944). Delirium, part I: Electroencephalographic data. *Archivs of Neurology and Psychiatry, 51,* 378–392.

Ron, M. A., & Logsdail, S. J. (1989). Psychiatric morbidity in multiple sclerosis: A clinical and MRI study. *Psychological Medicine, 19,* 887–895.

Rosch, E., Mervis, C. B., Gray, W. D., Johnson, D. M., & Boyes-Braem, P. (1976). Basic objects in natural categories. *Cognitive Psychology, 8,* 382–439.

Rose, F. C., & Symonds, C. P. (1960). Persistent memory defect following encephalitis. *Brain, 8,* 195–212.

Rose, S. (1997). *Lifelines: Biology, freedom, determinism.* London: Lane.

Rosene, D. L., & van Hoesen, G. (1977). Hippocampal afferents reach widespread areas of cerebral cortex and amygdala in the Rhesus monkey. *Science, 198,* 315–317.

Ross, E. D. (1980). Left medial parietal lobe and receptive language functions: Mixed transcortical aphasia after left anterior cerebral artery infarction. *Neurology, 30,* 144–151.

Ross, E. D. (1981). The Aprosodias: Functional-anatomic organization of the affective component of language in the right hemisphere. *Archives of Neurology, 38,* 561–569.

Ross, E. D. (1985). Modulation of affect and nonverbal communication by the right hemisphere. In M. M. Mesulam (Ed.), *Principles of behavioral neurology* (pp. 239–257). Philadeliphia: F. A. Davis Company.

Ross, E. D. (2000). Affective prosody and the aprosodias. In M. M. Mesulam (Ed.), *Principles of behavioral and cognitive neurology* (2nd ed., pp. 314–331). Oxford: Oxford University Press.

Ross, E. D., Jossman, P. B., Bell, B., Sabin, T., & Geschwind, N. (1975). Musical hallucinations in deafness. *Journal of the American Medical Association, 231*, 620–622.

Ross, E. D., & Mesulam, M. M. (1979). Dominant language functions of the right hemisphere?: Prosody and emotional gesturing. *Archives of Neurology, 36*, 144–148.

Ross, E. D., Orbelo, D. M., Burgard, M., & Hansel, S. (1998). Functional-anatomic correlates of aprosodic deficits in patients with right brain damage. *Neurology, 50*(Suppl. 4), A363.

Ross, E. D., & Stewart, R. M. (1981). Akinetic mutism from hypothalamic damage: Successful treatment with dopamine agonists. *Neurology, 31*, 1435–1439.

Rossi, A., Stratta, P., Gallucci, M., et al. (1988). Brain morphology in schizophrenia by magnetic resonance imaging (MRI). *Acta Psychiatrica Scandinavica, 25*, 223–231.

Rossi, G. F., & Rosadini, G. (1967). Experimental analysis of cerebral dominance in man. In C. H. Millikan & F. L. Darley (Eds.), *Brain mechanisms underlying speech and language* (pp. 167–184). New York: Grune and Stratton.

Rossion, B., Dricot, L., Devolder, A., Bodart, J. M., & Crommelonck, M. (2000). Hemispheric asymmetries for whole-based and part-based face processing in the human fusiform gyrus. *Journal of Cognitive Neuroscience, 12*, 793–802.

Rosvold, H. E., Mirsky, A. F., Sarason, I., Bransome, E. D. Jr., & Beck, L. H. (1956). A continous performance test of brain damage. *Journal of Consulting Psychology, 20*, 343–350.

Roth, B. (1980). *Narcolepsy and Hypersomnia*. New York: S. Karger.

Rothi, L. J. G., Kooistra, C., Heilman, K. M., & Mack, L. (1988). Subcortical ideomotor apraxia. *Journal of Clinical and Experimental Neuropsychology, 10*, 48.

Rothi, L. J. G., Raade, A. S., & Heilman, K. M. (1994). Localization of lesions in limb and buccofacial apraxia. In A. Kertesz (Ed.), *Localization and neuroimaging in neuropsychology* (pp. 407–427). New York: Academic Press.

Roudier, M., Marcie, P., Grancher, A. S., et al. (1998). Discrimination of facial indentity and of emotions in Alzheimer's disease. *Journal of Neurological Science, 154*, 151–158.

Roy, A. (1979). Some determinants of affective symptoms in epileptics. *Canadian Journal of Psychiatry, 24*, 554–556.

Royce, G. J. (1982). Laminar origin of cortical neurons which projects upon the caudate nucleus: A horseradish peroxidase investigation in the cat. *Journal of Comparative Neurology, 205*, 8–29.

Rubens, A. B. (1975). Aphasia with infarction in the territory of the anterior cerebral artery. *Cortex, 11*, 239–250.

Rubens, A. B., & Benson, D. F. (1971). Associative visual agnosia. *Archives of Neurology, 24*, 305–315.

Rubin, E., Drevets, W., & Burke, A. (1988). The nature of psychotic symptoms in senile dementia of Alzheimer's type. *Journal of Geriatric Psychiatry and Neurology, 1,* 16–20.

Rubins, J. L., & Friedman, E. D. (1948). Asymbolia for pain. *Archives of Neurology and Psychiatry, 60,* 554–573.

Rubinstein, S. Y. (1970). *Experimental methods of psychopathology and their clinical applications* [in Russian]. Moscow: Meditsina.

Ruff, R. L., & Russakoff, L. M. (1980). Catatonia with frontal lobe atrophy. *Journal of Neurology, Neurosurgery, and Psychiatry, 43,* 185–187.

Ruff, R. L., & Volpe, B. T. (1981). Environmental reduplication associated with right frontal and parietal lobe injury. *Journal of Neurology, Neurosurgery, and Psychiatry, 43,* 382–386.

Russel, W. R., & Espir, M. L. E. (1961). *Traumatic aphasia.* London: Oxford University Press.

Ryabova, E. E., Sluchevskiy, I. F., & Tonkonogy, J. M. (1964). Peculiarity of speech in patients with ataxic thinking and schizophasia [in Russian]. In E. N. Markova (Ed.), *Problems of psychiatry* (pp. 127–136). Leningrad: Meditsina.

Ryalls, J. (1986). An acoustic study of vowel production in aphasia. *Brain and Language, 29,* 48–67.

Ryalls, J. (1988). Concerning right-hemisphere dominance for affective language. *Archives of Neurology, 45,* 337–338.

Rylander, G. (1939). *Personality changes after operations on the frontal lobe.* London: Oxford University Press.

Saadah, E. S. M., & Melzack, R. (1994). Phantoms and congenital limb deficiency. *Cortex, 30,* 479–485.

Sackeim, H. A., Prohovnik, I., Moeller, J. R., Brown, R. P., Apter, S., Prudic, J., et al. (1990). Regional cerebral blood flow in mood disorders. I. Comparison of major depression and normal controls at rest. *Archives of General Psychiatry, 47,* 60–70.

Sacks, O. (1985). *The man who mistook his wife for a hat and other clinical tales.* New York: Summit Books.

Sakai, K., Hikosaka, O., Miyachi, S., Takino, R., Sasaki, Y., & Pütz, B. (1998). Transition of brain activation from frontal to parietal areas in visuomotor sequence learning. *Journal of Neuroscience, 18,* 1827–1840.

Sakata, H., Taira, M., Murata, A., & Mine, S. (1995). Neural mechanisms of visual guidance of hand action in the parietal cortex of the monkey. *Cerebral Cortex, 5,* 429–438.

Samelsohn, J. (1881). Zur Frage des Farbensinncentrums. *Centralblatt für die medicinische Wissenschaften, 29,* 850–853.

Sanchez-Longo, L. P., & Forster, F. M. (1958). Clinical significance of impairment of sound localization. *Neurology, 8,* 119–125

Sanchez-Longo, L. P., Forster, F. M., & Aut, T. L. (1957). A clinical test for sound localization and its application. *Neurology, 7,* 655–663.

Sandell, J. H., & Schiller, P. H. (1982). Effect of cooling area 18 cells on striate cortex in squirrel monkey. *Journal of Neurophysiology, 48,* 38–48.

Sanders, R. D., & Mathews, T. A. (1994). Hypergraphia and secondary mania in temporal lobe epilepsy. *Neuropsychiatry, Neuropsychology, and Behavioral Neurology, 7,* 114–117.

Sandson, T. A., Daffner, K. R., Carvalho, P. A., & Mesulam, M. M. (1991). Frontal lobe dysfunction following infarction of the left-sided medial thalamus. *Archives of Neurology, 48,* 1300–1303.

Sandyk, R., & Willis, G. L. (1992). Amine accumulation: a possible precursor of Lewy body formation in Parkinson's disease. *International Journal of Neuroscience, 66,* 61–74.

Sanford, H. S., & Bair, H. L. (1939). Visual disturbances associated with tumours of the temporal lobe. *Archives of Neurology and Psychiatry, 42,* 21–43.

Sano, K., Mayanagi, Y., Sekino, H., Ogashiva, M., & Ishigma, B. (1970). Results of stimulation and destruction of the posterior hypothalamus in man. *Journal of Neurosurgery, 33,* 689–707.

Santamaria, J., Blesa, R., & Tolosa, E. S. (1984). Confusional syndrome in thalamic stroke. *Neurology, 34,* 1618.

Satoh, K., Suzuki, T., Narita, M., et al. (1993). Regional blood flow in schizophrenia. *Psychiatry Research: Neuroimaging, 50,* 203–216.

Sawle, G. V., Hymas, N. F., Lees, A. J., et al. (1991). Obsessional slowness: Functional study with positron emission tomography. *Brain, 114,* 2191–2202.

Saxena, S., Bota, R. G., & Brody, A. L. (2001). Brain-behavior relationships in obsessive-compulsive disorder. *Seminar in Clinical Neuropsychiatry, 6*(2), 82–101.

Sayed, V. Z. A., Lewis, S. A., & Brittain, R. P. (1969). An electroencephalographic and psychiatric study of thirty-two insane murderers. *British Journal of Psychiatry, 115,* 1115–1124.

Saykin, A. J., Gur, R. C., Gur, R. E., et al. (1991). Neuropsychological function in schizophrenia: Selective impairment in memory and learning. *Archives of General Psychiatry, 48,* 618–624.

Scarone, S., Colombo, C., Livian, S., et al. (1992). Increased right caudate nucleus size in obsessive-compulsive disorder: Detection with magnetic resonance imaging. *Psychiatry Research, 45,* 115–121.

Schacter, D. L. (1994). Priming and multiple memory systems: perceptual mechanisims of implicit memory. In D. L. Scahchter & E. Tulving (Eds.), *Memory systems 1994* (pp. 233–268). Cambridge, MA: MIT Press.

Schacter, D. L. (1995). Implicit memory: A new frontier for cognintive neuroscience. In M. S. Gazzaniga (Ed.), *The cognitive neurosciences* (pp. 815–824). Cambridge, MA: MIT Press.

Schacter, D. L., & Bucjner, R. L. (1998). Priming and the brain. *Neuron, 20,* 185–195.

Schacter, D. L., Wang, P. L., Tulving, E., & Freeman, M. (1982). Functional retrograde amnesia: A quantitative case study. *Neuropsychologia, 20,* 523–532.

Schankweiler, D. (1966). Effect of temporal-lobe damage on perception of dichotically presented melodies. *Journal of Comparative Physiology and Psychology, 62,* 115–119.

Scheffer, D. G. (1954). *Hypothalamic (diencephalic) syndromes.* Moscow: Meditsin.

Scheller, H., & Seidemann, H. (1931–1932). Zur frague der optischraumlichen agnosie. *Monatsschrift für Psychiatri und Neurologie, 81,* 97–188.

Schenk, I., & Bear, D. (1981). Multiple personality and relative dissociative phenomena in patients with temporal lobe epilepsy. *American Journal of Psychiatry, 138,* 1311–1318.

Schilder, P. (1935). *The image and appearance of the human body.* London: Routledge and Kegan Paul.

Schilder, P., & Stengel., E. (1931). Das Krankheits bild der Schmertzasymbolie. *Zeitschrift für Neurologie und Psychiatrie, 129,* 250–279.

Schlanger, B. B., Schlanger, P., & Gerstmann, L. J. (1976). The perception of emotionally toned sentences by right hemisphere-damaged and aphasic patients. *Brain and Language, 3,* 393–406.

Schneider, C. (1929). Über Pickshe Krankheit. *Monatsschrift für Psychiatrie und Neurologie, 65,* 230–275.

Schneider, C. (1930). *Psychologie der schizophrenen.* Leipzig: Theme.

Schneider, C. (1959). *Clinical psychopathology* (5th ed.; M. W. Hamilton, Trans.). New York: Grune & Stratton.

Schnider, A., Bassetti, C., Gutbrod, K., & Ozboda, C. (1995). Very severe amnesia with acute onset after isolated hippocampal damage due to systemic lupus erythematous. *Journal of Neurology, Neurosurgery, and Psychiatry, 59,* 644–646.

Schonfield, S. M., Golbe, L. I., Sage, J. I., Safer, J. N., & Duvoisin, R. C. (1987). Computed tomography findings in progressive supranuclear palsy; correlation with clinical grade. *Movement Disorders, 2,* 263–278.

Schott, B., Mauguiére, F., Laurent, B., Serclerat, O., & Fischer, C. (1980). L'amnésie thalamique. *Revue Neurologique, 136,* 117–130.

Schreiner, C. E., Mendelson, J. R., & Sutter, M. L. (1992). Functional topography of cat auditory primary cortex: Representation of tone intensity. *Experimental Brain Research, 92,* 105–122.

Schulhoff, C., & Goodglass, H. (1969). Dichotic listening, side of brain injury and cerebral dominance. *Neuropsychologia, 7,* 149–160.

Schwab, R. S. (1953). A case of status epilepticus in petit mal. *Electroencephalography and Clinical Neurophysiology, 5,* 441–442.

Schwarcz, J. R., Theilgaard, A., Owen, D. R., & White, D. (1972). Stereotactic hypothalamotomy for behavior disorders. *Journal of Neurology, Neurosurgery, and Psychiatry, 35,* 356–359.

Schwartz, J. M., Stoessel, P. W., Baxter, L. R., Martin, K. M., & Phelps, M. E. (1996). Systematic changes in cerebral glucose metabolic rate after successful behavior modification treatment of obsessive-compulsive disorder. *Archives of General Psychiatry, 53,* 109–113.

Schwartz, M. F., Saffran, E. M., & Marin, O. S. M. (1980). The word order problem in agrammatism. I. Comprehension. *Brain and Language, 10,* 249–262.

Scott, S. K., Young, A. W., Calder, A. J., Hellawell, D. J., Aggleton, J. P., & Johnson, M. (1997). Impaired auditory recognition of fear and anger following bilateral amygdala lesions. *Nature, 385,* 254–257.

Scoville, W. B., & Milner, B. (1957). Loss of recent memory after bilateral hippocampal lesions. *Journal of Neurology, Neurosurgery, and Psychiatry, 20,* 11–21.

Seggern, H. von. (1881). Achromatopsie bei Homonymer Hemianopsie mit voller Sehscshärfe. *Klinische Monastschrift für Augenheilkunde, 71,* 101–104.

Selemon, L. D., & Goldman-Rakic, P. S. (1985). Longitudinal topography and interdigitation of corticostriatal projections in the rhesus monkey. *Journal of Neuroscience, 5,* 776–794.

Selnes, O. A., Knopman, D., Niccum, N., Rubens, A. B., & Larson, D. (1983). CT scan correlates of auditory comprehension deficit in aphasia: a prospective recovery study. *Neurology, 33,* 558–566.

Selnes, O. A., Rubens, A. B., Risse, G. L., & Levy, R. S. (1982). Transient aphasia with persistent apraxia: Uncommon sequelae of massive left-hemisphere stroke. *Archives of Neurology, 39,* 122–126.

Semenofv, S. F. (1965). *Visual agnosia and hallucination* [in Russian]. Kiev: Meditsina.

Semenza, C., & Zettin, M. (1988). Generating proper names: A case of selective inability. *Cognitive Neuropsychology, 5,* 711–721.

Sem-Jacobsen, C. W., & Torkildsen, A. (1960). Depth recording and electrical stimulation in the human brain. In E. R. Ramey & D. S. O'Doherty (Eds.), Electrical studies on the unanesthezide brain (pp. 275–290). New York: Hoeber.

Serafetinides, E. A. (1965). Aggressivness in temporal lobe epileptics and its relation to cerebral dysfunction and environmental factors. *Epilepsia, 6,* 33–42.

Seron, X., Vand der Kaa, M. A., Remitz, A., & Van der Linden, M. (1979). Pantomime interpretation and aphasia. *Neuropsychologia, 17,* 661–668.

Shah, S. A., Doraiswamy, P. M., Husian, M. M., Escalona, P. R., et al. (1992). Posterior fossa abnormalities in major depression: A controlled magnetic resonance imaging study. *Acta Psychiatrica Scandinavica, 85,* 474–479.

Shallice, T. (1981) Phonological agraphia and the lexical route in writing. *Brain, 104,* 413–429.

Shallice, T. (1994). Multiple levels of control processes. In C. Umilta & M. Moskovitch (Eds.), *Attention and performance XV: Conscious and unconsious information processing* (pp. 395–420). Cambridge, MA: MIT Press.

Shallice, T., & Burgess, P. (1996). The domain of supervisory processes and temporal organization of behavior. *Philosophical Transaction of Royal Society of London, 351,* 1405–1411.

Shallice, T., & Warrington, E. K. (1977). The possible role of selective attention in acquired dyslexia. *Neuropsychologia, 15,* 31–41.

Shallice, T., & Warrington, E. K. (1980). Single and multiple component central dyslectic syndromes. In M. Coltheart, K. Patterson, & J. C. Marshall (Eds.), *Deep dyslexia* (pp. 119–145). London: Routledge.

Shapiro, B. E., Grossman, M., & Gardner, H. (1981). Selective processing of deficits in brain damaged populations. *Neuropsychologia, 19*, 161–169.

Shelton, R. C., & Weinberger, D. R. (1986). X-ray computerized tomography studies in schizophrenia: A review and synthesis. In H. A. Nasrallah & D. R. Weinberger (Eds.), *The neurology of schizophrenia* (Vol. 1, pp. 207–250). Amsterdam: Elsevier Science Publisher B.V.

Shenton, M. E., Kikinis, R., Jolesz, F. A., et al. (1992). Abnormalities of the left temporal lobe and thought disorder in schizophrenia: A quantitative magnetic resonance imaging study. *New England Journal of Medicine, 327*(9), 604–612.

Shepherd, M. (1961). Morbid jealousy: Some clinical and social aspects of a psychiatric symptom. *Journal of Mental Science, 107*, 687–753.

Sher, P. K., & Brown, S. B. (1976). Gelastic epilepsy. *American Journal of Diseases in Childhood, 130*, 1126–1131.

Shergill, S. S., Brammer, M. J., Williams, S. C. R., Murray, R. M., & McGuire, P. K. (2000). Mapping auditory hallucinations in schizophrenia using functional magnetic resonance imaging. *Archives of General Psychiatry, 57*, 1033–1038.

Shikata, E., Tanaka, Y., Nakamura, H., Taira, M., & Sakata, H. (1996). Selectivity of parietal visual neurons in 3D orientation of surface of stereoscopic stimuli. *Neuroreport, 7*, 2389–2394.

Shlegel, S., & Kretzschmar, K. (1987). Computed tomography in affective disorder: I. Ventricular and sulcal measurements. *Biological Psychiatry, 22*, 4–14.

Shlegel, S., Maier, W., Philllip, M., et al. (1989). Computed tomography in depression: Association between ventricular size and psychopathology. *Psychiatry Research, 29*, 221–230.

Shmaryan, A. C. (1949). *Brain pathology and psychiatry* [in Russian]. Moscow: Medgiz.

Shore, D., Filson, R. C. R., Johnson, W. E., et al. (1989). Murder and assault arrests of White House cases; clinical and demographic correlates of violence subsequent to civil commitment. *American Journal of Psychiatry, 146*, 645–651.

Shukla, G. D., Srivastava, B., Katiar, B. C., et al. (1979). Psychiatric manifestations in temporal lobe epilepsy: A controlled study. *British Journal of Psychiatry, 135*, 411–417.

Shukla, S., Cook, B. L., Mukherjee, S., et al. (1987). Mania following head trauma. *American Journal of Psychiatry, 144*, 93–96.

Shuster, P., & Taterka, H. (1926). Beitrag zur Anatomie und Klinik des reinen Worttaubheit. *Zeitschrift für Neurologie und Psychiatrie, 125*, 498–538.

Signer, S., Cummings, J. L., & Benson, D. F. (1989). Delusions and mood disorders in patients with chronic aphasia. *Journal of Neuropsychiatry and Clinical Neuroscience, 1*, 40–45.

Signoret, J. L., Van Eeckhout, P., Poncet, M., & Castaigne, P. (1987). Aphasie sans amusie chez organiste aveugle. *Revue Neurologique, 143*, 172–181.

Silberman, E. K., Post, R. M., Nurnberger, J., Theodore, W., & Boulenger, J. P. (1985). Transient sensory, cognitive and affective phenomena in affective illness. *Brisith Journal of Psychiatry, 146*, 81–89.

Silberpfennig, J. (1941). Contribution to the problem of eye movements: III. Disturbances of ocular movements with pseudo-hemianopsia in frontal lobe tumors. *Confinia Neurologica, 4*, 1–13.

Silfverskiold, P., & Risberg, J. (1989). Regional cerebral blood flow in depression and mania. *Archives of General Psychiatry, 46*, 253–259.

Silva, J. A., & Leong, G. B. (1993). A case of organic Othello syndrome. *Journal of Clinical Psychiatry, 43*, 277.

Silva, S. G., & Marin, R. S. (1999). Apathy in neuropsychiatric disorders. *CNS Spectrum, (4)*, 31–50.

Sim, M., & Sussman, I. Alzheimer's disease: Its natural history and differential diagnosis. *Journal of Nervous and Mental Diseases, 135*, 489–499.

Simeon, D., Guralnik, O., Hazlett, E. A., Spiegel-Cohen, J., Hollander, E., & Buchsbaum, M. S. (2000). Feeling unreal: A PET study of depersonalization disorder. *American Journal of Psychiatry, 157*, 1782–1788.

Sims, A. (1988). *Symptoms in the mind: An introduction to descriptive psychopathology*. London: Saunders.

Sinyor, D., Amato, P., Kaloupek, D. G., Beccke, R., Goldenberg, M., & Coopersmith, H. (1986). Poststroke depression: relationship to functional impairment, coping strategies, and rehabilitation outcome. *Stroke, 17*, 1102–1107.

Sittig, O. (1921). Storungen un Verhalten gegenuber Farben bei Aphasischen. *Monatsschrift für Psychiatrie und Neurologie 49*, 63-68, 169–187.

Sittig, O. (1931). *Über Apraxie*. Berlin: Karger.

Sjögren, T., Sjögren, H., & Lindgren, A. G. H. (1952). Morbus Alzheimer and Morbus Pick. *Acta Psychiatrica et Neurologica Scandinavica, 82*(Suppl.), 1–152.

Slater, E., Beard, A. W., & Clithero, E. (1963). The schizophrenia-like psychosis of epilepsy. *British Journal of Psychiatry, 109*, 95–150.

Smith, D. M., & Atkinson, R. M. (1997). Mood disorders secondary to drugs and pharmacologic agents. *Seminars in Clinical Neuroscience, 2*, 285–295.

Smith, E. E., & Jonides, J. (1999). Storage and executive processes in the frontal lobe. *Science, 283*, 1657–1661.

Smith, J. M., Kucharski, L. T., Oswald, W. T., & Waterman, L. J. (1979). A systematic investigation of tradive dyskineasia in inpatients. *American Journal of Psychiatry, 136*, 918–922.

Snodgrass, J. G., & Corwin, J. (1988). Perceptual identification thresholds for 150 fragmented pictures from the Snodgrass and Vanderwart picture set. *Perceptual and Motor Skills, 67*(Suppl. 1), 3–36.

Snowdon, D. A., Greiner, L. H., Mortimer, J. A., Riley, K. R., Greiner, P. A., & Markesbery, W. R. (1997). Brain infarction and the clinical expression of Alzheimer disease. *Journal of the American Medical Association, 277,* 813–817.

Soechting, J. F., & Flanders, M. (1993). Parallel inderdependent channels for location and orientation in sensorimotor transformations for reaching and grasping. *Journal of Neurophysiology, 70,* 1137–1150.

Soechting, J. F., Gordon, A. M., & Engel, K. C. (1996). Sequential hand and finger movement: Typing and piano playing. In J. R. Bloedel, T. J. Ebner, & P. W. Steven (Eds.), *The acquisition of motor behavior in vertebrates* (pp. 343–360). Cambridge, MA: MIT Press.

Soma, Y., Sugishita, M., Kitamura, K., Maruyama, S., & Imanaga, H. (1989). Lexical agraphia in the Japanese language. *Brain, 112,* 1549–1561.

Soyka, M. (1998). Delusional jealousy and localized cerebral pathology. *Journal of Neuropsychiatry and Clinical Neuroscience, 10,* 472.

Speedie, L. J., & Heilman, K. M. (1982). Amnesic disturbance following infarction of the left dorsomedial nucleus of thalamus. *Neuropsychologia, 20,* 597–604.

Spence, S. A., Taylor, D. G., & Hirsh, S. R. (1995). Depressive disorder due to craniopharyngioma. *Journal of the Royal Society of Medicine, 88,* 637–638.

Sperry, R. W. (1952). Neurology and the mind-brain problem. *American Scientist, 40,* 291–312.

Sperry, R. W. (1981). Some effects of disconnecting the cerebral hemispheres, Nobel Lecture. Lex Prix Nobel. Stockholm: Almqvist & Wikslow.

Sperry, R. W., & Gazzaniga, M. S. (1967). Language following surgical disconnection of the hemispheres. In C. Millikan & F. Darley (Eds.), *Brain mechanisms underlying speech and language* (pp. 108–115). New York: Grune and Stratton.

Spinnler, H. (1999). Alzheimer's disease. In G. Dines & L. Pizzamiglio (Eds.), *Handbook of clinical and experimental neuropsychology* (pp. 699–746). Hove, East Sussex, UK: Psychology Press.

Spinnler, H., & Vignolo, L. A. (1966). Impaired recognition of meaningful sounds in aphasia. *Cortex, 2,* 337–348.

Spitz, M. C. (1991). Panic disorder and seizure patients: A diagnostic pitfall. *Epilepsia, 32,* 33–39.

Spreen, O., Benton, A. L., & Fincham, R. (1965). Auditory agnosia without aphasia. *Archives of Neurology, 133,* 84–92.

Spreen, O., & Strauss, E. (Eds.). (1998). *A compendium of neuropsychological tests* (2nd ed.). New York: Oxford University Press.

Sprofkin, B. E., & Sciarra, D. (1952). Korsakoff's psychosis associated with cerebral tumours. *Neurology, 2,* 427–434.

Squire, L. R. (1987). *Memory and brain.* New York: Oxford University Press.

Squire, L. R. (1994). Declarative and nondeclarative memory: multiple brain systems supporting learning and memory. In D. L. Schacter &

E. Tulving (Eds.), *Memory systems 1994* (pp. 203–232). Cambridge, MA: MIT Press.

Squire, L. R., & Knowlton, B. J. (1995). Learning about categories in the absence of memory. *Proceeding of the National Academy of Science U.S.A., 92,* 12470–12474.

Squire, L. R., Knowlton, B., & Musen, G. (1993). The structure and organization of memory. *Annual Revue of Psychology, 44,* 453–495.

Squire, L. R., & Moore, R. Y. (1979). Dorsal thalamic lesion in a noted case of human memory dysfunction. *Annals of Neurology, 6,* 503–506.

Squire, L. R., & Zola-Morgan, S. (1985). Neuropsychology of memory: New links between humans and experimental animals. In D. Olton, S. Corkin, & E. Gamzu (Eds.), *Memory dysfunction: an integration of animal and human research from preclinical and clinical perspectives* (pp. 137–139). New York: New York Academy of Science.

Srinivas, K., & Ogas, J. (1999). Disorders of somesthetic recognition: A theoretical review. *Neurocase, 5,* 83–93.

Standage, G. P., Benevento, L. A. (1983). The organization of connections between the pulvinar and visual area MT in macaque monkey. *Brain Research, Amsterdam, 262,* 288–294.

Standish-Barry, H. M. A. S., Bouras, M., Bridges, P. K., et al. (1982). Pneumoencephalographic and computerized axial tomography scan changes in affective disorder. *British Journal of Psychiatry, 141,* 614–617.

Stark-Adamec, C., Adamec, R. E., Graham, J. M., Hicks, R. C., & Brun-Meyer, S. E. (1985). Complexities in the complex partial seizures personality controversy. *Psychiatric Journal of the University of Ottawa, 10,* 231–236.

Starkstein, S. E., Boston, J. D., & Robinson, R. G. (1988) Mechanisms of mania after brain uninjury. *Journal of Nervous and Mental Diseases, 176,* 87–100.

Starkstein, S. E., Federoff, J. P., Price, T. R., Leiguarda, R. C., & Robinson, R. G. (1994). Neuropsychological and neuroradiologic correlates of emotional prosody comprehension. *Neurology, 44,* 515–522.

Starkstein, S. E., & Leiguarda, R. (1993). Neuropsychological correlates of brain atrophy in Parkinson's disease: A CT-scan study. *Movement Disorders, 1,* 51–55.

Starkstein, S. E., & Manes, F. (2000). Apathy and depression following stroke. *CNS Spectrum, 5*(3), 43–50.

Starkstein, S. E., Pearlson, G. D., Boston, J., & Robinson, R. G. (1987). Mania after brain injury: A controlled study of causative factors. *Archives of Neurology, 44,* 1069–1073.

Starkstein, S., Mayberg, H. S., Berthier, M. L., et al. (1989). Secondary mania: Neuroradiological, metabolic, and neuropsychological findings. *Neurology, 38*(Suppl. 1), 295.

Starkstein, S. E., Robinson, R. G., Berthier, M. L., et al. (1988). Differential mood changes following basal ganglia vs thalamic lesions. *Archives of Neurology, 45,* 725–730.

Starkstein, S. E., Robinson, R. G., & Berthier, M. L. (1992). Post-stroke hallucinatory delusional syndromes. *Neuropsychiatry, Neuropsychology, and Behavioral Neurology, 5*, 114–118.

Starkstein, S. E., Robinson, R. G., Honig, M. A., et al. (1989). Mood changes after right hemisphere lesions. *British Journal of Psychiatry, 155*, 79–85.

Starkstein, S. E., Robinson, R. G., & Price, T. R. (1987). Comparison of cortical and subcortical lesions in the production of poststroke mood disorder. *Brain, 110*, 1045–1059.

Starkstein, S. E., Robinson, R. G., & Price, T. R. (1988). Comparison of patients with and without poststroke major depression matched for size and location of lesion. *Archives of General Psychiatry, 45*, 247–252.

Starkstein, S. E., Vazquez, S., Migliorelli, R., Teson, A., Sabe, L., & Leiguarda, R. (1995). A single-photon emission computed tomographic study of anosognosia in Alzheimer's disease. *Archives of General Psychiatry, 52*, 415–420.

Starkstein, S. E., Vázquez, S., Petracca, G., Sabe, L., Migriorelli, R., Teson, A., & Leiguarda, R. (1994). A SPECT study of delusions in Alzheimer's disease. *Neurology, 44*, 2055–2059.

Startup, M. (1996). Insight and cognitive deficit in schizophrenia: Evidence for a curvilinear relationship. *Psychological Medicine, 26*, 1277–1281.

Stauder, K. H. (1934). Die toldliche katatonia. *Archiv für Psychiatrie und Nervenkrankheiten, 102*, 614–634.

Stauffenberg, W. von. (1918). Klinische und anatomische Beiträge zur Kenntnis der aphasischen, agnostischen and apraktischen Symptome. *Zietschrift Gesamte Neurologie und Psychiatrie, 93*, 71–212.

Steele, J. C. (1972). Progressive supranuclear palsy. *Brain, 95*, 693–704.

Steele, J. C., Richardson, J. C., & Olszewski, J. (1964). Progressive supranuclear palsy: A heterogenous degeneration involving the brain stem, basal ganglia and cerebellum with vertical gaze and pseudobulbar palsy, nuchal dystonia and dementia. *Archives of Neurology, 10*, 333–358.

Steffan, P. H. (1881). Beitrag zur Pathologie des Farbensinnes. *Graefes Archiv für Ophalmologie, 27*, 1–24.

Stein, J., & von Weizsacker. (1926). Über klinische sensibilitatsprufingen. *Deutsche Archiv für klinische Medizine, 151*, 230–253.

Stein, M. B., & Uhde, T. W. (1989). Infrequent occurrence of EEG abnormalities in panic disorder. *American Journal of Psychiatry, 146*, 517–520.

Steinhal, H. (1871), cited by Thiele, R. (1928). Aphasie, Apraxie, Agnosie. *Bumke Handbuch Geisteskrankheit.* Berlin: Springer.

Stengel, E. (1941). On the etiology of the fugue states. *Journal of Mental Science, 87*, 572–599.

Stengel, E. (1947). A clinical and psychological study of echo-reaction. *Journal of Mental Science, 93*, 598–612.

Stepien, L., & Serpinski, S. (1964). Impairment of recent memory after temporal lesions in man. *Neuropsychologia, 2*, 291–303.

Stern, K., & Dabcey, T. E. (1942). Glioma of the diencephalon in a manic patient. *American Journal of Psychiatry, 98,* 716–719.

Stertz, G. (1931). Üden Anteil des Zwischenhirns an der Symptomgestaltung organischer Rekrankungen des Zentralnervensystems: ein diagnostisch brauchbares Zwischenhirnsyndrom. *Deitsche Zeitschrift für Nervenheilkunde, 117,* 630–635.

Stiles-Davis, J., Janovsky, J., Engel, M., & Nass, R. (1988). Drawing ability in four young children with congenital unilateral brain lesions. *Neuropsychologia, 26,* 359–371.

Stillhard, G., Landis, T., Schiess, R., Regard, M., & Sialer, G. (1990). Bitemporal hypoperfusion in transient global amnesia: 99m-HM-PAO SPECT and neuropsychological findings during and after an attack. *Journal of Neurology, Neurosurgery, and Psychiatry, 53,* 339–342.

Stone, V. E., Baron-Cohen, S., & Knight, R. T. (1998). Frontal lobe contribution to theory of mind. *Journal of Cognitive Neuroscience, 10*(5), 640–656.

Stracciari, A., Ghidoni, E., Guarino, M., Poletti, M., & Pazzaglia, P. (1994). Post-traumatic retrograde amnesia with selective impairment of autobiographical memory. *Cortex, 30,* 459–468.

Strakowski, S. M., Wilson, D. R., Tohen, M., Woods, B. T., Douglass, A. W., & Stoll, A. L. (1993). Structural brian abnormalities in first-episode mania. *Biological Psychiatry, 33,* 602–609.

Strang, R. R. (1965). Imipramine in treatment of parkinsonism: A double-blind placebo study. *British Medical Journal, 2,* 33–34.

Strauss, I., & Keschner, M. (1935). Mental symptoms in cases of tumor of frontal lobe. *Archives of Neurology and Psychiatry, 33,* 986–1005.

Strauss, J. S., Carpenter, W. T., & Barko, J. J. (1974). The diagnosis and understanding of schizophrenia, part 3: Speculations on the process that underlie schizophrenic symptoms and signs. *Schizophrenia Bulletin, 11,* 61–75.

Street, R. F. (1931). *A gestalt completion test.* New York: Teachers College, Columbia University.

Strobos, R. J. (1961). Mechanisms in temporal lobe seizures. *Archives of Neurology, 5,* 48–57.

Strobos, R. R. J. (1953). Tumors of the temporal lobe. *Neurology, 3,* 752–760.

Stroop, J. R. (1935). Studies of interference in serial verbal reaction. *Journal of Experimental Psychology, 18,* 643–662.

Strub, R. I. (1989). Frontal lobe syndrome in patient with bilateral globus pallidus lesions. *Archives of Neurology, 46,* 1024–1027.

Strub, R. L., & Geschwind, N. (1983). Localization in Gerstmann syndrome. In A. Kertesz (Ed.), *Localization in neuropsychology* (pp. 295–321). New York: Academic Press.

Stryker, M. P. (1992). Elements of visual perception. *Nature, 360,* 301–302.

Stuss, D. T., Alexander, M. P., Lieberman, A., & Levine, H. (1985). An extraordinary form of confabulation. *Neurology,* 1166–1172.

Stuss, D. T., & Benson, D. F. (1984). Neuropsychological studies of the frontal lobes. *Psychological Bulletin, 95,* 3–28.

Stuss, D. T., & Benson, D. F. (1986). *The fronatal lobes*. New York: Raven Press.

Stuss, D. T., & Cummings, J. L. (1990). Subcortical vascular dementia. In J. L. Cummings (Ed.), *Subcortical dementia* (pp. 145–163). New York: Oxford University Press.

Suga, N. (1969). Classification of inferior collicular neurons of bats in term of responses to pure tones, FM sounds and noise bursts. *Journal of Physiology (London), 200,* 555–574.

Suga, N. (1977). Amplitue-spectrum representation in the Doppler-shifted-SF processing area of the auditory cortex of mustache bat. *Science, 196,* 64–67.

Suga, N. (1995). Processing of auditory information carried by species-specific complex sounds. In M. S. Gazzaniga (Ed.), *The cognitive neurosciences* (pp. 295–314). Cambridge, MA: MIT Press.

Suga, N., & Jen, P. H.-S. (1976). Disproportionate tonotopic representation for processing species-specific CF-FM sonar signals in the mustache bat auditory cortex. *Science, 194,* 542–544.

Sugase, Y., Yamane, S., Ueno, S., & Kawano, K. (1999). Global and fine information coded by simple neurons in the temporal visual cortex. *Nature, 400,* 869–873.

Sulkava, R. (1982). Alzheimer's disease and senile dementia of the Alzheimer type: A comparative study. *Acta Neurologica Scandinavica, 65,* 636–650.

Sultzer, D. L., Mahler, M. E., Mandelkern, M. A., et al. (1995). The relationships between psychiatric symptoms and regional cortical metabolism in Alzheimer's disease. *Journal of Neuropsychiatry and Clinical Neuroscience, 7,* 476–484.

Sunaert, S., Van Hecke, P., Marchal, G., & Orban, G. A. (1999). Motion-responsive regions of the human brain. *Experimental Brain Research, 127,* 355–370.

Sutherland, N. S. (1968). Outline of a theory of visual pattern recognition in animal and man. *Proceeding of the Royal Society of London, B, 171,* 297–317.

Swayze, V. W. II., Andreasen, A. C., Alliger, R. J., Yuh, W. T. C., & Ehrhardt, J. C. (1992). Subcortical and temporal structures in affective disorder and schizophrenia: A magnetic resonance imaging study. *Biological Psychiatry, 31,* 221–240.

Swayze, V. W., Andreasen, N. C., Alliger, R. J., et al. (1990). Structural brain abnormalities in bipolar affective disorder. *Archives of General Psychiatry, 47,* 1054–1059.

Swedo, S. E., Pietrini, P., Leonard, H. L., et al. (1992). Cerebral glucose metabolism in childhood-onset obsessive-compulsive disorder: Revisualization during pharmacotherapy. *Archives of General Psychiatry, 49,* 690–694.

Swedo, S. E., Shapiro, M. G., Grady, C. L., et al. (1989). Cerebral glucose metabolism in childhood onset obsessive-compulsive disorder. *Archives of General Psychiatry, 45,* 518–523.

Sweet, J. (1983). Confounding effect of depression on neuropsychological testing: Five illustrative cases. *Clinical Neuropsychology, 5,* 103–109.

Sweet, W. H., Talland, G. A., & Ervin, F. R. (1959). Loss of recent memory following section of the fornix. *Transactions of American Neurological Association, 84,* 876–882.

Swindell, C. S., Holland, A. L., Fromm, D., & Greenhouse, J. B. (1988). Characteristics of recovery of drawing ability in left and right brain-damaged patients. *Brain and Cognition, 7,* 16–30.

Swoboda, K., & Jenike, M. A. (1995). Frontal abnormalities in a patient with obsessive-compulsive disorder: The role of structural lesions in obsessive-compulsive behavior. *Neurology, 45,* 2130–2134.

Talland, G. A., Sweet, W. H., & Ballantine, H. T. (1967). Amnesic syndrome with anterior communicating artery aneurysm. *Journal of Nervous and Mental Diseases, 145,* 179–182.

Tamura, H., & Tanaka, K. (2001). Visual response properties of cells in ventral and dorsal parts of the macaque inferotemporal cortex. *Cerebral Cortex, 11,* 384–399.

Tanabe, H., Nashikawa, K., Nakagawa, Y., Ikeda, M., Yamamoto, H., Harada, K., et al. (1991). Memory loss due to tansient hypoperfusion in the medial temporal lobes, including hippocampus. *Acta Neurologica Scandinavica, 84,* 22–27.

Tanabe, H., Ikeda, M., Nakagawa, Y., et al. (1992). Gogi (word meaning) aphasia and semantic memory for words. *Higher Brain Function Research, 12,* 153–167.

Tanabe, H., Kazui, H., Ikeda, M., Nashikawa, K., Hashimoto, M., Yamada, N., et al. (1994). Slowly progressive amnesia without dementia. *Neuropathology, 14,* 105–114.

Tanaka, J. W., & Sengco, J. A. (1997). Features and their configuration in face recognition. *Memory and Cognition, 25*(50), 583–592.

Tanaka, K., Satto, H., Fukada, Y., & Moriya, M. (1990). Integration of form, texture and color information in the inferotemporal cortex of the macaque. In E. Iwai & M. Miskin (Eds.), *Vision memory and the temporal lobe* (pp. 101–109). New York: Elsevier.

Tanaka, Y., Hazama, H., Fukuhara, T., et al. (1982). Computereized tomography of the brain in manic-depressive patients: A controlled study. *Folia Psychiatrica et Neurologica, 36,* 137–144.

Taniwaki, T., Hokosawa, S., Goto, I., et al. (1992). Positron emission tomography (PET) in "pure akinesia." *Journal of Neurological Science, 107,* 34–39.

Tarachow, S. (1941). The clinical value of hallucinations in localizing the brain tumors. *American Journal of Psychiatry, 97,* 1434–1442.

Tardiff, K. (1983). A survey of assault by chronic patients in a state hospital system. In J. Lion & W. H. Reid (Eds.), *Assault within psychiatric facilities* (pp. 3–19). New York: Grune and Stratton.

Taylor, A., & Warrington, E. K. (1971). Visual agnosia: A single case report. *Cortex, 7,* 152–161.

Taylor, A. E., Saint-Cyr, J. A., Lang, A. E., & Kenny, F. T. (1986). Parkinson's disease and depression: A critical re-evaluation. *Brain, 109,* 279–292.

Taylor, D. C. (1969). Aggression and epilepsy. *Journal of Psychosomatic Research, 13,* 229–236.

Taylor, M. A. (1990). Catatonia: a review of a behavioral neurologic syndrome. *Neuropsychiatry, Neuropsychology, and Behavioral Neurology, 3,* 48–72.

Tennent, T. (1937). Discussion of mental disorder following head injury. *Proceedings of the Royal Society of Medicine, 30,* 1092–1093.

Terzian, H. (1964). Behavioral and EEG effects of intracarotid sodium amytal injection. *Acta Neurochirurgie (Wien), 12,* 230–239.

Terzian, H., & Dalle Ore, G. (1955). Syndrome of Kluver and Bucy reproduced in man by bilateral removals of the temporal lobes. *Neurology, 5,* 373–380.

Testa, J. A., Beatty, W. W., Gleason, B. A., Oebelo, B. A., & Ross, E. D. (2001). Impaired affective prosody in AD: Relationship to aphasic deficit and emotional behaviors. *Neurology, 57,* 1949–1955.

Teuber, H. L., Battersby, W. S., & Bender, M. B. (1960). *Visual fields defects after penetrating missle wounds of the brain.* Cambridge, MA: Harvard University Press.

Teuber, H. L., & Diamond, S. (1956). Effect of brain injury in man on binaural localization of sounds. Paper read at 27th Annual Meeting of the Eastern Psychological Association, Atlantic City, NJ.

Teuber, H. L., & Weinstein, S. (1956). Ability to discover hidden figures after cerebral lesions. *AMA Archives of Neurology and Psychiatry, 76,* 369–379.

Thomas, C. J., & Flemming, G. W. T. H. (1934). Lilliputian and Brobdingnagian hallucinations occurring simultaneously in a senile patient. *Journal of Mental Science, 80,* 94–102.

Thomas, J. E., Reagan, T. J., & Klass, D. W. (1977). Epilepsia partialis continua. *Archives of Neurology, 34,* 266–275.

Thompson, R. F. (1990). Neural mechanisms of classical conditioning in mammals. *Philosophical Transations of the Royal Society of London (Biology), 329,* 161–170.

Tippin, J., & Dunner, F. J. (1981). Biparietal infarctions in patient with catatonia. *American Journal of Psychiatry, 138,* 1386–1387.

Tisher, P. W., Holzer, J. C., Greenberg, M., et al. (1993, November–December). Psychiatric presentation of epilepsy. *Harvard Revue of Psychiatry,* 219–228.

Tissot, R., Constantinidis, J., & Richard, J. (1975). *La Maladie de Pick.* Paris: Masson.

Tittle, J. S., & Perotti, V. J. (1998). The perception of shape and curvedness from binocular stereopsis and structure from motion. *Perception and Psychophysics, 59,* 1167–1179.

Todd, J., & Dewhurst, K. (1955). The double: Its psycho-pathology and psychophysiology. *Journal of Nervous, Mental Diseases, 122,* 47–55.

Tognola, G., & Vignolo, L. A. (1980). Brain lesions associated with oral apraxia in stroke patients: A clinico-neuroradiological investigation with the CT scan. *Neuropsychologia, 18,* 257–272.

Tomlinson, B. E. (1977). The pathology of dementia. In C. E. Wells (Ed.), *Dementia* (2nd ed., pp. 113–153). Philadelphia: Davis FA.

Tonkonogy, J. (2001). White matter hyperintensity in elderly psychiatric patients with primary and secondary psychiatric disorder. In K. Maurer (Ed.), *International society for neuroimaging in psychiatry, ISNIP 2001.* Bern: Unversity Hospital of Clinical Psychiatry.

Tonkonogy, J., & Barreira, P. (1989). Obsessive-compulsive disorder and caudate-frontal lesion. *Neuropsychiatry, Neuropsychology, and Behavioral Neurology, 2*(3), 203–209.

Tonkonogy, J., & Moak, G. (1988). Alois Alzheimer on presenile dementia. *Journal of Geriatric Psychiatry and Neurology, 1,* 199–206.

Tonkonogy, J. M. (Ed.). (1968a). *Psychological experiment in psychiatric and neurological clinics* [in Russian]. Leningrad: Meditsina.

Tonkonogy, J. M. (1968b). *Stroke and aphasia* [in Russian]. Leningrad: Meditsina.

Tonkonogy, J. M. (1973). *Introduction to clinical neuropsychology* [in Russian]. Leningrad: Meditsina.

Tonkonogy, J. M. (1984). Impairment of pitch discrimination and phonem perception in aphasia. In *Proceeding of the 22nd Annual Meeting of Academy of Aphasia.* Santa Monica, CA.

Tonkonogy, J. M. (1986). *Vascular aphasia.* Cambridge, MA: MIT Press.

Tonkonogy, J. M. (1989). Recognition memory for tones: The importance of the left posterior-superior temporal region. *Abstracts of the 19th Annual Meeting of the Society for Neuroscience, 15*(1), 4.

Tonkonogy, J. M. (1991). Violence and temporal lobe lesion: Head CT and MRI data. *Journal of Neuropsychiatry and Clinical Neuroscience, 3,* 189–196.

Tonkonogy, J. M. (1997). *Brief cognitive neuropsychological examination.* Los Angeles: Western Psychological Services.

Tonkonogy, J. M., & Ageeva, A. N. (1961). On kinetic disorder of speech in a case with infarction in the territory of the left anterior cerebral artery [in Russian]. In G. B. Abramovich & G. Z. Levin (Eds.), *Problems of localization and localization diagnosis in psychiatry and neurology* (Vol. 21, pp. 41–54). Leningrad: Bechterev Insitute Press.

Tonkonogy, J. M., & Armstrong, J. (1988). Daignostic algorithms and clinical diagnostic thinking. In *Proceeding of the Symposium on the Engineering of Computer-based Medical Systems* (pp. 71–74). Minneapolis, MN: IEEE Engineering in Medicine and Biology Society.

Tonkonogy, J. M., Dorofeeva, S. A., & Meerson, Y. A. (1995). Auditory and visual working memory and posterior hemispheric lesions. *Journal of Neuropsychiatry and Clinical Neuroscience, 7,* 424–425.

Tonkonogy, J. M., & Gaulin, B. (1992). Anitconvulsants and behavior control in state hospital patients. *Hospital and Community Psychiatry,* Newsletter, 62–63.

Tonkonogy, J. M., & Geller, J. L. (1992). Hypothalamic lesions and intermittent explosive disorder. *Journal of Neuropsychiatry and Clinical Neuroscience, 4*, 45–50.

Tonkonogy, J. M., & Geller, J. L. (1999). Late-onset paranoid psychosis as a distinct clinicopathological entity: Magnetic resonance imaging data in elderly patients with paranoid psychosis of late onset and schizophrenia of early onset. *Neuropsychiatry, Neuropsychology, and Behavioral Neurology, 12*(4), 230–235.

Tonkonogy, J. M., & Goodglass, H. (1981). Language function: Foot of the third frontal gyrus and Rolandic operculum. *Neurology, 38*, 486–490.

Tonkonogy, J. M., Smith, T. W., & Barreira, P. J. (1994). Obsessive-compulsive disorder in Pick's disease. *Journal of Neuropsychiatry and Clinical Neuroscience, 6*, 176–180.

Tonkonogy, J. M., Vasserman, L. I., Dorofeeva, S. A., & Meerson, Y. A. (1977). *Diagnostic neuropsychological examination* [in Russian]. Leningrad: Bechterev Institute Press.

Torack, R. M., & Morris, J. C. (1988). The association of ventral tegmental area histopathology with adult dementia. *Archives of Neurology, 45*, 497–501.

Tranel, D., Damasio, A. R., & Damasio, H. (1988). Intact recognition of facial expression, gender, and age in patients with impaired recognition of face indentity. *Neurology, 38*, 690–696.

Traugott, N. N. (1959). About the peculiarities of auditory function in disorders of cortical region of auditory analyzer in children [in Russian]. *Problems of Physiological Acoustics, 4*, 201–207.

Traugott, N. N., & Kaidanova, S. I. (1975). *Auditory disturbances in sensory alaliya and sensory aphasia* [in Russian]. Leningrad: Nauka.

Treff, W. M., & Hempel, K. J. (1958). Die Zeldichte bei schizophrenenund klinisch gesunden. *Journal für Hirnforschung, 4*, 314–369.

Trescher, J. H., & Ford, F. R. (1937). Colloid cyst of the third ventricle. *Archives of Neurology and Psychiatry, 37*, 959–973.

Trillet, M., Croisile, B., Tourniaire, D., & Schott, B. (1990). Perturbations de l'activité motrice volotaire et lésions des noyaux caudés. *Revue Neurologique, 146*, 338–344.

Trimble, M. (1991). *The psychosis of epilepsy.* New York: Raven Press.

Trojanovski, J. Q., Green, R. C., & Levine, D. N. (1980). Crossed aphasia in dextral: A clinicopathological study. *Neurology, 30*, 709–713.

Trousseau, A. (1864). De l'aphasie, maladie decrite recemmentsons lenom improper d'aphamie. *Gazette des Hôpitaux, 37.*

Trubetzkoy, N. S. (1939/1969). *Grundzuge der Phonologie [Principle of Phonology].* Berkeley: University of California Press.

Ts'o, D. Y., & Roe, A. (1995). Functional compartmennets in visual cortex. In M. S. Gazzaniga (Ed.), *The cognitive neurosciences* (pp. 325–338). Cambridge, MA: MIT Press.

Tsunoda, T., & Oka, M. (1976). Lateralization of emotion in the human brain and auditory cerebral dominance. *Proceeding of the Japan Academy, 52,* 528–531.

Tucker, D. M., Watson, R. T., & Heilman, K. M. (1977). Discrimination and evocation of affectively intoned speech in patients with right parietal disease. *Neurology, 27,* 947–950.

Tuller, B. (1984). On categorizing aphasic speech errors. *Neuropsychologia, 22,* 547–557.

Tulving, E. (1995). Organization of memory: Quo vadis? In M. S. Gazzaniga (Ed.), *The cognitive neurosciences* (pp. 839–847). Cambridge, MA: MIT Press.

Turnbull, O. H., Carey, D. P., & McCarthy, R. A. (1997). The neuropsychology of object constancy. *Journal of International Neuropsychological Society, 3,* 288–298.

Tyler, H. R. (1968). Abnormalities of perception with defective eye movements (Balint's syndrome). *Cortex, 3,* 154–171.

Tzavaras, A., Hecaen, H., & Le Bras, H. (1970). Le probleme de la specificite du deficit de la reconnaissance du visage humain lors de lesions hemispheriques unilaterales. *Neuropsychologia, 8,* 403–417.

Uhl, F., Goldenberg, G., Lang, W., Lindinger, M., Steiner, M., & Deesce, L. (1990). Cerbral correlates of imamging colours, faces, and a map: II. Negative cortical DC potentials. *Neuropsychologia, 28,* 81–93.

Ullman, S. (1996). *High-level vision: Object recognition and visual cognition.* Cambridge, MA: MIT Press.

Ullman, S. (1999). Three-dimentional object recognition based on the combination of views. In M. J. Tarr & H. H. Bulthoff (Eds.), *Object recognition in man, monkey, and machine* (pp. 21–44). Cambridge, MA: MIT Press.

Ungerleider, L. G., & Mishkin, M. (1982). Two cortical visual systems. In D. J. Ingle, M. A. Goodale, & R. J. W. Mansfield (Eds., pp. 45–74), *Analysis of visual behavior.* Cambridge, MA: MIT Press.

Uytdenhoef, P., Portlange, P., Jacguy, J., et al. (1983). Regional cerebral blood flow and lateralized and hemispheric dysfunction in depression. *British Journal of Psychiatry, 143,* 128–132.

Van Bogaert, L. (1924). Syndrome Inférieur du noyau rouge, troubles psychosensoriels d'origine mésoceéphalique. *Revue Neurolgique, 40,* 417–423.

Van Bogaert, L. (1927). L'hallucinose pédonculaire. *Revue Neurologique, 43,* 608–617.

Van Essen, D. C., Felleman, D. J., DeYoe, E. A., Olavarria, J., & Knierim, J. J. (1990). Modular and hierrarchical organization of extrastriate visual cortex in the macaque monkey. *Cold Spring Harbor Symposium, Quantitative Biology, 55,* 679–696.

Van Horn, J. D., & McManus, I. C. (1992). Ventricular enlargement in schizophrenia: A meta-analysis of studies of the ventricular-brain ratio (VBR). *British Journal of Psychiatry, 160,* 687–697.

Varney, N. R. (1980). Sound recognition in relation to aural language comprehension in aphasic patients. *Journal of Neurology, Neurosurgery, and Psychiatry, 43,* 71–75.

Varney, N. R. (1984). Alexia for ideograms: Implications for Kanjii alexia. *Cortex, 20,* 535–542.

Verrey, D. (1888). Hemiachromatopsie droite absolute. *Archives D'Ophtalmologie* (Paris), *8,* 239–300.

Victor, M., Adams, R. D., & Collins, G. H. (1971). *The Wernickke-Korsakoff Syndrome: A clinical and pathological study of 245 patients, 82 with post-mortem examination.* Philadelphia: F.A. Davis Company.

Victor, M., Angevine, J. B., Mancall, E. L., & Fisher, C. M. (1961). Memory loss with lesions of the hippocampal formation. *Archives of Neurology, 5,* 244–263.

Victoroff, J. I., Benson, F., Grafton, S. T., Engel, J., & Mazziota, J. C. (1994). Depression in complex partial seizures. *Archives of Neurology, 51,* 155–163.

Vighetto, A., & Aimard, G. (1981). Les troubles specifique de l'utilization de l'espace de de/ambulation. *Journal des Agrégés, 14,* 325–334.

Vignolo, L. (1969). Auditiry agnosia: A review and report of recent evidence. In A. Benton (Ed.), *Contributions to clinical neuropsychology* (pp. 172–208). Chicago: Aldine.

Vilkki, J. (1985). Amnestic syndromes after surgery of anterior communicating artery aneurysm. *Cortex, 21,* 431–434.

Vix, E. (1910). Anatomischer befund zu dem in band 37 dieses Archivs veroeffentlichten Fall von transcortikaler sensorischer Aphasie. *Archiv für Psychiatrie und Nervenkrankheiten, 47,* 200–212.

Volavka, J. (1995). *Neurobiology of violence.* Washington, DC: American Psychiatric Press.

Volkow, N. D., Wolf, A. P., Van Gelder, P., et al. (1987). Phenomenological correlates of metabolic activity in 18 patients with chronic schizophrenia. *Neuroendocrinology, 144,* 151–158.

Volle, E., Beato, R., Levy, R., & Dubois, B. (2002). Forced collectionism after orbitofrontal damage. *Neurology, 58,* 488–490.

Volpe, B. T., & Hirst, W. (1983). Amnesia following the rupture and repair of an anrterior communicating artery aneurysm. *Journal of Neurology, Neurosurgery, and Psychiatry, 46,* 704–709.

Volpe, B. T., Sidris, J. J., Holtzman, J. D., Wilson, D. H., & Gazzaniga, M. S. (1982). Cortical mechanisms involved in praxia: Observations following partial and complete section of the corpus callosum in man. *Neurology, 32,* 645–650.

Von Cramon, D. Y., & Schuri, U. (1992). The septo-hippocampal pathways and their relevance to human memory: A case report. *Cortex, 28,* 411–422.

Von der Heydt, R. (1995). Form analysis in the visual cortex. In S. Gazzaniga (Ed.), *The cognitive neurosciences* (pp. 365–382). Cambridge, MA: MIT Press.

Von der Heydt, R., Peterhans, E., & Baumhartner, G. (1984). Illusory contours and cortical neuron responses. *Science, 224,* 1260–1261.

Von der Malsburg, C. (1973). Self-organization of orientation sensitive cells in striate cortex. *Cybernetic, 14,* 85–100.

Von Economo, C. (1931). *Encephalitis lethargica: Its sequelae and treatment.* (K. O. Newman, Trans.). New York: Oxford University Press.

Von Feuerbach, A. R. (1828). Aktenmassige darstellung merkwurdiger verbrechen. *Harper, 28,* 120–138.

Von Meyendorf, N. (1930). *Vom Lokalisationsproblems der artikulierten Sprache.* Leipzig: Barth.

Von Stockert, F. G. (1932). Subcortical demenz. *Archives of Psychiatry, 97,* 97–100.

Vuilleumier, P., Ghika-Schmid, F., Bogousslavsky, J., Assal, G., & Regli, F. (1998). Persistent recurrence of hypomania and prosoaffective agnosia in a patient with right thalamic infarct. *Neuropsychiatry, Neuropsychology, and Behavioral Neurology, 11*(1), 40–44.

Wagner, W. (1943). Anosognosie, Zeitrafferphaenomenon und Uhrzeitagnosie als Symptome der Stoerungen im rechten Parito-Occipitallapen. *Nervenarzt, 16,* 49–57.

Wald, A. (1947). *Sequential analysis.* New York: Academic Press.

Wall, M., Mielke, D., & Luther, S. J. (1986). Panic attacks and psychomotor seizures following right temporal lobectomy. *Journal of Clinical Psychiatry, 47*(4), 219.

Wall, M., Tuchman, M., & Mielke, D. (1985). Panic attacks and temporal lobe seizures associated with a right temporal lobe arterio-venous malformation: case report. *Journal of Clinical Psychiatry, 46*(4), 143–145.

Walsh, R. (1956). Orbitalhirn und Charakter. In E. Rehwald (Ed.), *Das Hirntrauma* (pp. 461–468). Stuttgart: Springer.

Walston, F., Blennerhassett, R. C., & Charlston, B. (2000). "Theory of mind," persecutory delusions and somatic marker mechanism. *Cognitive Neuropsychiatry, 5*(3), 161–174.

Ward, C. D. (1988). Transient feelings of compulsion caused by hemispheric lesions: Three cases. *Journal of Neurology, Neurosurgery, and Psychiatry, 51,* 266–268.

Warren, L. R., Butler, R. W., Katholi, C. R., McFarland, C. E., Crews, E. L., Halsey, J. H. Jr. (1984). Focal changes in cerebral blood flow produced by monetary incentive during a mental mathematic task in normal and depressed subjects. *Brain and Cognition, 3,* 71–75.

Warrington, E. K. (1975). The selelctive impairment of semantic memory. *Quarterly Journal of Experimental Psychology, 27,* 635–657.

Warrington, E. K. (1981). Concrete word dyslexia. *British Journal of Psychology, 72,* 175–196.

Warrington, E. K. (1986). Visual deficit associated with occipital lobe lesions in man. *Experimental Brain Research Supplementum, 11,* 247–261.

Warrington, E. K., & James, M. (1967). Tachistoscopic number estimation in patients with unilateral cerebral lesions. *Journal of Neurology, Neurosurgery, and Psychiatry, 30,* 468–474.

Warrington, E. K., & James, M. (1985). Visual object recognition in patients with right-hemisphere lesions: Axes or features. *Perception, 15,* 355–366.

Warrington, E.K., & James, M. (1988). Visual apperceptive agnosia: A clinico-anatomical study of three cases. *Cortex, 24,* 13–32.

Warrington, E. K., James, M., & Kinsbourne, M. (1966). Drawing disability in relation to the laterality of cerebral lesion. *Brain, 89,* 53–82.

Warrington, E. K., & Rabin, P. (1970). Perceptual matching in patients with cerebral lesions. *Neuropsychologia, 8,* 475–487.

Warrington, E. K., & Taylor, A. M. (1973). The contribution of the right parietal lobe to object recognition. *Cortex, 9,* 152–164.

Warrington, E. K., & Taylor, A. M. (1978). Two categorical stages of object recognition. *Perception, 7,* 695–705.

Watkins, E. S., & Oppenheimer, D. R. (1962). Mental disturbances after thalamolysis. *Journal of Neurology, Neurosurgery, and Psychiatry, 25,* 243–250.

Watson, R. T., & Heilman, K. M. (1979). Thalamic neglect. *Neurology, 29,* 690–694.

Watson, R. T., & Heilman, K. M. (1983). Callosal apraxia. *Brain, 106,* 391–403.

Watson, R. T., Valenstein, E., & Heiman, K. M. (1981). Thalamic neglect: The possible role of the medial thalamus and nucleus reticularis of thalamus in behavior. *Archives of Neurology, 38,* 501–507.

Waxman, S. G., & Geschwind, N. (1975). The interictal behavior syndrome of temporal lobe epilepsy. *Archives of General Psychiatry, 32,* 1580–1586.

Wechsler, A. F. (1977). Presenile dementia presenting as dementia. *Journal of Neurology, Neurosurgery, and Psychiatry, 40,* 303–305.

Wechsler, A. F., Verity, M., Rosenschein, S., Fried, I., & Scheibel, A. B. (1982). Pick's disease. *Archives of Neurology, 39,* 287–290.

Wechsler, D. (1955). *Wechsler Adult Intelligence Scale.* New York: The Psychological Corporation.

Weilburg, J. B., Bear, D. M., & Sachs, G. (1987). Three patients with concomitant panic attacks and seizure disorder: Possible clue to the neurology of anxiety. *American Journal of Psychiatry, 144,* 1053–1056.

Weilburg, J. B., Mesulam, M., Weintraub, J., Buonanno, F., Jenike, M., & Stakes, J. W. (1989). Focal striatal abnormalities in a patient with obsessive-compulsive disorder. *Archives of Neurology, 46,* 233–235.

Weilburg, J. B., Schachter, S., Sachs, G. S., Worth, J., Pollack, M. H., Ives, J. R., et al. (1993). Focal paroxysmal EEG during atypical panic attacks. *Journal of Neuropsychiatry and Clinical Neuroscience, 5,* 50–55.

Weinberger, D. R., Berman, K. F., & Zec, R. F. (1988). Physiological dysfunction of dorsolateral prefrontal cortex in schizophrenia: I. Regional cerebral blood flow (rCBF) evidence. *Archives of General Psychiatry, 45,* 609–615.

Weinberger, D. R., & Wyatt, R. J. (1982). Brain morphology in schizophrenia: In vivo studies. In F. A. Henn & H. A. Nasrallah (Eds.), *Schizophrenia as a brain disease* (pp. 148–175). New York: Oxford University Press.

Weinstein, E. A., & Cole, M. (1963). Concepts of anosopagnosia. In L. Halpern (Ed.), *Problems of dynamic neurology* (pp. 254–273). Jerusalem: Jerusalem Post Press.

Weinstein, E. A., & Kahn, R. L. (1952). Nonaphasic misnaming (paraphasia) in organic brain disease. *Archives of Neurology and Psychiatry, 67,* 72–79.

Weinstein, E. A., Kahn, R. C., & Slate, W. H. (1955). Withdrawal, inattention, and pain asymbolia. *Archives of Neurology and Psychiatry, 74,* 245–248.

Weinstein, S., Vetter, R. J., & Sersen, E. A. (1970). Phantoms following breast amputations. *Neuropsychologia, 8,* 185–197.

Weintraub, S., Rubin, N. P., & Mesulam, M. M. (1990). Primary progressive aphasia: Longitudinal course, neuropsychological profile, and language features. *Archives of Neurology, 47,* 1329–1335.

Weintraub, S., & Mesulam, M. M. (1993). Four neuropsychological profiles in dementia. In H. Spinnler & F. Boller (Eds.), *Handbook of neuropsychology* (Vol. 8, pp. 253–282). Amsterdam: Elsevier.

Weiss, A. P., & Jenike, M. A. (2000). Late-onset obsessive-compulsive disorder: A case series. *Journal of Neuropsychiatry and Clinical Neuroscience, 12,* 265–268.

Wellman, H. M. (1990). *The child theory of mind.* Cambridge, MA: MIT Press.

Weniger, G., Irie, E., Exner, C., & Ruther, E. (1997). Defective conceptualization of emotional expressions during T2 signal enhancement of the right amygdala. *Neurocase, 3,* 259–266.

Wenk, G. L., & Olton, D. S. (1987). Basal forebrain cholinergic neurons and Alzheimer's Disease. In J. T. Coyle (Ed.), *Animal models of dementia: A synaptic neurochemical perspective* (pp. 81–100). New York: Alan R. Liss.

Wernicke, C. (1874). *Der Aphasische Symptomencomplex.* Breslau, Prussia: Cohn und Weigert.

Wernicke, C. (1881). *Lehrbuch der Gehirhkrankheiten.* Berlin: Th. Fisher and Kassel.

Wernicke, C. (1895). Zwei falle von Rindenlasion. *Arbeiten Aus die Psychiatrische Klinic In Breslau, 2,* 33–53.

Wernicke, C. (1906). *Fundamentals of psychiatry.* Leipzig, Germany: Theime.

Wernicke, C., & Friedlander, C. (1893). A case of deafness as a result of bilateral lesions of the temporal lobe. In G. H. Eggert (Ed.), *Wernicke's work on aphasia* (pp. 164–172). New York: Mouton.

Wertheim, N., & Botez, M. I. (1961). Receptive amusia: A clinical analysis. *Brain, 84,* 19–30.

Weston, M. J., & Whitlock, F. A. (1971). The Capgras syndrome following head injury. *British Journal of Psychiatry, 119,* 25–31.

Wexler, B. E., Giller, E. L. Jr., & Southwick, S. (1991). Cerebral laterality, symptoms, and diagnosis in psychotic pataients. *Biological Psychiatry, 29,* 103–116.

Whalen, P. J. (1998). Fear, vigilance, and ambiguity: Initial neuroimaging studies of the human amygdala. *Current Directions in Psychological Science, 7*(6), 177–188.

Whitaker, H. (1976). A case of the isolation of the language function. In H. Whitaker & H. A. Whitaker (Eds.), *Studies in neurolinguistics* (Vol. 2, pp. 261–292). New York: Academic Press.

White, J. C., & Cobb, S. (1955). Psychological changes associated with giant pituitary neoplasms. *Archive of Neurology and Psychiatry, 74*, 383–396.

Whitehouse, P. J., Proce, D. L., Struble, R. G., Clark, A. W., Coyle, J. T., & DeLong, M. R. (1982). Alzheimer's disease and senile dementia: Loss of neurons in the basal forebrain. *Science, 215*, 1237–1239.

Whiteley, A., & Warrington, E. K. (1977). Prosopagnosia: A clinical, psychological and anatomical study of three patients. *Journal of Neurology, Neurosurgery, and Psychiatry, 40*, 395–435.

Whiteley, A. M., & Warrington, E. K. (1978). Selective impairment of topographical memory: A single case study. *Journal of Neurology, Neurosurgery, and Psychiatry, 41*, 575–578.

Whitlock, F. A., & Siskind, M. M. (1980). Depression as a major symptom of multiple sclerosis. *Journal of Neurology, Neurosurgery, and Psychiatry,* 861–865.

Whitman, S., Coleman, T. E., Patmon, C., Desai, B. T., Cohen, R., & King, L. N. (1984). Epilepsy in prison: Elevated prevalence and no relationship to violence. *Neurology, 34*, 775–782.

Whitty, C. M., Duffield, J. E., Tow, P. M., et al. (1952). Anterior cingulotomy in the treatment of mental disease. *Lancet, 1*, 475–481.

Whitty, C. W. M., & Lishman, W. A. (1996). Amnesia in cerebral disease. In C. W. M. Whitty & O. L. Zangwill (Eds.), *Amnesia* (pp. 321–634). London: Buttreworths.

Widen, L., Bergstrom, M., Blomqvist, G., et al. (1981). Glucose metabolism in patients with schizophrenia: Emission computed tomography measurement with 11-C glucose. *Cerebral Blood Flow Metabolism, 1*(Suppl. 1), S455.

Wiesel, F. A., Wik, G., Sjoegren, I., et al. (1987). Regional brain glucose metabolism in drug free schizophrenic patients and clinical correlates. *Acta Psychiatrica Scandinavica, 76*, 628–641.

Wilbrand, H. (1884). *Ophtalmiatrische Beitrage zur Diagnostik der Gehirn-Krankheiten.* Wiesbaden, Germany: Bergmann.

Wilbrand, H. (1887). *Die Seelenblindheit at Herderscheinung und ihre Beziehungen zur homonymen Hemianopsie, zur Alexie und Agraphie.* Wiesbaden, Germany, J. F. Bergmann.

Wilbrand, H. (1892). Ein fall von Seelenblindheit und Hemianopsie mit Sectionsbefund. *Deutsche Zeitschrift für Nervenheilkunde, 2*, 361–387.

Wilcox, J. A. (1991). Cerebellar atrophy and catatonia. *Biological Psychiatry, 29*, 733.

Williams, M. (1970). *Brain damage and mind.* Baltimore: Penguin Books.

Williamson, P., Pelz, D., Merskey, H., Morrison, S., & Conlon, P. (1991). Correlation of negative symptoms in schizophrenia with frontal lobe parameters on magnetic resonance imaging. *British Journal of Psychiatry, 159*, 130–134.

Willis, T. (1664). *Cerebri anatomie*. London: Martzer and Alleftry.

Wilson, F. A. W., O'Scalaidhe, S. P., & Goldman-Rakic, P. S. (1993). Dissociation of object and spatial processing domain in primate prefrontal cortex. *Science, 260,* 1955–1958.

Wilson, M. (1957). Effects of circumscribed cortical lesions upon somesthetic and visual discrimination in the monkey. *Journal of Comparative Physiology and Psychology, 50,* 630–635.

Wilson, S. A. K. (1908). A contribution to study of apraxia. *Brain, 31,* 164–216.

Wimmer, H., & Perner, J. (1983). Beliefs about beliefs: Representation and constraining function of wrong beliefs in young children's understanding of deception. *Cognition, 35,* 245–275.

Winokur, G., Pfol, B., & Tsuang, M. (1987). A 40-year follow-up of hebephrenic-catatonic schizophrenia. In N. Miller & G. Cohen (Eds.), *Schizophrenia and aging* (pp. 52–60). New York: Guilford Press.

Wolfe, G. I., & Ross, E. D. (1987). Sensory aprosodia with left hemiparesis from subcortical infarction: Right hemisphere analogue of sensory-type aphasia with right hemiparesis. *Archives of Neurology, 44,* 661–671.

Wolkin, L. I., Jaeger, J., Brodie, J. D., et al. (1985). Persistence of cerebral metabolic abnormalities in chronic schizophrenia as determined by positron emission tomography. *American Journal of Psychiatry, 142,* 564–571.

Wolpert, I. (1924). Die simultanagnosie: Storung der Gesamtauffassung. *Zeitschrift für die gesamte Neurologie und Psychiatrie, 93,* 397–415.

Wong, A. H. C., & Meier, H. M. R. (1997). Case report: Delusional jealousy following right-sided cerebral infarct. *Neurocase, 3,* 391–394.

Woodard, J. S. (1962). Concentric hyaline inclusion body formation in mental disease: Analysis of twenty seven cases. *Journal of Neuropathology and Experimental Neurology, 21,* 442–449.

Woodruff, P. W. R. (2004). Auditory hallucinations: Insights and questions from neuroimaging. *Cognitive Neuropsychiatry, 9*(1/2), 73–91.

Woods, B. T., Schoene, W., & Keisley, L. (1982). Are hippocampal lesions sufficient to cause lasting amnesia? *Journal of Neurology, Neurosurgery, and Psychiatry, 45,* 243–248.

Wortis, S. B., & Pfeiffer, A. Z. (1948). Unilateral auditory-spatial agnosia. *Journal of Nervous and Mental Diseases, 108,* 181–186.

Wszolek, Z. K., Pfeiffer, R. F., Bhatt, M. H., et al. (1992). Rapidly progressive autosomal dominant parkinsonism and dementia with pallido-pontal-nigral degeneration. *Annual Review of Neurology, 32,* 312–320.

Wu, J. C., Gillin, J. C., Buchsbaum, M. S., et al. (1992). The effect of sleep deprivation on brain metabolism of depressed patients. *American Journal of Psychiatry, 149,* 538–543.

Wu, S., Schenkenberg, T., Wing, A. M., & Osborn, A. G. (1981). Cognitive correlates of diffuse cerebral atrophy determined by computed tomography. *Neurology, 31,* 1180–1184.

Yamadory, A., Osumi, Y., Masuhara, S., & Okubo, M. (1977). Preservation of singing in Broca's aphasia. *Journal of Neurology, Neurosurgery, and Psychiatry, 40,* 196–221.

Yaryura-Tobias, J. A., & Neziroglu, F. (1975). Violent behavior, brain dysrhythmia and glucose dysfunction: a new syndrome. *Journal of Orthomolecular Psychiatry, 4,* 182–188.

Yates, W. R., Jacoby, C. G., & Andreasen, N. C. (1987). Cerebellar atrophy in schizophrenia and affective disorder. *American Journal of Psychiatry, 144,* 465–467.

Yeterain, E. H., & Van Hoesen, G. W. (1978). Cortico-striate projections in the rhesus monkey: The organization of certain cortico-caudate connections. *Brain Research, 139,* 43–63.

Yhar, M. D. (1984). Parkinsonism. In L. P. Rowland (Ed)., *Merrit's textbook of neurology* (7th ed., pp. 526–537). Philadelphia: Lee and Febiger.

Yoshimura, M. (1983). Cortical changes in the parkinsonian brain: A contribution to the delineation of "diffuse Lewy body disease." *Journal of Neurology, 229,* 17–32.

Young, A. W., Flude, B. M., & Ellis, A. W. (1991). Delusional misidentification incident in a right hemisphere stroke patient. *Behavioural Neurology, 4,* 81–87.

Young, D. A., Davila, R., & Scher, H. (1993). Unawareness of illness and neuropsychological performance in chronic schizophrenia. *Schizophrenia Research, 10,* 117–124.

Young, M. P. (1995). Open questions about the neural mechanisms of visual pattern recognition. In S. Gazzaniga (Ed.), *The cognitive neurosciences* (pp. 463–474). Cambridge, MA: MIT Press.

Young, M. P., & Yamane, S. (1992). Sparse population coding of faces in the inferotemporal cortex. *Science, 256,* 1327–1331.

Yuasa, T., Homa, Y., Takahashi, H., Mori, S., & Nayashi, H. (1987). Progressive supranuclear palsy with pure akinesia as initial symptom. *Shinkei Naika, 26,* 460–467.

Zaidel, D., & Sperry, R. W. (1977). Some long-term effects of cerebral commissurotomy in man. *Neuropsychologia, 15,* 193–203.

Zandi, T., Cooper, M., & Garrison, L. (1992). Facial recognition: A cognitive study of elderly demented patients and normal older adults. *International Psychogeriatrics, 4,* 215–221.

Zarit, S. & Kahn, R. L. (1974). Impairment and adaptation in chronic disabilities: Spatial inattention. *Journal of Nervous and Mental Disease, 159,* 63–72.

Zeigarnik, B. V. (1961). *The pathology of thinking* [in Russian]. Moskow: Moskow State University Press.

Zeki, S. M. (1990). A century of cerebral achromatopsia. *Brain, 113,* 1721–1777.

Zilbovicius, M., Boddaert, N., Belin, P., Poline, J., Remy, P, Mangin, J., et al. (2000). Temporal lobe dysfunction in childhood autism: A PET study. *American Journal of Psychiatry, 157,* 1988–1993.

Zola, S. (2000). Amnesia: I. Neuroanatomic and clinical issues. In J. F. Farah & T. E. Feinberg (Eds.), *Patient-based approaches to cognitive neuroscience* (pp. 275–290). Cambridge, MA: MIT Press.

Zola-Morgan, S., Squire, L. R., & Amaral, D. (1986). Human amnesia and the medial temporal region: Enduring memory impairment following a bilateral lesion limited to the CA1 field of the hippocampus. *Journal of Neuroscience, 6,* 2950–2967.

Index

Abstract attitude, 7
Abstract language, 6
Abulia. *See* Avolition
Acalculia, 100
Achromatopsia
  clinical features of, 91–92
  historical description of, 90
  metamorphopsia with, 188
  occipito-temporal lesions in, 96
Acquired immunodeficiency
    syndrome (AIDS), 659
Action agnosia
  anatomical aspects of, 170–172,
    185
  apperceptive, 166–167
  associative, 168–170
  card sorting test with, 179
  complex action recognition in,
    166–167
  conventional action recognition
    in, 163–165
  gestalt images in, 172–175
  object alternation test with, 178
  patterns of order in, 181–184
  recurrent figures in, 181
  sequence recognition in, 177–178
  simple features in, 165

simultanagnosia, 166, 170
  visuomotor sequential procedures
    in, 175–177
Action recognition
  complex, 166–167
  conventional, 163–165
  simple features in, 165
Activities of daily living, with social
    apraxia, 326–327
Acute confusional state, 608, 617–618
ADD. *See* Attention deficit disorder
ADHD. *See* Attention deficit
    hyperactivity disorder
Affective flattening, 503–504
Age, old, hallucinations in, 213–215
Aggression, pathological
  anatomical aspects of, 588
  frontal lobe in, 597
  seizure activity in, 590
  sociopsychological problems
    arising in, 586
Agnosia, 32–33. *See also specific agnosia*
Agnosia of depth, 100–102
Agnosia of person, 222–223
Agnosia of sequences, evaluation of,
    681–682
Agnosia of shape, 25–29

Agnosia of space, dementia with, 628
Agnosia of time, dementia with,
    628–629
Agrammatism, motor
    in Broca's aphasia, 346
    posterior aphasia with, 364
Agraphia, 140. *See also specific
    agraphias*
    alexia with, 414
    clinical aspects of, 415–418, 422
    description of, 406–407
    musical alexia as, 425
Agraphic alexia, 408–409
Ahylognosia, 129
AIDS. *See* Acquired
    immunodeficiency syndrome
AIDS dementia, 659
Akinesia. *See also specific akinesias*
    brain information processing in,
        524–527
    types of, 514
Akinetic mutism
    anatomical aspects of, 520–521
    clinical aspects of, 517
Alcoholism, amnestic disorders
    caused by, 4, 428
Alertness
    in dementia, 621
    fluctuating, 507
Alexia. *See also specific alexias*
    agraphia with, 414
    anatomical aspects of, 412–415
    clinical aspects of, 407–412
    description of, 406–407
Alienation
    body part, 138–139
    in color agnosia, 92–93
    of word meaning, 349–350, 356–357,
        365, 373
Alloesthesia
    optic, 133, 189
    somatic, 146
    tactile, 133
    with visuospatial agnosia, 99
Alogia subscale, 503
Alzheimer's disease
    agnosias with, 628
    aphasia with, 376–377

apraxia with, 638
atrophy localization in, 637
cortical atrophy with, 639–640
cortical lesions with, 640–642
delusions with, 289
dementia from, 621–622, 632–634
hallucinations from, 213–214
lesion localization in, 634
memory with, 634
senile *vs.* presenile onset of, 633
vascular pathology in, 642–644
Amnesia. *See also* Amnestic disorders;
    Psychogenic amnesia;
    Retrograde amnesia
    anterograde, 438, 446–447
    dissociative, 268
    with frontal lobe lesions, 453–454
    isolated, 450–451
    reduplicative, 437, 452–453
    transient global, 437–438, 451–452
Amnesia of Charcot-Wilbrand. *See*
    Visual imagery loss
Amnestic aphasia, 344
Amnestic color blindness, 91
Amnestic disorders
    alcoholism causing, 4, 428
    evaluation of, 681, 684
    lesion localizations in, 454
    self-image disorders with, 265–268
Amnestic Korsakoff's syndrome. *See*
    Korsakoff's syndrome
Amorphognosia, 129
Amphetamines, panic disorder from,
    569
Amusia
    anatomical aspects of, 423–425
    early description of, 4, 419
    types of, 420–421
Amygdala
    bilateral ablation of, 592
    depression's location in, 16
    lesions of
        emotion recognition and, 251–252
        rage attacks with, 592–594
    in mood disorders, 605
    neuronal reactions of, 581
    in panic disorder, 570–571
Amygdalotomy, 594

Anger
  as basic emotion, 585
  hunger with, 596–597
  pathological, 586
Angle differentiation
  exposition time experiments with,
    69–71
  increasing interstimuli intervals in,
    68–69
  with parietal lobe lesions, 58
Anhedonia subscale, 503
Anomia, 344
  color, 93, 96–97
  in frontotemporal dementia, 638
  syndrome localization with, 15–16
Anomic aphasia, 344
Anomic-sensory aphasia, 365
Anosognosia
  in bipolar disorder, 153–155
  brain information processing and,
    155–157
  hemianopic, 150–151
  lesion localization in, 148, 156
  for pain, 152
  in schizophrenia, 153–155
  somatoagnosia as, 137
  symptoms of, 147
Anosognosia of aphasia, 151–152
Anosognosia of blindness, 4, 150
Anosognosia of deafness, 151
Anosognosia of delusions, 153
Anosognosia of dementia, 155
Anosognosia of hallucinations, 153
Anosognosia of hemiplegia, 4,
    148–150
Anosognosia of paralysis, 14
Anoxia, delirium with, 613
Anterior aphasia
  anatomical aspects of, 389–393
  articulation disturbances in,
    346–347
  comprehension disturbances with,
    349–350
  expressive speech disturbances in,
    341–342
  naming disturbances with, 343–344
  oral movement disturbances
    with, 347

phonological level disturbances
    with, 344–345, 357–358
  reading and writing disturbances
    with, 348–349
  repetition disturbances with,
    347–348
  word-finding disturbances with,
    342–343
Anterior cingula
  in mood disorders, 605
  in OCD, 581
Anterior transverse gyrus,
    hallucinations with, 194
Anterograde amnesia, Korsakoff's
    syndrome with, 438, 446–447
Anticonvulsants
  panic disorder treatment with, 573
  rage attack treatment with, 591–592
Antidepressants, hypotheses on
    efficacy of, 554
Anxiety
  cognitive evaluation with, 600
  disorders, 567
  in normal conditions, 566
Apathy
  anatomical aspects of, 504–509
  brain information processing in,
    524–527
  clinical aspects of, 503–504
  definition of, 501
  early description of, 501–502
  frontal lobe injury causing, 4
  lesion localization with, 509
  with thalamic lesions, 506
Aphasia
  in Alzheimer's disease, 376–377
  anosognosia of, 151–152
  apraxia without, 315
  brain information processing in,
    379–389
  Broca's, 6
  cerebral dominance in, 404
  classification of, 339–341
  dementia with, 375, 630–631
  early descriptions of, 335–338
  evaluation of, 680
  historical understanding of, 5
  lesion size and, 6

Aphasia (*continued*)
  localization schemes in, 340
  phonological level disturbances in, 379–382
  in Pick's disease, 376–377
  in schizophrenia, 377–378
  semantic level disturbances in, 382–383
  slowly progressive isolated, 640
  symptoms of, 6
  syntax processing in, 388–389
  terminology of, 341
  Wernicke's, 12
  working memory in, 384, 388–389
Aphemia, 3, 341
Aphemie, 2
Apperceptive agnosia, 24. *See also specific agnosia*
Apractognosia, 222, 302
Apraxia. *See also specific apraxia*
  with Alzheimer's disease, 638
  without aphasia, 315
  brain information processing disturbances in, 301–305
  definition of, 157
  finger-hand position, 297–298
  with frontal lobe lesions, 319–321
  gait, 296, 321
  lesion localization with, 314–324
  topographical, 105
Apraxia of axial body movements, 295
Apraxia of simple sequences, evaluation of, 682–683
Apraxic agraphia
  anatomical aspects of, 417
  clinical aspects of, 415
Aprosodia, 238
Argentophilic cytoplasmatic inclusions, 635
Arteriosclerotic changes, depression with, 541–542
Articulation
  conversation with, 353–354
  disturbances of, 346–347
Articulation aphasia
  anatomical aspects of, 393–395
  expressive speech in, 352

single articulation production with, 346–347
  in Wernicke-Lichtheim schema, 341
Artificial intelligence, principles of, 8
Asperger's syndrome, theory of mind deficits in, 258
Asponteneity, anatomical aspects of, 504–505
Associative agnosia. *See also specific agnosia*
  early categorization of, 24
  semantic disturbances in, 29–30
Astasia-abasia, 295
Astereognosis. *See* Tactile agnosia
Asymbolia
  early description of, 5, 221
  tactile, 129
Ataxic thinking, 377
Atherosclerosis, infarctions from, 640
Athymhormia, 508
Atopagnosia, 132
Atrophy. *See also* Cortical atrophy
  in Alzheimer's disease, 637
  cerebral, 661
  in hippocampal formations, 455
Attention
  in brain information processing, 484
  flexibility of, 498–499
  focus of, 487
  lesion localization in disturbances of, 499
  scheduling, 484
  span, 497
Attentional alexia
  anatomical aspects of, 412–414
  clinical aspects of, 408
Attention deficit disorder (ADD), 498
Attention deficit hyperactivity disorder (ADHD), 498
Attitude, abstract, 7
Audible thoughts, 193
Auditory agnosia
  apperceptive, 115
  associative, 114–115

brief sound signals with, 123–125
cortical deafness with, 115–116
definition of, 113
for object sounds, 113–114
perceptive, 115
sound filtration in, 116
sound frequency in, 117–121
sound patterns in, 117
sound sequence differentiation
    with, 121–123
of speech sounds, 369–370
tone differentiation in, 118–119
Auditory hallucinations
anatomical aspects of, 193–198
complex verbal, 193
elementary, 192
musical, 193, 198–199
Auditory illusion, 190
Auditory space agnosia
clinical aspects of, 127–128
lesion localization in, 129
sound localization in, 126–127
Aura
excitatory lesions in, 19
intellectual, 579
psychic, 580
Autism, theory of mind deficits in,
    257–258
Autoscopic (heautoscopic)
    hallucinations, 142
Autotopagnosia
autoscopic hallucinations in,
    142
body part alienation in, 138–139
body part naming in, 138
body part space relations in,
    143–144
clinical aspects of, 138
finger agnosia in, 139–140
FOP in, 142
Gerstmann syndrome in,
    139–141
lesion localization in, 145–146
phantom limb in, 143
somatic illusions in, 143
somatoagnosia as, 137
Avocalia, 420

Avolition
anatomical aspects of, 504–509
brain information processing in,
    524–527
clinical aspects of, 503–504
definition of, 501
early description of, 501–502
lesion localization with, 509
self-image underactivation with,
    269
Awareness
with delirium, 609
delusions underlain by self,
    280–287
of hemianopia, 150–151
Axial body movements, apraxia
    of, 295

Babinski's sign, 649
Balint's syndrome
anatomical aspects of, 489
brain information processing in,
    485–488
clinical aspects of, 485
Bar-press phase recordings, 581
Basal forebrain, Korsakoff's
    syndrome in, 443–444
Basal ganglia lesions
agnosia with, 252
negative symptoms with,
    507–508
in OCD, 576
Bilateral lesions
cortical deafness with, 125–126
topographical disorientation with,
    106–108
visual imagery loss with, 112
Binswanger's disease, 651–654
Bipolar disorder
anosognosia in, 153–155
delirium with, 613
glucose metabolism with,
    550–552
mania in, 556
white matter hyperintensity in,
    546–547
Blepharospasms, 517

Blindness
  amnestic color, 91
  anosognosia of, 4, 150
  cortical, 22, 31–32
  mind, 30
  psychic, 22
  pure word, 407, 412–413
  word, 4
Blood flow, with depression, 550–552
BNCE. *See* Brief Neuropsychological
    Cognitive Examination
Body
  alienation of parts of, 138–139
  movements, apraxia of axial, 295
  naming of parts of, 138
  Pick's, 635
  recognition of, 137
  space relations, 143–144
Body image, 261
Boston Aphasia Diagnostic
    Examination, methodology of,
    676–677
Boston Naming Test, 674
Bradykinesia, 514
Bradyphrenia, subcortical dementia
    as, 644–645
Brain damage, negative effect of, 18
Brain function, localization of, 1
Brain information processing
  in akinesia, 524–527
  anosognosia and, 155–157
  in apathy, 524–527
  in aphasia, 379–389
  in apraxia, 301–305
  attention disturbances in, 484
  in avolition, 524–527
  in Balint's syndrome, 485–488
  compensatory mechanisms in,
    17–18
  in constructional apraxia, 310–314
  in delirium, 616–620
  hallucinations and, 215–217
  in illusion, 190–191
  lesion size in, 17–18
  modularity in, 483
    conventional and
      unconventional tasks in, 10–13

criticisms of, 10
  general concept of, 8–10
  localization of operations in,
    13–15
  social agnosia with, 260–261,
    270–271
  in social delusions, 283–287
  theory of mind disturbances in,
    260–261
  topographical disorientation in,
    105–106
  unilateral visual neglect in, 492–493
  visual
    pathways of, 44–45
    stages of, 62–63
Brain stem dementia, 645
Brain stem lesion, visual
    hallucination in, 208
Brain tumors
  dementia with, 658
  depression with, 531
  diencephalic epilepsy from, 572
  hallucinations frequency from,
    212
  musical hallucinations from, 198
  visual hallucinations from, 202
Brief Neuropsychological Cognitive
    Examination (BNCE)
  clinical syndromes assessment for,
    685–688
  comprehension and naming
    subtest of, 680
  constructional praxis subtest of,
    681
  dementia progression testing with,
    687–688
  for Huntington's disease profile,
    649
  incomplete pictures subtest of,
    683
  methodology of, 679
  number tracking subtest of,
    682–683
  orientation subtest of, 680
  presidential memory subtest of,
    681
  for priming disturbances, 457

shifting set subtest of, 681–682
similarities subtest of, 684
working memory subtest of, 684
Brief tests, 677
Brobdingnagian hallucinations, 188
Broca, 2–3, 335–338
Broca's aphasia, 341. *See also* Anterior
     aphasia
   anatomical aspects of, 389–393
   language disturbances in, 404–406
   lesion size in, 17
   motor agrammatism with, 346
   phonological level disturbances in,
       379–381
   in Rolandic operculum, 392–393
   sentence formation with, 343
   transient forms of, 6
Broca's area, transient aphasia and, 6
Brodmann's area, aphasia in, 390
Bromocriptine, 515
Buccofacial apraxia
   characteristics of, 296–297
   facial and tongue movements
       with, 347
   posterior aphasia with, 365

Callosal lesions
   astereognosis from, 134
   limb apraxia with, 322
Capgras syndrome, 237, 278–279
Capsulotomy, 582, 584
Carbamazepine, rage attack
       treatment with, 591
Carbon monoxide poisoning, 28
Cardiac arrhythmias, panic disorder
       with, 569
Cardiac infarction, delirium with, 613
Cardiopulmonary failure, delirium
       with, 613
Card sorting test, 179
Catatonia
   anatomical aspects of, 521–523
   clinical aspects, 518
   early descriptions of, 519
   sub-syndromes of, 518–519
Categorization
   of associative agnosia, 24

evaluation of, 684
   with frontal lobe lesions, 472
   object, top-down processing in,
       82–84
Category Test, executive functions
       testing with, 670
Caudate lesions, in OCD, 577
Center of concepts, 3
Central agraphia, 416
Central alexia
   anatomical aspects of, 414–415
   clinical aspects of, 408–409
Central gyrus, lesion of, 321
Cerebral atrophy, schizophrenia
       with, 661
Cerebral dominance, in aphasia,
       404
Cerebral edema, delirium with, 613
Cerebri limbus, 602
Cerebrovascular diseases
   delirium with, 613
   depression with, 541–543
   vascular dementia with, 641
Charles Bonnet syndrome, 209
Checking rituals, 579
Cingulotomy, 581
Circuitry. *See also* Dorsolateral
       prefrontal cortex circuit
   in artificial intelligence, 8
   definition of, 16–17
   emotional, 602–603
Circumscribed large lesions, 18–19
de Clerambault's syndrome, 277
Clinical syndromes assessment,
       BNCE for, 685–688
Clinicians, role of, 1
Clinico-anatomical approach, 4
Clonazepam, 516
Cocaine, panic disorder from, 569
Cognitive assessment tests, 642
Cognitive disorder
   in dementia, 623
   with mood disorders, 601
   pattern analysis for, 1
Cognitive impairment
   in dementia, 623
   evaluation of, 684–685

Color
   apperceptive agnosia compensated
      with, 28
   recall of, 110
   test of, 179
Color agnosia
   color alienation in, 92–93
   color anomia with, 93
   color sensory aphasia with, 93
   emotion with, 93–94
   historical descriptions of, 90–91
   occipito-temporal lesions in,
      96–97
   scene recognition in, 93–95
   spatial relations with, 93–94
Color anomia
   color agnosia with, 93
   occipito-temporal lesions in, 96–97
Color aphasia
   color agnosia with, 93
   occipito-temporal lesions in, 96–97
Color vision, neural correlates of, 95
Communication
   language in, 335
   of modules, 9
Compensatory mechanisms
   in apperceptive agnosia, 28
   lesion size with, 17–18
Completion operations, disturbances
   in, 87–88
Complex features. *See* Features
Comprehension
   with aphasia, 349–350
   with dementia, 638
   disturbances of, 355
   of speech, 354–355
   test of, 680
   verbal, 674
   in word deafness, 369–371
Compulsion
   definition of, 574–575
   transient, 576
Computed tomography (CT)
   clinico-anatomical studies with, 7
   on OCD, 583
   of panic disorder, 573
Computer chips, 17

Conduction aphasia, 341
   anatomical aspects of, 399–400
   development of, 249
   phonological level disturbances
      in, 379
   transcortical aphasia with, 367–368
Confabulations, in Korsakoff's
   syndrome, 449–450
Confusional state
   acute, 608, 617–618
   delirium with, 613
Constructional apraxia, 100
   brain information processing
      disturbances, 310–314
   clinical aspects of, 308
   definition of, 308
   evaluation of, 681
   for geometric drawings, 309–310
   lesion localization in, 315–316
Continuous performance test, 497
Contours
   filtration of, 495–496
   recognition of overlapping, 38
Conventional information
      processing
   in action agnosia, 163–165
   in emotional agnosia, 240–242
   in modules, 10–13
   visual object agnosia with, 49–50
   in vocabulary of actions, 305–307
Conversation, 353–354, 356, 365, 369
Coronary artery disease, depression
   with, 544
Cortex. *See also* Dorsolateral
      prefrontal cortex circuit
   central, equipotentiality of, 6
   inferior-posterior prefrontal,
      prosopagnosia with, 235
   prefrontal, working memory
      domains in, 475
Cortical atrophy
   Alzheimer's disease with, 639–640
   with Huntington's disease, 648
   in primary depression, 547–549
Cortical blindness
   stages of, 31–32
   in visual agnosia, 22

Cortical deafness, 115–116
  lesion localization, 125–126
Cortical lesions
  Alzheimer's disease with, 640–642
  extended, 60
  mania from, 563
  visual object agnosia with, 60
Cortico-subcortical circuitry, 16
Cortico-subcortical lesion, aphasia
    from, 389
Cotard's syndrome, 281–282
Creutzfeldt-Jakob disease
  cortical atrophy with, 639
  dementia from, 622
CT. *See* Computed tomography

Deafness. *See also* Word deafness
  anosognosia of, 151
  auditory agnosia with, 115–116
  lesion localization with, 125–126
  musical hallucinations with, 199
  types of, 339
Deception, in autism, 257
Decision making
  by physicians, 690
  simple and complex features
    in, 88
Decline, general intellectual, 5
Decomposition, complex feature
    recognition with, 78–79
Deep agraphia
  anatomical aspects of, 418
  clinical aspects of, 417
Deep dyslexia
  anatomical aspects of, 414–415
  clinical aspects, 409–410
  reading and writing disturbances
    in, 407
Degenerative diseases, hallucinations
    from, 213–215
Degraded pictures, 41
Dehydration, delirium with, 613
Déjà pensé, 580
Déjà vu, 201
Delirium
  anatomical aspects of, 613–614
  awareness with, 609

brain information processing in,
    616–620
clinical aspects of, 608
definition of, 607
delusions with, 610
dementia's differentiation with,
    607, 611–612, 621
detachment with, 609
diseases with, 613
hallucinations with, 610
hyperactive and hypoactive,
    608–611, 617–620
illusions with, 610
manic, 506
memory with, 610–611
mood swings with, 611
from occipito-temporal lesions,
    614–615
oneiroid state with, 612–613
from parietal lobe lesions, 614–615
REM sleep in, 618–620
sleep-wake cycle with, 616–617
speech with, 610
from subcortical lesion, 616
thalamocortical relay neurons in,
    616
Delusions. *See also* Persecutory
    delusions; Somatic delusions
anosognosia of, 153
brain information processing
    disturbances with, 283–287
Capgras, 237, 278–279
classification of, 273
of control, 283
definition of, 272
dementia with, 631–632, 633, 665
of doubles, 237
grandiose, 222, 280
of guilt, 281
hallucinations with, 284
jealous, 276–277
lesion localization in, 288
of mind control loss, 282–283
misidentification syndromes as,
    277–278
nihilistic, 281–282
primary, 272, 289

Delusions (*continued*)
  right hemisphere origin of, 288
  secondary, 272, 289–290
  of self image, 281–283
  social, 273
  social agnosia underlaying, 273–279
  white matter hyperintensities
    with, 653
Dementia. *See also specific dementia*
  agnosia of space with, 628
  agnosia of time with, 628–629
  alertness in, 621
  in Alzheimer's disease, 621–622,
    632–634
  anatomical aspects of, 632
  anosognosia of, 155
  aphasia with, 375, 630–631
  in Binswanger's disease, 652
  as bradyphrenia, 644–645
  cognitive impairment degrees in,
    623
  cortical, 632
  course of, 621
  definition of, 622
  delirium with, 607, 611–612, 621
  delusions with, 631–632, 633, 665
  descriptions of, 621
  executive disturbances with, 645
  frontotemporal, 634–638
  hallucinations with, 631–633, 665
  with Huntington's disease, 622,
    646–650
  language with, 630–631, 663
  lesion localization with, 664
  with Lewy bodies, 622, 657–658
  memory disturbances with,
    627–628, 645
  mental processing slowness with,
    645, 665
  mood changes in, 626, 633
  motor apraxia with, 629–630
  multi-infarct, 289
  occupational functioning
    disturbed by, 662
  from Parkinson's disease, 622,
    656–657
  personality changes in, 626

Pick's disease with, 634–638
plaque's effect on, 643
posterior cortical atrophy with,
  639–640
progression testing on, 687–688
progressive supranuclear palsy in,
  645–647
with schizophrenia, 621, 659–662
self-environment relationship in,
  626–627
semantic, 372
senile, 299
social agnosia and apraxia with,
  623–626
subcortical, 644
subcortical lesions in, 650
types of, 622, 688
visual object agnosia with, 629,
  663–664
Dementia praecox, 659
Dementia Rating Scale
  methodology of, 677
  vascular disorders studied with,
    642
Depersonalization
  anatomical aspects of, 263
  clinical aspects of, 262
Depression
  apathy and avolition *vs.*, 504
  with arteriosclerotic changes,
    541–542
  clinical aspects of, 531–532
  with coronary artery disease, 544
  cortical atrophy in, 547–549
  cortical blood flow with, 549–552
  delirium with, 613
  with drugs, 544
  with endocrine disorders, 543–544
  with epilepsy, 531, 533, 545
  from frontal lobe tumors, 533–537
  glucose metabolism with, 549–550
  with Huntington's disease, 540–541
  lateral ventricle enlargement in,
    547–549
  from left hemisphere lesions,
    537–538
  lesion localization in, 554

limbic system in, 553
with mesodiencephalic lesions, 543
with multiple sclerosis, 532
with Parkinson's disease, 539–540
with pharmacological agents, 544
primary, 531
from right hemisphere lesions, 538
secondary, 531
situation assessment with, 599
from stroke, 533–534, 542–543, 545
symptoms of, 531
with systemic medical conditions, 544
from temporal lobe tumors, 532–533
thalamic blood flow with, 552
with tumors, 531
with white matter hyperintensities, 541–542
Depression, in amygdala, 16
Depth, agnosia of, 100–102
Derealization
anatomical aspects of, 263
clinical aspects of, 262
Detachment, with delirium, 609
Detection thresholds, in filtration, 35–36
Diagnostic algorithms, 688–690
Diagnostic and Statistical Manual of Mental Disorders (DSM-IV)
on delirium, 608
on dementia, 621–622
hallucinations in, 191
on intermittent explosive disorder, 587
on OCD, 574
on panic disorder, 567
self-image disturbances in, 137
Diagnostic evaluations
imaging in, 667
neuropsychological testing with, 668
Diagnostic process, stages of, 673
Diencephalic autonomic seizures, 572–573
Diencephalic lesions, mania from, 560. *See also* Mesodiencephalic lesions

Direction, in motion recognition disturbances, 162
Disgust, recognition of, 238
Disorientation. *See also* Topographical disorientation
right-left, 140–141
visual-spatial
2-D to 3-D transfer in, 101–102
space features in, 101
space orientation in, 100–101
syndromes with, 99–100
Dissociative amnesia, 268
Dissociative fugue, 265–266
Dissociative identity disorder, 264–265
Distinct personality profile, seizure disorders with, 270
Distraction, overcoming, 13
DLPFC circuit. *See* Dorsolateral prefrontal cortex circuit
Dominance, cerebral, 404
Dopamine, production of, 657
Doppelganger, 142
Dorsolateral prefrontal cortex circuit (DLPFC circuit)
functional role of, 526
with negative symptoms in schizophrenia, 510–514
Drawing
of geometric figures, 309–310
motor schema for, 312
of sequences of, 460–461
unilateral neglect in, 492
Dreamy state
delirium with, 612–613
hallucinations with, 200–201
Dressing apraxia
clinical symptoms of, 294–295
in right hemisphere, 315
Drive-emotion-speech activation system, in schizophrenic patients, 512
Drowsiness, 612
Drugs
delirium induced by, 613
depression with, 544
hallucinations induced by, 212–213

Drugs (*continued*)
  hypersensitivity to, 568
  panic disorder with, 569
  parkinsonism induced by, 515–516
DSM-IV. *See Diagnostic and Statistical Manual of Mental Disorders*
Dynamic aphasia, 340, 351–352
Dysarthria, 244
Dyscontrol, episodic
  characteristics of, 586
  minimal brain dysfunction in, 587
Dysexecutive syndrome, 468
Dyslexia. *See also* Deep dyslexia; Surface dyslexia
  neglect, 408
  types of, 407
Dysprosody, motor, 347

"*Echo de pensées,*" 193
Edema, cerebral, 613
EEG. *See* Electroencephalogram
Efferent apraxia, 302
Effron's test
  figures in, 74
  as shape discrimination test standard, 73
Egosyntonic repetitive behavior, 575–576
Ekphorization, of information, 430
Electrical scheme, 16
Electrical stimulation, visual hallucinations from, 204–205
Electroencephalogram (EEG)
  diagnostic evaluations with, 667
  in motiveless homicide, 590
  in panic disorder, 569–570
  in rage attacks, 590
Elementary auditory hallucinations, 192
Elementary visual illusions, 188
Elementary visual sensations, loss of, 63
Emotion
  action activation/inhibition by, 529–530
  anger as basic, 585
  basic words of, 601

brain circuitry of, 602–603
  color agnosia with, 93–94
  functional role, 599–600
  language of, 529, 601
  program transmission, 604–605
  reciprocal programs in, 603–604
  recognition of, 237–238, 251–252
  rigidity of, 530
  in social gnosis, 285
Emotional agnosia
  apperceptive, 240
  associative, 239–240
  basal ganglia lesions with, 252
  as communication disorder, 237
  conventional information processing disturbances in, 240–242
  development of, 249
  neuropsychological testing in, 238–239
  right *vs.* left hemisphere involvement in, 245–251
  stroke with, 246–248
  unconventional information processing disturbances in, 242–243
Employment
  dementia's impact on, 662
  with Huntington's disease, 649–650
  with social apraxia, 327–328
Empty euphoria, 597
Empty speech, 638
Encephalitic lethargica, 516
Encephalitis, dementia with, 658
Encephalitis subcorticalis chronica progressiva, 651
Endocrine disorders, depression with, 543–544
Engrams, motor, 302–305
Epilepsy
  delirium with, 613
  depression with, 531, 533, 545
  excitatory lesions in, 19
  negative symptoms of, 502
  panic disorder and, 567
  positive symptoms of, 502
  temporal lobe

distinct personality profile with, 270
fear in, 571
fugue states with, 267
personality changes caused by, 5
rage attacks and, 588–589
tonical hyperactivity in, 286
Episodic dyscontrol
characteristics of, 586
minimal brain dysfunction in, 587
Episodic memory, 428
Equipotentiality, of central cortex, 6
Ergotonic triangle, 595, 599
Erotomania, 277
Erythropsia, metamorphopsia with, 188
Euphoria
empty, 597
fatuous, 556
Excitatory lesions, 19–20
Executive disturbances
dysexecutive syndrome as, 468
evaluation of, 669
with subcortical dementia, 645
Executive functions testing, 669–772
Extended test batteries, 675
Extracampine hallucinations, 200
Eye movements
in Balint's syndrome, 486
rapid, 618–620

Face
individuality of, 228–230
recognition of, 223
Facial akinesia. *See* Oral-facial akinesia
Facial mask, 516
Facial Recognition Test, 674–675
Facultas signatrix, 22
False belief task
autism and, 257–258
theory of mind testing with, 255–256
Fatal catatonia, 519
Fatuous euphoria, 556
Faux pas task, 255–256

Fear
as ictal symptom, 571
recognition of, 238
Features
complex
in decision making, 88
decomposition recognition methods with, 78–79
differentiation of, 73–75
general shape assessment with, 76
invariant point recognition with, 78
neural correlates of, 72–73
visual working memory for, 474–476
vocabulary of, 77
in decision making, 88
simple
in action agnosia, 165
in decision making, 88
differentiation of, 65–68
neural correlates in analysis of, 64–65
use of, 76–77
space, 101
spatial relations between, 80
Feedback projections, 81–82
Feedforward projections, 81–82
Feeling of presence (FOP), 142
Festination, 516
Fever, delirium with, 613
Figure. *See also* Geometric figures
in Effron's test, 74
incomplete, 40–42
recurrent, 181
Filtration agnosia, 34
Filtration of signal from noise
contour, 495–496
sound, 116
visual, 33, 35–36
Finger agnosia, 138–140, 146–147
Finger-hand position apraxia, 297–298
Finger movements, 299–300
Fixed test batteries, 675
Florid mental status, 608

Focus of attention, 487
Fodor, 8
FOP. *See* Feeling of presence
Forced normalization, 590–591
Forced thinking, 579–580
Fornix
    damage to, 453
    Korsakoff's syndrome in, 442
Fragment completion task, 456
Fregoli syndrome, 278
Frequency
    hallucinations, 212
    of object properties, 84–87
    sound, 117–121
Frontal lobe
    injuries to, 4
    in mania, 557–558
    in pathological aggression, 597
    in theory of mind tasks, 259
Frontal lobe lesions
    amnesia with, 453–454
    apraxia with, 319–321
    categorization difficulties from,
        472
    motor aprosodia with, 253
    negative symptoms with, 504–506
    OCD with, 578–580
    social agnosia with, 331
    somatic delusions from, 145
    transcortical motor aphasia with,
        395–397
    unilateral neglect in, 494
    visual object agnosia with, 55–56
Frontal lobe tumors
    depression from, 533–537
    Korsakoff's syndrome with,
        444–446
Frontotemporal dementia, 634
    anomia in, 638
    language with, 637
    parkinsonism with, 635
Fugue states
    dissociative, 265–266
    epileptic history with, 267
    Korsakoff's syndrome with, 437
    psychogenic, 267
    self-image in, 265
Functional status assessment, 685

Gage, Phineas, 4, 324–326
Gait
    with parkinsonism, 514–515
    with pure akinesia, 516
Gait apraxia, 296, 321
Gaze fixation, 486
Gedankenlautwerden, 193
Gegenhalten, 518
Gelb-Goldstein Color Sorting Test,
        179
Generalized extended lesions, 18–19
Geometric figures
    constructional apraxia with,
        309–310
    visual working memory for, 474
Geon, 79
Gerstmann syndrome, 139–141, 416
Gestalt
    agnosia of action with, 172–175
    visual, 25
Gestaltblindheit, 25
Gestures, symbolic, 295
Gliosis, 639–640
Global aphasia
    anatomical aspects of, 402–403
    clinical signs of, 373–374
Globus pallidus, lesions of, 507–508
Glucose metabolism
    with bipolar disorder, 550–552
    with depression, 549–550
God, in grandiose delusions, 280
Grandiose delusion, 222, 280
Grandiosity, 222
Gray matter lesions, Alzheimer's
        disease with, 634
Guilt, delusions of, 281
Gustatory hallucinations, 210
Gyrus
    anterior transverse, 194
    central, 321

Hallucinations. *See also* Auditory
        hallucinations; Visual
        hallucinations
    agnosia and, 216–217
    from Alzheimer's disease, 213–214
    anosognosia of, 153
    autoscopic, 142

bidirectional sensory information
    processing and, 217–218
brain information processing in,
    215–217
from brain tumors, 202, 212
Brobdingnagian, 188
categorization of, 191–192
definition of, 191
from degenerative diseases, 213–215
delirium with, 610
delusions with, 284
dementia with, 631–633, 665
drug induced, 212–213
electrical stimulation with,
    204–205
gustatory, 210
Lilliputian, 188
narcolepsy with, 208
from occipital lobe lesions, 211
olfactory, 209–210
ophthalmologic lesions with, 209
paroxysmal activity and, 218–219
primary, 212
seizures with, 203
sensory systems and, 215
stroke with, 206–207
from temporal lobe pathology, 210
tonical hyperactivity with, 286
Halstead-Reitan Test Batteries
    executive functions testing with,
        670
    lesion localization revealed by, 6–7
    methodology of, 676
Head injury
    delirium with, 613
    dementia with, 622, 658
Hearing problems, hallucinations
    with, 193
Hebephrenic schizophrenia, 556
Hemianopia, unawareness of, 150–151
Hemianopic anosognosia, 150–151
Hemihypesthesia, 371
Hemiparesis, 614
Hemiplegia, anosognosia of, 4,
    148–150
Hepatic encephalopathy, delirium
    with, 613
Hippocampal formations

atrophy in, 455
Korsakoff's syndrome in, 440–442
Hippocampal lesion, visual object
    agnosia with, 53
Hippocampus, preservation of, 637
HIV. See Human immunodeficiency
    virus
Homicide, motiveless, 590
Hooper Visual Organization Test, 674
Human immunodeficiency virus
    (HIV), 622
Hunger, anger with, 596–597
Huntington's disease
    BNCE profile with, 649
    cortical atrophy with, 648
    dementia with, 622, 646–650
    depression from, 540–541
    hallucinations from, 214–215
Hyperactive delirium, 608–611,
    618–620
Hyperphagia, in rage attacks, 596–597
Hypersexual activity, 54
Hypersomnia, with thalamic lesions,
    507
Hyperthyroidism, panic disorder
    with, 569
Hypnagogic hallucinations, 201
Hypnopompic hallucinations, 201
Hypoactive delirium, 608–611, 617–618
Hypochondriasis
    delusion proportions of, 155
    OCD vs., 575
Hypofrontality, 510, 513
Hypomanic episode, 555
Hypoperfusion, 636
Hypophonia, 244
Hypothalamic rage, 596–597
Hypothalamus, in rage attacks,
    594–596

Ictal EEG, 570
Ideational apraxia
    with Alzheimer's disease, 638
    with complex action, 298–299
    definition of, 292
    hand and finger movements in,
        299–300
    kinetic limb, 300–301

Identity disorder, dissociative, 264–265
Ideographic alexia, 412
Ideomotor apraxia
    with Alzheimer's disease, 638
    clinical aspects of, 293–295
    definition of, 292
Illusion
    auditory, 190
    brain information processing in, 190–191
    definition of, 187–188
    with delirium, 610
    lesion localization of, 189
    of movement, 190
    somatic, 143
    visual, 188–189
Imaging. See also Computed tomography; Magnetic resonance imaging; Positron emission tomography
    in clinico-anatomical studies, 7–8
    in diagnostic evaluations, 667
Imperception
    social agnosia and, 221
    visual agnosia and, 22
Incomplete pictures, 457–458
Infamy, 3
Infections, delirium with, 613
Inferior-posterior prefrontal cortex, prosopagnosia with, 235
Insight
    lack of, 449–450
    loss of, 13
    in OCD, 585
Instrumental amusia, 420–421
Insula lesions, aphasia from, 392
Intellectual ability, general, 5
Intellectual aura, 579
Intelligence, artificial, 8
Interictal scalp EEG, 569
Intermetamorphosis syndrome, 278
Intermittent explosive disorder, 587
Interstimuli intervals, angle differentiation experiments with, 68–69
Intoxication, delirium with, 613

Invariant features, recognition with, 78
Ischemic penumbra, 18

Jacksonian seizures, 218
Jamais vu, 201
Jargonaphasia, 362
Jealousy, delusional, 276–277

Kinesthetic apraxia, 301–302
Kinetic apraxia, 302
Kinetic limb apraxia, 293, 300–301
Kluver-Bucy syndrome, 592–593
Korsakoff's syndrome
    anterograde amnesia with, 438, 446–447
    basal forebrain in, 443–444
    clinical aspects of, 433–434
    confabulations in, 449–450
    diseases with, 435
    fornix in, 442
    frontal lobe tumors in, 444–446
    fugues with, 437
    hippocampal formations in, 440–442
    mammillary bodies in, 438–440
    memory disturbances in, 434
    multiple personality disorder with, 437
    psychogenic amnesia with, 437
    reduplicative paramnesia in, 452–453
    reduplicative paramnesia with, 437
    retrograde amnesia with, 438, 447–448
    thalamic medial dorsal nuclei in, 438–440
    transient global amnesia with, 437–438, 451–452
    Wernicke's disease with, 436–437

Labile paraphasia, 345
Lacunar state, 650
Language
    abstract, 6
    with aphasia, 404–406
    communication with, 335

dementia's effect on, 630–631, 663
of emotion, 529, 601
with frontotemporal dementia, 637
information processing modules
for, 11
motor aprosodia related
disturbances of, 244–245
with schizophrenia, 377–378
working memory for, 476
Late-onset paranoid psychosis
(LOPP), 660
Late paraphrenia, 273–279
Lateral ventricle enlargement, in
primary depression, 547–549
L-dopa, 515
Leborgne, 2, 335–338
Left hemispheric lesions
depression from, 537–538
in emotional agnosia, 245–251
limb apraxia with, 314
mania with, 560–562
unilateral visual neglect in, 493
Lesion. See also specific lesion
size of
aphasia and, 6
compensatory mechanisms with,
17–18
types of, 18–20
Lewy bodies dementia, 622, 657–658
Lexical agraphia
anatomical aspects of, 418
clinical aspects of, 417
Lilliputian hallucinations, 188
Limb apraxia, 293–295. See also Kinetic
limb apraxia
anatomical aspects of, 314
lesion localization in, 319–320,
322–323
Limbic system
in depression, 553
emotion in, 602
Linear discriminant analysis, 689
Literal paraphasia, 342, 344–345
Lobectomy, recent memory with, 472
Localization
historical understanding of, 1–4
of operations, 13–15

strict, 6–7
of syndromes, 15–16
LOPP. See Late-onset paranoid
psychosis
Luria-Nebraska Neuropsychological
Battery, methodology of,
675–676

Macaca fuscata, 570
Macropsia, 188
Macrosomatoagnosia, 143
Magnetic resonance imaging (MRI)
clinico-anatomical studies with, 7
on OCD, 583
of panic disorder, 573
Mammillary bodies, Korsakoff's
syndrome in, 438–440
Mania
clinical aspects of, 555
from cortical lesions, 563
from diencephalic lesions, 560
eroto-, 277
etiology of, 556
frontal lobe in, 557–558
frontotemporal lesions in, 559
functional brain abnormalities
with, 565
primary, 564–566
programs of, 603–604
right vs. left hemisphere in,
560–562
secondary, 555
situation assessment with, 600
structural brain abnormalities
with, 564
from subcortical lesions, 560
temporal lobe in, 558–559
white matter hyperintensity with,
566
Manic delirium, with thalamic
lesions, 506
Manic episode. See Bipolar disorder;
Hypomanic episode; Mania
Melokinetic apraxia, 292–293
Memory. See also Modular memory;
Working memory
in Alzheimer's disease signs, 634

Memory (*continued*)
    declarative and nondeclarative,
        428–429
    definition of, 427
    with delirium, 610–611
    dementia's effect on, 627–628, 645
    distributed, 17
    episodic, 428
    evaluation of, 681
    explicit and implicit, 429–430
    in Korsakoff's syndrome, 434
    lobectomy with recent, 472
    long-term, 431–433
    operational, 8
    procedural, 429, 463
    prototypes in, 459
    with schizophrenia, 659
    semantic, 428, 430–431
Mental processing
    florid status of, 608
    slowness of, 645, 665
    undivided, 1–2
Mesencephalic regions, visual
        hallucination in, 208
Mesodiencephalic lesions
    depression with, 543
    panic disorder with, 567, 572–573
Metamorphopsia, 188. *See also*
        Intermetamorphosis
        syndrome
Micropsia, 188
Microsomatoagnosia, 143
Migraines, delirium with, 613
Mind. *See* Theory of mind
Mind-blindness, 30
Mind reading, 260
Mini-Mental State Examination, 642,
        678–679
Minus tissue, 18
Mirrored neurons, 14
Mirror-tracing task, 464
Mitgehen, 518
Mixed anterior-posterior aphasia.
        See Global aphasia; Mixed
        transcortical aphasia
Mixed transcortical aphasia, 374–375,
        403

Modularity and Mind (Fodor), 8
Modular memory, 429
    anatomical aspects of, 462
    priming disturbances in, 456–461
    role of, 455–456
Modules
    in artificial intelligence, 8
    in brain information processing,
        483
    communication of, 9
    conventional and unconventional
        tasks of, 10–13
    criticisms of, 10
    general concept of, 8–10
    independence of, 10
    for language, 11
    operation localization of, 13–15
    for visual object agnosia, 61
Monkeys, visual discrimination tasks
        in, 51
Mood disorders
    cognitive impairments with, 601
    emotional rigidity from, 530
    lesion sites in, 605
    social agnosia and, 606
Mood swings
    with delirium, 611
    in dementia, 626, 633
Moria, 556
Motion recognition disturbances
    anatomical aspects of, 160–163
    clinical aspects of, 158
    direction in, 162
    speed in, 158–160
    terminology of, 157
    time acceleration in, 158–160
Motor agrammatism
    in Broca's aphasia, 346
    posterior aphasia with, 364
Motor amusia
    anatomical aspects of, 423
    clinical aspects of, 420–421
Motor aphasia, 341
Motor apraxia. *See also* Ideomotor
        apraxia
    definition of, 291
    dementia with, 629–630

early descriptions of, 291–293
social apraxia's similarity to,
    329–330
Motor aprosodia
abnormal prosody *vs.*, 244
clinical aspects of, 244
as communication disorder, 237
development of, 249
early description of, 243
frontal lobe lesions in, 253
language disturbances related to,
    244–245
Motor dysprosody, 341, 347
Motor engrams, 302–305
Motor prosody, posterior aphasia
    with, 365
Movement
body, 295
eye, 486, 618–620
hand and finger, 299–300
illusions with, 190
oral, 347
stereotyped, 575
MRI. *See* Magnetic resonance
    imaging
Multi-infarct dementia, delusions
    in, 289
Multimodal sequences, working
    memory for, 477–478
Multiple personality disorder
clinical aspects of, 264–265
Korsakoff's syndrome with, 437
Multiple sclerosis
dementia with, 658
depression with, 532
Muscular rigidity, 514–515
Musical agnosia
apperceptive, 421–422
associative, 421
Musical alexia
as agraphia, 425
clinical aspects of, 422
Musical hallucinations, 193,
    198–199
Muteness, types of, 339. *See also*
    Akinetic mutism
My-ness, 136

Naming
with aphasia, 343–344
with autotopagnosia, 138
muteness, 339
with posterior aphasia, 363
test of, 674, 680
Narcolepsy, visual hallucination
    with, 208
Negative symptoms
classification of, 503, 511
DLPFC circuit dysfunction with,
    510–514
of epilepsy, 502
with frontal lobe lesions, 504–506
with globus pallidus lesions,
    507–508
of schizophrenia, 502, 510–514
speech with, 504
with subcortical lesions, 506
Neglect dyslexia, 408. *See also*
    Unilateral visual neglect
Neuritique plaques, 643
Neurofibrillary tangles, 643
Neuroleptic-induced parkinsonism,
    515–516
Neurons
of amygdala, 581
mirrored, 14
thalamocortical relay, 616
Neuropsychological testing
brain imaging's correlations with,
    667
diagnostic evaluation with, 668
in emotional agnosia, 238–239
Neurotransmitter hypothesis, 554
Nihilistic delusions, 281–282
Noise. *See also* Filtration of signal
    from noise
contours in, 495–496
delayed presentation of, 37
signal similar to, 496
signal simultaneously presented
    with, 33–37
Nonlinear discriminant analysis,
    689
Normal individuals, data on, 668
Normalization, forced, 590–591

Normative data, 668, 691
Number cancellation test, 497

Object
  categorization of, 82–84
  common properties of, 62
  exposition time of, 39–40, 54, 69–71
  individuality of, 228–230
  partially occluded, 683–684
  sounds, 113–114
  visual working memory for, 474
Object alternation test, 178
Object recognition
  decomposition in, 78–79
  invariant features in, 78
  neural correlates of, 44–45
  spatial relations in, 80
  touch in, 129
  unilateral visual neglect in, 492
Obsessive-compulsive disorder
    (OCD)
  anterior cingula in, 581
  basal ganglia in, 576
  caudate lesions in, 577
  checking rituals in, 579
  clinical aspects of, 574
  CT of, 583
  definition of, 574–575
  déjà pensé in, 580
  forced thinking in, 579–580
  frontal lobe lesions in, 578–580
  insight in, 585
  late-onset, 578
  lesion localization in, 584
  MRI of, 583
  PET scan data on, 583
  pica with, 577–578
  primary, 583
  subcortical connections in, 582
  transient compulsions in, 576
Occipital lesion
  hallucinations from, 211
  prosopagnosia with, 230–232
  topographical disorientation with,
    108–109
  unilateral neglect in, 494
  visual object agnosia with, 44–49

Occipital lobe
  unimodal sequences and, 476–477
  visual hallucination from, 202
Occipito-temporal lesions
  color agnosia with, 96–97
  delirium from, 614–615
  transcortical sensory aphasia with,
    401
Occupational function
  dementia's impact on, 662
  with Huntington's disease, 649–650
  with social apraxia, 327–328
OCD. See Obsessive-compulsive
    disorder
Old age, hallucinations in, 213–215
Olfactory hallucinations, 209–210
Oneiroid state, delirium with, 612–613
Operational memory, in artificial
    intelligence, 8
Operations
  in artificial intelligence, 8
  completion, 87–88
  distribution of, 13
  localization of, 13–15
Ophthalmologic lesions, visual
    hallucinations with, 209
Optic alloesthesia, 133, 189
Optic aphasia. See also Anomia
  early descriptions of, 24
  semantic disturbances in, 30–31
  syndromes with, 15–16
Optic ataxia, 486
Oral apraxia, 296–297
Oral-facial akinesia, 516
Oral movement disturbances, 347
Orbitofrontal lesion, social apraxia
    from, 332
Orbitofrontal syndrome,
    pathological aggression with,
    597
Order, shifting patterns of, 181–184
Organology, 8
Orientation
  with dementia, 638
  map, 104–105
  of self, 104
  in space, 100–101

test of, 680
topographical, 490–491
visual, 491
working memory for, 478–480

Pain, anosognosia for, 152
Palinopsia, 200
Palsy. *See* Progressive supranuclear
        palsy, anatomical aspects of
Panic disorder
    amygdala's role in, 570–571
    autonomic symptoms of, 568
    brain imaging of, 573
    clinical aspects of, 567
    with drugs, 569
    EEG in, 569–570
    epilepsy and, 567
    lesion localization in, 574
    with medical conditions, 569
    medication hypersensitivity in, 568
    with mesodiencephalic lesion, 567,
        572–573
    with pheochromocytoma, 569
    with seizures, 567–568, 572–573
    temporal lobe's role in, 570–571
    treatment of, 573
Pantomimic apraxia, 296
Paralysis, anosognosia of, 14
Paranoid delusions, 272. *See also*
        Late-onset paranoid psychosis
Pareidolia, 189
Parietal lobe lesion
    apraxia with, 316–319
    auditory space agnosia with, 129
    delirium from, 614–615
    depth agnosia with, 102
    emotional agnosia from, 245
    somatic delusions from, 145
    tactile agnosia from, 133–134
    unilateral neglect in, 494
    visual object agnosia with, 56–59
Parkinsonian type of akinesia, 514
Parkinsonism
    anatomical aspects of, 520
    frontotemporal dementia with, 635
    primary, 514–515
    secondary, 515–516

Parkinson's disease
    dementia from, 622, 656–657
    depression with, 539–540
    hallucinations from, 215
Paroxysmal activity
    hallucinations and, 218–219
    in temporal lobe, 598
Partial intellectual disturbance, 5
Patterns
    analysis of, 1
    of order, 181–184
    of sound, 117
Pelopsia, 189
Penumbra, ischemic, 18
Peppery mask, 34
Perceptual closure, 41
Peripheral agraphia, 415–416
Peripheral alexia, 412–414
Peripheral nervous system lesion,
        phantom limb phenomenon
        from, 146
Perivascular gliosis, 640
Persecutory delusions
    anatomical, 275–276
    auditory hallucinations with, 284
    clinical aspects of, 273–274
    delirium with, 610
    theory of mind mechanisms with,
        258
Personality changes. *See also* Multiple
        personality disorder
    in dementia, 626
    epilepsy, temporal lobe, causing, 5
    frontal lobe injury causing, 4
Personality profile, 270
PET. *See* Positron emission
        tomography
Phantom limb, 143
Pharmacological agents
    depression with, 544
    hypersensitivity to, 568
Pheochromocytoma, panic disorder
        with, 569
Phonemes, 379
Phonetic disintegration syndrome,
        341
Phonetic sensory aphasia, 369

Phonological agraphia
  anatomical aspects of, 418
  clinical aspects of, 417
Phonological analysis, 371
Phonological disturbances, 344–345,
    357–358, 379–382
Photographs, recognition of, 28
Physicians
  decision-making process of, 690
  role of, 1
Pica, 577–578
Pick's body, 635
Pick's disease
  aphasia in, 376–377
  cortical and subcortical atrophy
    with, 636
  dementia from, 621–622, 634–638
  perfusion patterns with, 636
Pictures
  degraded, 41
  incomplete, 457–458
Pitch differentiation, in aphasia, 385
Pituitary adenoma, 573
Plaque, dementia's severity effected
    by, 643
Pneumonia, delirium with, 613
Polypsia, 189
Positive snout, 649
Positive symptoms
  of epilepsy, 502
  of schizophrenia, 503
Positron emission tomography (PET)
  clinico-anatomical studies with, 7
  on OCD, 583
  of panic disorder, 573
Posterior aphasia
  articulation in, 365
  comprehension disturbances
    with, 355
  conversational speech with, 356
  lesion localization in, 397–400
  motor agrammatism with, 364
  motor prosody with, 365
  naming with, 363
  nonverbal level disturbances with,
    359, 385–387
  phonological level disturbances
    with, 357–358

syntactic rules in, 359–361
  verbal level disturbances with,
    358–359
  Wernick's aphasia in, 355
  word-finding difficulties with,
    362
Prefrontal cortex, working memory
    domains in, 475
Presidential Memory Test, 628
Priming, 429
  anatomical aspects of, 462
  definition of, 456
  disturbances of, 456–461
Procedural memory, 429, 463
Processing. *See* Brain information
    processing; Top-down
    processing
Program
  reciprocal, 603–604
  transmission of, 604–605
Progressive supranuclear palsy
  anatomical aspects of, 520
  cognitive performance with,
    646
  pseudodementia of, 645
  subcortical dementia in, 645–647
Projections, neural correlates of,
    81–82
Prosody, abnormal, motor
    aprosodia *vs.*, 244
Prosopagnosia, 106
  anatomical aspects of, 230–235
  apperceptive, 225–226
  associative, 226–227
  clinical aspects of, 224
  historical description of, 223–224
  individuality with, face and object,
    228–230
  visual object agnosia's lesion
    overlap with, 237
Prototypes, in memory, 459
Pseudodementia, 645
Pseudo-hallucinations, 201–202
Psychic aura, 580
Psychic blindness, 22
Psychogenic amnesia
  Korsakoff's syndrome with, 437
  self image in, 265, 267–268

Psychometric system
    clinical data based, 672–673
    normative data based, 668
Psychomotor retardation, clinical
        aspects of, 517
Pure akinesia
    anatomical aspects of, 520
    clinical aspects of, 516–517
Pure alexia, 407
Pure word blindness, 407, 412–413
Pure word deafness, 341
Pursuit-motor tracking task, 463

Rage
    cognitive evaluation with, 600
    definition of, 530
Rage attacks, 586
    amygdala lesions in, 592–594
    anticonvulsant treatment of,
        591–592
    clinical aspects of, 586–587
    EEG data on, 590
    episodic dyscontrol in, 586
    forced normalization in, 590–591
    hyperphagia in, 596–597
    hypothalamus' role in, 594–596
    lesion localizations in, 598
    lesion studies of, 592–594
    seizures' similarities with, 589
    temporal lobe epilepsy and,
        588–589
Rapid eye movement (REM), 618–620
RAT. *See* Reticular activation system
Reading disturbances
    with anterior aphasia, 348–349
    with deep dyslexia, 407
Reading, mind, 260
Reciprocal programs, 603–604
Recognition. *See also* Action
        recognition; Motion
        recognition disturbances;
        Object recognition
    body, 137
    complex feature, 78–79
    emotion, 237–238
    facial, 223, 674–675
    fear, 238
    invariant point, 78

overlapping contour, 38
photograph, 28
scene, 93–95
sequence, 177–178
signal, 8
unilateral neglect in, 492
Recordings
    bar-press phase, 581
    single-cell, 14
    subdural, 570
Recurrent figures, 181
Reduplicative paramnesia,
        Korsakoff's syndrome with,
        437, 452–453
Reitan Trail Making Test, 642
REM. *See* Rapid eye movement
Repetition
    in anterior aphasia, 347–348
    egosyntonic, 575–576
    priming, 457
    in transcortical sensory aphasia, 368
Reticular activation system (RAT),
        617–618
Retrograde amnesia
    dementia with, 627
    Korsakoff's syndrome with, 438,
        447–448
Revisualization, loss of, 109–110
Right hemisphere
    constructional apraxia in, 316
    delusions origin in, 288
    depression from, 538
    dressing apraxia in, 315
    in emotional agnosia, 245–251
    mania in, 560–562
    social agnosia in, 271
    unilateral visual neglect in, 493
Rolandic operculum
    in articulation aphasia, 393–394
    Broca's aphasia in, 392–393

SANS. *See* Scale for the Assessment of
        Negative Symptoms
SAPS. *See* Scale for the Assessment of
        Positive Symptoms
Satiety-hunger feelings, 596
Scale for the Assessment of Negative
        Symptoms (SANS), 503, 511

Scale for the Assessment of Positive Symptoms (SAPS), 503, 511
Scenes, recognition of, 93–95
Scenic hallucinations, 200
Schizophrenia. *See also* Delusions
  adolescent-onset, 660
  anosognosia in, 153–155
  cerebral atrophy in, 661
  delirium with, 613
  dementia from, 621, 659–662
  DLPFC dysfunction in, 510–514
  drive-emotion-speech activation system in, 512
  in elderly patients, 659
  hallucinations with, 153
  hebephrenic, 556
  hypofrontality in, 510, 513
  language disturbances in, 377–378
  memory with, 659
  negative symptoms of, 502, 510–514
  neuroanatomical differences in, 514
  positive symptoms of, 503
  theory of mind deficits with, 258
  ventricular brain ratios in, 510–511
  white matter hyperintensity with, 662
Schneider, 25–27
Scientists, role of, 1
Seizures
  distinct personality profile with, 270
  fear generation in, 571
  forced thinking before, 579–580
  hallucinations with, 194, 203, 218–219
  Jacksonian, 218
  metamorphopsia with, 188
  multiple personality disorder with, 264
  panic disorder with, 567–568, 572–573
  in pathological aggression, 590
  rage attacks' similarities with, 589
  self-image underestimation with, 269–270
  violence during, 588

Self-awareness, delusions underlain by, 280–287
Self, environment's relationship with, 626–627
Self-image
  in amnestic disorders, 265–268
  definition of, 261
  delusion of socially related, 281–283
  delusions of, 281–283
  overestimation of, 268–269
  somatic *vs.* social, 261
  in somatoagnosia, 136–137
  underactivation of, 269
  underestimation of, 269–270
Semantic aphasia, 371–372
Semantic dementia, 372
Semantic disturbances
  in aphasia, 382–383
  in associative agnosia, 29–30
  in optic aphasia, 30–31
Semantic memory, 428, 430–431
Senile dementia, ideational apraxia in, 299
Senility, Alzheimer's onset time in, 633
Sensorimotor procedural learning, disturbances of, 463–466
Sensory amusia
  anatomical aspects of, 423–425
  clinical aspects of, 421
Sensory aphasia, 340–341
Sensory aprosodia, 9
Sensory systems
  bidirectional information processing of, 217–218
  hallucinations and, 215
Sentence formation, with Broca's aphasia, 343
Sentence length, motor agrammatism's effect on, 364
Sentence muteness, 339
Sequence
  agnosia of, 681–682
  apraxia of, 682–683
  drawing, 460–461
  multimodal, 477–478
  recognition, 177–178

sound, 121–123
unimodal, 476–477
Sequential statistical analysis, 689
Sexual activity
    hyper, 54
    with mania, 555
Shape
    apperceptive object agnosia of,
        25–29
    discrimination test, 73
    general assessment of, 75–76
Shifting, concept of, 179
Shyness, 244
Signal. *See also* Filtration of signal
        from noise
    attention disturbances in detection
        of, 495
    delayed presentation of, 37
    noise similar to, 496
    noise simultaneously presented
        with, 33–37
    processing brief, 123–125
    recognition of, 8
Signal/noise ratio, 33
Simple features. *See* Features
Simple signs test, 673–674
Simultanagnosia
    anatomical aspects of, 170
    Balint's syndrome with, 488
    early description of, 166
Single-cell recording, mirrored
        neuronal activity observed
        by, 14
Sleep-wake cycles
    with delirium, 616–617
    disturbances of, 607
    REM sleep in, 618–620
    reversal of, 612
Slowly progressive isolated aphasia,
    640
Social agnosia, 21, 136
    amnestic disorders with, 265–268
    brain information processing
        disturbances in, 260–261,
        270–271
    definition of, 222
    delusions underlain by, 273–279

dementia with, 623–626
depersonalization and
        derealization with, 262–263
    frontal lobe involvement in, 259
    frontal lobe lesions in, 331
    mood disorders and, 606
    multiple personality disorders
        with, 264–265
    self-image in, 261
    social apraxia *vs.*, 221
    tests of, 624–625
    theory of mind with, 254–255
Social apraxia
    activities of daily living with,
        326–327
    anatomical aspects of, 331–333
    definition of, 324
    dementia with, 623–626
    disorganization with, 329–330
    early description of, 324–326
    employment with, 327–328
    general cognition in, 328
    motor apraxia's similarity to,
        329–330
    social agnosia *vs.*, 221
    social problem solving with, 327
    tests of, 624–625
    vocabulary of social actions in,
        330–331
Social cognition, 221
Social delusions, 273, 283–287
Somatic alloesthesia, 146
Somatic delusions
    classification of, 273
    lesion localization in, 145
Somatic illusions, 143
"Somatic Myself." *See* Somatoagnosia
Somatoagnosia. *See also* Anosognosia;
        Autotopagnosia
    definition of, 4
    macro- and micro-, 143
    self-image in, 136–137
    types of, 137
Somatopsyche, 137
Sound
    brief signal processing and, 123–125
    filtration of, 116

Sound (*continued*)
frequency, 117–121
localization of, 126–127
object, 113–114
patterns of, 117
sequence differentiation, 121–123
tone of, 118–119
Sound muteness, 339
Space
body part relations in, 143–144
features of, 101
orientation in, 100–101
position in, 478–480
Space-time agnosia, test of, 680
Spatial agraphia
anatomical aspects of, 418
clinical aspects of, 415–416
Spatial alexia, 100
Spatial apraxia, 302
Spatial relation
color agnosia with, 93–94
object recognition with, 80
Speech
arrested, 609
comprehension of, 354–355
conversational, 353–354, 356, 365, 369
with delirium, 610
empty, 638
expressive, 341–342, 352, 353–354, 366–367, 370
with negative symptoms, 504
patterns of, 117
working memory for, 476
Speech akinesia
clinical aspects, 517–518
definition of, 504
Speech disorders localization-3, 2
Speed, in motion recognition disturbances, 158–160
Spelling agraphia
anatomical aspects of, 418
clinical aspects of, 416
Standard paraphasia, 345
Stereotyped movements, 575
Stool incontinence, dementia with, 631

Strange men, hallucinations with, 199
Stroke
depression after, 533–534, 542–543, 545
emotional agnosia from, 246–248
social apraxia from, 332
visual hallucination from, 206–207
Stroop Test, 13, 671
Subcortical connections, in OCD, 582
Subcortical dementia
as bradyphrenia, 644–645
in progressive supranuclear palsy, 645–647
Subcortical diseases, depression with, 538–541
Subcortical gliosis, 639
Subcortical lesions, 322
aphasia from, 389–392
delirium from, 616
in dementia, 650
mania from, 560
negative symptoms with, 506
unilateral neglect in, 494
in vascular dementia, 650
Subdural recording, 570
Substantia nigra, dopamine in, 657
Suicide, from mood disorders, 530
Superior temporal sulcus, action recognition in, 164–165
Supervisory activating system, 468
Supervisory attention system, 484
Surface agraphia
anatomical aspects of, 418
clinical aspects of, 417
Surface dyslexia, 407
anatomical aspects of, 414
clinical aspects of, 410–411
Symbolic gesture apraxia, 295
Symbolic understanding, 30
Synesthesia, 133
Syntax
disturbances, 342
rules, in posterior aphasia, 359–361
in transcortical sensory aphasia, 366

working memory in process of, 388–389

Systemic medical conditions, depression with, 544

Tactile agnosia
  apperceptive, 130
  associative, 130–131
  early descriptions of, 4
  historical descriptions of, 129
  lesion localization in, 133–135
  object recognition in, 129
  stages of, 132–133
Tactile alloesthesia, 133
Tactile aphasia, 344
Tactile asymbolia, 129
Tactile extinction, 132
Tau protein, 635
Telegraph boy, 167–168
Telegraph style, 346
Telescopy, 189
Temporal lobe
  in mania, 558–559
  in mood disorders, 605
  in panic disorder, 570–571
  paroxysmal activity in, 598
  rage attacks and, 588–589
  unimodal sequences and, 476–477
  visual hallucinations from, 202
Temporal lobe epilepsy
  distinct personality profile with, 270
  fear in, 571
  fugue states with, 267
  personality changes caused by, 5
  rage attacks and, 588–589
  tonical hyperactivity in, 286
Temporal lobe injuries, delusions with, 289–290
Temporal lobe lesions
  apraxia with, 316
  auditory hallucinations with, 195–196
  auditory space agnosia with, 129
  delusion with, 288
  emotional agnosia with, 245
  hallucinations from, 210

motion recognition disturbances with, 160–162
  prosopagnosia with, 230–235
  self-image underestimation with, 269–270
  somatic delusions from, 145
  topographical disorientation with, 108–109
  visual imagery loss with, 112
  visual object agnosia with, 49–55
Temporal lobe seizure, hallucinations with, 194
Temporal lobe tumors
  delusions with, 275
  depression from, 532–533
Temporo-occipital lesion, visual object agnosia with, 44–49
Test batteries, 675. *See also specific test*
Textures, contours in, 495–496
Thalamic dementia, 650, 656
Thalamic lesions, negative symptoms with, 506–507
Thalamic medial dorsal nuclei, Korsakoff's syndrome with, 438–440
Thalamocortical relay neurons, in delirium, 616
Theory of mind
  Asperger's syndrome and, 258
  autism and, 257–258
  brain information processing disturbances with, 260–261
  frontal lobe involvement in, 259
  schizophrenia and, 258
  with social action agnosia, 254–255
  tests of, 255–256
Theta activity, dreamy state with, 613
Thoughts
  audible, 193
  disorders of, 378–379
  withdrawal of, 282–283
Thromboembolism, infarctions from, 640
Time
  acceleration of, 158–160
  agnosia of, 628–629
  object exposition, 39–40, 54, 69–71

Tinnitus, as hallucination, 193
Token Test, 674
Tone differentiation, 118–119
Tonical hyperactivity
   development of, 285
   hallucinations with, 286
Top-down processing
   object categorization with, 82–84
   property frequencies in, 84–87
Topographical agnosia, 105–106
Topographical apraxia, 105
Topographical disorientation
   brain information processing
      disturbances in, 105–106
   familiar space in, 103
   landmarks in, 106
   lesion location in, 106–109
   map orientation in, 104–105
   self-orientation in, 104
   syndromes with, 102–103
   as visuospatial agnosia, 99
Topographical orientation, unilateral
   neglect in, 490–491
Tourette's syndrome, 576
Tractotomy, subcaudate, 582
Trail Making Test, executive
   functions testing with, 670
Transcortical motor aphasia, 341
   anatomical aspects of, 395–397
   articulation aphasia with, 352
   conversational speech with, 365
   dynamic, 351–352
Transcortical sensory aphasia, 341
   anatomical aspects of, 400–401
   anomic-sensory aphasia with, 365
   conduction aphasia with, 367–368
   expressive speech in, 366–367
   repetition in, 368
   syntax in, 366
   word alienation in, 365
Transient compulsion, 576
Transient global amnesia, Korsakoff's
   syndrome with, 437–438,
   451–452
Tumors. *See* Brain tumors; Frontal
   lobe tumors; Temporal lobe
   tumors

Twilight states
   self-image in, 265
   studies of, 266–267

Unconventional information
      processing
   in agnosia, 32–33
   in emotional agnosia, 242–243
   in modules, 10–13
   in visual object agnosia, 50–55
   in vocabulary of actions, 307–308
Unilateral visual neglect
   anatomical aspects of, 493–494
   in brain information processing,
      492–493
   in drawing, 492
   early description of, 490
   in object recognition, 492
   in topographical orientation,
      490–491
   in visual orientation, 491
Unimodal sequences, working
      memory for, 476–477
Uremia, delirium with, 613
Urinary incontinence, dementia
   with, 631

Valproic acid, rage attack treatment
   with, 591
Vascular dementia
   in Alzheimer's disease, 642–644
   anatomical aspects of, 640–642
   among dementia types, 622
   subcortical lesions in, 650
Ventral simultanagnosia, 170
Ventricular brain ratio, in
      schizophrenic patients, 510–511
Ventromedial hypothalamus, 595–596
Verbal comprehension, 674
Verbal paraphasia, 342, 344–345,
   362–363
Viewing position, disturbances in,
   42–44
Visual agnosia. *See also* Visual object
      agnosia
   basal ganglia lesions with, 252
   historical description of, 22–23

of partially occluded object,
683–684
visual imagery loss from, 109
Visual gestalt, 25
Visual hallucinations
anatomic aspects of, 202–209
types of, 199–202
Visual imagery loss
clinical features of, 109–110
lesions with, 112–113
object perception with, 110–111
from visual agnosia, 109
Visual object agnosia
apperceptive, 24–29
associative, 24, 29–30
compensation in, 28
completion operations with, 87–88
dementia with, 629, 663–664
disturbance types in, 89
lesions with
extended cortical, 60
frontal lobe, 55–56
hippocampal, 53
occipital, 44–49
parietal lobe, 56–59
posterior temporo-occipital,
44–49
temporal lobe, 49–55
module for, 61
prosopagnosia's lesion overlap
with, 237
recognition in
angle of, 58
exposition time in, 39–40
incomplete figure, 40–42
novel objects, 24–25
overlapping contours in, 38
process of, 23–24
shape, 25–29
signal and noise presentation in,
33–37
unconventional view in, 42–44
simple features
analysis of, 64–65
differentiation of, 65–68
unconventional information
processing in, 50–55

Visual orientation, 491
Visual systems, ventral *vs.* dorsal, 51
Visual working memory
angle differentiation experiments
with, 68–69
for complex features, 474–476
Visuomotor sequential procedures,
learning of, 175–177
Visuospatial agnosia
disorientation in
immediate space, 99–102
topographical, 99, 102–109
early descriptions of, 4
Vitamin deficiency, delirium with,
613
Vocabulary of actions
conventional information
processing in, 305–307
motor engrams and, 302–305
social, 330–331
unconventional information
processing in, 307–308

Wakefulness, 612
WCST. *See* Wisconsin Card Sorting
Test
Wechsler Adult Intelligence Scale
cognitive assessment with, 642
role of, 669
Weigl-Goldstein-Scheerer Color-
Form Sorting Test, 179
Wernicke-Lichtheim model
aphasias in, 341
Kleist's classification system *vs.*, 339
Wernicke's aphasia
information processing module
in, 12
Korsakoff's syndrome with,
436–437
language disturbances in, 404–406
lesion localization in, 397–398
phonological level disturbances in,
379–382
in posterior aphasia, 355
in Wernicke-Lichtheim model,
341
Western Aphasia Battery, 642

White matter
chronic ischemic changes in, 642
lesions of, Alzheimer's disease
with, 634
White matter hyperintensities
Binswanger's disease with, 651
in bipolar disorder, 546–547
depression with, 541–542
late-onset delusions with, 653
with mania, 566
with schizophrenia, 662
Wisconsin Card Sorting Test (WCST)
executive functions testing with,
670
lesion localization revealed by, 6–7
shifting concept in, 179
Withdrawal syndromes
delirium with, 613
hallucinations with, 213
Wolpert's simultanagnosia, 166, 170
Word
alienation from, 349–350, 356–357,
365, 373
blindness, 4, 407, 412–413
emotion's basic, 601
finding disturbances, 342–343, 362
muteness, 339
Word deafness
anatomical aspects of, 398–399
comprehension disorders with,
369–371

phonetic sensory aphasia as, 369
pure, 341
Working memory. *See also* Visual
working memory
in aphasia, 384, 388–389
in artificial intelligence, 8
auditory, 470–471
central executive part of, 467–
469
definition of, 466
function of, 467
for language, 476
lesion localization with, 481
multimodal, 471–474, 477–478
in prefrontal cortex, 475
slave systems of, 469–470
for space position and orientation,
478–480
for speech, 476
test of, 684
unimodal, 470, 476–477
visual, 471–474
Wortblindheit, 4
Writing disturbances
with anterior aphasia, 348–349
with deep dyslexia, 407

Yarbus test, 486

Zeitrafferphenomen, 158
Zoopsia, 213